Comprehensive Approach to Adult Congenital Heart Disease

Anita Sadeghpour • Majid Kyavar
Azin Alizadehasl
Editors

Comprehensive Approach to Adult Congenital Heart Disease

Springer

Editors
Anita Sadeghpour, MD, FACC, FASE
Rajaie Cardiovascular Medical and Research Center
Iran University of Medical Science
Tehran
Iran

Azin Alizadehasl, MD, FACC
Rajaie Cardiovascular Medical and Research Center
Iran University of Medical Science
Tehran
Iran

Majid Kyavar, MD, FACC
Rajaie Cardiovascular Medical and Research Center
Iran University of Medical Science
Tehran
Iran

Additional material to this book can be downloaded from http://extras.springer.com

ISBN 978-1-4471-6382-4 ISBN 978-1-4471-6383-1 (eBook)
DOI 10.1007/978-1-4471-6383-1
Springer London Heidelberg New York Dordrecht

Library of Congress Control Number: 2014945750

Printed on acid-free paper

Springer is part of Springer Science+Business Media (www.springer.com)

To
My husband, Ramin, and my daughter, Ariana
Anita Sadeghpour, MD, FACC, FASE

My wife, Zohre, and my daughters, Elnaz and Parinaz
Majid Kyavar, MD, FACC

My husband, Rasoul, and my daughter, Armita
Azin Alizadehasl, MD, FACC

and
To our parents, colleagues, and patients

Foreword

Medicine in the Middle East dates back to at least 3000 BC, with ancient Persia being a center of learning. Thus, it is fitting that modern Iran continues that tradition with this textbook, *Comprehensive Approach to Adult Congenital Heart Disease*. Written by a group of Iranian scholars, primarily led by Anita Sadeghpour and Azin Alizadehasl, but with contributions from their Iranian colleagues as well, this book achieves in prose and videos exactly what its title says: a comprehensive discussion of congenital heart disease. The text rivals Western publications in accuracy and completeness. Beginning with discussions of epidemiology, embryology and fetal circulation, and normal and abnormal anatomy, the chapters continue through a detailed discourse of each congenital defect, including its clinical presentation, diagnostic workup, and treatment. Cardiac lesions are logically presented under headings of left to right shunts, cyanotic defects, valvular and vascular lesions, and a miscellaneous group. Between the detailed text and the many videos, readers will gain a thorough appreciation of congenital heart defects that now affect more adults than children. On a personal note, knowing the authors, I congratulate them in completing this text and demonstrating that medicine has the power to transcend divisive intrusions and unite doctors throughout the world in our common goal of caring for our patients.

IN, USA — Douglas P. Zipes, MD

Preface

The past half century had witnessed remarkable improvement in the survival of patients with congenital heart disease (CHD). A recent estimate shows that, for the first time in history, there are more adults living with CHD than children. That in combination with the current low surgical mortality rates has led to the belief that in the next decade, 1 in 150 young adults will probably have some form of CHD. Moreover, the complexity of the numerous lesions and the multitude of challenges that adult CHD patients face call for a multidisciplinary approach to care. This is indeed the essence of good adult CHD practice and the very focus of this training/educational book.

This book can serve as a forum for all cardiologists and cardiology trainees seeking further opportunities to immerse themselves in the fascinating and ever-evolving field of adult CHD. This book, which presents some unique cases of complex lesions, whether corrected or non-corrected, endeavors to create a balance between the introduction of diagnostic tools such as history/physical examination, electrocardiography, chest X-ray, echocardiography, computed tomography, cardiovascular magnetic resonance imaging, and catheterization on the one hand and the introduction of treatment choices on the other hand such that the reader can have the best possible guidance in the diagnosis and management of adult CHD. In addition, this book offers a comprehensive account of patients and their diagnostic and treatment modalities from the first presentation to the latest follow-up.

There is no doubt, however, that this book has its own limitations and shortcomings, which will be hopefully addressed in the future editions, thanks to your invaluable support, contribution, and guidance.

Tehran, Iran — Anita Sadeghpour, MD, FACC, FASE
Tehran, Iran — Majid Kyavar, MD, FACC
Tehran, Iran — Azin Alizadehasl, MD, FACC

Acknowledgments

We gratefully acknowledge Professor Douglas P. Zipes, MD, distinguished professor in Indiana University School of Medicine, our great mentor, without whom none of this would have been possible. We also appreciate the invaluable contributions of our colleagues, who played significant roles in the creation and improvement of this text. Many thanks are also due to the following individuals for their assistance: Grant Weston and Liz Pope (of Springer Publishing Company), Farshad Amouzadeh, Shahnaz Sheikh, Dr. Amirhossein Mohammad Alian, Dr. Samad Golzari, Abolfazl Abdi, and Amir Hossein Mirkamal.

Tehran, Iran — Anita Sadeghpour, MD, FACC, FASE
Tehran, Iran — Majid Kyavar, MD, FACC
Tehran, Iran — Azin Alizadehasl, MD, FACC

Contents

Contributors

Nehzat Akiash, MD Rajaie Cardiovascular Medical and Research Center, Department of Cardiology, Tehran, Iran

Azin Alizadehasl, MD, FACC Echocardiography Lab, Department of Cardiology, Rajaie Cardiovascular Medical and Research Center, Iran University of Medical Science, Tehran, Iran

Abolfath Alizadeh Diz, MD Electrophysiology Lab, Department of Cardiology, Rajaie Cardiovascular Medical and Research Center, Iran University of Medical Science, Tehran, Iran

Alireza Alizadeh Ghavidel, MD Cardiac Surgery Ward, Department of Cardiac Surgery, Rajaie Cardiovascular Medical and Research Center, Iran University of Medical Science, Tehran, Iran

Rasoul Azarfarin, MD, FACC Cardiac Anesthesiology Ward, Department of Anesthesiology, Rajaie Cardiovascular Medical and Research Center, Iran University of Medical Science, Tehran, Iran

Mitra Chitsazan, MD Rajaie Cardiovascular Medical and Research Center, Department of Cardiology, Tehran, Iran

Shadi Faghihi, MD Rajaie Cardiovascular Medical and Research Center, Department of Cardiology, Tehran, Iran

Arash Hashemi, MD Erfan General Hospital, Department of Cardiology, Tehran, Iran

Majid Kyavar, MD, FACC Cardiovascular Imaging Ward, Department of Cardiology, Adult Congenital Heart Disease Clinic, Rajaie Cardiovascular Medical and Research Center, Iran University of Medical Science, Tehran, Iran

Mohammad Mahdavi, MD Pediatric Ward, Department of Pediatric Cardiology, Rajaie Cardiovascular Medical and Research Center, Iran University of Medical Science, Tehran, Iran

Arya Mani, MD, FACC Cardiovascular Genetics Program, Yale University, New Haven, CT, USA

Shabnam Mohammadzadeh, MD Moheb General Hospital, Department of Cardiology, Tehran, Iran

Maryam Moradian, MD Department of Pediatric Cardiology, Rajaie Cardiovascular Medical and Research Center, Iran University of Medical Science, Tehran, Iran

Mohammad Esmaeil Rezaei, MD Rajaie Cardiovascular Medical and Research Center, Department of Cardiology, Tehran, Iran

Anita Sadeghpour, MD, FACC, FASE Echocardiography Lab, Department of Cardiology, Adult Congenital Heart Disease Clinic, Rajaie Cardiovascular Medical and Research Center, Iran University of Medical Science, Tehran, Iran

Abbreviations

ACE	Angiotensin converting enzyme
ACHD	Adult congenital heart disease
AF	Atrial fibrillation
Aft	Atrial flutter
AI	Aortic insufficiency
ALCAPA	Anomalous left coronary artery from the pulmonary artery
AO	Aorta
AR	Aortic valve regurgitation
ASD	Atrial septal defect
AV	Atrioventricular
AVR	Aortic valve replacement
AVSD	Atrioventricular septal defect
BAV	Bicuspid aortic valve
CCTGA	Congenitally corrected transposition of the great arteries
CFI	Color flow imaging
CHD	Congenital heart disease
CHF	Congestive heart failure
CMR	Cardiac magnetic resonance
CoA	Coarctation of the aorta
CS	Coronary sinus
CT	Computed tomography
CXR	Chest X-ray
DCRV	Double-chambered right ventricle
ECG	Electrocardiogram
EDV	End-diastolic volume
EF	Ejection fraction
ESV	End-systolic volume
FC	Functional class
HF	Heart failure
HHT	Hereditary hemorrhagic telangiectasia
HLHS	Hypoplastic left heart syndrome
ICD	Implantable cardioverter-defibrillator
IVC	Inferior vena cava
IVS	Intact ventricular septum
JVP	Jugular venous pulse/pressure
LA	Left atrium
LAO	Left anterior oblique

LAVV	Left atrioventricular valve
LPA	Left pulmonary artery
LSB	Left sternal border
LV	Left ventricle
LVEDd	LV end-diastolic dimension/diameter
LVESd	LV end-systolic dimension/diameter
LVOT	Left ventricular outflow tract
MAPCA	Major aortopulmonary collateral artery
MPA	Main pulmonary artery
MR	Mitral regurgitation
MRI	Magnetic resonance imaging
MS	Mitral stenosis
NYHA	New York Heart Association
PA	Pulmonary atresia or pulmonary artery
PAH	Pulmonary arterial hypertension
PAPVC	Partial anomalous pulmonary venous connection
PAVMs	Pulmonary arteriovenous malformations
PDA	Patent ductus arteriosus
PFO	Patent foramen ovale
PH	Pulmonary hypertension
PR	Pulmonary valve regurgitation
PS	Pulmonary stenosis
PV	Pulmonary valve
PVC	Premature ventricular contraction
PVn	Pulmonary vein
PVnS	Pulmonary vein stenosis
PVR	Pulmonary vascular resistance
Qp	Pulmonary blood flow
Qs	Systemic blood flow
RA	Right atrium
RAO	Right anterior oblique
RBBB	Right bundle branch block
RPA	Right pulmonary artery
RV	Right ventricle
RVOT	Right ventricular outflow tract
SV	Stroke volume
SVASD	Sinus venosus atrial septal defect
SVC	Superior vena cava
SVR	Systemic vascular resistance
TA	Tricuspid atresia or truncus arteriosus
TAPVC	Total anomalous pulmonary venous connection
TCPC	Total cavopulmonary connection
TDI	Tissue Doppler imaging
TEE	Transesophageal echocardiogram
TGA	Transposition of the great arteries
TOF	Tetralogy of Fallot
TR	Tricuspid regurgitation
TS	Tricuspid stenosis

TTE	Transthoracic echocardiography
TV	Tricuspid valve
VA	Ventriculoarterial
Vo_2	Oxygen consumption
VSD	Ventricular septal defect
VT	Ventricular tachycardia
2D	Two dimensional
2DE	Two-dimensional echocardiography
3D	Three dimensional
3DE	Three-dimensional echocardiography

List of Videos

Video 30.1 Transthoracic echocardiography in 4 chamber view showing main ventricle with LV morphology (DILV), receiving two separate atrioventricular valves (WMV 356 kb)

Video 30.2 Transthoracic echocardiography in parasternal long axis view showing DILV and transposition of great arteries (WMV 325 kb)

Video 30.3 Trans esophageal echocardiography in transgasteric short axis and long axis view showing main ventricle with LV morphology (DILV) and Aorta arises from the rudimentary anterior chamber (MPG 1,200 kb)

Video 30.4 Trans esophageal echocardiography in transgasteric short axis and long axis view showing main ventricle with LV morphology (DILV) and Aorta arises from the rudimentary anterior chamber (MPG 1,258 kb)

Video 30.5 Trans esophageal echocardiography in long axis view demonstrating transposition of great arteries and severe pulmonary stenosis (MPG 1,108 kb)

Video 32.1 Abdominal situs solitus (Aorta at the left and IVC at the right of the vertebra) in subcostal 2D echocardiography study as a part of segmental sequential approach (MPG 550 kb)

Video 32.2 Transthoracic echocardiography in 4 apical chamber view showing atrial situs solitus, L-loop ventricle and atrioventricular discordance (MPG 686 kb)

Video 32.3 Transthoracic echocardiography in 4 apical chamber view showing atrial situs solitus, L-loop ventricle and atrioventricular discordance (MPG 894 kb)

Video 32.4 L-loop ventricle in short axis view (MPG 890 kb)

Video 32.5 Parallel great arteries in off axis view associated with ventriculoarterial connection (WMV 328 kb)

Video 32.6 CCTGA, VSD, and PS: Vertical laying the intra ventricular septum, presence of VSD and PS and also laying the aorta in anterior position in lateral injection. In addition aorta is located on morphological trabeculated RV (WMV 1,310 kb)

Video 32.7 CCTGA, VSD, and PS: Vertical laying the intra ventricular septum, presence of VSD and PS and also laying the aorta in anterior position in lateral injection. In addition aorta is located on morphological trabeculated RVE (WMV 1,610 kb)

Video 33.1 Parasternal long axis view showing anterior located right ventricle (RV) associated with transposed great arteries and anterior located aorta (AO) (MPG 1,388 kb)

Video 33.2 Parasternal long axis view showing anterior located right ventricle (RV) associated with transposed great arteries and anterior located aorta (AO) (MPG 1,896 kb)

Video 33.3 Parasternal short axis view demonstrating dilated aorta (AO), hypoplastic pulmonary artery and anterior located AO associated with ASD (MPG 1,224 kb)

Video 33.4 Apical 4 chamber view showing D-Loop ventricle associated with a large VSD (MPG 1,556 kb)

Video 33.5 CMR reliably demonstrates the ventricular and arterial looping besides the ventricular size and function (AVI 3,887 kb)

Video 33.6 Transthoracic echocardiography in 4 chamber view showing pulmonary venous chamber drains to the morphologic RV and systemic venous chamber o the left ventricle with no obstruction in 2D study (WMV 1,006 kb)

Video 33.7 Transthoracic echocardiography in 4 chamber view showing pulmonary venous chamber drains to the morphologic RV and systemic venous chamber o the left ventricle with no obstruction in 2D study (WMV 738 kb)

Video 33.8 Patent systemic venous chamber with no leakage as demonstrated in right hand contrast injection (WMV 308 kb)

Video 33.9 Patent systemic venous chamber with no obstruction in SVC anastomosis. SVC anastomosis is patent if contrast injected into a peripheral arm vein promptly enters the SVA, In obstruction at the SVC, azygous or other collaterals to IVC will cause contrast to first enter the IVC and then to SVA (WMV 1,425 kb)

Video 34.1 Transesophageal echocardiography showing circular structure which is cross section of the lateral tunnel with significant stagnant flow through it (WMV 96 kb)

Video 34.2 Transesophageal echocardiography reveals patent SVC and IVC anastomosis an the whole Fontan circuit (MPG 2,612 kb)

Video 34.3 Transesophageal echocardiography reveals patent SVC and IVC anastomosis an the whole Fontan circuit (MPG 784 kb)

Video 34.4 Transesophageal echocardiography reveals patent SVC and IVC anastomosis an the whole Fontan circuit (MPG 2,428 kb)

Video 34.5 CMR in a patient with lateral tunnel denotes significant stasis with no thrombosis (WMV 247 kb)

Video 35.1 Oval shape opening of the Bicuspid Aortic valve (BAV) in parasternal short-axis view, note the evaluation was done in systole (AVI 3,618 kb)

Video 35.2 Transesophageal echocardiography showing thickened and calcified BAV in short axis view (WMV 628 kb)

Video 35.3 The catheter course is arterial; injection was performed in aortic root and showed doming of AV cusps due to bicuspid aortic valve (WMV 422 kb)

Video 35.4 Quadricuspid aortic valve in short axis and long axis transesophageal echocardiography associated with significant aortic regurgitation (WMV 544 kb)

Video 35.5 Quadricuspid aortic valve in short axis and long axis transesophageal echocardiography associated with significant aortic regurgitation (WMV 333 kb)

Video 36.1 Parasternal long-axis view showing a discrete fibrous ring encircling the left ventricular (LV) outflow tract with extension to the anterior MV leaflet (white arrows) (MPG 3,592 kb)

Video 36.2 2D and color Doppler study in apical 5 chamber view demonstrating the discrete subaortic membrane resulting turbulent flow in LVOT, Color flow Doppler study is helpful for identifying the level of stenosis. In the subaortic stenois turbulent flow originate from the LVOT rather than either the AV annulus or above the AV (MPG 3,662 kb)

Video 36.3 2D and color Doppler study in apical 5 chamber view demonstrating the discrete subaortic membrane resulting turbulent flow in LVOT, Color flow Doppler study is helpful for identifying the level of stenosis. In the subaortic stenois turbulent flow originate from the LVOT rather than either the AV annulus or above the AV (MPG 3,314 kb)

Video 36.4 Transesophageal echocardiography in long-axis view demonstrating fibromuscular ridge encircling the left ventricular (LV) outflow tract (white arrow) with extension to the anterior MV leaflet and aortic valve (MPG 1,436 kb)

Video 36.5 Typical LVOT narrowing in subaortic stenosis in left ventriculography (WMV 1,426 kb)

Video 37.1 Color flow Doppler study is helpful for identifying the level of the stenosis. In the supra aortic stenois turbulent flow originate above the AV (MPG 2,576 kb)

Video 37.2 Transthoracic 2D and color Doppler study in apical 5 chamber view showing a discrete membrane above the Aortic valve (AV) that turbulent flow begins above the AV (MPG 2,674 kb)

Video 37.3 Transthoracic 2D and color Doppler study in apical 5 chamber view showing a discrete membrane above the Aortic valve (AV) that turbulent flow begins above the AV (MPG 2,674 kb)

Video 38.1 Transthoracic echocardiography in suprasternal view showing the site of the CoA (AVI 9,529 kb)

Video 38.2 Transesophageal echocardiography showing the CoA site in proximal of descending thoracic Aorta with a systolic turbulent flow in color Doppler study (WMV 297 kb)

Video 38.3 Transesophageal echocardiography showing the CoA site in proximal of descending thoracic Aorta with a systolic turbulent flow in color Doppler study (AVI 2,496 kb)

Video 39.1 Transthoracic echocardiography in short axis view showing aneurysmal dilation of right sinus of Valsalva with protrusion to the RVOT (AVI 4,942 kb)

Video 39.2 Transesophageal echocardiography in short axis view revealed a "windsock" dilatation of the right sinus of Valsalva which is ruptured to the RA and color flow imaging showing continuous systolic-diastolic flow (MPG 2,606 kb)

Video 39.3 Transesophageal echocardiography in short axis view revealed a "windsock" dilatation of the right sinus of Valsalva which is ruptured to the RA and color flow imaging showing continuous systolic-diastolic flow (MPG 2,308 kb)

Video 39.4 Transesophageal echocardiography in long axis view revealed a "windsock" dilatation of the right sinus of Valsalva which is ruptured to the RVOT (white arrow) and associated VSD (yellow arrow) and color flow imaging showing continuous turbulent systolic-diastolic flow drains to the RVOT (AVI 2,145 kb)

Video 39.5 Transesophageal echocardiography in long axis view revealed a "windsock" dilatation of the right sinus of Valsalva which is ruptured to the RVOT (white arrow) and associated VSD (yellow arrow) and color flow imaging showing continuous turbulent systolic-diastolic flow drains to the RVOT (AVI 3,903 kb)

Video 39.6 Aortic root injection revealed rupture sinus of Valsalva to the right ventricle (MPG 3,650 kb)

Video 40.1 Transthoracic echocardiography in short axis view showing divided mitralorifice into two components (DOMV) (AVI 9,086 kb)

Video 41.1 Isolated mitral valve cleft as 2D defect in anterior mitral leaflet in four chamber transesophageal echocardiography (MPG 3,316 kb)

Video 41.2 The same patient with isolated mitral valve cleft as 2D defect in anterior mitral leaflet and color flow imaging confirm the diagnosis and associated mitral regurgitation (AVI 6,344 kb)

Video 42.1 2D echocardiography imaging of dome shaped and stenotic pulmonary valve in both transthoracic and transesophageal echocardiography (MPG 1,260 kb)

Video 42.2 2D echocardiography imaging of dome shaped and stenotic pulmonary valve in both transthoracic and transesophageal echocardiography (AVI 4,265 kb)

Video 42.3 2D echocardiography imaging of dome shaped and stenotic pulmonary valve in transesophageal echocardiography arch view image study (AVI 4,004 kb)

Video 42.4 2D echocardiography imaging of dome shaped and stenotic pulmonary valve in transesophageal echocardiography arch view image study (AVI 2,923 kb)

Video 42.5 Injection was done by venous catheter at later view and in the hypertrophied RV that showing doming in PV leaflets and post stenotic dilation (WMV 656 kb)

Video 42.6 Percutaneous valvuplasty was done and balloon perforation was occurred as a rare complication (WMV 922 kb)

Video 44.1 Left PA origin stenosis detected in 2D echocardiography (WMV 375 kb)

Video 44.2 The same patient with left PA origin stenosis by CFI study (WMV 391 kb)

Video 45.1 Transthoracic echocardiography in 4 chamber shows an anomalous hypertrophied muscle bundle in mid portion of right ventricle (AVI 3,012 kb)

Video 45.2 Transthoracic echocardiography short axis view showing anomalous hypertrophied muscle bundle in mid portion of right ventricle suggestive of double-chamber RV (MPG 810 kb)

Video 45.3 Transthoracic echocardiography short axis view showing anomalous hypertrophied muscle bundle in mid portion of right ventricle suggestive of double-chamber RV (MPG 1,020 kb)

Video 45.4 Transesophageal echocardiography reveals anomalous hypertrophied muscle bundle in mid portion of right ventricle suggestive of double-chamber RV with turbulent flow (MPG 1,450 kb)

Video 45.5 Transesophageal echocardiography reveals anomalous hypertrophied muscle bundle in mid portion of right ventricle suggestive of double-chamber RV with turbulent flow (MPG 1,272 kb)

Video 45.6 Typicall perimembranous VSD which is found in more than 75 % of patients with DCRV (AVI 2,293 kb)

Video 45.7 Injection at lateral view in RV shows RV muscle band at mid portion. Also contrast passage from LV to RV in recirculation is seen via VSD (WMV 1,038 kb)

Video 46.1 Parasternal long axis view showing a highly mobile redundant tissue attached to the mitral valve (MV) suggestive of accessory tissue mitral valve (ATMV) (WMV 606 kb)

Video 46.2 Large redundant accessory tissue mitral valve (ATMV) may appear as a cystic mass in transesophageal echocardiography (WMV 419 kb)

Video 46.3 Accessory tissue mitral valve (ATMV) in long axis view of transesophageal echocardiography (WMV 438 kb)

Video 47.1 Transthoracic echocardiography in 4 chamber view showing that all of the TV chordae tendinea attach to a single papillary muscle (MPG 954 kb)

Video 47.2 Trans esophageal echocardiography in RV inflow- out flow imaging of the same patient reveal, all of the TV chordae tendinea attach to a single dominant papillary muscle (MPG 678 kb)

Video 49.1 Huge left main coronary artery in transthoracic echocardiography short axis view (MPG 1,024 kb)

Video 49.2 Off axis transthoracic echocardiography showing coronary artery fistulae with aneurysmal formation and continuous turbulent flow which drains to the right ventricle (RV) (AVI 2,547 kb)

Video 49.3 Off axis transthoracic echocardiography showing coronary artery fistulae with aneurysmal formation and continuous turbulent flow which drains to the right ventricle (RV) (MPG 1,864 kb)

Video 49.4 Off axis transthoracic echocardiography showing coronary artery fistulae with aneurysmal formation and continuous turbulent flow which drains to the right ventricle (RV) (MPG 2,682 kb)

Video 49.5 Left coronary angiography showing aneurysmal dilatation of left main and left anterior descending coronary artery with fistulization to the right ventricle (WMV 803 kb)

Video 50.1 Transthoracic echocardiography in parasternal and 4 chamber view showing cortriatriatum with a small opening and significant smoky pattern (WMV 146 kb)

Part I

Basic Principles and Practical Issues in Recognition and Evaluation of Congenital Heart Disease

Epidemiology, Definition, and Classification of Adult Congenital Heart Disease

1

Anita Sadeghpour and Azin Alizadehasl

Keywords

Adult congenital heart disease (ACHD) • Epidemiology • Prevalence • Simple complexity of CHD • Moderate complexity of CHD • Great complexity of CHD

Epidemiology and Definition of Adult Congenital Heart Disease

Congenital heart malformations are the most common cluster of birth defects [1]. *Congenital cardiovascular disease (CHD) is defined as an anomaly in the cardiocirculatory structures or function that is present at birth time, even if it is diagnosed much later*. The exact incidence of congenital heart malformations is difficult to define precisely, partly because of difficulties in definition. *Birth prevalence of CHD is overall presumed to be about 0.8 %, although this does not take into consideration local differences and the two most common cardiac abnormalities: the congenital, functionally bicuspid aortic valve and the prolapse of the mitral valve. There is a variation in the incidence of CHD between 1.2 and 17 per 1,000* [2, 3].

In the United States, now, there are more patients over 20 years old with CHD than under that age. The number of patients is rising to a rate of 5 % per year, with 1–1.3 million people in the United States. Extraordinary improvement in the survival rate of patients with adult congenital heart disease (ACHD) has happened during the past half century. Survival to adulthood is better because of improved fetal diagnoses, advances in neonatal and childhood intensive care, improved surgical techniques, early complete surgical repair, and lower perioperative morbidity and mortality rate [2, 4–6]. Developments in diagnostic, interventional, and critical care services have resulted in the survival rate of about 90 % of these children to adulthood. *In fact, it is now predictable that for the first time in history, there are more adults living with CHD than children. Given new surgical mortality rate of less than 5 %, one would suppose that in the next decade, nearly 1 in 150 young adults will have some degree of CHD. In particular, there are a considerable number of young adults with single-*

A. Sadeghpour, MD, FACC, FASE (✉)
Echocardiography Lab, Department of Cardiology, Adult Congenital Heart Disease Clinic, Rajaie Cardiovascular Medical and Research Center, Iran University of Medical Science, Tehran, Iran
e-mail: anita.sadeghpour@gmail.com, asadeghpour@rhc.ac.ir

A. Alizadehasl, MD, FACC
Echocardiography Lab, Department of Cardiology, Rajaie Cardiovascular Medical and Research Center, Iran University of Medical Science, Tehran, Iran
e-mail: alizadeasl@gmail.com, alizadeasl@rhc.ac.ir

A. Sadeghpour et al. (eds.), *Comprehensive Approach to Adult Congenital Heart Disease*,
DOI 10.1007/978-1-4471-6383-1_1,

ventricle physiology, systemic right ventricles, and complex intracardiac baffles who are now entering adult life cycle and starting families [6–8].

Marelli et al. [9] showed the prevalence of CHD increased for children and adults from 1985 to 2000 and also revealed a shift in the patients living with CHD to those older than 18 years of age. In 2000, there were approximately equal numbers of adults and children with severe CHD. *The median age of all patients with severe CHD was 11 years in 1985, but 17 years in 2000. However, the prevalence of significant CHD in adults increased by 85 %. In this research, at all ages, the most common malformations were conotruncal anomalies and atrioventricular canal defects (AVCD) for severe CHD and atrial septal defect (ASD) and ventricular septal defect (VSD) for other CHD. The authors revealed that ASD was the most common congenital disease in adults.* Consistent with what has been available in children, conotruncal anomalies, containing tetralogy of Fallot (TOF), were the most common significant congenital lesions in adults.

Altogether, the most common anomalies seen in patients with adult CHD are ASD, coarctation of the aorta, pulmonary stenosis, aortic stenosis, Ebstein's anomaly, TOF, and corrected transposition, and other common defects in adults are double-outlet RV, postoperative atrioventricular canal, subaortic stenosis, abnormal mitral valve, primum ASD, and single ventricle [4, 10, 11].

So, given a prevalence of 0.3 % in CHD within a world population of about 4.4 billion adults, a total number of 13 million adult CHD survivors globally can be estimated. These patients are being followed up in more than 15,000 hospitals and medical clinics around the globe. Nevertheless, a large number of them, equal to 30–60 %, are lost to follow-up and only a small percentage of ACHD patients appear to be receiving specialized care [5, 11].

Variations in mortality between industrialized countries and the Third World are significant and interesting (3 % vs. 20 %). *Overall mortality rate of CHD decreased by 40 % between 1979 and 1997. However, the annual hospitalization rate of adults with CHD has more than doubled in the United States between 1998 and 2005. Also during this period of time, hospitalization for adults with complex CHD increased up to 60 %* [12]. In one report, there were over 84,000 adult CHD hospital admissions in the United States during 2007 [13]. Seventeen thousand (20 %) patients were admitted with heart failure. *Fifty-four percent were women. The most common abnormalities noted were ASD, VSD, and aortic valve abnormalities. The mean interval of hospital stay among these patients was 7.6 days.* The patients admitted with heart failure had three times the risk of death, compared with the adult CHD patients admitted during the same time period without heart failure. Other comorbidities were common and contained arrhythmias, pulmonary artery hypertension, and renal failure.

Unfortunately, all countries in the world are not training enough physicians to deal with caring for patients with adult CHD [13–15]. In addition, we have a major problem with patients' shift from infancy to adult care and with the setting in which to do it. In a total population of 360 ACHD patients over the age of 19 in a Canadian study [14], 47 % of the patients were transferred successfully to adult care.

Sex differences in the incidence of CHD at birth time are very well recognized. ASD, mitral valve prolapse, Ebstein's anomaly, patent ductus arteriosus, and common atrium show a strong female dominance, while aortic valve stenosis, aortic coarctation, transposition of the great arteries, pulmonary and tricuspid atresia, and TOF occur more frequently in males [3, 15, 16].

The medical management of adults with CHD will continue to be a challenge because the numbers of the variety of these patients increase on a yearly basis, while the expertise and personnel remain limited and focused upon a very few specialized centers [2, 4, 10]. More higher risk of some major cardiac complications in males with CHD may explain the increased in mortality rate in men. Regional and local differences in quality of life between CHD patients have been described, and methodological variances may play a significant role and also sociocultural differences warrant more attention. Socioeconomic consequences in CHD patients such as lower education, more joblessness, and fewer connections might have a different impact on quality of life in different countries and cultures [4, 17–20]. While race and culture are often difficult to differentiate from socioeconomic and other lifestyle issues, genetic factors certainly may play a role in the ethnic and racial differences of CHD. *In Asia, interestingly, relatively more right-sided and less left-sided lesions have been informed in previous studies* [2, 20–23]. In a large European investigation of over 4,000 ACHD patients from 24 countries, it was revealed that men are more likely to die from CHD than women [16]. Regarding the type of lesion and age, it was found that the accumulative mortality rate within 5 years was greater in the man (4 %) than in the woman (3 %) population. However, meaningfully more men in this cohort study were smokers (90.8 % vs. 81.5 % women), which was shown to be a risk factor for higher mortality rate [16, 17].

A difference in the seasonal mortality of CHD patients was detected in a study of 231 deaths among 8,595 CHD patients, though without achieving statistical significance [11]. A tendency was seen with the highest cardiac mortality in fall (32.7 % vs. 22.3 %, 23.2 %, and 21.8 % in winter, spring, and summer, respectively). Per season, the modes of death were equally disseminated [18]. This seasonal difference in mortality can be described by climatic factors, psychosocial factors, behavior changes, or concomitant infections. In the two reported studies by Zomer et al. [18, 22], over 25 % of cardiac mortality rate was preceded by infection.

Geographical and regional differences in CHD incidence and prevalence can be described by variations in socioeconomic status, education, urbanism, climatic issues, ethnicity, and patient-related factors like comorbidities, culture, lifestyle, and healthcare activities [20–24].

Classification of Adult Congenital Heart Disease

Based on the need for the delivery of appropriate healthcare and pattern of visit, ACHD patients have been categorized as simple (Table 1.1)*, moderate* (Table 1.2)*, and great complexity* (Table 1.3). *Adult patients with simple CHD can frequently be attended to in the general medical community. Adults with CHD of moderate complexity must be seen regularly at adult CHD centers, and those with high-grade complexity should be seen periodically at local ACHD centers* [6–8]. *A study of general adult cardiologists in a recent study by Fernandes et al.* [5]. *revealed that only a small percentage of ACHD patients appear to be receiving specific care in accordance with the American College of Cardiology (ACC) Guidelines for the Management of ACHD (2008).* The study confirmed that the overwhelming majority of general

Table 1.1 Adult patients with simple congenital heart disease

Native disease*
Isolated congenital aortic valve disease
Isolated congenital mitral valve disease (e.g., except parachute valve, cleft leaflet)
Small atrial septal defect
Isolated small ventricular septal defect (no associated lesions)
Mild pulmonary stenosis
Small patent ductus arteriosus
Repaired conditions
Previously ligated or occluded ductus arteriosus
Repaired secundum or sinus venosus atrial septal defect without residua
Repaired ventricular septal defect without residua

Modified from Warnes et al. [6]

*These patients can usually be cared for in the general medical community

Table 1.2 Adults with congenital heart disease of moderate complexity

Conduits, valved or nonvalved*
Cyanotic congenital heart (all forms)
Double-outlet ventricle
Eisenmenger syndrome
Fontan procedure
Mitral atresia
Single ventricle (also called double inlet or outlet, common, or primitive)
Pulmonary atresia (all forms)
Pulmonary vascular obstructive disease
Transposition of the great arteries
Tricuspid atresia
Truncus/hemitruncus arteriosus
Other abnormalities of atrioventricular or ventriculoarterial connection not included above (i.e., crisscross heart, isomerism, heterotaxy syndromes, ventricular inversion)

Modified from Warnes et al. [6]

*These patients should be seen regularly at adult congenital heart disease centers

Table 1.3 Adults with congenital heart disease of great complexity

Aorto-left ventricular fistulas*
Anomalous pulmonary venous drainage, partial or total
Atrioventricular septal defects (partial or complete)
Coarctation of the aorta
Ebstein's anomaly
Significant right ventricular outflow tract (infundibular) obstruction
Ostium primum atrial septal defect
Patent ductus arteriosus (not closed)
Pulmonary valve regurgitation (moderate to severe)
Sinus of Valsalva fistula/aneurysm
Sinus venosus atrial septal defect
Subvalvular or supravalvular AS (except HOCM)
Tetralogy of Fallot
Ventricular septal defect with:
Absent valve or valves
Aortic regurgitation
Coarctation of the aorta
Mitral disease
Right ventricular outflow tract obstruction
Straddling tricuspid/mitral valve
Subaortic stenosis

Modified from Warnes et al. [6]

*These patients should be seen periodically at regional adult congenital heart disease center

adult cardiologists (95 %) provided care to patients with adult CHD, with approximately half reporting caring for at least one patient with complex CHD. *Almost all the respondents (99.0 %) stated the desire for further information regarding the care of adults with CHD.* The most desired and anticipated means for receiving this information were continuing medical education programs (56.1 %) and Web-based resources (54.6 %).

References

1. Hoffman JL. Incidence of congenital heart disease. I. Postnatal incidence. Pediatr Cardiol. 1995;16:103–13.
2. Bernier PL, Stefanescu A, Samoukovic G, et al. The challenge of congenital heart disease worldwide: epidemiologic and demographic facts. Semin Thorac Cardiovasc Surg Pediatr Card Surg Annu. 2010;13(1):26–34. doi:10.1053/j.pcsu.2010.02.005.
3. Bonow R, Mann D, Zipes D, et al. Braunwald's heart disease a textbook of cardiovascular medicine. 9th ed. Philadelphia: Elsevier Saunders; 2012. p. 517.
4. Mulder BJM. Epidemiology of adult congenital heart disease: demographic variations worldwide. Neth Heart J. 2012;20(12):505–8.
5. Fernandes S, Pearson D, Rzeszut A, et al. Adult congenital heart disease incidence and consultation. Am Coll Cardiol. 2013;61(12):1303–4. doi:10.1016/j.jacc.2013.01.005.
6. Warnes CA, Liberthson R, Danielson GK, et al. Task Force 1: the changing profile of congenital heart disease in adult life. J Am Coll Cardiol. 2001;37:1170–5.
7. Williams R, Pearson G, Barst R, et al. Report of the National Heart, Lung and Blood Institute Working Group on research in adult congenital heart disease. J Am Coll Cardiol. 2006;47:701–7.
8. Warnes C, Williams R, Bashore T, et al. ACC/AHA 2008 guidelines for the management of adults with congenital heart disease: a report of the American College of Cardiology/American Heart Association Task Force on Practice Guidelines. J Am Coll Cardiol. 2008;52(23):e143–263. doi:10.1016/j.jacc.2008.10.001.
9. Marelli AJ, Mackie AS, Ionescu-Ittu R, et al. Congenital heart disease in the general population: changing prevalence and age distribution. Circulation. 2007;115(2):163–72.
10. Care of the Adult with Congenital Heart Disease. Presented at the 32nd Bethesda Conference, Bethesda, Maryland, Oct 2–3, 2000. J Am Coll Cardiol. 2001;37(5):1161–98.
11. Vis JC, Velde ET, Schuuring MJ, et al. Wanted! 8000 heart patients: identification of adult patients with a congenital heart defect lost to follow-up. Int J Cardiol. 2011;149(2):246–7. doi:10.1016/j.ijcard.2011.02.019.
12. Niwa K, Perloff JK, Webb GD, et al. Survey of specialized tertiary care facilities for adults with congenital heart disease. Int J Cardiol. 2004;96(2):211–6.
13. Rodriguez 3rd FH, Moodie DS, Parekh DR, et al. Outcomes of hospitalization in adults in the United States with atrial septal defect, ventricular septal defect, and atrioventricular septal defect. Am J Cardiol. 2011;108(2):290–3.
14. Sable C, Foster E, Uzark K, et al. Best practices in managing transition to adulthood for adolescents with congenital heart disease: the transition process and medical and psychosocial issues: a scientific statement from the American Heart Association. Circulation. 2011;123(13):1454–85.
15. Perloff JK. Congenital heart disease in adults: a new cardiovascular subspecialty. Circulation. 1991;84:1881–90. doi:10.1161/01.CIR.84.5.1881.
16. Engelfriet P, Mulder BJM. Gender differences in adult congenital heart disease. Neth Heart J. 2009;17(11):414–7. doi:10.1007/BF03086294.
17. Engelfriet PM, Drenthen W, Pieper PG, et al. Smoking and its effects on mortality in adults with congenital heart disease. Int J Cardiol. 2008;127(1):93–7. doi:10.1016/j.ijcard.2007.05.008.
18. Zomer AC, Vaartjes I, Uiterwaal CS, et al. Circumstances of death in adult congenital heart disease. Int J Cardiol. 2012;154(2):168–72. doi:10.1016/j.ijcard.2010.09.015.

19. Boneva RS, Botto LD, Moore CA, et al. Mortality associated with congenital heart defects in the United States: trends and racial disparities, 1979–1997. Circulation. 2001;103:2376–81. doi:10.1161/01.CIR.103.19.2376.
20. Van der Bom T, Bouma BJ, Meijboom FJ, et al. The prevalence of adult congenital heart disease, results from a systematic review and evidence based calculation. Am Heart J. 2012;164(4):568–75.
21. Gilboa SM, Salemi JL, Nembhard WN, et al. Mortality resulting from congenital heart disease among children and adults in the United States, 1999 to 2006. Circulation. 2010;122(22):2254–63. doi:10.1161/CIRCULATIONAHA.110.947002.
22. Zomer AC, Vaartjes I, Uiterwaal CS, et al. Social burden and lifestyle in adults with congenital heart disease. Am J Cardiol. 2012;109(11):1657–63. doi:10.1016/j.amjcard.2012.01.397.
23. Verheugt CL, Uiterwaal CS, Velde ET, et al. Gender and outcome in adult congenital heart disease. Circulation. 2008;118(1):26–32. doi:10.1161/CIRCULATION/AHA.107.758086.
24. Kovacs AH, Sears SF, Saidi AS. Biopsychosocial experiences of adults with congenital heart disease: review of the literature. Am Heart J. 2005;150(2):193–201. doi:10.1016/j.ahj.2004.08.025.

Embryology

2

Azin Alizadehasl and Maryam Moradian

Keywords
Embryology • Congenital heart disease • Heart tube • Angiogenic cells

Most congenital heart defects lead to abnormal cardiac development, yet there is surprisingly little known about the central processes that occur in the heart. During the first 20 days of growth, the human embryo has no any obvious cardiovascular structure. In the second month, the heart structure and great vessels finished their growth process. This wonderful developmental course transforms isolated angiogenic cell islands into a 4-chambered apparatus. Throughout this transformation, the single heart tube begins to beat at the 23rd day of development, and by 30 days blood circulates in all parts of the embryo.

The cardiovascular system comprises the heart and vessels. The embryonic development of any organ, including the heart, is controlled by complex processes: cell growth, migration, death, differentiation, and adhesion. The precursors of the cardiovascular system are angiogenic cell clusters. Initially, these clusters shape twin tubular structures, which by 22 days of development attach in the midline on the ventral side of the embryo to shape up a single, slightly bent heart tube. Before cardiac looping, segments of the heart can be identified, including the sinus venosus and also the atrium (left and right atria), the primitive ventricle (left ventricle), the bulbus cordis (right ventricle), and the truncus arteriosus (aorta and pulmonary arteries). At around 22 days, the heart tube initiates to fold ventrally and turn toward the right side, whereas the caudal atrial portion begins to bend in a posterosuperior direction (looping). Looping brings the future left ventricle leftward and the future right ventricle rightward. In order to separate the systemic and pulmonary circulations, the original single-chamber heart begins to be partitioned. The development of endocardial cushions at both atrioventricular and also conotruncal junctions starts at 26 days and leads to the septation of the heart. The superior and inferior cushions joined each other by the 5th week, resulting in a right (tricuspid) and left (mitral) atrioventricular orifice. The appearance of septum of the atria initiates at 30 days with the downward growth of the septum primum, which leaves an open ostium primum. However, the ostium primum is subsequently obliterated due

A. Alizadehasl, MD, FACC (✉)
Echocardiography Lab, Department of Cardiology, Rajaie Cardiovascular Medical and Research Center, Iran University of Medical Science, Tehran, Iran
e-mail: alizadeasl@gmail.com, alizadeasl@rhc.ac.ir

M. Moradian, MD
Department of Pediatric Cardiology, Rajaie Cardiovascular Medical and Research Center, Iran University of Medical Science, Tehran, Iran
e-mail: maryam_moradian2008@yahoo.com, m.moradian@rhc.ac.ir

A. Sadeghpour et al. (eds.), *Comprehensive Approach to Adult Congenital Heart Disease*,
DOI 10.1007/978-1-4471-6383-1_2, © Springer-Verlag London 2014

to the fusion of the septum primum along with the endocardial cushions. Meanwhile, the ostium secundum shapes up within the septum primum. At the end of the process, the septum secundum grows downward and lies at the right side of the septum primum, but an interatrial opening (i.e., the foramen ovale) remains until birth. The interventricular septum formation is the result of the dilation of two primitive ventricles (right and left conus swellings) with the opposition of the medial walls. At the distal portion of the cardiac tube, the bulbus cordis divides into subaortic and subpulmonary muscular conuses; the subpulmonary conus lengthens and the subaortic conus resorbs, allowing the aorta to transfer posteriorly and to attach to the left ventricle [1–4].

In 1942, Kramer theorized that there are three embryological areas: the conus, the truncus, and finally the pulmonary arterial sections. Every segment grows the two opposing edges of the endocardial tissue; the opposite pairs of the edges and those shapes up various segments encounter to make a septum separating the two outflow tracts and the aortopulmonary trunks [5]. The aortopulmonary septum is created by the rims separating the 4th (upcoming aortic arch) and the 6th (upcoming pulmonary arteries) aortic arches. Then, the truncus ridges are fashioned in the area where the semilunar (future aortic and pulmonic) valves are intended to be shaped, thereby forging the septum in the middle of the ascending aortic trunk and the main pulmonary artery [5].

Atria

The atria of the developed heart can originate from more than one source. The appendages of the left and right atria (trabeculated portions) are shape up by the primitive atria, while the smooth posterior parts of the right and left atria are created by the union of the venous vessels. The posterior side of the left atrium is made by a combination of the pulmonary veins; on the other hand, the posterior smooth part of the right atrium originated from the sinus venosus. Then, the embryonic sinuatrium is separated into the left and right atria by developing downward from the roof of the septum primum toward the atrioventricular canal, fusing with the cushions. Numerous perforations develop in the anterosuperior part of the septum primum. Thereafter, there is a superior enfolding of the roof of the atria, which has traditionally been called the septum secundum. The remnant of the septum primum makes the fossa ovalis.

The union of the endocardial cushions anteriorly and posteriorly splits the atrioventricular canal into tricuspid and mitral inlets. The inferior part of the atrial septum and superior part of the ventricular septum and portions of the septal leaflet of the tricuspid valve and also the anterior leaflet of the mitral valve are formed by the endocardial cushions. The posterior leaflet of the mitral valve predominantly develops from a piece of the atrioventricular myocardium that protrudes into the lumen of the ventricle. The integrity of the intra-atrial septum depends on the growth of the septum primum and the superior enfolding and appropriate combination of the endocardial cushions. Atrial septal defects are the result of deficits in the development of this course [1, 3, 7].

Ventricles

The division of the ventricles occurs as the cephalic development of the main ventricular septum results in its union with the endocardial cushions and the infundibular or conus septum. There are two mechanisms for intraventricular septal defects. These defects may occur due to a deficiency in septal substance, malalignment in the components of the septum in different levels, discontinuation of their fusion, or sometimes the formation of a long conus, splitting the septal components. Isolated simple defects are possibly the result of the first mechanism, whereas ventricular septal defects in tetralogy of Fallot and transposition complexes are a consequence of the latter two mechanisms [1–3, 7].

Pulmonary Veins

The pulmonary vein is documented as a canal entering the atrial component adjacent to the atrioventricular junction. After the closure of the interventricular communication, the pulmonary veins transfer to the roof of the left atrium. This communicates with the splanchnic plexus, forming pulmonary venous drainage into the left atrium. However, anomalous pulmonary venous connections to the umbilicovitelline (portal) venous system or to the cardinal system (superior vena cava) result from the failure of the common pulmonary vein to develop or to establish communications to the splanchnic plexus [5–8].

Great Arteries

While the six aortic arches appear consecutively, some parts of the arch system and dorsal aorta disappear at different times during embryogenesis. The first, second, and fifth groups of the paired arches regress totally. The proximal parts of the 6th arch develop the right and left pulmonary arteries, and the distal left 6th arch develops the ductus arteriosus. The third aortic arch makes the connection between the internal and external carotid arteries, and the left 4th arch becomes the arterial portion between the left carotid and subclavian arteries. Then, the proximal part of the right subclavian artery is formed by the right fourth arch. An abnormality in the regression of the arch system in a number of sites can create a wide variety of arch anomalies, for example, a failure of regression usually results in a double aortic arch malformation [6, 7].

Abnormal Development

Anomalies can result from deficiencies in this basic developmental pattern. For example, a double-inlet left ventricle is detected when the tricuspid orifice does not align over the right ventricle or when the various forms of persistent truncus arteriosus are caused by the failure of the truncus to divide into the main pulmonary artery and the aorta. The double-outlet anomalies of the right ventricle are created by the failure of either the subpulmonary or the subaortic conuses to resorb, or the resorption of the subpulmonary instead of the subaortic conus may give rise to the transposition of the great arteries [5–8].

References

1. Bird GL, Jeffries HE, Licht DJ, et al. Neurological complications associated with the treatment of patients with congenital cardiac disease: consensus definitions from the Multi-Societal Database Committee for Pediatric and Congenital Heart Disease. Cardiol Young. 2008;18 Suppl 2:234.
2. Thorne S, Mac Gregor A, Nelson-Piercy C. Risks of contraception and pregnancy in heart disease. Heart. 2006;92:1520.
3. Becker AE, Anderson RH. Cardiac embryology. In: Nora JJ, Talao A, editors. Congenital heart disease: causes and processes. New York: Futura; 1984. p. 339–58.
4. Benson DW, et al. New understanding in the genetics of congenital heart disease. Curr Opin Pediatr. 1996;8:505–11.
5. Abdulla R, Blew GA, Holterman MJ. Cardiovascular embryology. Pediatr Cardiol. 2004;25:191–200.
6. Bockman ED. Effect of neural crest on the development of the heart and arch arteries in the chick. Am J Anat. 1987;180:332–41.
7. Bonow RO, Mann DL, Zipes DP, Libby P, eds. Braunwald's Heart Disease: A Textbook of Cardiovascular Medicine. 9th ed. Philadelphia, Pa: Saunders Elsevier; 2011.
8. Perloff J, Marelu A. Perloff's clinical recognition of congenital heart disease. 6th ed. Philadelphia: Elsevier Saunders; 2012.

Fetal Circulation

3

Maryam Moradian

Keywords
Embryology • Fetal circulation • Congenital heart disease • Heart tube

In the fetal circulation, unlike in the adult circulation, the placenta provides gas and metabolite exchange. And in addition, the right and left ventricles are in a parallel circuit, rather than in a series circuit of a newborn or an adult. The ductus venosus, foramen ovale, and ductus arteriosus are three cardiovascular structures that are unique to the fetus and are important for maintaining this parallel circulation.

Enriched with oxygen and nutrients, blood travels from the placenta to the liver through the umbilical vein (Fig. 3.1a, b). About less than half of this saturated blood goes in the hepatic circulation, and the remainder of this blood bypasses the liver via the ductus venosus and reaches the right atrium (RA) via the inferior vena cava (IVC) (Fig. 3.2a, b).

A functional sphincter regulates the flow of blood through the ductus venosus at the level of the umbilical vein. During the periodic contractions of the uterus, this sphincter closes, preventing sudden overloading of the heart.

M. Moradian
Department of Pediatric Cardiology,
Rajaie Cardiovascular Medical and Research Center,
Iran University of Medical Science, Tehran, Iran
e-mail: maryam_moradian2008@yahoo.com,
m.moradian@rhc.ac.ir

In the IVC, the oxygenated blood from the placenta mixes with the deoxygenated blood recurring from the lower part of the fetal body. It thereafter enters the RA and favorably flows into the left atrium (LA) via the foramen ovale. This shunt allows normal development of the LA and the left ventricle (LV) because the development of the cardiac chambers is dependent on the flow of blood through them. In the RA, a small amount of blood mixes with the desaturated blood from the superior vena cava (SVC) and preferentially traverses the tricuspid valve into the right ventricle (RV). However, due to the high pressure in the lungs, just a small portion of the blood passes through the pulmonary circulation and reaches the LA via the pulmonary veins. A significantly larger part flows through the ductus arteriosus and goes into the descending aorta and thus directly into the large (systemic) circulation system to perfuse the inferior part of the fetal body (Fig. 3.3).

The left atrial blood enters the left ventricle and then to the ascending aorta (Fig. 3.4).

Consequently, the upper part of the fetal body, containing the coronary arteries, cerebral arteries, and superior extremity arteries, is perfused with blood that has a faintly higher PO2. Only a small volume of blood continues down via the isthmus to the descending aorta, mixing with the blood

A. Sadeghpour et al. (eds.), *Comprehensive Approach to Adult Congenital Heart Disease*,
DOI 10.1007/978-1-4471-6383-1_3, © Springer-Verlag London 2014

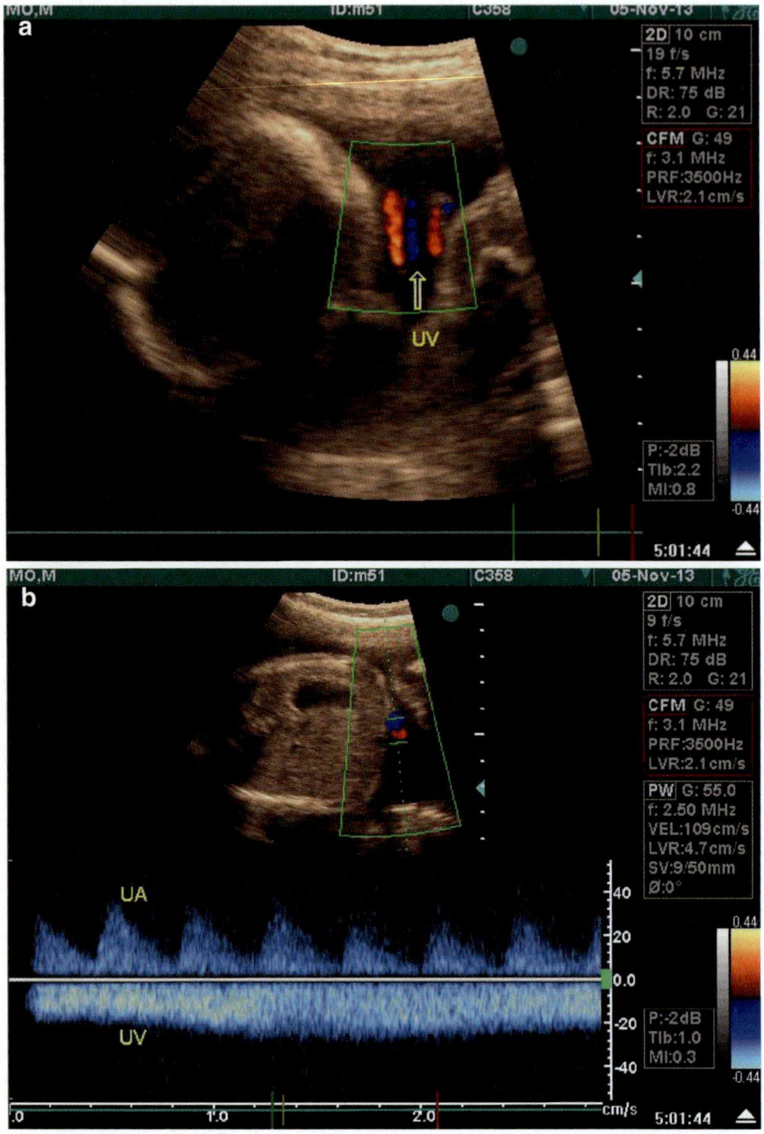

Fig. 3.1 (**a**) Two-dimensional fetal echocardiography, showing an oblique view of the umbilical cord with two arteries and a vein. (**b**) Doppler echocardiography, showing normal flow in the umbilical vein and umbilical artery. *UV* umbilical vein, *UA* umbilical artery

that has been shunted through the ductus arteriosus. Next, it perfuses the lower portion of the body and finally returns to the placenta through the two umbilical arteries.

In the fetus, it is not possible to separate the output of the left and right heart sides because of the intracardiac and extracardiac shunts, and the output of RV is about 1.3 times of LV output. Thus, in the fetus due to the shunt-dependent circulation, combined two ventricular outputs (CVO) are evaluated. About 45 % of CVO is directed to the placental circulation with only 8 % of CVO entering the pulmonary circulation.

After birth, the transition from fetal to newborn life involves the closure of the circulatory shunts and acute variations in pulmonary and systemic vascular resistance [1–3].

Transitional Circulation

At birth, as the transition to postnatal life begins, many changes occur in the fetal cardiovascular system. The elimination of the low-resistance placental circulation leads to a dramatic fall in the venous return, and the closure of the ductus

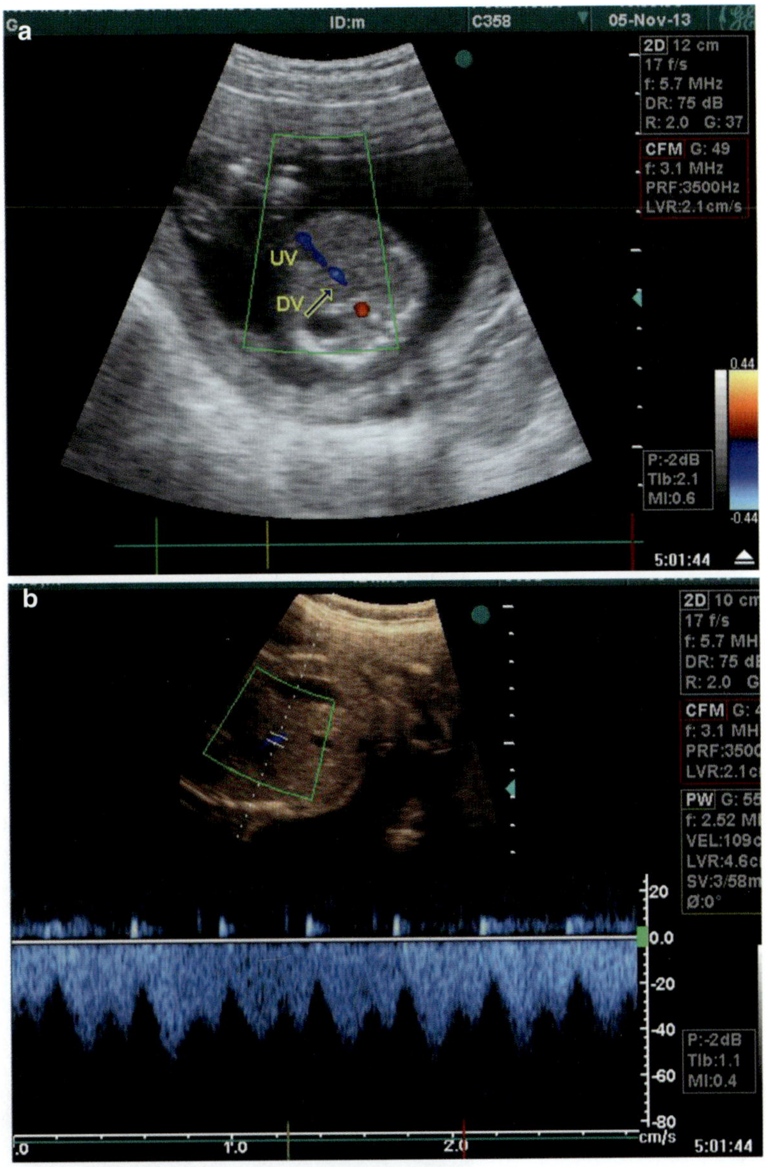

Fig. 3.2 (**a**) Transverse view of the fetal abdomen, showing the umbilical vein and a ductus venosus. (b) Doppler echocardiography, showing normal flow in the ductus venosus. *UV* umbilical vein, *DV* ductus venosus

venosus takes place during the third to the tenth day after birth. Moreover, not only does systemic vascular resistance increase but also pulmonary vascular resistance falls and pulmonary blood flow increases in consequence of an expansion in the lungs. Concomitant with the fall in pulmonary vascular resistance, the shunt in the level of the ductus arteriosus becomes bidirectional, and when the pulmonary vascular resistance becomes lesser than systemic vascular resistance, the shunt over the ductus arteriosus reverses and also becomes left to right. The exact mechanism of ductal closure is not known, but the increase in neonatal blood oxygen and reduction in PGE2, produced in the placenta, lead to the constriction of the smooth muscle within the duct. Functional closure is then followed by anatomical closure, eventually becoming the ligamentum arteriosum by endothelial and fibrous tissue proliferation.

The rise in the pulmonary blood flow leads to an increase in the pulmonary venous return to the LA. Also, the closure of the ductus venosus results in a reduction in the venous return to

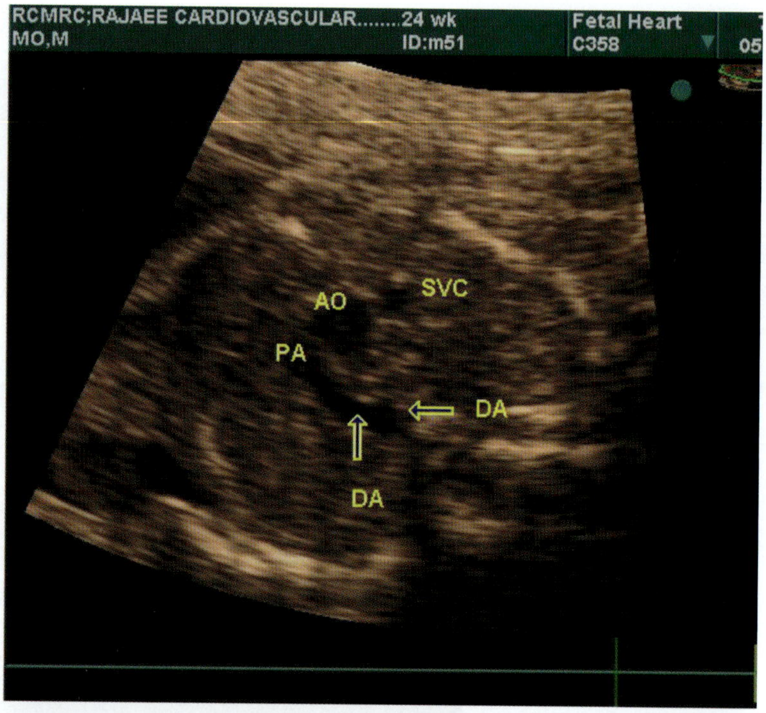

Fig. 3.3 Three-vessel view, showing a ductus arteriosus *DA* (*vertical arrow*) extending to the descending aorta *DA* (*horizontal arrow*). *PA* pulmonary artery, *AO* aorta, *SVC* superior vena cava

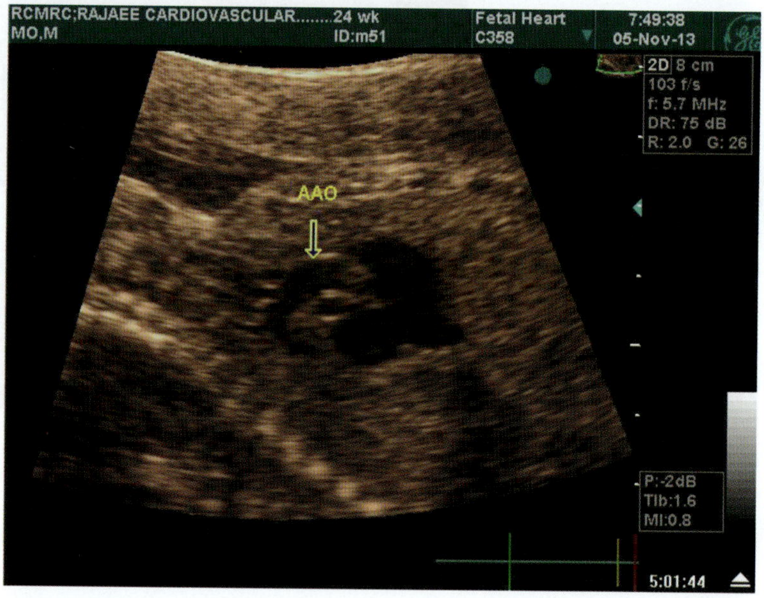

Fig. 3.4 Longitudinal views of the ascending aorta and aortic arch. *AAO* ascending aorta

the RA. Accordingly, LA pressure and volume increase sufficiently to push the septum primum against the septum secundum. This initial closure of the foramen ovale happens within minutes to hours after birth. The anatomical closure of the foramen ovale happens later via tissue proliferation during the first year, though it may remain probe patent. The umbilical arteries develop to umbilical ligaments attached to the internal iliac arteries above to the superior vesical arteries. The ductus venosus becomes a fibrous band named ligamentum venosum, which is seen in continuation with the ligamentum teres (obliterated left-sided umbilical vein) [3, 4].

Neonatal Circulation

In postnatal life, cardiopulmonary adaptation to extrauterine life should be made. Gas exchange should be transferred to the lungs when the neonate takes the first breath. Meanwhile, the pulmonary circulation initiates and the right and left hearts become completely independent of each other. During the first week of life, pulmonary vascular resistance drops from the high fetal level to the low adult level. Over the first weeks of life, the renovation of the pulmonary vasculature, containing the thinning of the vascular smooth muscles and recruitment of new vessels, takes place. This drop in pulmonary vascular resistance affects the timing of the clinical appearance of many congenital heart defects like ventricular septal defect. The left to right shunt through the ventricular septal defect will rise as pulmonary vascular resistance falls. As a result, in the first few days of life, no murmur may be heard and the child would be asymptomatic. If pulmonary vascular resistance does not drop normally after birth, pulmonary arterial pressure will not fall to the normal postnatal level. This phenomenon, persistent pulmonary hypertension of the newborn (PPHN), may result from some conditions such as meconium aspiration and also perinatal asphyxia. In PPHN, the shunt flow through the ductus arteriosus or foramen ovale remains right to left and leads to cyanosis.

In specific congenital heart defects, the patency of the foramen ovale and ductus arteriosus that does not completely close at birth plays an important role. In some of these lesions, this patency could be lifesaving, as is the case in severe coarctation and transposition of great arteries.

The muscle mass and the wall thickness of the LV and RV are equal at birth. After birth, pulmonary vascular resistance drops in consequence of an expansion in the lungs, and systemic vascular resistance rises as a result of placental removal. The RV wall, therefore, starts to thin.

Initially, the newborn's cardiac output is extremely high (near 350 ml/kg/min). Nevertheless, during the first two months of life, it falls to near 150 ml/kg/min and then slowly decreases to the adult level (near 75 ml/kg/min). Also high percentage of fetal hemoglobin (HbF) may interfere with oxygen delivery, so an augmented cardiac output is needed for a sufficient oxygen supply. Synthesis of HbF decreases after the newborn period and by 6–12 months of age is substituted by adult hemoglobin, causing a better oxygen delivery to the organs. This change in the oxygen delivery is believed to result in the gradual reduction in the cardiac output [3, 5–7].

References

1. Rudolph AM. Congenital cardiovascular malformations and the fetal circulation. Arch Dis Child Fetal Neonatal. 2010;95:132–6.
2. Ellis H. Anatomy of fetal circulation. Anaesth Intensive Care Med. 2005;6(3):73.
3. Sachdeva R. Atrial septal defects In: Allen HD, Driscoll DJ, Shaddy RF, Feltes TF, editors. Moss and Adams's heart disease in infants, children. 8th ed. Philadelphia: Lippincott Williams & Wilkins; 2013. p. 672–88.
4. Drose JA. Embryology and physiology of the fetal heart In: Drose JA, editor. Fetal echocardiography. 2nd ed; Philadelphia: Saunders; 2010. p. 1–12.
5. Bernstein D. Developmental biology of the cardiovascular system. In: Kligman RM, Stanton BF, Schor NF, St. Geme III JW, Behrman RE, editors. Nelson text book of pediatrics. 19th ed. Philadelphia: Saunders; 2011. p. 1527–9.
6. Friedman AH, Fahey JT. The transition from fetal to neonatal circulation: normal responses and implications for infants with heart disease. Semin Perinatol. 1993;17(2):106–21.
7. Bonow R, Mann D, Zipes D, Libby P. Braunwald's heart disease: a textbook of cardiovascular medicine. 9th ed. Philadelphia: Elsevier Saunders; 2011. p. 1435–50.

Normal Cardiac Anatomy

4

Anita Sadeghpour

Keywords
Normal anatomy • Left ventricle (LV) • Right ventricle (RV) • Right atrium (RA) • Left atrium (LA) • Crista terminalis (CT) • Chiari network • Coronary sinus (CS) • Isomerism • Situs solitus

Diagnosis of congenital heart disease (CHD) requires a thorough understanding of normal cardiac anatomy. In fact, the recognition of 'abnormal' anatomy relies on the definition of '*normal*' anatomy.

Normally, most of the major systems develop in a midline position with bilateral mirror-image symmetry. *The cardiovascular, respiratory, and digestive systems later become asymmetric and are characterized by their situs or position in the body.* So, it is not uncommon to observe the associated anomalies of abdominal viscera in cardiac malposition.

A. Sadeghpour, MD, FACC, FASE
Echocardiography Lab,
Department of Cardiology,
Adult Congenital Heart Disease Clinic,
Rajaie Cardiovascular Medical
and Research Center, Iran University of Medical
Science, Tehran, Iran
e-mail: anita.sadeghpour@gmail.com,
asadeghpour@rhc.ac.ir

Common Definitions and Abbreviations in Congenital Heart Disease

To use a uniform clinical language in the context of CHD, the following definitions and abbreviations have been suggested [1–7]:

Cardiac position means the location of the heart in the thorax and is categorized as left sided (levocardia), right sided (dextrocardia), or midline (mesocardia).

Cardiac malposition refers to an abnormal location of the heart or when the location is abnormal relative to the abdominal viscera.

Situs refers to the site, position, sidedness, and handedness.

Situs should be determined separately for the abdominal viscera, atria, ventricles, and great arteries as:

Solitus (normal, usual), which may be abbreviated as (S)

Inversus (mirror image, reverse), which may be abbreviated as (I)

Ambiguus (uncertain or indeterminate), which may be abbreviated as (A)

Cardiac situs refers to the position of the morphologic right atrium, independent of the

A. Sadeghpour et al. (eds.), *Comprehensive Approach to Adult Congenital Heart Disease*,
DOI 10.1007/978-1-4471-6383-1_4, © Springer-Verlag London 2014

direction of the apex, ventricles, or great arteries.

Heterotaxy denotes an abnormal arrangement and describes the complex abnormalities of visceral and atrial situs such as isomerism.

Isomerism means the symmetric morphology of the structures that normally are not symmetric, such as similarity between the right and left atrial appendages and the right and left lung and bronchi.

Right isomerism refers to the morphologic bilateral right sidedness of the atrial appendages, bronchi, and lungs, all of which should have normal different lateralization. This condition is u*sually associated with asplenia (rudimentary spleen or* absence of spleen).

Left isomerism refers to the morphologic bilateral left sidedness of the atrial appendages, bronchi, and lungs and is usually associated with polysplenia.

Ventricular looping (situs) refers to the right or left bending (loop) of the straight heart tube of the embryo and is designated as the *D-loop ventricle (D) or L-loop (inversus) ventricle (L).*

D-loop (solitus) ventricle means that the morphologic right ventricular inflow lies to the right of the morphologic left ventricle and is the normal rightward bending of the embryonic heart tube.

L-loop (inversus) ventricle means that the morphologic right ventricular inflow lies to the left of the morphologic left ventricle and is the leftward bending of the embryonic heart tube.

Great arteries situs is categorized as:

Solitus (S)
Inversus (I)
Ambiguus or anterior transposition/malposition (A)
D-loop transposition/malposition (D)
L-loop transposition/malposition (L)

Concordant means agreeing or appropriate connection.

Discordant means not agreeing or inappropriate connection.

Atrioventricular concordance means the appropriate connection of the morphologic right atrium to the morphologic right ventricle and is associated with the appropriate connection of the morphologic left atrium to the morphologic left ventricle.

Each of the atrioventricular valves is determined according to the morphologic ventricle to which it is attached.

Ventriculoarterial concordance means the appropriate connection of the morphologic right ventricle to the pulmonary artery and the appropriate connection of the morphologic left ventricle to the aorta.

Concordant ventricular looping that agrees with the visceroatrial situs is D-loop in situs solitus and L-loop in situs inversus.

Infundibulum (conus) is a subpulmonary ventriculoarterial segment in a normal heart.

Transposition of the great arteries refers to a condition in which the great arteries connect to a discordant ventricle (ventriculoarterial discordance). The aorta arises from the right ventricle and the pulmonary trunk arises from the left ventricle.

Malposition of the great arteries refers to a condition in which there is an abnormal spatial relationship between the great arteries (aorta and the pulmonary artery).

The great arteries can be malposed without associated transposition as long as the ventriculoarterial concordance is maintained.

Normal Anatomy

A normal heart is a left-sided heart with a leftward-pointing apex and is located in the middle mediastinum [4, 7]. *Normal cardiac location that refers to the position of* most of the cardiac mass is levoposition (Fig. 4.1). *Cardiac orientation that refers to the base-to-apex axis is leftward pointing*. The apex is directed leftward, anteriorly, and inferiorly. *Usually these two*, i.e., *cardiac location and cardiac orientation, go together.*

The cardiac size can be measured radiographically as the ratio between the maximal transverse diameters of the heart divided by the maximal width of the thorax. This ratio is called the cardiothoracic ratio and is normally 50 % or less in adults (Fig. 4.2).

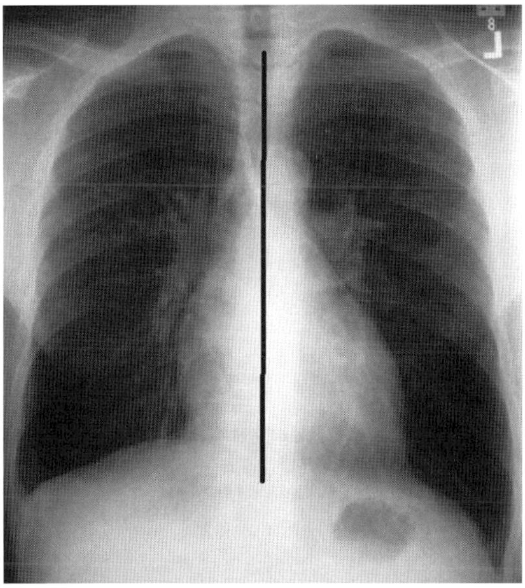

Fig. 4.1 Standard posteroanterior chest X-ray, showing a normal heart, which is a left-sided heart with a leftward-pointing apex

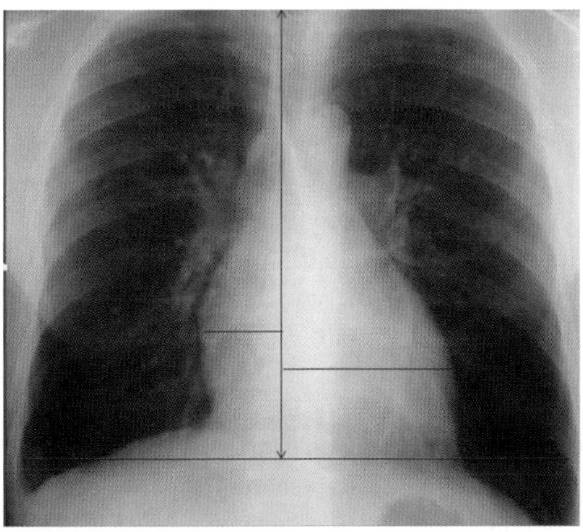

Fig. 4.2 Cardiothoracic ratio measurement as the ratio between the maximal transverse diameters of the heart divided by the maximal width of the thorax

Situs Solitus

Situs solitus means normal cardiac situs and is associated with normal abdominovisceral situs. It is noteworthy that *cardiac situs* is determined by the position of the morphologic right atrium.

Usually atrial situs and abdominal situs are concordant.

Visceral situs is determined by the position of the liver, stomach, aorta, and inferior vena cava. The spleen and pancreas are normally located on the same side of the vertebral column as the stomach.

In the abdominal situs solitus, the stomach is left sided, the liver is right sided, and the aorta lies to the left and the inferior vena cava (IVC) lies to the right of the spine. The atrial situs is reliably predicted by bronchial morphology. In the situs solitus, the right and left bronchi are asymmetric as the right bronchus is relatively straight and short and the left bronchus is relatively long and curved (Fig. 4.3). The right bronchus is trilobed and concordant with the right lung and the left bronchus is bilobed and concordant with the left lung [4–7].

Interestingly, the level of the hemidiaphragm is determined by the location of the cardiac apex, not by the location of the liver. Therefore, normally the left hemidiaphragm is lower than the right hemidiaphragm.

The plain chest X-ray yields valuable and unique information since it not only establishes the cardiac location, base-to-apex axis, and positions of the liver and stomach but also discloses bronchial morphology (Fig. 4.4).

Normal Heart

A diagnostic approach to CHD needs a systematic sequential approach. The sequential segmental approach begins with the identification of the atrial and abdominal situs, followed by the determination of the three segments, *the atria, ventricles, and great arteries*, and the two connections, *atrioventricular and ventriculoarterial connections*.

As a rule, the heart chambers are recognized based on their morphology rather than their position. So, the approach to CHD requires a thorough knowledge of cardiac anatomy.

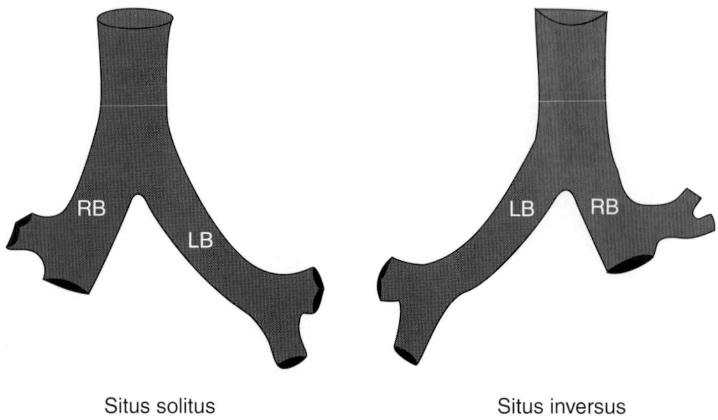

Fig. 4.3 Asymmetric right and left bronchi in situs solitus: a relatively straight and short right bronchus and a relatively long and curved left bronchus. *RB* right bronchus, *LB* left bronchus

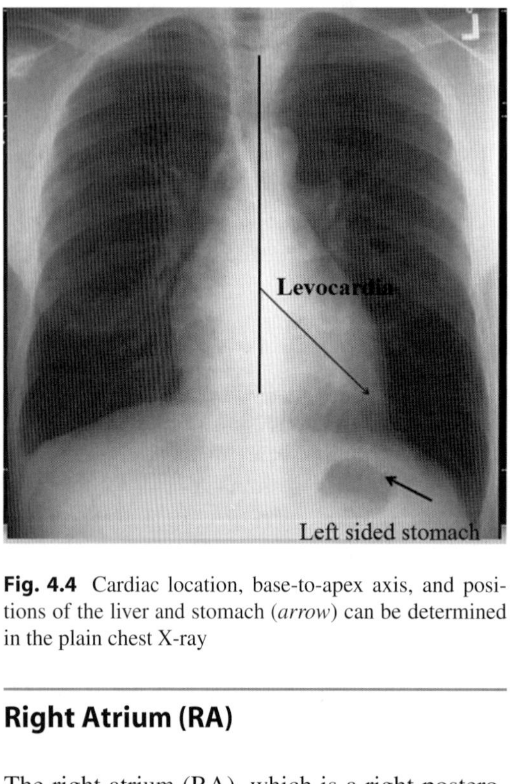

Fig. 4.4 Cardiac location, base-to-apex axis, and positions of the liver and stomach (*arrow*) can be determined in the plain chest X-ray

Right Atrium (RA)

The right atrium (RA), which is a right posterolateral chamber, receives the systemic venous blood return from the inferior and superior venae cavae and the coronary venous blood return from the coronary sinus. One of the morphologic characteristics of the RA is a large pyramidal, wide-based appendage with irregular arrangement of the pectinate muscles (Fig. 4.5). The RA receives the blood of the inferior and superior venae cavae from the posterior aspect.

The RA has a unique morphology with several important landmarks, including the CT, Eustachian valve, Thebesian valve, and Chiari network [8–11]. The coronary sinus and the inferior vena cava connect to the inferior wall of the RA. The Eustachian valve guards the orifice of the inferior vena cava (Fig. 4.6), whereas the ostium of the coronary sinus is guarded by the Thebesian valve (Fig. 4.7).

The Chiari network is a reticulated filamentous structure in the RA which originates from the Eustachian valve and connects to the different parts of the right atrium [8, 12, 13]. It is a normal variant and results from the incomplete reabsorption of the right sinus venosus valve. It has been found in approximately 2 % of the general population with little clinical consequence in some studies although the correlation with persistent patent foramen ovale (PFO) and paradoxical embolism has been suggested (Figs. 4.8 and 4.9).

Crista terminalis (CT) which is a prominent C-shaped ridge of the muscle separates the smooth-walled sinus venarum part of the RA from the trabeculated atrial appendage [9, 14].

The CT is located at the junction of the RA appendage and the smooth muscle part of the RA. The CT varies in size and can be misdiagnosed as an RA mass in transthoracic echocardiography (Figs. 4.10 and 4.11).

The most prominent feature of the interatrial septum is the fossa ovalis,[4] which contains a horseshoe-shaped rim (limbus). The limbus thickness averages between 4 and 8 mm in adolescents and adults (Fig. 4.11). From the embryological view, the fossa ovalis valve represents the septum primum and the limbus represents the septum secundum.

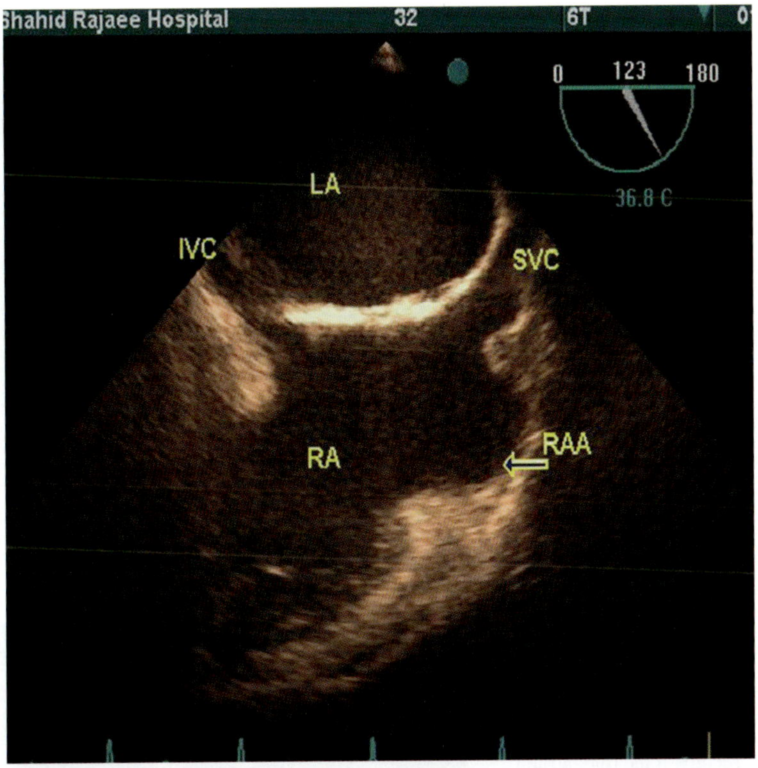

Fig. 4.5 Right atrial appendage (*arrow*), which is a large pyramidal, wide-based appendage with irregular arrangement of the pectinate muscles. *LA* left atrium, *IVC* inferior vena cava, *SVC* superior vena cava, *RAA* right atrium appendage

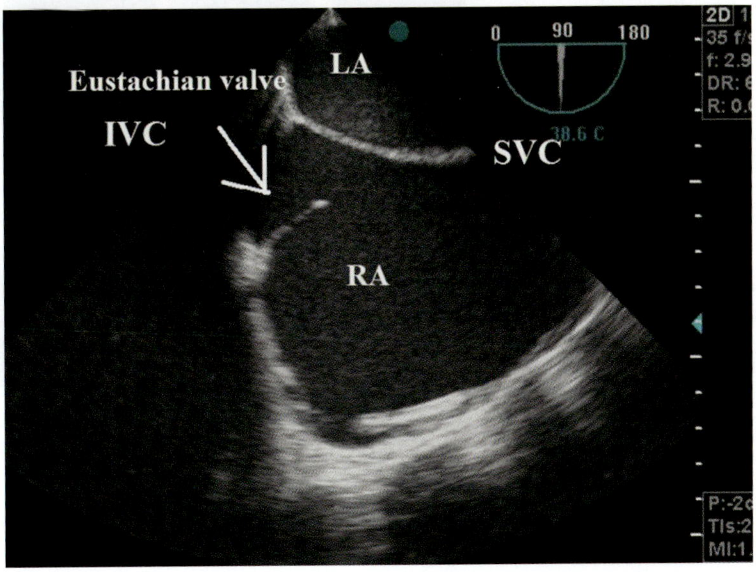

Fig. 4.6 Eustachian valve (*arrow*), guarding the inferior vena cava orifice. *LA* left atrium, *IVC* inferior vena cava, *SVC* superior vena cava, *RAA* right atrium appendage

Left Atrium (LA)

The LA is a posterior chamber that usually receives the blood return from the four pulmonary venous drainages. Except for the LA appendage (LAA), the bulk of the LA is smooth walled, with no evidence of pectinate muscles or CT [5, 7].

The LAA is a fingerlike structure containing small pectinate muscles (Fig. 4.12).

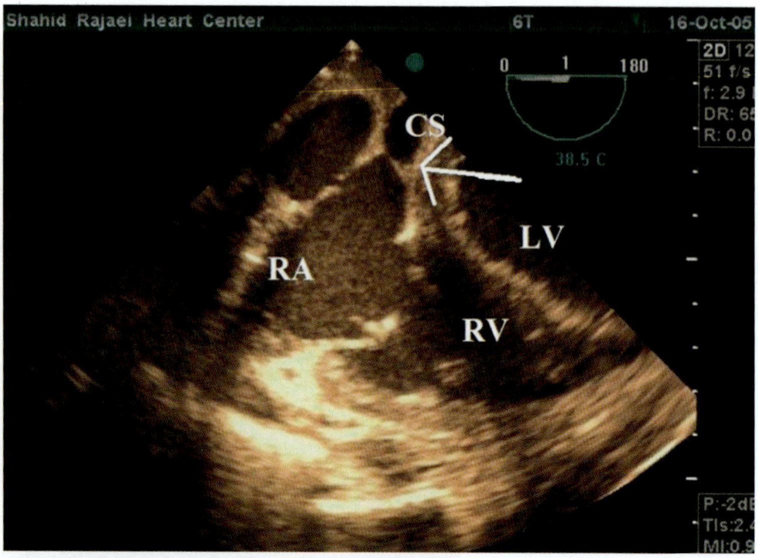

Fig. 4.7 Thebesian valve (*arrow*), guarding the ostium of the coronary sinus. *CS* coronary sinus, *LV* left ventricle, *RA* right atrium, *RV* right ventricle

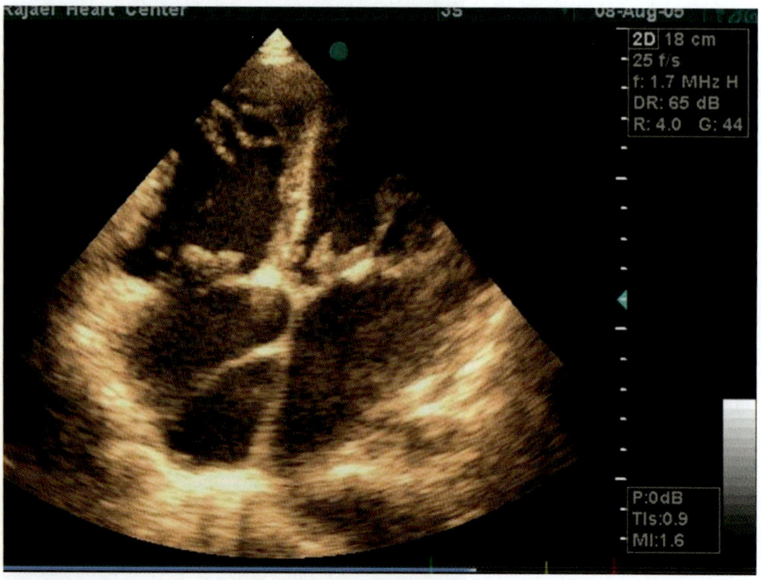

Fig. 4.8 Four-chamber view in transthoracic echocardiography, showing the Chiari network, which is a reticulated filamentous structure in the right atrium

Determination of Ventricle

Morphologic determination of a ventricle should be preceded by a definition of a ventricle. Based on the 50% rule, a chamber can be termed "ventricle" if it receives 50 % or more of the inlet, even if this inlet is an imperforate fibrotic membrane and is situated over a small right ventricle (RV), as is the case in tricuspid atresia. Note that a chamber need not have an outlet in order to be termed "ventricle" [6, 15, 16].

Right Ventricle (RV)

The RV is the most anteriorly located chamber. It lies behind the sternum and wraps around the left ventricle (LV).

The RV is divided into three components:

1. Inlet portion, which supports and surrounds the tricuspid valve.
2. Apical portion, which is quite thin and vulnerable to iatrogenic perforation by pacemaker electrodes and cardiac catheters. The RV apex has a typical coarse trabeculation.

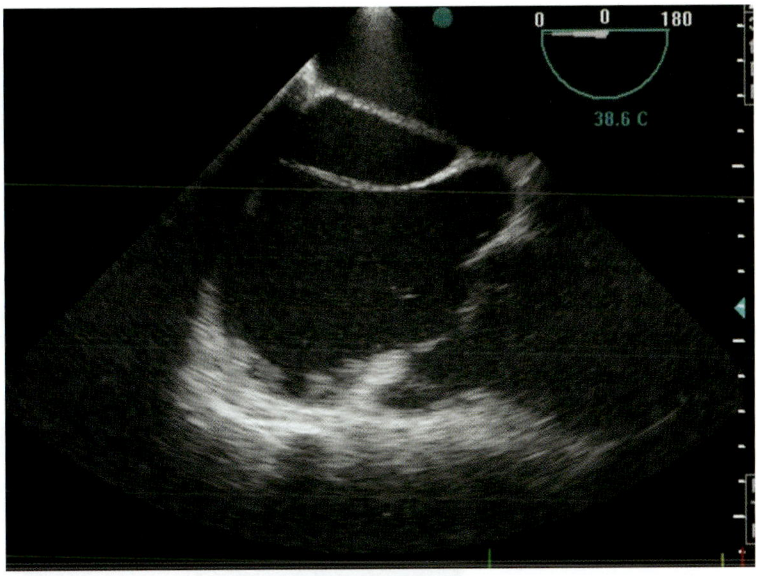

Fig. 4.9 Chiari network in the right atrium in transesophageal echocardiography

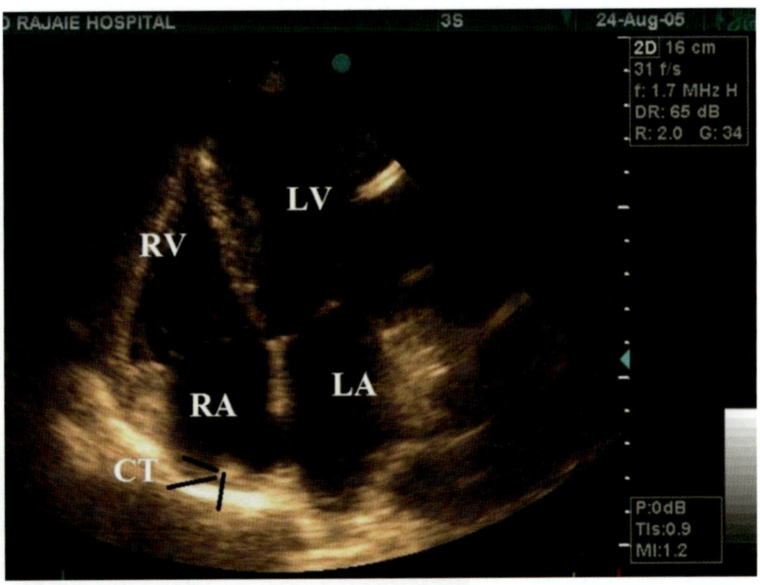

Fig. 4.10 Crista terminalis (*arrow*) in four-chamber view in transthoracic echocardiography. *LV* left ventricle, *RV* right ventricle, *RA* right atrium, *LA* left atrium, *CT* crista terminalis

3. Outlet portion, which is a tubular muscular structure (pulmonary infundibulum or conus) and supports the pulmonary valve leaflets.

The RV is characterized by:

1. Crescent shape in short-axis cross-sectional view
2. Coarse septal surface heavy trabeculations
3. Presence of the moderator band, which is a muscle bundle with extension to the right ventricular free wall
4. Infundibulum (the crista supraventricularis)
5. Tricuspid-pulmonary discontinuity

Left Ventricle (LV)

The LV is a conical structure characterized by:

1. Apical fine trabeculations and remarkably thin myocardium at the LV apex
2. Smooth septal surface with no papillary muscle attachment to the left side of the interventricular septum
3. Mitral-aortic fibrous continuity
4. Presence of two papillary muscles named "posteromedial" and "anterolateral" papillary muscles at the mid-ventricular level

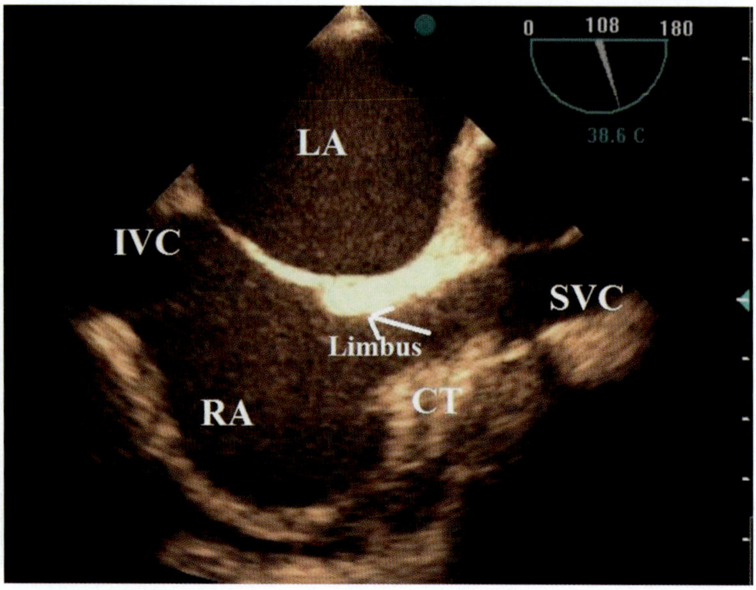

Fig. 4.11 Transesophageal bicaval view, showing the interatrial septum (*arrow*) and the fossa ovalis, which contains a horseshoe-shaped rim (limbus). *IVC* inferior vena cava, *SVC* superior vena cava, *RA* right atrium, *CT* crista terminalis

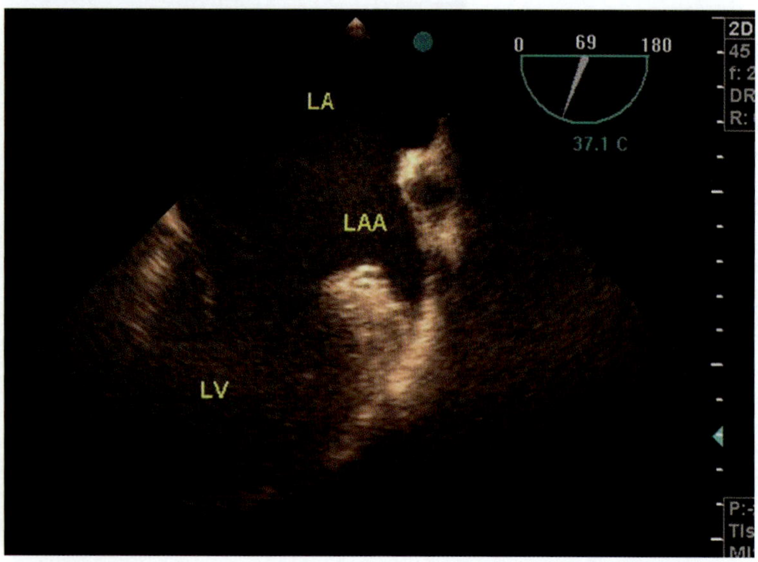

Fig. 4.12 Left atrial appendage anatomy in transesophageal echocardiography as a fingerlike structure containing small pectinate muscles. *LA* left atrium, *LAA* left atrium appendage, *LV* left ventricle

5. Similar distances from the mitral annulus to the apex and the aortic annulus to the apex, except in the atrioventricular septal defect, in which the inflow length is shorter than the outflow length

Morphologic landmarks [4, 5, 7, 8] for the identification of the cardiac ventricle are depicted in Table 4.1 and Figs. 4.13 and 4.14.

Atrioventricular Valves

The atrioventricular valves connect the atria to the underlying ventricles and are labeled according to their ventricle morphology. [The tricuspid valve always attaches to the morphologic RV and the mitral valve (MV) to the morphologic LV.]

Mitral Valve

The MV apparatus consists of five components: annulus, leaflets, commissures, papillary muscles, and chordae tendineae. Normally, the functioning MV depends on the perfect interaction between all these components.

The mitral annulus, which is the region of the attachment of the left atrium to the valve leaflets, plays an important role in the proper functioning of the MV. It demonstrates nonplanar saddle morphology (Fig. 4.15).

The MV has two leaflets with different appearances and complex anatomies. The anterior mitral leaflet (aortic leaflet) has shorter attachment compared to the posterior mitral leaflet (mural leaflet) and comprises about one third of the mitral annulus circumferences. The posterior mitral leaflet has three scallops separated by indentation and is recognized as P1, P2, and P3 scallops [8, 17–21]. The free edge of the anterior mitral leaflet is continuous without any indentation and is artificially based on the corresponding P1, P2, and P3 scallops. The anterior mitral valve has been divided into A1, A2, and A3 scallops (Figs. 4.16 and 4.17).

Table 4.1 Morphologic landmarks for the identification of the cardiac ventricles

Left ventricle (LV)	Right ventricle (RV)
Fine apical trabeculations	Coarse apical trabeculations
Smooth septal surface	Coarse septal surface
Presence of two papillary muscles	Presence of the moderator band
Receives the mitral valve	Receives the tricuspid valve
No mitral valve chordal insertion to the septal surface of LV	Chordal insertion of tricuspid septal leaflet to the septal surface of RV
Circular in cross section	Crescentic in cross section
Mitral-aortic continuity	Tricuspid-pulmonary discontinuity

Tricuspid Valve

The tricuspid valve has three unequally sized leaflets, anterior leaflet, posterior leaflet, and septal leaflet, the anterior one being usually the largest one. The septal leaflet has a distinguishing feature with its direct attachment to the interventricular septum. The tricuspid valve components are almost similar to those of the MV, but with greater variability.

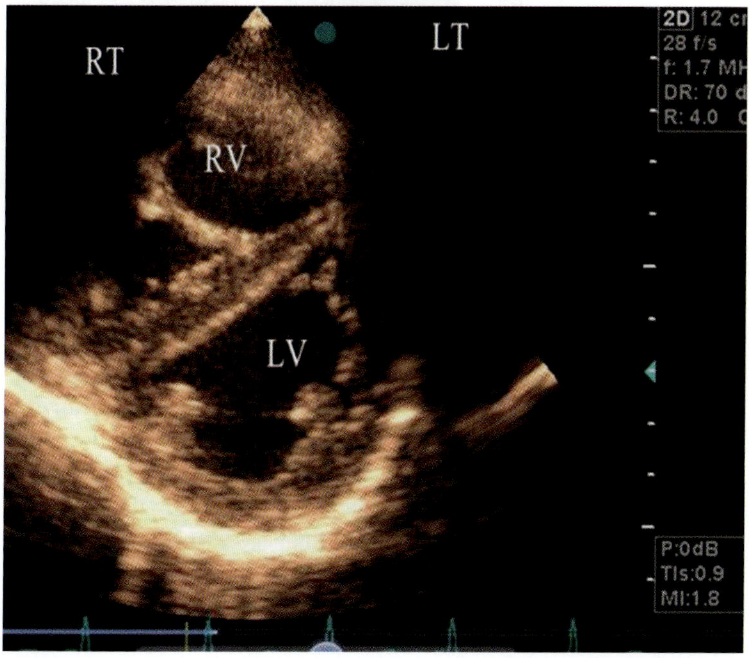

Fig. 4.13 Short-axis view of the ventricles, demonstrating the moderator band in the right ventricle. *RT* right, *LT* left, *RV* right ventricle, *LV* left ventricle

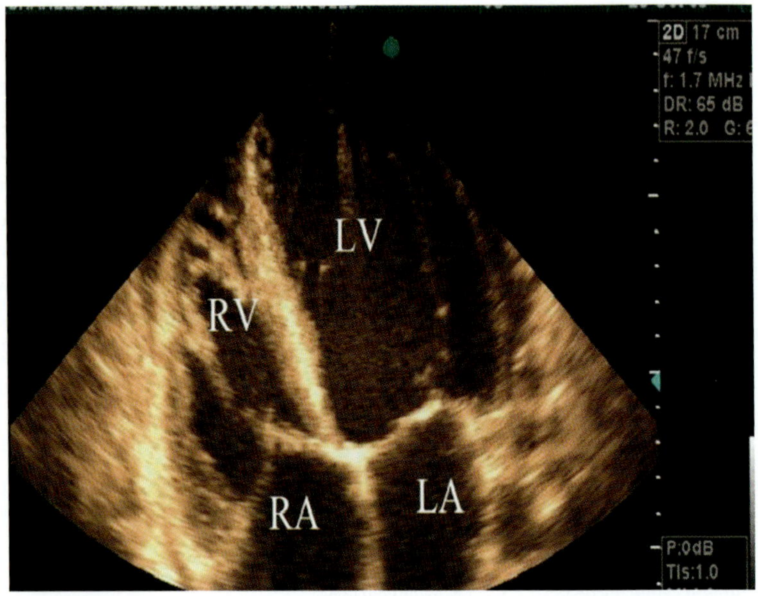

Fig. 4.14 Four-chamber view in transthoracic echocardiography, demonstrating landmarks for the determination of the ventricles. *RV* right ventricle, *LV* left ventricle, *RA* right atrium, *LA* left atrium

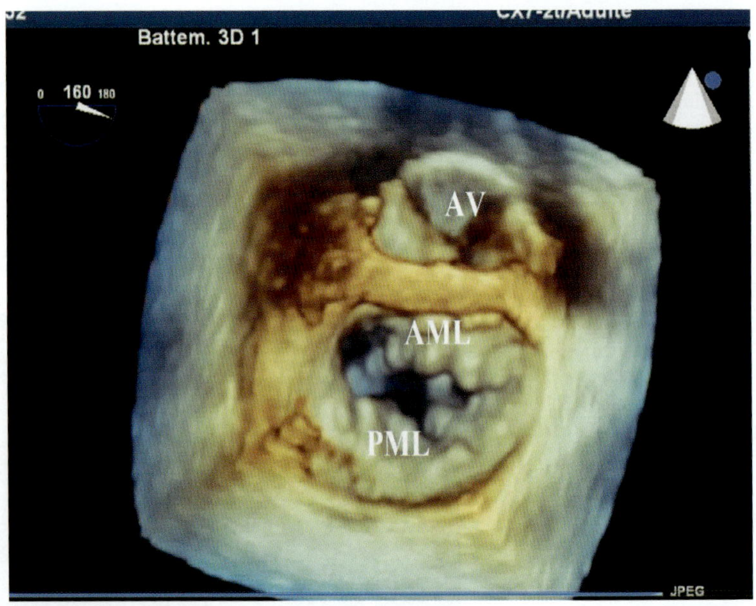

Fig. 4.15 Mitral valve and mitral annulus morphology in three-dimensional transesophageal echocardiography. *AV* aortic valve, *AML* anterior mitral leaflet, *PML* posterior mitral leaflet

Semilunar Valves (Aortic Valve, Pulmonary Valve)

The semilunar valves, i.e., aortic valve and pulmonary valve, connect the ventricle to an associated great artery. The great arteries (pulmonary artery and aorta) are specified simply by their arterial branches. The semilunar valves are determined by their associated great arteries as the pulmonary valve for the pulmonary artery and the aortic valve for the aorta.

Interestingly, the aortic and pulmonary valves are anatomically identical. The semilunar valves are normally tricuspid with no discrete annulus (Fig. 4.18).

In the normal relationship, the pulmonary trunk is to the left of and lies anterior to the ascending aorta. In congenital heart disease, the determination of the relationship between the aorta and the pulmonary artery is of vital importance [5, 8].

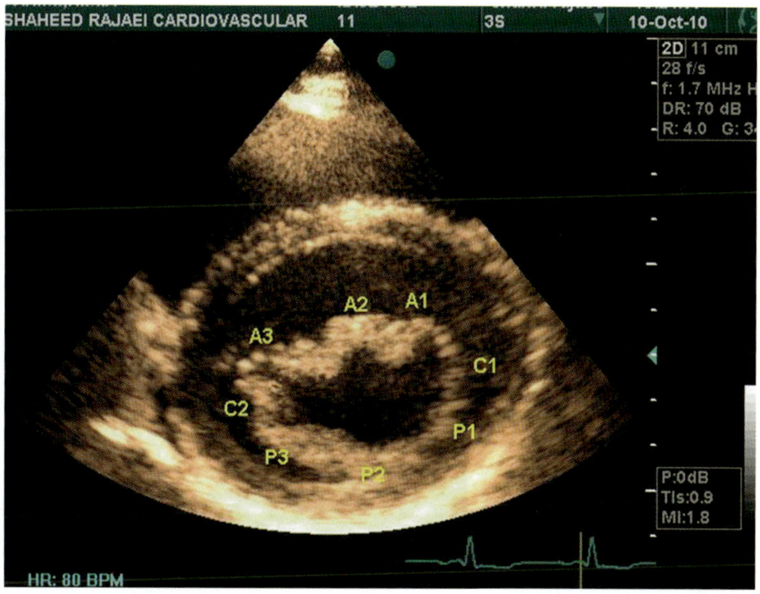

Fig. 4.16 Short-axis view of the mitral valve, demonstrating the mitral valve scallops in two-dimensional transthoracic echocardiography. *A1* anterolateral scallop, *A2* anteromiddle scallop, *A3* anteromedial scallop, *P1* posterolateral scallop, *P2* posteromiddle scallop, *P3* posteromedial scallop, *C1* lateral commissure, *C2* medial commissure

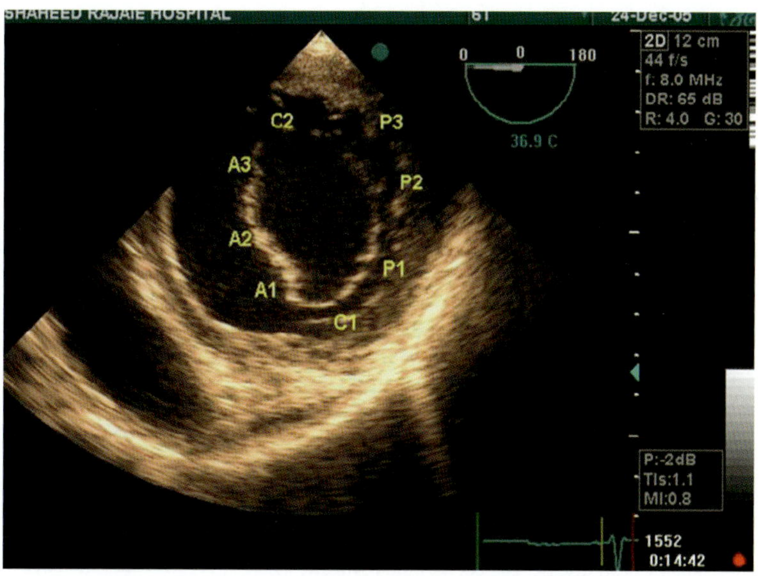

Fig. 4.17 Short-axis view of the mitral valve, demonstrating the mitral valve scallops in two-dimensional transesophageal echocardiography. *A1* anterolateral scallop, *A2* anteromiddle scallop, *A3* anteromedial scallop, *P1* posterolateral scallop, *P2* posteromiddle scallop, *P3* posteromedial scallop, *C1* lateral commissure, *C2* medial commissure

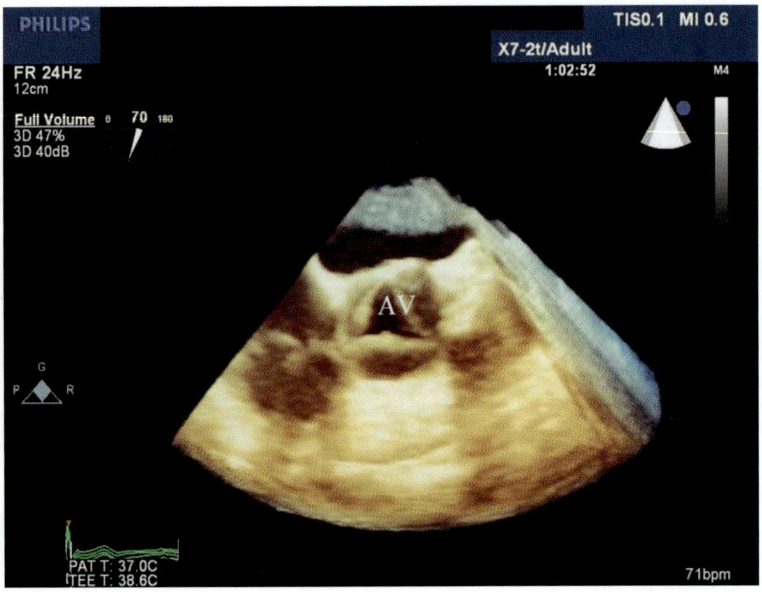

Fig. 4.18 Normal tricuspid aortic valve by three-dimensional transesophageal echocardiography. *AV* aortic valve

References

1. Van Praagh R. Terminology of congenital heart disease. Glossary and commentary. Circulation. 1977;56: 139–43.
2. Anderson RH, Macartney FJ, Shinebourne EA, et al. Terminology. In: Paediatric cardiology. Edinburgh: Churchill Livingstone; 1987. p. 65.
3. Van Praagh R, Weinberg PM, Smith SD, et al. Malpositions of the heart. In: Moss AJ, editor. Heart disease in infants, children and adolescents. 4th ed. Baltimore: Williams & Wilkins; 1989.
4. Perloff JK, Child JS, et al. Congenital heart disease in adults. 3rd ed. Philadelphia: Saunders Elsevier; 2009.
5. Driscoll HD. Moss and Adams' heart disease in infants, children, and adolescents: including the fetus and young adults. 7th ed Allen. Copyright ©2008 Philadelphia: Lippincott Williams & Wilkins.
6. Snider AR, Serwer GA, Ritter SB. Echocardiography in pediatric heart disease. 2nd ed. St. Louis: Mosby; 1997.
7. Perloff JK, Marelu A. Perloff's clinical recognition of congenital heart disease. 6th ed. Philadelphia: Saunders Elsevier; 2013.
8. Saremi F, Krishnan S. Cardiac conduction system: anatomic landmarks relevant to interventional electrophysiologic techniques demonstrated with 64-detector CT. Radiographics. 2007;27(6):1539–65.
9. Sanchez-Quintana D, Anderson RH, Cabrera JA, et al. The terminal crest: morphological features relevant to electrophysiology. Heart. 2002;88:406–11.
10. Anderson RH, Brown NA. The anatomy of the heart revisited. Anat Rec. 2007;246:1–7.
11. Wilcox BR, Cook AC, Anderson RH. Surgical anatomy of the heart. Cambridge: Cambridge University Press; 2004. p. 11–82.
12. Loukas M, Sullivan A, Tubbs R, et al. Chiari's network: review of the literature. Surg Radiol Anat. 2010;32(10):895–901.
13. Schneider B, Hofmann T, Justen MH, et al. Chiari's network: normal anatomic variant or risk factor for arterial embolic events? J Am Coll Cardiol. 1995; 26(1):203–10.
14. Mckay T, Thomas L. Prominent crista terminalis and Eustachian ridge in the right atrium: Two dimensional (2D) and three dimensional (3D) imaging. Eur J Echocardiogr. 2007;8(4):288–91.
15. Van Praagh R, David I, Van Praagh S. What is a ventricle? The single ventricle trap. Pediatr Cardiol. 1982;2:79.
16. Anderson RH, et al. The univentricular atrioventricular connection: getting to the root of a thorny problem. Am J Cardiol. 1984;54:822.
17. Anderson RH, Frater RW. How can we best describe the components of the mitral valve? J Heart Valve Dis. 2007;15:736–9.
18. Muresian H. The clinical anatomy of the mitral valve. Clin Anat. 2009;22(1):85–98.
19. Levine RA, Handschumacher MD, Sanfilippo AJ, et al. Three-dimensional echocardiographic reconstruction of the mitral valve, with implications for the diagnosis of mitral valve prolapse. Circulation. 1989; 80:589–98.
20. Lancellotti P, Moura L, Pierard LA, et al. European Association of Echocardiography recommendations for the assessment of valvular regurgitation. Part 2: mitral and tricuspid regurgitation (native valve disease). Eur J Echocardiogr. 2010;11(4):307–32.
21. Baharestani B, Sadeghpour A, Ghaffari Nejad. The principles of the mitral valve repair associated with echocardiographic evaluation. 1st edn. Omran Publication: IRAN; 2011.

Abnormal Cardiac Anatomy 5

Anita Sadeghpour

Keywords
Congenital Heart Disease (CHD) • Abnormal Cardiac Anatomy • Levocardia • Dextrocardia • Mesocardia

In this chapter, we will review the four types of cardiac malpositions:

1. Dextrocardia with visceroatrial situs inversus (situs inversus totalis) with the mirror-image position of the heart
2. Dextrocardia with visceroatrial situs solitus
3. Levocardia with visceroatrial situs inversus
4. Mesocardia

Besides the abnormality of the atrioventricular and ventriculoarterial valve, we will focus on the overriding and straddling types and definition.

Cardiac Malposition

Four types of cardiac malpositions have been defined [1–3]:

1. Dextrocardia with visceroatrial situs inversus (situs inversus totalis) with the mirror-image position of the heart
2. Dextrocardia with visceroatrial situs solitus
3. Levocardia with visceroatrial situs inversus (Fig. 5.1)
4. Mesocardia (midline heart)

A. Sadeghpour, MD, FACC, FASE
Echocardiography Lab, Department of Cardiology, Adult Congenital Heart Disease Clinic, Rajaie Cardiovascular Medical and Research Center, Iran University of Medical Science, Tehran, Iran
e-mail: anita.sadeghpour@gmail.com, asadeghpour@rhc.ac.ir

Dextrocardia

Dextrocardia implies the right-sided location of the heart and is categorized according to the following three conditions:

1. Dextroposition refers to the displaced heart to the right chest, mostly due to the abnormality in the right lung (such as absence of normal lung volume) or due to the space-occupying left-sided mass.
2. Dextroversion refers to a right-pointing apex associated with atrioventricular discordance with an increased rate of CHD.
3. Situs inversus totalis refers to the mirror-image position of the heart.

Mesocardia refers to a midline heart usually with situs solitus and bulboventricular loop as a variation of normal; however, in a midline heart with L-bulboventricular looping, abdominal and atrial inversus major congenital malformations occur.

For comprehensive clinical and pathologic segmental analyses, the following six segments should be addressed independently [4–7]:

- Systemic and pulmonary veins
- Abdominal and atrial situs (Fig. 5.2)
- AV connection
- Ventricular looping
- VA connection
- Great artery looping

The AV connection should be evaluated as concordant or discordant, absent, atretic, and

A. Sadeghpour et al. (eds.), *Comprehensive Approach to Adult Congenital Heart Disease*, DOI 10.1007/978-1-4471-6383-1_5, © Springer-Verlag London 2014

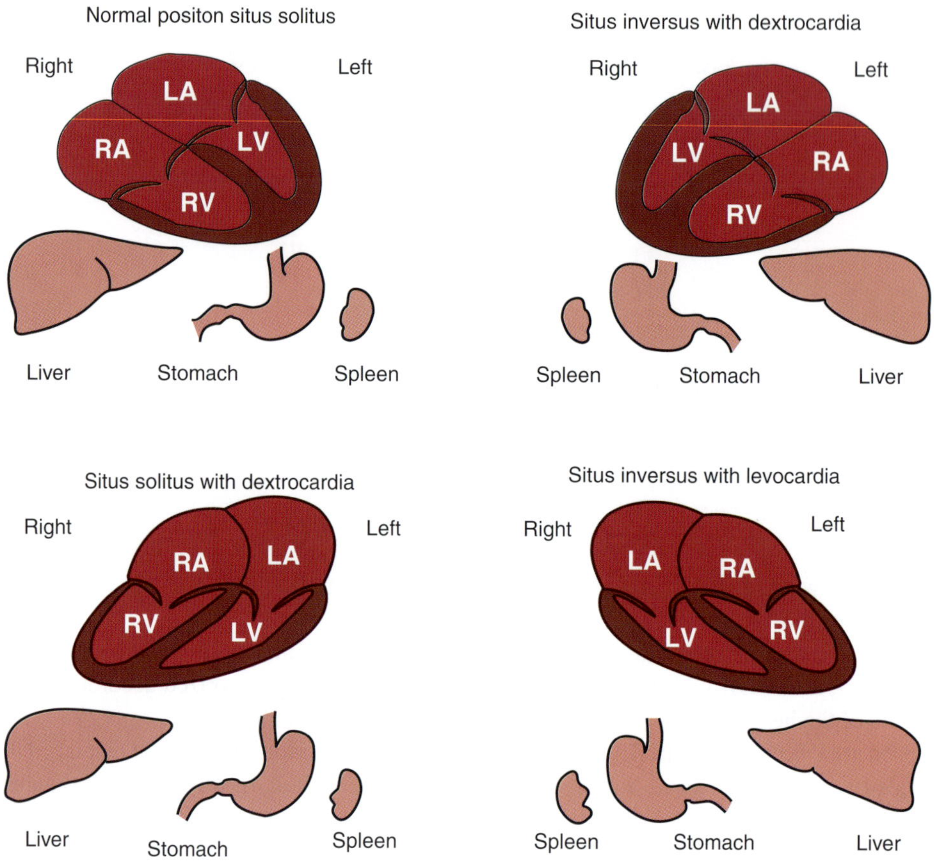

Fig. 5.1 Illustrating the three cardiac malpositions compared to the normal heart (With permission from Perloff and Marelli [2])

common inlet AV valve, double inlet AV valve, crisscross AV valve, and overriding AV valve.

When both atria connect with only one ventricular chamber, a univentricular AV connection applies.

Straddling of the AV valve refers to the chordae tendineae and papillary muscle apparatus and indicates anomalous insertion of the chordae tendineae to the contralateral ventricle.

It can involve the tricuspid or mitral valve or both, and based on the severity of the straddling, it has been categorized as the following three types: A, B, or C, depending on the straddling chordae insertion.

Type A is defined as the chordae attached to the opposite side of the ventricular septum crest (within the upper 1 cm).

Type B is defined as abnormal attachment of the chordae to the opposite side of the interventricular septum more than upper 1 cm.

Type C is defined as the abnormal attachment of the chordae to the opposite interventricular wall or opposite papillary muscle of the contralateral ventricle (Figs. 5.3, 5.4, 5.5, and 5.6) [8].

After determining the AV valve morphology (Fig. 5.7), connection, and abnormality, the great artery position and connections should be determined. The ventriculoarterial connection is concordant or discordant. The normal heart is characterized by a right posterior aorta:

It is important to note that the key to the diagnosis of CHD is an appreciation of the sequential segmental approach. The sequential

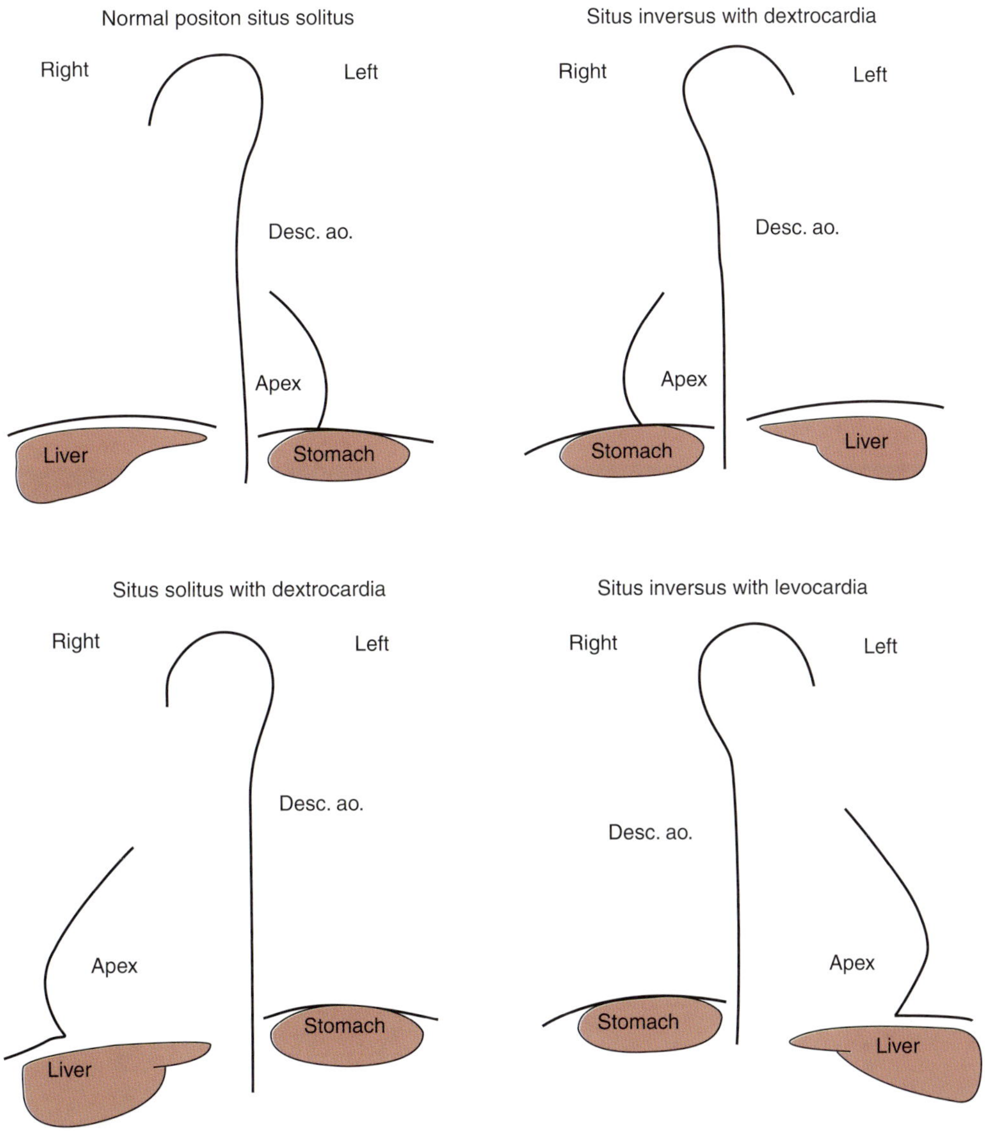

Fig. 5.2 Demonstrating the abdominal and cardiac situs relationship based on the radiographic projection in the chest X-ray. *Desc. ao* descending aorta(With permission from Perloff and Marelli [2])

segmental approach is a systematic and standard approach for both simple and complex CHD. Generally, the sequential segmental approach consists of the following steps: cardiac position and orientation, visceroatrial situs, ventricular position (ventricular looping), and the great artery position (looping). Thereafter, the atrioventricular and ventriculoarterial connections are analyzed in terms of connections and relations [7–11]. The sequential segmental approach has been discussed in the echocardiography chapter.

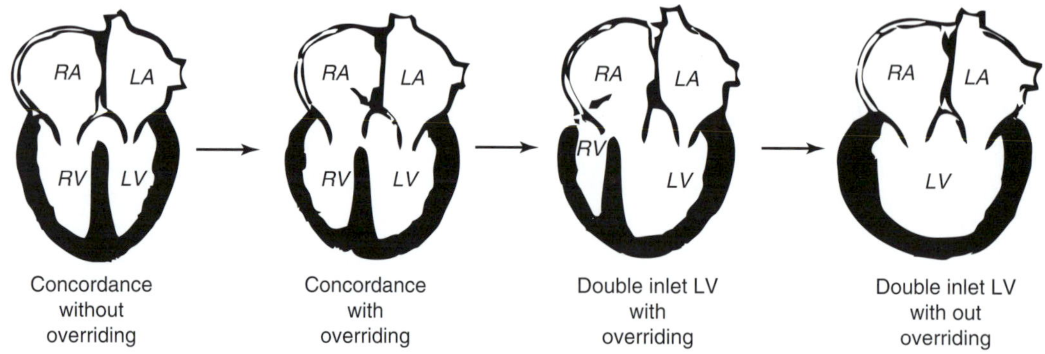

Fig. 5.3 Demonstrating overriding atrioventricular valve which is an abnormality of AV valve alignment

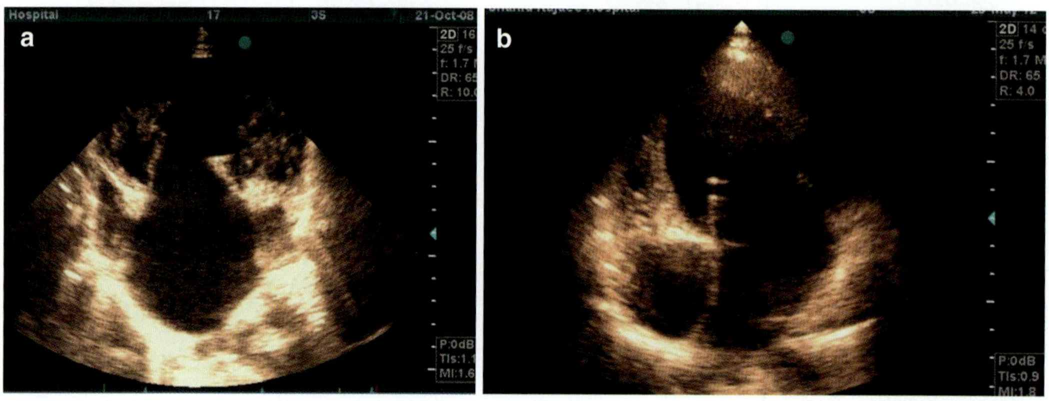

Fig. 5.4 (**a**, **b**) Showing common AV valve associated with common atrium and atretic right AV valve (tricuspid atresia)

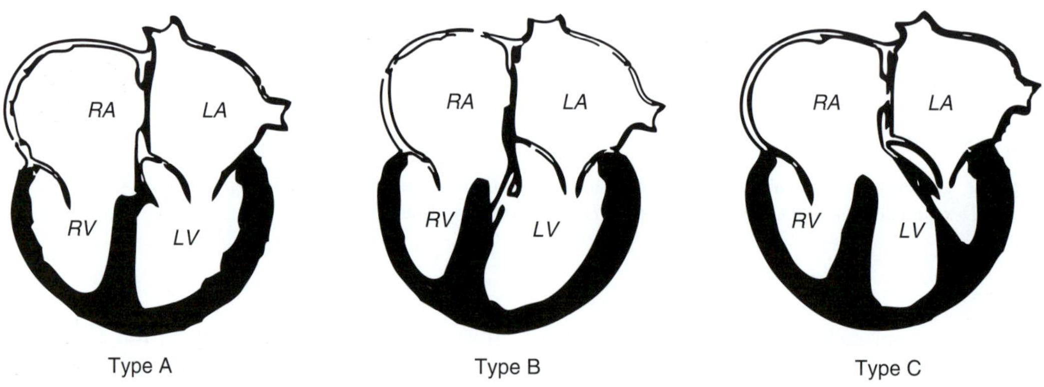

Fig. 5.5 Straddling of the AV valve categorized as types A, B, C

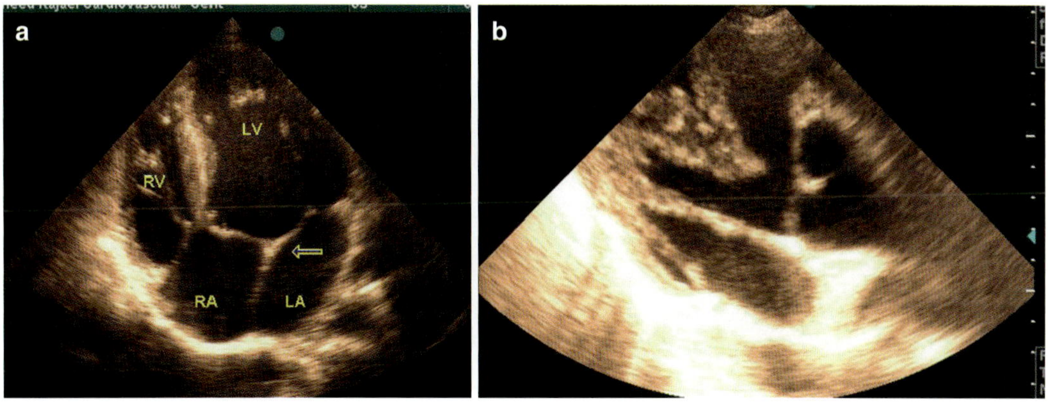

Fig. 5.6 (**a**, **b**) Overriding AV valves versus overriding ventriculoarterial valves

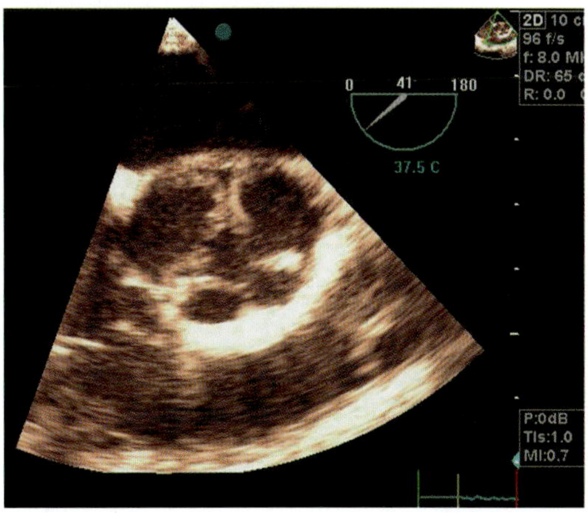

Fig. 5.7 Quadricuspid aortic valve resulting in aortic regurgitation

References

1. Perloff JK. The clinical recognition of congenital heart disease. 5th ed. Philadelphia: WB Saunders; 1994. p. 300–25.
2. Perloff JK, Marelli AJ. Perloff's clinical recognition of congenital heart disease. 6th ed. Philadelphia: WB Saunders Elsevier; 2013.
3. Perloff JK, Child J, et al. Congenital heart disease in adults. 3rd ed. Philadelphia: Saunders Elsevier; 2009.
4. Otto CM, editor. The practice of clinical echocardiography. 3rd ed. Philadelphia: W. B. Saunders/Elsevier; 2007. p. 1083–109.
5. Eidem BW, Cetta F, Oleary P. Echocardiography in pediatric and adult congenital heart disease. Philadelphia: Lippincott Williams & Wilkins; 2010.
6. Bonow RO, Mann DL, Zipes DP, Libby P. Braunwald's heart disease: a textbook of cardiovascular medicine. 9th ed. London: Elsevier Health Sciences; 2011. p. 1435–50.
7. Snider AR, Serwer GA, Ritter SB. Echocardiography in pediatric heart disease. 2nd ed. St. Louis: Mosby; 1997.
8. Allen HD, Driscoll DJ, Shaddy RE. Moss and Adams' heart disease in infants, children, and adolescents: including the fetus and young adults. 7th ed. Philadelphia: Lippincott Williams & Wilkins; 2008.
9. Warnes CA, American Heart Association. Adult congenital heart disease, AHA clinical series. Chichester: Wiley; 2009.
10. Warnes C, Williams RG, Bashore TM, et al. ACC/AHA, guidelines for the management of adults with congenital heart disease. JACC. 2008; 52(23):e143–263.
11. Baumgartner H, Bonhoeffer P, De Groot N, et al. ESC guidelines for the management of grown-up congenital heart disease (new version 2010). Eur Heart J. 2010;31:2915–57.

6 Cyanosis

Majid Kyavar and Anita Sadeghpour

Keywords
Cyanotic congenital heart disease • Hyperviscosity syndrome • Erythrocytosis • Cyanosis • Therapeutic phlebotomy

Definition and Classification

Cyanosis in adults with congenital heart disease (CHD) should not be regarded simply as a bluish discoloration of the tissues secondary to arterial oxygen desaturation. It is a multisystem involvement affecting most body systems, including hematologic, gynecologic, endocrine, vascular, renal, respiratory, and central nervous systems, as well as digits, long bones, and bilirubin kinetics. One of the most important manifestations of cyanosis is the hyperviscosity syndrome, which results from secondary erythrocytosis in response to low systemic arterial oxygen saturation [1, 2].

M. Kyavar, MD, FACC
Cardiovascular Imaging Ward,
Department of Cardiology,
Adult Congenital Heart Disease Clinic,
Rajaie Cardiovascular Medical and Research Center,
Iran University of Medical Science, Tehran, Iran
e-mail: kiavar0049@gmail.com, kiavar@rhc.ac.ir

A. Sadeghpour, MD, FACC, FASE (✉)
Echocardiography Lab, Department of Cardiology,
Adult Congenital Heart Disease Clinic,
Rajaie Cardiovascular Medical and Research Center,
Iran University of Medical Science, Tehran, Iran
e-mail: anita.sadeghpour@gmail.com,
asadeghpour@rhc.ac.ir

Cyanosis usually is apparent when arterial oxygen saturation (SaO_2) drops to <85 % or the absolute level of deoxyhemoglobin in the capillary bed exceeds 5 g/100 mL blood [1].

According to the underlying pathophysiology, cyanosis can be categorized as central or peripheral.

Central cyanosis: It refers to marked arterial oxygen desaturation resulting from the shunting or mixing of the arterial and venous circulation. The magnitude of mixing and the amount of pulmonary blood flow correlate with the severity of desaturation and cyanosis. Arterial oxygen desaturation may be caused by decreased inhaled oxygen (as in high altitudes), impaired pulmonary function (as in pulmonary edema), or more commonly admixing of desaturated systemic venous blood into the saturated pulmonary circulation through a bidirectional or reversed shunt due to an anatomical communication between the systemic and pulmonary circulations at the atrial, ventricular, or arterial level. Central cyanosis may also occur when nonfunctional hemoglobin is present such as in methemoglobinemia or sulfhemoglobinemia [1, 2].

Peripheral cyanosis: It occurs due to a decreased blood flow following peripheral vasoconstriction. This condition is most often seen in cold, shock, congestive heart failure, and peripheral vascular

A. Sadeghpour et al. (eds.), *Comprehensive Approach to Adult Congenital Heart Disease*,
DOI 10.1007/978-1-4471-6383-1_6, © Springer-Verlag London 2014

disease. Anemic patients may not appear blue despite low SaO_2, while polycythemic patients appear blue with higher SaO_2 [1, 2].

Cyanotic Heart Disease

The congenital heart defects that result in central cyanosis comprise a heterogeneous group of lesions which can be categorized on the basis of different underlying anatomy and pathophysiology as the following five Ts: transposition of the great arteries, tetralogy of Fallot, tricuspid atresia, truncus arteriosus, and total anomalous pulmonary venous return and the following two Es – Ebstein anomaly and Eisenmenger physiology as well as critical pulmonary stenosis or atresia and functionally single ventricle [1].

Also, these cardiac defects based on the pulmonary blood flow have been divided as those with:

1. Restricted pulmonary blood flow in the presence of an obstruction across the pulmonary outflow tract
2. Increased pulmonary blood flow in the absence of such an obstruction, which eventually leads to the development of pulmonary arterial hypertension and the Eisenmenger physiology

Adaptive Mechanisms

Cyanosis results in adaptive mechanisms to enhance oxygen transport and delivery to the tissues. Chronic hypoxemia induces erythropoietin production by interstitial fibroblasts in the kidneys, which in turn stimulates red blood cell production in the bone marrow and subsequently improves the oxygen-carrying capacity of the arterial circulation. This physiologic response improves tissue oxygenation at the cost of a higher hematocrit level; this desirable adaptive response is called secondary erythrocytosis. In secondary erythrocytosis, there is an isolated increase in the red blood cell mass in response to a stimulus like as systemic arterial oxygen desaturation in cyanotic CHD. Platelet counts are usually in the low range of normal or thrombocytopenic.

Erythrocytosis has been categorized as compensated and decompensated. Compensated erythrocytosis indicates an adequate rise in the red blood cell mass and the hemoglobin concentration to offset tissue hypoxemia, which leads to the normalization of erythropoietin levels. Decompensated erythrocytosis reflects the failure of this equilibrium, as a result of which the rise in the erythropoietin level and erythrocyte mass continues.

Rightward shift of the oxyhemoglobin dissociation curve and increase in cardiac output are other adaptive mechanisms in response to tissue hypoxia [3].

Cardiovascular manifestation varies based on the underlying pathophysiology. In general, cyanotic patients have significantly higher mortality rates than acyanotic patients [4]. Factors affecting the outcome of the patients include the underlying anatomy/pathophysiology, palliative procedures, and cyanotic complications.

Cyanotic Complications

Cyanosis and secondary erythrocytosis affect the entire organ systems.

Hematologic Complications

- *Hyperviscosity syndrome:* Blood viscosity, which is directly related to the red blood cell mass, is increased in patients with central cyanosis due to secondary erythrocytosis [5]. Hyperviscosity symptoms include headache; faintness; dizziness; fatigue; altered mentation; tinnitus; blurred vision; paresthesia of fingers, toes, and lips; muscle pain; and weakness (classified as moderate when they interfere with some activities and severe when they interfere with most activities) [3]. Hyperviscosity symptoms are unlikely in an iron-replete patient with hematocrit <65 %, while hyperviscosity syndromes may be seen at a hematocrit level of <65 % in the presence of iron deficiency, as a common finding in cyanotic adult patients undergoing frequent phlebotomies or excessive bleeding. Blood viscosity is determined by a complex interplay of a number of variables.

- *Thrombosis/bleeding:* Hemostatic abnormalities are common in cyanotic patients with erythrocytosis and have been reported in up to 20 % of patients. These included quantitative and qualitative abnormalities in platelets (thrombocytopenia and thrombasthenia) and coagulation pathways. Vitamin K-dependent clotting factors (factors II, VII, IX, and X), factor V, and the largest von Willebrand multimers are reduced, while fibrinolytic activity increases. Laboratory investigation reveals elevated prothrombin and partial thromboplastin times. However, these hemostatic abnormalities do not protect patients against thrombotic complications.

Spontaneous bleeding is usually minor, superficial, and self-limiting (leading to dental bleeding, epistaxis, easy bruising, skin petechiae, and menorrhagia). However, it can also be moderate or life threatening such as intracranial, gastrointestinal, and postoperative bleeding or hemoptysis. Hemoptysis is the most common major bleeding event and has been reported in up to 100 % of patients with the Eisenmenger physiology. Although it is an external manifestation of an intrapulmonary hemorrhage, it does not reflect the extent of parenchymal bleeding [6].

Thrombosis is caused by coagulation abnormalities, stasis of blood in dilated chambers and vessels, atherosclerosis and/or endothelial dysfunction, presence of thrombogenic material (e.g., conduits), and arrhythmias. Laminated thrombi in large, partially calcified and aneurysmal pulmonary arteries [7, 8] are common and occur in up to 30 % of patients with central cyanosis, especially in association with female gender, low oxygen saturation, older age, biventricular dysfunction [9, 10].

- *Iron deficiency:* In adults, iron deficiency is most often a result of inappropriate phlebotomies, whereas in children, iron deficiency is due to abnormal diet or malnutrition.

Central Nervous System Complications

Cerebrovascular accidents may be caused by thromboembolic events (paradoxical emboli), cerebral hemorrhage, and microcytosis due to iron deficiency anemia, endothelial dysfunction, and traditional atherosclerotic risk factors. The severity of secondary erythrocytosis is not predictive of the development of central nervous system complications [11]. While iron deficiency-induced microcytosis due to inappropriate phlebotomies is the strongest independent risk factor for cerebrovascular events [12], dehydration in the setting of diarrhea or vomiting is one of the aggravating factors in cerebral venous thromboses.

Paradoxical emboli may be caused by either supraventricular arrhythmias or transvenous leads or catheters. As a result, air filters in peripheral and central venous lines are recommended to prevent paradoxical emboli through a right-to-left shunt.

Renal Complications

Renal dysfunction is common and is due to the functional and structural abnormalities of the kidneys. Renal dysfunction can cause proteinuria, hyperuricemia, or renal failure. Hyperuricemia is common and is believed to mainly result from decreased renal reabsorption of uric acid rather than from overproduction due to red blood cell turnover and erythrocytosis. Urate nephropathy and uric acid nephrolithiasis are the consequences of hyperuricemia.

Rheumatologic Complications

Hyperuricemia is commonly seen in the wake of increased red blood cells/hemoglobin turnover and also impaired urate filtration by the kidneys [13].

Rheumatologic complications include:

- Gouty arthritis
- Hypertrophic osteoarthropathy
- Kyphoscoliosis

In cyanotic patients, the clinical manifestations of gout are similar to those with primary gout, although the management somewhat differs between them.

The treatment of hyperuricemia in asymptomatic cyanotic adults is not recommended.

If symptomatic gouty arthritis occurs, treatment with probenecid or sulfinpyrazone, allopurinol, or a combination of these drugs is recommended. Acute gouty arthritis usually responds to colchicine; however, the major limitation is dehydration caused by vomiting and diarrhea.

Arthralgia and bone pain affect up to one third of cyanotic patients and are believed to be secondary to hypertrophic osteoarthropathy. Moreover, it has been postulated that in patients with right-to-left shunting, megakaryocytes released from the bone marrow bypass the lungs. These megakaryocytes are entrapped in the systemic arterioles and capillaries and stimulate the release of the platelet-derived growth factor and the proliferation of the local cells, leading to new osseous formation with periostitis and subsequent arthralgia and bone pain. Recently, it has been suggested that clubbed fingers and hypertrophic osteoarthropathy both share a common pathogenesis.

Gastrointestinal Complications

Due to an increased concentration of unconjugated bilirubin, cyanotic patients are prone to develop calcium bilirubinate gallstones. Calcium bilirubinate gallstones may be complicated by cholecystitis/choledocholithiasis.

Infection

Infectious complications include endocarditis, cerebral abscess, and pneumonia. A brain abscess should be suspected in a cyanotic patient with a combination of fever and new-onset or different headache or new neurologic symptoms.

Arrhythmias

Both supraventricular and ventricular arrhythmias may be seen in cyanotic patients.

Coronary Arteries

Patients with central cyanosis have dilated coronaries with no obstruction [14].

Recent investigations have also demonstrated severe endothelial dysfunction in cyanotic patients due to increased shear stress, reflected by the marked impairment of endothelium-dependent vasodilation [15]. Consequently, chronic tissue hypoxia, increased blood viscosity, and endothelial dysfunction denote profound consequences on microcirculation, myocardial function, and function of the other organ systems. Hypocholesterolemia is much more frequent in cyanotic CHD patients by comparison with atherosclerosis.

Diagnostic Work-Up

- Particular attention should be paid to hyperviscosity symptoms and bleeding/ischemic complications.
- Oxygen saturation must be measured with pulse oximetry at rest for at least 5 min, and exercise capacity should be assessed on a regular basis, preferably with a 6-min walk test.
- Blood work-up should include complete blood count, mean corpuscular volume (MCV), serum ferritin (serum iron, transferrin, and transferrin saturation may be required for earlier detection of iron deficiency), creatinine, serum uric acid, clotting profile, and brain natriuretic peptide (BNP) or pro-BNP. Folic acid and vitamin B12 should also be measured if MCV is normal or elevated in the presence of low serum ferritin.

Laboratory Investigation

- Coagulation parameters should be investigated. The plasma volume is reduced due to secondary erythrocytosis, and the amount of sodium citrate must be adjusted to hematocrit if hematocrit is >55 %.
- Hematocrit is determined with automated electronic particle counts. (Microhematocrit centrifugation results in falsely high hematocrit due to plasma trapping.)

- Glucose level can be reduced. (There is an increase in in vitro glycolysis, which results from the increased number of red blood cells.)

Indications for Intervention

Risk and benefit must be expertly contemplated. A cyanotic patient without pulmonary artery hypertension/Eisenmenger syndrome must be periodically evaluated for any procedure that may improve quality of life and reduce morbidity or for eligibility for physiological repair.

Medical Therapy

Arrhythmias: Sinus rhythm should be maintained whenever possible. Anti-arrhythmic therapy must be individualized [medications, ablation, and epicardial pacemaker (PM)/implantable cardioverter-defibrillator (ICD)]. Anti-arrhythmic therapy is extremely difficult in this patient group. Drug therapy should be initiated with particular carc and generally in a hospital. Transvenous leads must be avoided. Catheter ablation for cyanotic adult CHD patients should be done at centers with experienced staff expert in the complex anatomy and distinctive arrhythmia in these complex congenital heart defects (level of evidence: B) [16, 17].

Therapeutic phlebotomy: It should only be performed in the presence of moderate/severe hyperviscosity symptoms due to secondary erythrocytosis (hematocrit >65 %) and in the absence of dehydration and iron deficiency. Concomitant isovolumic fluid replacement (750–1,000 mL of isotonic saline while removing 400–500 mL of blood) should be undertaken.

Iron supplementation: It should be performed in the presence of iron deficiency (MCV <80 fL) and carefully followed (rebound effect).

Routine anticoagulation/aspirin: The currently available data do not support any benefit of routine anticoagulation/aspirin in cyanotic patients to prevent thromboembolic complications. However, there is an increased risk of bleeding.

- *Indication for Anticoagulation*
  - Atrial flutter/fibrillation [target international normalized ratio (INR) = 2–2.5; higher target INR in the presence of a mechanical valve]

Hemoptysis: It requires chest X-ray, followed by chest computed tomography (CT) scan if there is an infiltrate. Bronchoscopy puts the patient at risk and seldom provides useful information.

Appropriate therapy for hemoptysis episodes includes:

- Discontinuation of:
  - Aspirin
  - Nonsteroidal anti-inflammatory agents
  - Oral anticoagulants
- Treatment of hypovolemia and anemia
- Reduction of physical activity
- Suppression of nonproductive cough

However, in refractory intrapulmonary hemorrhage/hemoptysis, selective embolization of the bronchial arteries may be required.

Hyperuricemia: Asymptomatic hyperuricemia does not need any medical treatment.

Acute gouty arthritis: It is treated with oral or intravenous colchicine, probenecid, and anti-inflammatory drugs. Particular caution is required due to the risk of renal failure and bleeding with these medications. Uricosuric (e.g., probenecid) or uricostatic agents (e.g., allopurinol) have been shown to reduce recurrent attacks of gouty arthritis in cyanotic patients.

Home oxygen therapy: It has pulmonary vasodilatory effects and may play a beneficial role in increasing arterial oxygen saturation. Nonetheless, its clinical indications and outcomes are not clear yet [18].

Follow-Up

All cyanotic patients should be evaluated with follow-up visits every 6–12 months in a specialized adult congenital heart center including:

- Comprehensive evaluation of the underlying heart disease; systematic review of potential systemic complications of cyanosis, especially hyperviscosity symptoms; change in exercise tolerance; change in the oxygen saturation level; and prophylaxis against endocarditis, influenza, and pneumococcal infections

Table 6.1 Risk reduction strategies in patients with cyanotic congenital heart disease

Prophylactic measures are the mainstay of care to avoid complications
The following exposures/activities should be avoided
Pregnancy
Iron deficiency and anemia (no routine, inappropriate phlebotomies to maintain a predetermined hemoglobin)
Dehydration
Infectious disease: annual influenza vaccination, Pneumovax (every 5 years)
Cigarette smoking, recreational drug abuse including alcohol
Transvenous PM/ICD leads
Strenuous exercise
Acute exposure to heat (sauna, hot tub/shower)
Other risk reduction strategies include
Use of an air filter in an intravenous line to prevent air embolism
Consultation of an adult CHD cardiologist before the administration of any agent and performance of any surgical/interventional procedure
Prompt therapy of upper respiratory tract infections
Cautious use or avoidance of agents that impair renal function
Contraceptive advice

- Blood work-up (complete blood count, ferritin, clotting profile, renal function, and uric acid)
- Regular Doppler echocardiographic studies
- Education about risk reduction strategies (Table 6.1)

Additional Considerations

- *Exercise/sports:* Moderate to severe strenuous exercise should be avoided in all cyanotic patients.
- *Air flight:* Commercial air travel is well tolerated [19, 20]. Risk reduction strategies include avoidance of travel and non-travel-related stress, dehydration, alcoholic drinks, and measures to prevent deep vein thrombosis.
- *Exposure to high altitude:* Acute exposure to high altitudes (>2,500 m) should be avoided. Gradual ascent (e.g., cable car) up to 2,500 m may be tolerated.
- *Pregnancy:* Pregnancy results in conspicuous maternal and fetal complications in cyanotic patients without pulmonary hypertension. Oxygen saturation (>85 %) and hemoglobin (<20 g/L) prior to pregnancy have been shown to be the strongest predictors for live birth [21]. However, pregnancy is contraindicated in patients with the Eisenmenger syndrome.
- *Infective endocarditis prophylaxis:* It is recommended in all patients with cyanotic CHD [16, 17].

References

1. Bonow RO, Mann DL, Zipes DP, Libby P, eds. Braunwald's Heart Disease: A Textbook of Cardiovascular Medicine. 9th ed. Philadelphia, PA: Saunders Elsevier; 2011.
2. Gatzoulis MA, Webb GD, Broberg CS, Uemura H. Cases in adult congenital heart disease. Philadelphia: Churchill Livingstone; 2010.
3. Oechslin E. Hematological management of the cyanotic adult with congenital heart disease. Int J Cardiol. 2004;97 Suppl 1:109–15.
4. Engelfriet P, Boersma E, Oechslin E, Tijssen J, Gatzoulis MA, Thile'n U, Kaemmerer H, Moons P, Meijboom F, Popelova' J, Laforest V, Hirsch R, Daliento L, Thaulow E, Mulder B. The spectrum of adult congenital heart disease in Europe: morbidity and mortality in a 5 year follow-up period. The Euro Heart Survey on adult congenital heart disease. Eur Heart J. 2005;26:2325–33.
5. Broberg CS, Bax BE, Okonko DO, Rampling MW, Bayne S, Harries C, Davidson SJ, Uebing A, Khan AA, Thein S, Gibbs JS, Burman J, Gatzoulis MA. Blood viscosity and its relationship to iron deficiency, symptoms, and exercise capacity in adults with cyanotic congenital heart disease. J Am Coll Cardiol. 2006;48:356–65.

6. Daliento L, Somerville J, Presbitero P, Menti L, Brach-Prever S, Rizzoli G, Stone S. Eisenmenger syndrome. Factors relating to deterioration and death. Eur Heart J. 1998;19:1845–55.
7. Broberg CS, Ujita M, Prasad S, Li W, Rubens M, Bax BE, Davidson SJ, Bouzas B, Gibbs JS, Burman J, Gatzoulis MA. Pulmonary arterial thrombosis in Eisenmenger syndrome is associated with biventricular dysfunction and decreased pulmonary flow velocity. J Am Coll Cardiol. 2007;50:634–42.
8. Silversides CK, Granton JT, Konen E, Hart MA, Webb GD, Therrien J. Pulmonary thrombosis in adults with Eisenmenger syndrome. J Am Coll Cardiol. 2003;42:1982–7.
9. Niwa K, Perloff JK, Kaplan S, Child JS, Miner PD. Eisenmenger syndrome in adults: ventricular septal defect, truncus arteriosus, univentricular heart. J Am Coll Cardiol. 1999;34:223–32.
10. Perloff JK, Hart EM, Greaves SM, Miner PD, Child JS. Proximal pulmonary arterial and intrapulmonary radiologic features of Eisenmenger syndrome and primary pulmonary hypertension. Am J Cardiol. 2003;92:182–7.
11. Perloff JK, Marelli AJ, Miner PD. Risk of stroke in adults with cyanotic congenital heart disease. Circulation. 1993;87:1954–9.
12. Ammash N, Warnes CA. Cerebrovascular events in adult patients with cyanotic congenital heart disease. J Am Coll Cardiol. 1996;28:768–72.
13. Perloff JK. Systemic complications of cyanosis in adults with congenital heart disease. Hematologic derangements, renal function, and urate metabolism. Cardiol Clin. 1993;11:689–99.
14. Fyfe A, Perloff JK, Niwa K, et al. Cyanotic congenital heart disease and coronary artery atherogenesis. Am J Cardiol. 2005;96:283.
15. Oechslin E, Kiowski W, Schindler R, Bernheim A, Julius B, Brunner-La Rocca HP. Systemic endothelial dysfunction in adults with cyanotic congenital heart disease. Circulation. 2005;112:1106–12.
16. Baumgartner H, Bonhoeffer P, De Groot NM, et al. ESC Guidelines for the management of grown-up congenital heart disease (new version 2010). Task Force on the Management of Grown-up Congenital Heart Disease of the European Society of Cardiology (ESC); Association for European Paediatric Cardiology (AEPC); ESC Committee for Practice Guidelines (CPG). Eur Heart J. 2010;31(23):2915–57.
17. Warnes CA, Williams RG, Bashore TM, et al. ACC/AHA 2008 guidelines for the management of adults with congenital heart disease: a report of the American College of Cardiology/American Heart Association Task Force on Practice Guidelines (Writing Committee to Develop Guidelines on the Management of Adults With Congenital Heart Disease). Developed in Collaboration With the American Society of Echocardiography, Heart Rhythm Society, International Society for Adult Congenital Heart Disease, Society for Cardiovascular Angiography and Interventions, and Society of Thoracic Surgeons. J Am Coll Cardiol. 2008;52(23):e143–263.
18. Walker F, Mullen MJ, Woods SJ, Web GD. Acute effects of 40% oxygen supplementation in adults with cyanotic congenital heart disease. Heart. 2004;90:1073.
19. Broberg CS, Uebing A, Cuomo L, Thein SL, Papadopoulos MG, Gatzoulis MA. Adult patients with Eisenmenger syndrome report flying safely on commercial airlines. Heart. 2007;93:1599–603.
20. Harinck E, Hutter PA, Hoorntje TM, Simons M, Benatar AA, Fischer JC, de Bruijn D, Meijboom EJ. Air travel and adults with cyanotic congenital heart disease. Circulation. 1996;93:272–6.
21. Presbitero P, Somerville J, Stone S, Aruta E, Spiegelhalter D, Rabajoli F. Pregnancy in cyanotic congenital heart disease. Outcome of mother and fetus. Circulation. 1994;89:2673–6.

Congestive Heart Failure in Adults with Congenital Heart Disease

7

Azin Alizadehasl

Keywords
Adult congenital heart disease • Heart failure • Heart and heart-lung transplantation

Epidemiology and Etiology

Congenital heart disease (CHD) has an incidence rate of around eight cases per 1,000 live births. A growing number of affected infants live to childhood and eventually to adulthood; it, therefore, seems reasonable to assume that adults with CHD might have heart failure (HF). However, rather than developing HF as a result of myocyte loss (such as myocardial infarction) or intrinsic anomalies in myocardial apparatuses (such as inherited cardiomyopathies), HF in CHD may develop in consequence of prolonged abnormalities in cardiac pressure, flow, volume, and tension. Surgeries sometimes improve these dynamics but rarely cause an increase in the "degree" of HF (transiently), for example, due to perioperative stress and neurohormonal activation [1–3].

Pathophysiology and Clinical Findings

HF can develop at different ages. Nowadays, fetal echocardiography allows the diagnosis of intrauterine cardiac failure. The fundamental findings of fetal HF are decreased fetal movements, scalp edema, ascites, and pericardial effusion. In preterm newborns, especially those of less than 1,500 g birth weight, the persistent patency of the ductus arteriosus is the most common reason for HF. *In full-term newborns, the hypoplastic left heart syndrome, aortic coarctation, tachyarrhythmia, and myocarditis are the important causes of HF. Beyond the age of 1–2 weeks, when reduced pulmonary vascular resistance permits considerable left-to-right shunting, the main reasons for HF are atrioventricular septal defect (AVSD), ventricular septal defect (VSD), transposition of the great arteries (TGA), truncus arteriosus (TA), and also total anomalous pulmonary venous connection (TAPVC). For infants younger than 1 year, cardiac anomalies account for 80–90 % of patients with known congestive heart failure (CHF).* Nevertheless, in older infants, HF is frequently due to an acquired disease or is a complication of cardiac surgical procedures. The acquired category comprises rheumatic heart disease, infective endocarditis,

A. Alizadehasl, MD, FACC
Echocardiography Lab, Department of Cardiology, Rajaie Cardiovascular Medical and Research Center, Iran University of Medical Science, Tehran, Iran
e-mail: alizadeasl@gmail.com, alizadeasl@rhc.ac.ir

A. Sadeghpour et al. (eds.), *Comprehensive Approach to Adult Congenital Heart Disease*,
DOI 10.1007/978-1-4471-6383-1_7, © Springer-Verlag London 2014

and hematological and nutritional diseases as well as persistent arrhythmias [3–5].

Interestingly, one previous study reported that there are no statistical differences between dilated cardiomyopathy and HF in adult CHD patients in terms of serum norepinephrine levels; however, epinephrine levels tend to be higher in all levels of functional capacity impairment in adults with CHD [5].

More information is now known about the other fundamental features of the HF syndrome such as exercise and activity limitation. Adults with cyanotic cardiac disease have major limitations in their oxygen uptake in exercise, such as adult patients with the Fontan physiology and also adults with a repaired atrial septal defect (ASD), surgically corrected transposition of the great arteries (d-TGA), congenitally corrected transposition of the great arteries (CCTGA), repaired tetralogy of Fallot (TOF), and also the Ebstein anomaly that was studied by Fredriksen PM, et al. previously [6]. They showed all these six groups had mean peak VO2 <22 ml/kg/min and mean peak VO2 was as low as 16 ml/kg/min in the Fontan patients, a character similar to that of patients with ischemic or dilated cardiomyopathy with New York Heart Association (NYHA) functional class III. Of course this appears typical of the HF syndrome as is currently perceived; this is limited to exercise capacity relating with the abnormalities of skeletal muscle resulting in cardiac pathology rather than the measures of central hemodynamics [6–8].

According to the American College of Cardiology and American Heart Association (ACC/AHA) Guidelines (2008) for Adults with CHD, typical adult CHD substrates for late HF in adult CHD patients are as follows [9]:

1. Severe aortic stenosis and/or regurgitation, bicuspid aortic valve and its variants, subvalvular or supravalvular pathologies, and also superimposed coarctation
2. Severe congenital mitral stenosis (MS) or mitral regurgitation (MR)
3. Unoperated ASD or partial AVSD
4. CCTGAs
5. d-TGA after the Mustard or Senning operation, in which the morphological right ventricle (RV) is the systemic ventricle
6. TOF with early era surgery, long-standing shunt, or severe pulmonary regurgitation
7. Single ventricle physiology
8. Fontan operation

Many CHD patients tend to experience a combination of persistent volume and pressure overload. Issues that predispose to the creation of late HF contain abnormal anatomy, surgical sequelae, and also progression of basic pathology. Also as we mentioned before, neurohormonal activation is common in adults with HF due to CHD like HF of all other types, and neurohormonal stimulation in such patients relates to the common measures of disease severity like functional class, exercise ability, and also ventricular dysfunction. The activation of each neurohormonal system rises in a stepwise manner through the NYHA functional class, whereas the plasma levels of natriuretic peptides, norepinephrine, and endothelin-1 increase even in asymptomatic patients [4–8].

Some congenital defects will lead to higher degrees of exercise limitation, HF symptoms, and neurohormonal stimulation than others. For example, those with cyanotic cardiac disease have poorer peak oxygen consumption and higher plasma levels of some neurohormones than matched patients with acyanotic heart disease, and also patients with the Fontan circulation seem to have poor exercise capacity and high NYHA class. Lesion-specific differences that develop HF may be important and certainly need more evaluation. Furthermore, neurohormonal levels are known to decrease, infrequently to normal, after reparative surgery. Among patients with TOF, those who have experienced palliative surgery are believed to have higher neurohormonal activation than those who have had repair [7–9].

The distinction between left-sided and right-sided HF in CHD patients is less obvious in infants than in older children or adults. Conversely, augmented filling or raised pressure of the right ventricle in infants reduces left ventricular compliance excessively compared with older infants or adults and gives rise to signs of both systemic and pulmonary venous congestions [5–9].

Paraclinic, Prevention, and Treatment

Care of infants or adults with HF following CHD must include careful consideration of the underlying structural or functional disorders. The general aims of management are to achieve an increase in cardiac performance, to augment peripheral perfusion, and to lessen pulmonary and systemic venous congestion. In many conditions, medical treatment cannot control the effects of the abnormal loads forced by a host of CHD. In these situations, cardiac diagnosis and interventional catheter or operative interventions may be immediately required [8, 10–13].

Of course CHF is not common in CHD practice, although the prevention of myocardial dysfunction is a common concern. The adult patient with CHD may develop HF in the presence of a substrate (e.g., myocardial dysfunction and valvular regurgitation) and a precipitant (e.g., sustained arrhythmia, pregnancy, hyperthyroidism, and obesity). Patients prone to CHF include those with long-standing volume loads (e.g., valvular regurgitation and left-to-right shunts) and those with a primary depression of the myocardial function (e.g., systemic right ventricles and ventricles damaged during surgery, or because of the late treatment of ventricular overload). Cardiac magnetic resonance imaging (MRI) to evaluate ventricular anatomy, dimensions, function, myocardial perfusion, and also ischemia in adults with unrepaired or repaired CHD (e.g., after atrial switch procedures) may be useful [14–20].

The cause of brain natriuretic peptide (BNP) production is ventricular wall stress. Accordingly, BNP has been revealed to be high not only in patients with HF and left ventricular (LV) systolic dysfunction but also in patients with significant diastolic dysfunction or RV dysfunction. Also, BNP can rise in cyanotic cardiac disease without sign or symptom of HF or myocardial dysfunction. Also BNP levels can aid in the emergency department in the diagnosis of HF and can be a predictor of cardiac events; however, their role in outpatient diagnosis, decision making, and clinical follow-up of HF in CHD remains unclear. Serial measurements of BNP in patients with risk for the creation and development of HF like patients with single ventricle anatomy may be beneficial in guiding interventional management [17].

Treatment depends on a clear understanding of the elements contributing to decompensation and addressing each of the treatable components. The greatest success is achieved when the main elements can be eliminated. When this is not possible, standard palliative adult HF regimens are applied and may include angiotensin-converting-enzyme (ACE) inhibitors, beta-blockers, angiotensin receptor blockers, diuretics, resynchronization pacing, transplantation, or other novel therapies [9, 14–17].

The role of such mentioned medical treatments in the prevention or management of HF has been evaluated only in small groups of CHD patients. For example, one report on the use of ACE inhibitors in adults undergoing the Mustard procedure revealed no significant change in the MRI parameters of RV volume and ejection fraction or of measured exercise capability [16–20].

And for beta-blockers, this class of drug is usually used to control supraventricular arrhythmias and hypertension in the treatment of CHD patients rather than to inhibit the pathophysiological sympathetic activation. Of course there are little reported systematic trials of beta-blocker use in adults with CHD for the particular treatment of HF, though there are some data from the pediatric literature about the use of these agents in children with severe CHF. Also *aldosterone blockade with spironolactone was reported to have improved the protein-losing enteropathy syndrome in a small number of Fontan operation patients* [9, 11–16].

Heart and Heart-Lung Transplantation

CHD accounts for 40 % of pediatric heart transplants but only 2 % of adult heart transplants.

According to the ACC/AHA Guidelines (2008) for Adults with CHD, the class I criteria for heart and heart-lung transplantation are as follows (in summary) [9]:

1. Patients with CHD and HF who may need heart transplantation must be assessed and managed in tertiary care centers with proficiency in the

management of both CHD and heart transplantation (level of evidence: C).

2. Patients with CHD and HF or respiratory failure who may need lung or heart-lung transplantation must be studied and managed in tertiary care centers with medical and surgical expertise in the management of CHD and also lung or heart-lung transplantation (level of evidence: C).

Patients with established and long-standing HF may have high pulmonary vascular resistance. Therefore, the donor's right-sided HF may ensue if the heart is suddenly located proximal to such resistant pulmonary vascular bed. Pharmacologically modulation of pulmonary vascular hemodynamics with pulmonary vasodilators during catheterization helps to forecast the outcome after heart transplantation. *In most transplant centers, a fixed pulmonary vascular resistance index of 6 units or more or transpulmonary gradient more than 15 mmHg that does not reduce by vasodilator therapy (such as oxygen, nitric oxide, or dobutamine) is contraindication to lone heart transplantation.*

Other contraindications to heart transplantation according to the ACC/AHA Guidelines (2008) for Adults with CHD are as follows [9]:

Active infections, Positive serology for human immunodeficiency virus(HIV) or hepatitis C virus, Severe metabolic disorders, multiple severe congenital lesions, Multiorgan failure, Active malignancies, Cognitive and behavioral disorder that restricts the compliance

Heart-lung transplantation is regularly held in reserve for patients with non-correctable or previously repaired CHD associated with significant pulmonary vascular diseases such as single ventricle physiology or significant LV dysfunction with concomitant pulmonary vascular disease. When a simple cardiac lesion is present (e.g., ASD, VSD, and patent ductus arteriosus), the cardiac anomaly can frequently be repaired in lung transplantation time. However, with more complex cardiac lesions, combined heart and lung transplantation is generally most suitable [9, 21, 22].

Adult CHD heart transplant recipients have a mean survival of 11 years, like patients with other forms of heart disease. Patients who have had Fontan surgery are likely to have worse outcomes, presumably because they have multiorgan disease. About one third of heart-lung transplants are done for CHD. Survival is about 50 % at 3 years, about 20 % in 10 years after heart-lung transplantation, and better in the presence of Eisenmenger syndrome [9, 17–21].

References

1. Francis GS. Pathophysiology of chronic heart failure. Am J Med. 2001;110(Suppl 7A):37S–46.
2. The SOLVD Investigators. Effect of enalapril on mortality and the development of heart failure in symptomatic patients with reduced left ventricular ejection fractions. N Engl J Med. 1992;327:685–91.
3. McMurray JJ, Stewart S. Epidemiology, etiology and prognosis of heart failure. Heart. 2000;83:596–602.
4. McDonagh TA. Asymptomatic left ventricular dysfunction in the community. Curr Cardiol Rep. 2000;2:470–4.
5. Metra M, Nodari S, D'Aloia A, et al. Effects of neurohormonal antagonism on symptoms and quality-of-life in heart failure. Eur Heart J. 1919;1998: B25–35.
6. Fredriksen PM, Veldtman G, Hechter S, et al. Aerobic capacity in adults with various congenital heart diseases. Am J Cardiol. 2001;87:310–4.
7. Chua TP, Ponikowski P, Harrington D, et al. Clinical correlates and prognostic significance of the ventilatory response to exercise in chronic heart failure. J Am Coll Cardiol. 1997;29(7):1585–90.
8. Coats AJ. The "muscle hypothesis" of chronic heart failure. J Mol Cell Cardiol. 1996;28:2255–62.
9. Warnes CA, Williams RG, Thomas M, et al. ACC/AHA 2008 guidelines for the management of adults with congenital heart disease. Circulation. 2008;52(23): e143-e263.
10. The CONSENSUS Trial Study Group. Effects of enalapril on mortality in severe congestive heart failure. Results of the Cooperative North Scandinavian Enalapril Survival Study (CONSENSUS). N Engl J Med. 1987;316:1429–35.
11. Hechter SJ, Fredriksen PM, Liu P, et al. Angiotensin-converting enzyme inhibitors in adults after the Mustard procedure. Am J Cardiol. 2001;87:660–3.
12. Lester SJ, Mc Elhinney DB, Viloria E, et al. Effects of losartan in patients with a systemically functioning morphologic right ventricle after atrial repair of transposition of the great arteries. Am J Cardiol. 2001;88:1314–6.
13. Hopkins WE, Kelly DP. Angiotensin-converting enzyme inhibitors in adults with cyanotic congenital heart disease. Am J Cardiol. 1996;77:439–40.
14. Laer S, Mir TS, Behn F, et al. Carvedilol therapy in pediatric patients with congestive heart failure:

a study investigating clinical and pharmacokinetic parameters. Am Heart J. 2002;143:916–22.
15. Shaddy RE. Beta-blocker therapy in young children with congestive heart failure under consideration for heart transplantation. Am Heart J. 1998;136:19–21.
16. Shaddy RE, Tani LY, Gidding SS, et al. Beta-blocker treatment of dilated cardiomyopathy with congestive heart failure in children: a multi-institutional experience. J Heart Lung Transplant. 1999;18: 269–74.
17. Troughton RW, Prior DL, Pereira JJ, et al. Plasma B-type natriuretic peptide levels in systolic heart failure: importance of left ventricular diastolic function and right ventricular systolic function. J Am Coll Cardiol. 2004;43:416–22.
18. Hunt SA, Abraham WT, Chin MH. ACC/AHA 2005 guideline update for the diagnosis and management of chronic heart failure in the adult: a report of the American College of Cardiology/American Heart Association Task Force on Practice Guidelines (Writing Committee to update the 2001 Guidelines for the Evaluation and Management of Heart Failure). J Am Coll Cardiol. 2005;46:e1–82. 202.
19. Pignatelli RH, Mc Mahon CJ, Chung T, et al. Role of echocardiography versus MRI for the diagnosis of congenital heart disease. Curr Opin Cardiol. 2003;18:357–65. 203.
20. Tulevski II, van der Wall EE, Groenink M, et al. Usefulness of magnetic resonance imaging dobutamine stress in asymptomatic and minimally symptomatic patients with decreased cardiac reserve from congenital heart disease (complete and corrected transposition of the great arteries and subpulmonic obstruction). Am J Cardiol. 2002;89:1077–81.
21. Williams RV, Ritter S, Tani LY, et al. Quantitative assessment of ventricular function in children with single ventricles using the Doppler myocardial performance index. Am J Cardiol. 2000;86:1106–10.
22. Vanderheyden M, Goethals M, Verstreken S, et al. Wall stress modulates brain natriuretic peptide production in pressure overload cardiomyopathy. J Am Coll Cardiol. 2004;44:2349–54.

Infective Endocarditis in Congenital Heart Disease

8

Azin Alizadehasl and Anita Sadeghpour

Keywords
Infective Endocarditis • Congenital Heart Disease • Echocardiography • Prophylaxis

Epidemiology and Incidence of Infective Endocarditis in Adults with Congenital Heart Disease

In recent decade, significant improvement in the long-term survival of adult patients with congenital heart disease (CHD) has given rise to a risk of late complications such as infective endocarditis (IE). The frequency of IE in adults with CHD exceeds tenfold that of the normal population, so a definition of the high-risk groups, a high diagnostic warning, and careful indication of antibiotics to these patients are health-care issues of vital importance [1].

Interestingly, the epidemiological profile of IE has undergone change in recent years. While affected patients commonly had rheumatic heart disease in the past, CHD is now predominant in Europe and the USA [2]. On the other hand, the population of patients with adult CHD has noticeably increased over the past decades and is presently estimated at 1.2 million in Europe [3]. The incidence of IE ranges from 3 to 10 episodes/100,000 person-years in the general population [2]. The prevalence of CHD in patients with IE has been defined to be between 2 and 18 % [4–6].

Although the prognosis of IE is more desirable in CHD compared with acquired heart disease, mortality still continues to remain high, with a reported variety between 4 and 10 % [7, 8]. Some simple lesions such as the secundum type of atrial septal defect and pulmonary valve stenosis seem to carry a low risk of IE [2]. Nevertheless, the incidence of IE in various congenital defects has yet to be fully investigated. For example, ventricular septal defect is frequently regarded as a high-risk defect, but a prospective research of these patients suggested that IE is mainly related to concomitant valve disease rather than to the septal defects [9].

Filippo et al. [10] studied 153 episodes of IE and reported that the mean age of CHD patients affected with IE has been higher in recent years.

Verheugt et al. [11], interestingly, studied the occurrence of IE in a population of 10,210 patients

A. Alizadehasl, MD, FACC (✉)
Echocardiography Lab, Department of Cardiology, Rajaie Cardiovascular Medical and Research Center, Iran University of Medical Science, Tehran, Iran
e-mail: alizadeasl@gmail.com, alizadeasl@rhc.ac.ir

A. Sadeghpour, MD, FACC, FASE
Echocardiography Lab, Department of Cardiology, Adult Congenital Heart Disease Clinic, Rajaie Cardiovascular Medical and Research Center, Iran University of Medical Science, Tehran, Iran
e-mail: anita.sadeghpour@gmail.com, asadeghpour@rhc.ac.ir

A. Sadeghpour et al. (eds.), *Comprehensive Approach to Adult Congenital Heart Disease*,
DOI 10.1007/978-1-4471-6383-1_8, © Springer-Verlag London 2014

with CHD and found an incidence of IE of 1.1 per 1,000 patient-years. Their study confirmed the augmented risk in these patients compared with 1.7–6.2 per 100,000 patient-years in the general population [12]. The study also approved the particularly low risk of patients with pulmonary valve stenosis and secundum type of atrial septal defect when these conditions are not associated with additional lesions. The highest risk was seen in pulmonary atresia with ventricular septal defect (hazard ratio [HR] = 16.7), followed not only by other complex lesions like congenitally corrected transposition of the great arteries and single ventricular heart defect (HR = 7.1 and 6.1) but also by simple diseases such as bicuspid aortic valve and ventricular septal defect (HR = 6.3 and 6.8).

Table 8.1 Primary reasons for revision of the IE prophylaxis in the guidelines

IE is much more likely to result from frequent exposure to bacteremias associated with daily activities than from bacteremia caused by a dental, GI tract, or GU tract procedure
Prophylaxis may prevent an exceedingly small number of cases of IE, if any, in individuals who undergo a dental, GI tract, or GU tract procedure
The risk of antibiotic-associated adverse events exceeds the benefit, if any, from prophylactic antibiotic therapy
Maintenance of optimal oral health and hygiene may reduce the incidence of bacteremia from daily activities and is more important than prophylactic antibiotics for a dental procedure to reduce the risk of IE

From Wilson et al. [27]

Prevention, Etiology, and Diagnosis of Infective Endocarditis in Adults with Congenital Heart Disease

The Filippo study [10] demonstrated that dental problems are the leading cause of IE with a significant variety of pathological organisms (with multiple species of *Streptococcus*). Also, the incidence of cutaneous causative infections has risen (5–17 %) with different types of *Staphylococcus* in recent decades. In that study, negative blood cultures diminished (from 20 to 7 %; *p* value = 0.03), and Streptococci were the most common causal organisms.

The incidence of severe heart failure and cardiovascular complications in CHD patients with IE has lessened recently. Early surgery was more common in earlier years with a drop, albeit not significantly, in overall mortality. In his study, the incidence of early mortality was 7.2 % as opposed to the varying rates of 10–25 % in the literature. *This improvement in early survival may be a result of earlier and more effective surgical management as reported in the literature* [13, 14].

For the diagnosis of IE, echocardiography plays a crucial role. To date, no study has assessed the sensitivity and specificity of transthoracic and transesophageal echocardiography in the diagnosis of IE in a group of patients with complex congenital malformations. In general, transthoracic echocardiography (TTE) is useful in the detection of vegetation, but frequently, the sensitivity is too low to rule out the absence of vegetation given the difficulty in the imaging of shunts and conduits and complexity in the anatomy combined with differentiating vegetation from dysplastic abnormal valves in adult CHD patients. Sometimes, careful comparison of valve anatomies and function with previous recordings is needed to detect differences.

Also of particular importance in the detection of IE in adolescents and adults is transesophageal echocardiography (TEE) for the assessment of the thoracic aorta, valved conduits, and ventricular outflow tracts and for the imagining of the entire ventricular septum (Table 8.1).

TEE may help to obtain prognostic information or to study IE and IE-related complications and may be more sensitive and specific than TTE in these patients. Be that as it may, TEE sometimes fails to image the lesions in patients with complex cardiac malformations. *The diagnosis of IE should, thus, rely on the Duke criteria other than echocardiography in complex lesions, shunts, and conduits* [15, 16].

TEE is indicated in adult CHD, if a TTE study is equivocal or when there is a complex congenital heart anatomy or a valve prosthesis in which transthoracic windows may be inadequate [17–25].

In order to decrease the risk of IE, the following recommendations are worth considering:

1. *Maintenance of oral hygiene and regular dental visit is significant.*
2. *Uninfected and hygienic measures in manipulation of venous catheters and any invasive procedures should be taken into account.*
3. *Adult CHD patients must be discouraged from receiving piercings and tattoos.*
4. *Antibiotic prophylaxis should be prescribed for patients with the highest risk of IE experiencing the highest-risk procedures* [25, 26].
5. *Physicians should bear in mind that the cyanotic patients with right-to-left shunts have the opportunity of "paradoxical" systemic embolization, which renders them at risk of stroke. Air filters should be utilized in order to avoid the injection of air bubbles.*

On the other hand, based on previous studies [2, 26], *transient bacteremia happens not only after dental procedures but often in the setting of daily routine actions like tooth brushing or chewing.* Due to the lack of efficient signs for the efficacy of antibiotic prophylaxis and the expected enormous number of patients that may require management to prevent one single event of IE, *it is now commended by expert consensus to limit antibiotic prophylaxis to patients with very high risk of IE experiencing the highest-risk procedures, namely, patients with previous IE, patients with prosthetic cardiac valves or prosthetic materials used for cardiac valves repair, and patients with CHD: (A) cyanotic CHD without previous surgical repair or with residual defects, shunts, or implanted conduits; (B) CHD after repair with prosthetic materials whether positioned by surgery or by a percutaneous method, till 6 months after the procedure; and (C) persistence of a residual defect at the site of the embedding of a prosthetic material or device following any cardiac surgery or a percutaneous procedure* (Table 8.2, 8.3 and 8.4) [2–26].

The recommendation has also been restricted to dental procedures requiring manipulation of the gingival or periapical area of the teeth or perforation of the oral mucosa. Antibiotics are not suggested for the respiratory tract as well as for gastrointestinal, genitourinary, dermatological, and musculoskeletal procedures except for an established infection [2–26].

Table 8.2 Cardiac conditions associated with the highest risk of adverse outcome from infective endocarditis for which prophylaxis with dental procedures is reasonable

Condition	Congenital-specific condition*
Previous infective endocarditis	Unrepaired cyanotic CHD, including palliative shunts and conduits[a]
Prosthetic cardiac valve or prosthetic material used for cardiac valve repair	Completely repaired congenital heart defect with prosthetic material or device, whether placed by surgery or by catheter intervention, during the first 6 months after the procedure
	Repaired CHD with residual defects at the site or adjacent to the site of a prosthetic patch or prosthetic device that inhibit endothelialization
	Cardiac transplant recipients who develop cardiac valvulopathy

By Modified from Wilson et al. [27]

Except for the conditions listed above, antibiotic prophylaxis is no longer recommended for any other form of CHD

*Prophylaxis is reasonable because endothelialization of prosthetic material occurs within 6 months after the procedure

[a]*CHD* indicates congenital heart disease

Table 8.3 Dental procedures for which endocarditis prophylaxis is reasonable for patients in Table 2

All dental procedures that involve manipulation of gingival tissue or the periapical region of teeth or perforation of the oral mucosa
The following procedures and events do not need prophylaxis: routine anesthetic injections through noninfected tissue, taking dental radiographs, placement of removable prosthodontic or orthodontic appliances, adjustment of orthodontic appliances, placement of orthodontic brackets, shedding of deciduous teeth, and bleeding from trauma to the lips or oral mucosa

From Wilson et al. [27]

Cultures should be obtained before the beginning of antibiotic therapy in order to find the causative organism [25, 26].

In summary, it should be highlighted that our knowledge of IE in patients with CHD is still limited as systematic reviews are few, mostly retrospective, and profoundly affected by selection bias. Patients with CHD and physicians should always be alert of the risk of IE. Any clinical

Table 8.4 Regimens for a dental procedure

		Regimen: single dose 30–60 min before procedure	
Situation	Agents	Adults	Children
Oral	Amoxicillin	2 g	50 mg/kg
Unable to take oral medication	Ampicillin or cefazolin or ceftriaxone	2 g IM or IV 1 g IM or IV	50 mg/kg IM or IV 50 mg/kg IM or IV
Allergic to penicillins or ampicillin (oral)	Cephalexin[a, b] or clindamycin or azithromycin or clarithromycin	2 g 600 mg 500 mg	50 mg/kg 20 mg/kg 15 mg/kg
Allergic to penicillins or ampicillin and unable to take oral medication	Cefazolin or ceftriaxone[a] or clindamycin	1 g IM or IV 600 mg IM or IV	50 mg/kg IM or IV 20 mg/kg IM or IV

From Wilson et al. [27]
IM intramuscular, *IV* intravenous
[a]Cephalosporins should not be used in an individual with a history of anaphylaxis, angioedema, or urticaria with penicillins or ampicillin
[b]Or other first- or second-generation oral cephalosporin in equivalent adult or pediatric dosage

doubt must prompt careful assessment, including echocardiography and blood culture, in order to provide so early diagnosis as possible and to let effective management.

References

1. Moreillon P, Que YA. Infective endocarditis. Lancet. 2004;363:139–49.
2. Habib G, Hoen B, Tornos P, et al. ESC Committee for Practice Guidelines. Guidelines on the prevention, diagnosis, and treatment of infective endocarditis (new version 2009): the Task Force on the Prevention, Diagnosis, and Treatment of Infective Endocarditis of the European Society of Cardiology (ESC). Eur Heart J. 2009;30:2369–413.
3. Moons P, Engelfriet P, Kaemmerer H, et al. Delivery of care for adult patients with congenital heart disease in Europe: results from the Euro Heart Survey. Eur Heart J. 2006;27:1324–30.
4. Michel PL, Acar J. Native cardiac disease predisposing to infective endocarditis. Eur Heart J. 1995;16(Suppl B):2–6.
5. De Gevigney G, Pop C, Delahaye JP. The risk of infective endocarditis after cardiac surgical and interventional procedures. Eur Heart J. 1995;16(Suppl B):7–14.
6. Roder BL, Wandall DA, Espersen F, et al. Neurologic manifestations in Staphylococcus aureus endocarditis: a review of 260 bacteremic cases in nondrug addicts. Am J Med. 1997;102:379–86.
7. Li W, Somerville J. Infective endocarditis in the grown-up congenital heart (GUCH) population. Eur Heart J. 1998;19:166–73.
8. Niwa K, Nakazawa M, Tateno S, et al. Infective endocarditis in congenital heart disease: Japanese national collaboration study. Heart. 2005;91:795–800.
9. Gabriel HM, Heger M, Innerhofer P, et al. Long-term outcome of patients with ventricular septal defect considered not to require surgical closure during childhood. J Am Coll Cardiol. 2002;39:1066–71.
10. Di Filippo S, Delahaye F, Semiond B, et al. Current patterns of infective endocarditis in congenital heart disease. Heart. 2006;92:1490–5.
11. Verheugt CL, Uiterwaal CSPM, Van der Velde E, et al. Turning with congenital heart disease: prediction of infective endocarditis based on a very large population. Eur Heart J. 2011. doi:10.1093/eurheartj/ehq485. Published online ahead of print 8 January 2011.
12. Hoen B, Alla F, Selton-Suty C, et al. Changing profile of infective endocarditis: results of a 1-year survey in France. JAMA. 2002;288:75–81.
13. Fisher MC. Changing risk factors for pediatric infective endocarditis. Curr Infect Dis Rep. 2001;3:333–6.
14. Martin JM, Neches WH, Wald ER. Infective endocarditis: 35 years of experience at a children's hospital. Clin Infect Dis. 1997;24:669–75.
15. Aly AM, Simpson PM, Humes RA. The role of transthoracic echocardiography in the diagnosis of infective endocarditis in children. Arch Pediatr Adolesc Med. 1999;153:950–3.
16. Greaves K, Mou D, Patel A, et al. Clinical criteria and the appropriate use of transthoracic echocardiography for the exclusion of infective endocarditis. Heart. 2003;89:273–5.
17. Mylonakis E, Calderwood SB. Infective endocarditis in adults. N Engl J Med. 2001;345:1318–30.
18. Child JS, Perloff JK, Kubak B. Infective endocarditis: risks and prophylaxis. In: Perloff JK, Child JS, editors. Congenital heart disease in adults. Philadelphia: W.B. Saunders; 1998. p. 129–43.
19. Bayer AS, Bolger AF, Taubert KA, et al. Diagnosis and management of infective endocarditis and its complications. Circulation. 1998;98:2936–48.

20. Fowler VG, Durack DT. Infective endocarditis. Curr Opin Cardiol. 1994;9:389–400.
21. Horstkotte D, Follath F, Gutschik E, et al. Guidelines on prevention, diagnosis and treatment of infective endocarditis executive summary; the task force on infective endocarditis of the European Society of Cardiology. Eur Heart J. 2004;25:267–76.
22. Dodo H, Child JS. Infective endocarditis in congenital heart disease. Cardiol Clin. 1996;14:383–92.
23. Child JS. Echo-Doppler and color-flow imaging in congenital heart disease. Cardiol Clin. 1990;8:289–313.
24. Krivokapich J, Child JS. Role of transthoracic and transesophageal echocardiography in diagnosis and management of infective endocarditis. Cardiol Clin. 1996;14:363–82.
25. Warnes C, Williams RG, Bashore TM, et al. ACC/AHA 2008 guidelines for the management of adults with congenital heart disease. J Am Coll Cardiol. 2008;52(23):1890–947.
26. Baumgartner H, Bonhoeffer P, De Groot NM, ESC Committee for Practice Guidelines (CPG), et al. ESC guidelines for the management of grown-up congenital heart disease (new version 2010). Eur Heart J. 2010;31:2915–57.
27. Wilson W, Taubert KA, Gewitz M, Lockhart PB, Baddour LM, Levison M, et al. Prevention of infective endocarditis: guidelines from the American Heart Association: a guideline from the American Heart Association Rheumatic Fever, Endocarditis, and Kawasaki Disease Committee, Council on Cardiovascular Disease in the Young, and the Council on Clinical Cardiology, Council on Cardiovascular Surgery and Anesthesia, and the Quality of Care and Outcomes Research Interdisciplinary Working Group. Circulation 2007;116:1736–54. Erratum in: Circulation 2007;116:e376–7.

Chest Radiography in Congenital Heart Disease

9

Anita Sadeghpour and Arash Hashemi

Keywords
Congenital heart disease • Chest radiography • Pulmonary vasculature • Shunt vascularity • Chest X-ray

Abdominal and Cardiac Position

The first step in chest X-ray interpretation is to determine the position of the heart, base-to-apex axis, and abdominal situs. *In a normal heart with visceral situs solitus, the heart is positioned left sided with a leftward-pointing base-to-apex axis, the stomach is left sided, the liver is right sided, the aorta lies to the left, and the inferior vena cava lies to the right of the spine* (Fig. 9.1). One should pay close attention to the bronchial pattern as it is very useful in the identification of a patient's situs. In situs solitus, the right and left bronchi are asymmetric; the right bronchus is relatively straight and short and the left bronchus is relatively long and curved. *Normally, the left hemidiaphragm is seen lower than the right hemidiaphragm due to the left-sided cardiac apex.*

The determination of the abdominocardiac or visceroatrial situs is very important because situs solitus with dextroversion or situs inversus with levocardia has a strong association with complex congenital heart disease. Situs inversus totalis with dextrocardia or mirror- image dextrocardia carries a low incidence of congenital heart disease. When cardiac dextroversion is associated situs solitus,

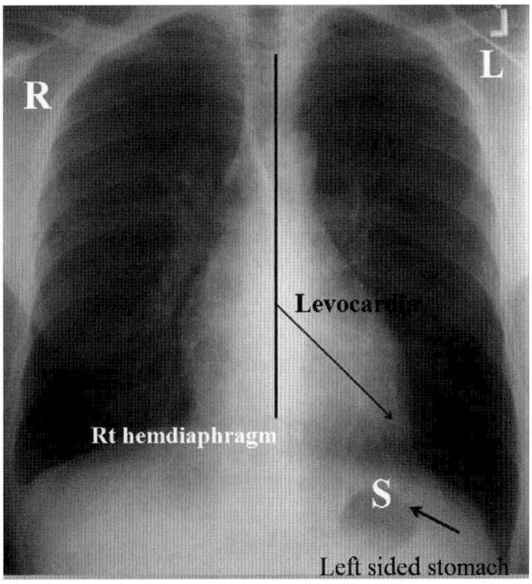

Fig. 9.1 Cardiac location, base-to-apex axis, and positions of the liver and stomach can be determined in the plain chest X-ray. *S* stomach

A. Sadeghpour, MD, FACC, FASE (✉)
Echocardiography Lab, Department of Cardiology, Adult Congenital Heart Disease Clinic, Rajaie Cardiovascular Medical and Research Center, Iran University of Medical Science, Tehran, Iran
e-mail: anita.sadeghpour@gmail.com, asadeghpour@rhc.ac.ir

A. Hashemi, MD
Department of Cardiology, Erfan General Hospital, Tehran, Iran

A. Sadeghpour et al. (eds.), *Comprehensive Approach to Adult Congenital Heart Disease*, DOI 10.1007/978-1-4471-6383-1_9, © Springer-Verlag London 2014

congenitally corrected transposition of the great arteries, which is associated with ventricular septal defect and pulmonary stenosis, will be the common cardiac malposition finding. Dextrocardia should be distinguished from dextroposition, in which the heart is located within the right thorax but its apex points to the patient's left [1–4].

Cardiac Chamber Size

The estimation of the cardiac chamber size is another important step in the interpretation of congenital heart disease patient's X-ray. The cardiothoracic ratio (CT ratio) is the widest diameter of the heart in comparison to the widest internal diameter of the rib cage, and any ratio >50 % is considered an increased CT ratio. It is rewarding to identify an increase in the cardiac size and chambers (left atrium, right atrium, and left ventricle or right ventricle solely or in combination) responsible for the increase in the CT ratio.

Shunt Vascularity

The criteria for shunt vascularity in chest X-ray that are only seen when the pulmonary-to-systemic flow is >1.5–1 are as follows:

1. *Loss of normal distribution of vascular markings and a uniform vascularity pattern (Normally the lower lobe has dominant vascular markings.)*
2. *Prominent right descending pulmonary artery with diameters >17 mm*
3. Pulmonary artery marking larger than its adjacent bronchus (Fig. 9.2)

There are some potential sites of error as pregnancy, anemia, thyrotoxicosis, and pulmonary arteriovenous fistula may exhibit the same changes.

Pulmonary Vasculature

The pulmonary vasculature is another issue that should be addressed individually after shunt vascularity, and sufficient heed should be paid to pulmonary venous patterns, signs of increased pulmonary venous pressures, pulmonary artery,

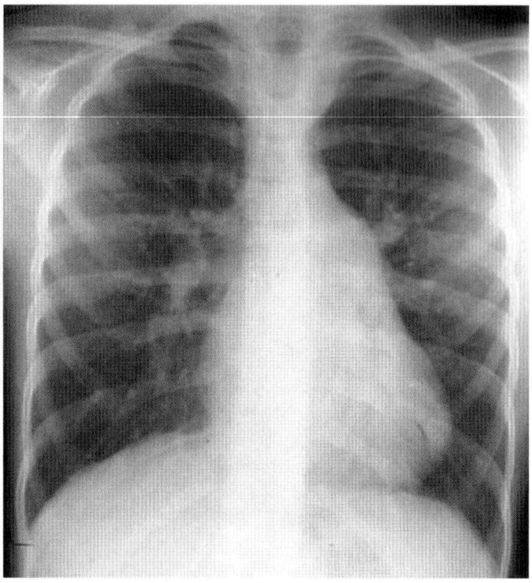

Fig. 9.2 Prominent main pulmonary artery, shunt vascularity, right ventricular enlargement, and small aortic knob, all in favor of atrial septal defect

and search for any post stenotic dilation. Five states can be seen in the pulmonary vasculature: normal, pulmonary venous hypertension, pulmonary arterial hypertension, increased flow, and decreased flow.

The determination of these patterns requires a close scrutiny of the right descending pulmonary artery (which should normally be <17 mm in diameter) as well as the distribution of the flow in the lungs at two sites: the upper versus the lower lobes and the central versus the peripheral lobes [4].

Usually in the standing position, due to the effect of the gravity, the blood flow to the bases is more than that to the apices. Also, there should be tapering of the vessels from the central part toward the peripheral part.

Venous hypertension is present when the right descending pulmonary artery is >17 mm and the upper lobe vessels size is equal to or greater than the size of the lower lobe vessels (which is called cephalization).

Pulmonary arterial hypertension is present when the right descending pulmonary artery is >17 mm in diameter and the main pulmonary artery is prominent. With an increase in pulmonary artery pressures, there may be a rapid cutoff in the size of the peripheral vessels in comparison with the size of the central vessels, and the central

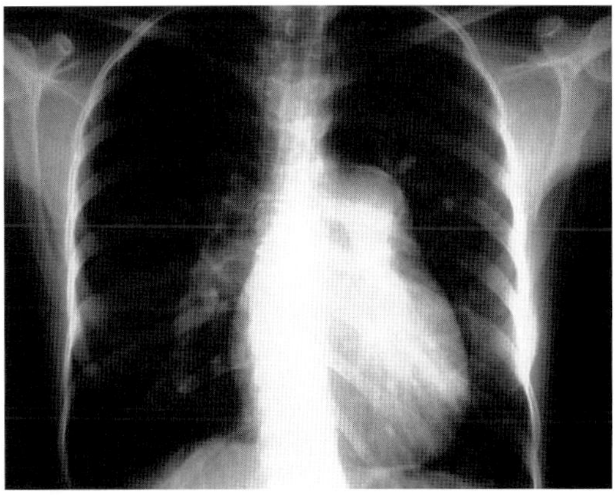

Fig. 9.3 Right ventricular enlargement, prominent main pulmonary artery, and peripheral vessel pruning suggestive of pulmonary atrial hypertension

vessels may seem to be too large for the size of the peripheral vessels (this pattern is called pruning Fig. 9.3).

Increased flow is seen when the right descending pulmonary artery is >17 mm in diameter, but there is normal and preserved distribution of the flow and gradual tapering from the center to the periphery.

Decreased flow is very hard to diagnose, but the presence of small hila and reduction in normal blood vessels may point toward it [5].

The aforementioned steps should be followed by a close inspection of the ribs (looking for subcostal notching), deviations in the trachea, foreign bodies, diaphragm, thymic shadow, costophrenic spaces, general shape of the heart, and presence or absence of pulmonary fluids.

Chest X-Ray Patterns in Specific Conditions

Conditions with Increased Pulmonary Vascularity

Atrial Septal Defect

Evidence of shunt vascularity in chest X-ray can be seen in shunt ratios >1.5/1. In shunt vascularity, the increased pulmonary vasculature is seen from the center to the periphery as well as in the upper and lower lobes. Nevertheless, the size of the upper lobe vessels is smaller than the lower lobe vessels, which is contrast to pulmonary venous hypertension.

Although the left atrium is normal in size, there is right atrial and right ventricular enlargement, both of which are best seen in lateral views. The chest X-ray film is often, but not always, abnormal in patients with significant atrial septal defect. The central pulmonary arteries are characteristically enlarged, with pulmonary plethora indicating an increased pulmonary flow. A small aortic knuckle, which reflects a chronically low cardiac output, is characteristic of atrial septal defect [4, 6].

Ventricular Septal Defect

In ventricular septal defect with significant left-to-right shunting, there is evidence of shunt vascularity and left atrial and left ventricular enlargement. The aorta is usually normal in size. In patients with ventricular septal defect and significant pulmonary arterial hypertension, the pulmonary artery segment is prominent, and the pulmonary vascular markings are diminished at the periphery of the lung [4, 7, 8].

Atrioventricular Septal Defect

Similar to atrial septal defect, an increased cardiothoracic ratio with prominent right atrium and right ventricle and increased pulmonary vascular marking is expected. If there is significant mitral regurgitation, there may be left ventricular and left atrial [4] enlargement.

Patent Ductus Arteriosus

Chest X-ray may have variable features regarding the severity and duration of the disease. A small duct produces a normal chest X-ray, whereas in more than moderate-sized ducts, patients develop cardiomegaly, enlarged left atrium and left ventricle, prominent main pulmonary artery, and shunt vascularity, in favor of left-to-right shunts, prominent peripheral pulmonary vasculature, and prominence of the ascending aorta (and possibly aortic arch). Adults with patent ductus arteriosus may exhibit linear calcification at the site of the ductus [4, 9, 10].

If the Eisenmenger syndrome develops, its findings with a prominent aortic knuckle are expected.

It should be noted that punctuate calcification at the site of a closed ductus is a normal finding.

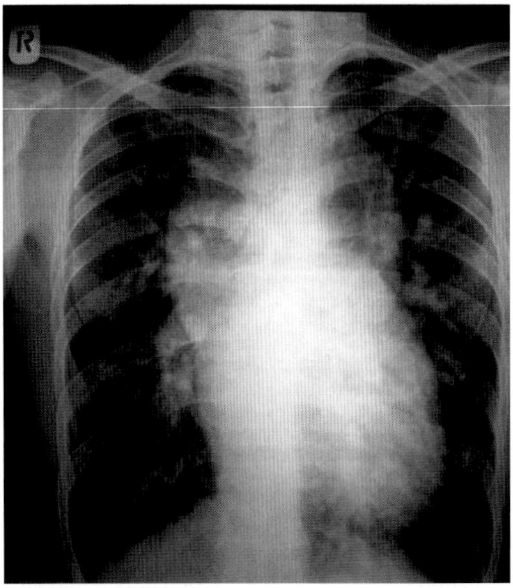

Fig. 9.4 The "snowman sign" or the "figure-of-eight sign," associated with shunt vascularity and right-sided cardiac chamber enlargement in total anomalous pulmonary venous drainage

Total and Partial Anomalous Pulmonary Venous Return

Total and partial anomalous pulmonary venous return has a distinctive pattern in chest X-ray. A *left-sided dilated vertical vein, prominent innominate vein on the top, and right-sided superior vena cava all together give form to a specific image called the "snowman sign"* (Fig. 9.4). In this distinct image, an enlarged right atrium forms the body of the snowman. Another name for this image is the "figure-of-eight sign" [4, 10].

Also, there is shunt vascularity, in favor of left-to-right shunting and enlargement of the right side of the heart due to volume overload. In newborns with total anomalous pulmonary venous return and obstructed pulmonary venous return, chest X-ray may show evidence of pulmonary edema.

In partial anomalous pulmonary venous return, an anomalous pulmonary vein originates from the right lung, curves in the right heart border, and usually continues from the mid part of the lung all the way through to the costophrenic angle. These *characteristic features resemble a Turkish sword called "scimitar," hence the term the "scimitar sign"* (Fig. 9.5) [11].

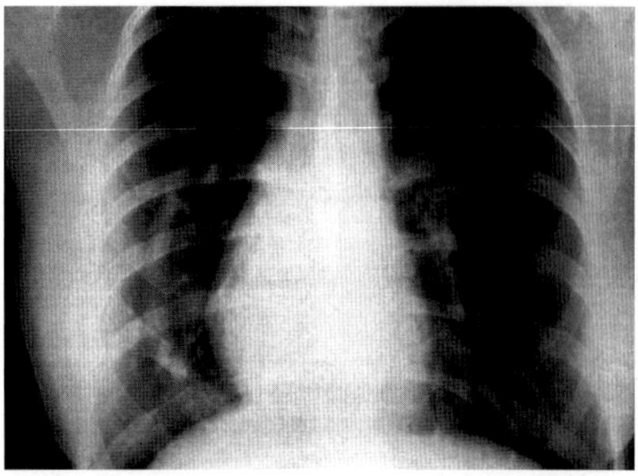

Fig. 9.5 An anomalous right pulmonary vein parallel to the right atrium named the "scimitar sign." Dextrocardia is often associated with the scimitar syndrome

Complete Transposition of the Great Arteries

The pulmonary artery is obscured by the aorta on frontal chest radiographs. This malposition, in association with stress-induced thymic atrophy and hyperinflated lungs, results in the apparent narrowing of the superior mediastinum on radiographs, the most consistent sign of transposition of the great arteries. *Accordingly, in dextro-transposition of the great arteries, an enlarged heart can be seen in conjunction with a narrow pedicle, giving the so-called "egg-on-a-string" appearance.* This is because the superior mediastinum appears narrow owing to the anteroposterior relationship between the transposed great vessels and the radiological absence of the thymus [12, 13].

Adult patients with this disease usually have undergone some sort of corrective surgery at some point in the past. After atrial switch operation, there is typically a narrow vascular pedicle plus an oblong cardiac silhouette, which is called the "egg-on-side pattern." In lateral views, an anteriorly located aorta may occupy the retrosternal space. In patients with a history of the arterial switch procedure and the Rastelli procedure, the chest X-ray is usually normal except for sternal wires or conduit calcification in the latter.

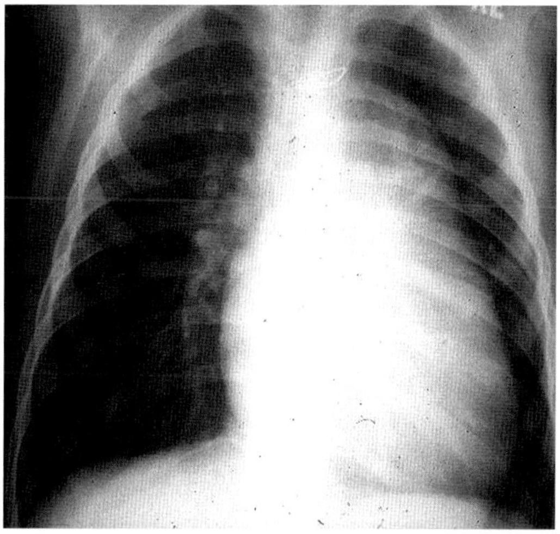

Fig. 9.6 The "waterfall appearance," in favor of congenitally corrected transposition of the great arteries

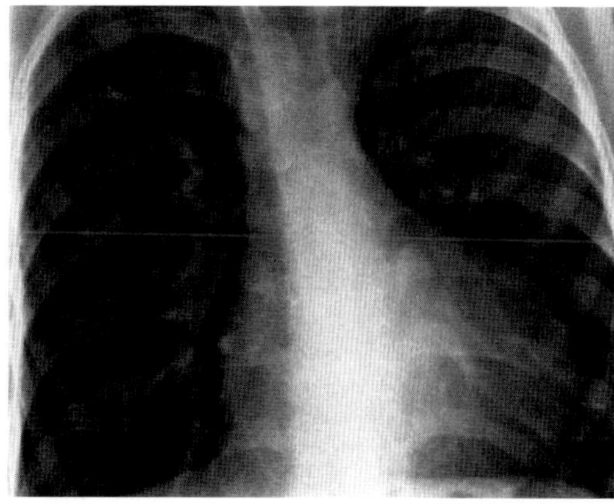

Fig. 9.7 Tetralogy of Fallot, hypovascularized lungs, small central pulmonary artery, and right ventricular enlargement, named "boot-shaped heart" or "Coeur en sabot"

Congenitally Corrected Transposition of the Great Arteries

The left supracardiac borders have a smooth convexity, and there is absence of the normal pulmonary artery segment. There is a left-sided ascending aorta, and the main pulmonary trunk is medially displaced. Furthermore, the right pulmonary hilum is prominent and is elevated in comparison to the left side. *The right pulmonary artery appears to have a high takeoff because of an absent aortic shadow, giving rise to a unique image called the "waterfall appearance"* (Fig. 9.6).

Truncus Arteriosus

There is an increased CT ratio with pulmonary arterial hypertension patterns, concave pulmonary artery segment, enlarged left atrium, and unusual high hilar areas. A right-sided aortic arch is seen in approximately half of the patients. The superior mediastinum is widened.

Conditions with Decreased Pulmonary Vascularity

Tetralogy of Fallot

There is a prominent right ventricle, resulting in the upward displacement of the apex and creating a concavity in the region of the right ventricular outflow tract, which is underdeveloped. *In addition, the pulmonary vasculature is diminished. This combination gives rise to a classic "boot-shaped heart" or "Coeur en sabot" appearance* (Fig. 9.7). There may be a right-sided aortic arch in approximately 25 % of cases [4, 10, 11]. It is important to look for indentation in the trachea to locate it. The ascending aorta is usually prominent.

Pulmonary Atresia with Ventricular Septal Defect

A normal-sized heart with a prominent right ventricle and upward displacement of the apex and reduced pulmonary artery markings is the rule. There may be a right-sided aortic arch.

Tricuspid Atresia

In patients with tricuspid atresia, it is expected to see levocardia, left-sided aortic arch (in 75 % of patients), and situs solitus. The CT ratio and the pulmonary vasculature are dependent on the amount of the pulmonary blood flow and accompanying conditions (Fig. 9.8), but usually a flat or concave pulmonary artery is seen. If there is a small atrial septal defect, the right atrium is enlarged [4, 10, 11]. However, if there is a large atrial septal defect, a normal or slightly enlarged right atrium is expected.

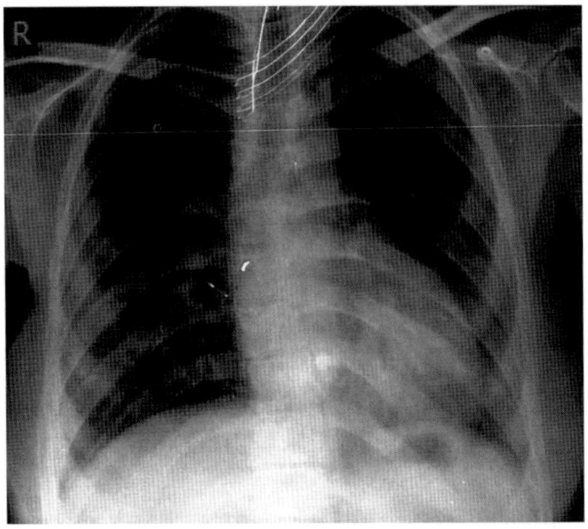

Fig. 9.8 Small right heart chambers with diminished lung vascularity

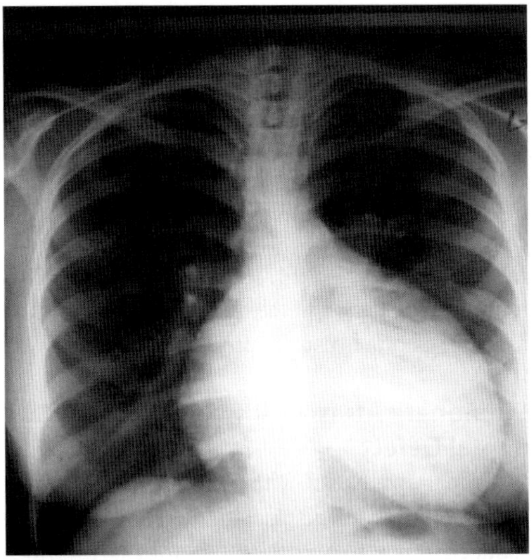

Fig. 9.9 Giant right atrium and atrialized right ventricle, associated with hypovascularized lungs

The Ebstein Anomaly

Enlarged right atrium and atrialized right ventricle and the resulting rightward convexity in addition to a dilated infundibulum produce a characteristic "water bottle" or "box-shaped heart" appearance (Fig. 9.9). Some degrees of cardiomegaly are always expected, and the aorta and the pulmonary trunk are both inconspicuous. The pulmonary vasculature is normal to diminished [4, 10, 11].

Pulmonary Hypertension/Eisenmenger Syndrome

Radiologic hallmarks of the Eisenmenger syndrome are dilated central pulmonary arteries with rapid tapering of the peripheral pulmonary vasculature, called vascular pruning [4, 10, 11]. If pulmonary hypertension is long lasting, there may be calcification in the pulmonary artery. In patients with the Eisenmenger syndrome, patent ductus arteriosus calcification in the duct can be seen.

If the patient's original disease is ventricular septal defect or patent ductus arteriosus, the CT ratio is normal to mildly increased. Nevertheless, if the atrial septal defect is responsible for the patient's condition due to right atrial and right ventricular dilation, the CT ratio is markedly increased and there is an inconspicuous aorta.

Conditions with Normal Pulmonary Artery Vascularity

Aortic Stenosis

In congenital cases, cardiomegaly due to right ventricular enlargement, upward displacement of the apex, and various degrees of pulmonary edema is usual. In non-congenital cases, there is marked cardiomegaly due to left ventricular hypertrophy, and there may be some degrees of post-stenotic dilation in the ascending aorta. In these cases, the pulmonary vasculature is usually normal.

In cases of subaortic stenosis, the chest X-ray usually is not helpful. In cases of supravalvular stenosis, in distinction with subvalvular and valvular stenosis, there is no dilation in the ascending aorta.

Coarctation of the Aorta

The most helpful radiographic sign *in aortic coarctation is "rib notching," which is erosion caused by increased pressures in the intercostal blood vessels in the posterior ribs. This phenomenon is usually seen in the 3rd thorough the 9th ribs and does not involve the 1st and the 2nd ribs. It can be unilateral or bilateral and usually is in the outer third of the ribs and has a sclerotic margin.*

Other signs include pre- and post-stenotic dilation in the aorta and the left subclavian

artery and indentation at the site of coarctation called the "figure-of-three sign." This figure is matched by "reverse 3" or "E" sign in the barium-filled esophagus [4, 10–12].

Other features may include a dilated aorta proximal to the coarctation site and convexity of the ascending aorta in the proximal 1/3 part.

Pulmonary Stenosis

Chest X-ray is variable in regard to concomitant conditions and patients' age. In neonates with an intact ventricular septum, there is diminished pulmonary vascular marking as well as right ventricular prominence. If the lesion is mild to moderate in intensity, a normal chest X-ray with normal heart size and normal pulmonary vasculature is expected, but there may be post-stenotic dilation in the main and left pulmonary arteries. If the lesion is severe, right-sided enlargement is detected both in the right ventricle and in the right atrium. In such cases, in which the severity is advanced, pulmonary vascular marking is diminished [4, 10, 11].

In cases of dysplastic pulmonary valve stenosis, the same findings are expected except for lack of post-stenotic dilation even in the case of severe obstruction. Due to the accompanying pulmonary lymphangiectasia, there may be the "ground-glass appearance," mimicking pulmonary venous obstruction.

Congenital Mitral Stenosis

Increased CT ratio and cardiomegaly due to enlarged left atrium and left ventricle is seen.

Cor Triatriatum

The chest X-ray pattern is highly dependent on the severity of the obstructive lesion and can vary from normal in mild cases to pulmonary edema in patients with significant lesions.

Malposition of Cardiac Lesions

Dextrocardia

The condition in which the heart has been shifted rightward by external causes is called dextroposition. Mixed dextrocardia indicates dextrocardia with atrioventricular discordance. Mirror-image dextrocardia refers to patients with situs inversus. If the apex of the heart is toward the right, it is dextrocardia; toward the left is levocardia; and toward the middle is mesocardia.

In plain chest X-ray, the confirmation of the patient's situs requires that the radiologist look for gastric bubbles as well as liver and tracheal segmentation. It is important to note that the abdominal organs' situs and their relation with the cardiac chambers will affect the likelihood of congenital heart defects [2].

Situs inversus totalis is when a patient has mirror-image dextrocardia with the gastric bubble on the right side and liver on the left side.

Miscellaneous Cardiac Lesions

Congestive Cardiac Failure

Based on the etiology, the chest X-ray pattern may vary widely. In cases of idiopathic congestive cardiac failure or non-cardiac-induced congestive cardiac failure, increased CT ratio, degrees of pulmonary venous hypertension patterns, fluid within the horizontal and oblique fissures, prominent Kerley B lines (indicative of lymphatic engorgement), and pleural effusion and/or pericardial effusion are expected.

Partial or Complete Absence of Pericardium

It is very hard to diagnose this condition solely based on plain chest X-ray. Magnetic resonance imaging (MRI) can prove extremely useful in this condition. The findings include prominent dilation of the left atrial appendage, cardiomegaly, and cardiac silhouette marking levoposition, faded heart borders on the right side, very prominent main pulmonary artery, and borderline irregularities in the upper left heart border. However, the most important finding is that there is a portion of the lung tissue between the main pulmonary artery and the aorta. This so-called "tongue-of-tissue sign" is the most common sign seen in patients with both complete and partial absence of the pericardium [14, 15].

References

1. Leung AKC, Robson WLM. Dextrocardia with sinus solitus. CMAJ. 2006;175(3):244.
2. Perloff J, Marelu A. Perloff's clinical recognition of congenital heart disease. 6th ed. Philadelphia: WB Saunders Elsevier; 2013.
3. Otto CM, editor. The practice of clinical echocardiography. 3rd ed. Philadelphia: W. B. Saunders/Elsevier; 2007.
4. Bonow, Mann, Zipes, Libby. Braunwald's Heart Disease: A Textbook of Cardiovascular Medicine, 9th edition, 2011.
5. Webb G, Gatzoulis M. Atrial septal defects in the adult: recent progress and overview. Circulation. 2006; 114:1645–53.
6. Webb G, Gatzoulis M. Congenital heart disease for the adult cardiologist atrial septal defects in the adult recent progress and overview. Circulation. 2006;114:1645–53.
7. Singh VN, Sharma RK, et al. Ventricular septal defect imaging. Medscape online version. 2010.
8. Moodie DS. Diagnosis and management of congenital heart disease in the adult. Cardiol Rev. 2001;9(5): 276–81.
9. George Hartnell. Chief editor: Lin EC. Patent ductus arteriosus imaging online version of Medscape, 2012.
10. Warnes C, Williams RG, Bashore TM, et al. ACC/AHA, guidelines for the management of adults with congenital heart disease. JACC. 2008;52(23):2008.
11. Allen HD, Driscoll DJ, Shaddy RE. Moss and Adams' heart disease in infants, children, and adolescents: including the fetus and young adults. 7th ed. Philadelphia: Lippincott Williams & Wilkins; 2008.
12. IJland MM, Tanke RB. Images in cardiovascular medicine aortic coarctation. Circulation. 2009;120: 1294–5.
13. McMahon C, Singleton E. Plain radiographic diagnosis of congenital heart disease. GRAPHIC
14. Abbas AE, Appleton CP, Liu PT, Sweeney JP. Congenital absence of the pericardium: case presentation and review of literature. Int J Cardiol. 2005;98(1): 21–5.
15. Gatzoulis MA, Munk MD, Merchant N, Van Arsdell GS, McCrindle BW, Webb GD. Isolated congenital absence of the pericardium: clinical presentation, diagnosis, and management. Ann Thorac Surg. 2000;69(4): 1209–15.

10 Syndromic Congenital Heart Diseases

Arya Mani and Azin Alizadehasl

Keywords
Syndromic congenital heart disease • Genetic • Chromosomal anomalies
Syndromic cardiovascular diseases

Introduction

The aggregate role of genetic factors in the etiology of congenital heart defects (CHD) is evident by the high prevalence of syndromes that clusters CHD with several extracardiac abnormalities. These syndromes are either caused by contiguous syndrome due to large deletions or duplications or by mutations in transcription factors that regulate development of the heart and several other organs. Often, the CHD defects are associated with abnormalities of facial structures and the musculoskeletal system. The pleiotropic effects of these genetic abnormalities, however, result in significant diversity in the phenotypes of within the general population and even within individual families [1–4].

Down Syndrome

Trisomy 21 (Down syndrome) is one the most common causes of CHD and mental retardation with a frequency of 1/700 living births. Clinical features include short hands, facial anomalies, and high rate of single palmar crinkle, neonatal hypotonia, gastrointestinal malformations, and also cardiovascular disease that affects approximately 50 % of patients. The genetic abnormality in most cases is caused by isochromosome duplication (dup21q) and in rare cases is the result of a fusion between two heterologous chromatids, known as Robertsonian translocation. These chromosomal changes are of both paternal and maternal origin and their rate increases with aging of the parents. Cardiac deformities include atrioventricular canal defect, atrial and ventricular septal defects, and also tetralogy of Fallot [4–8]. Cardiovascular disease is a major cause of mortality in these patients followed by respiratory obstructive disorders, immune system diseases, and infectious diseases [9, 10].

A. Mani, MD, FACC
Cardiovascular Genetics Program, Yale University, New Haven, CT, USA

A. Alizadehasl, MD, FACC (✉)
Echocardiography Lab, Department of Cardiology, Rajaie Cardiovascular Medical and Research Center, Iran University of Medical Science, Tehran, Iran
e-mail: alizadeasl@gmail.com, alizadeasl@rhc.ac.ir

A. Sadeghpour et al. (eds.), *Comprehensive Approach to Adult Congenital Heart Disease*,
DOI 10.1007/978-1-4471-6383-1_10,

Noonan-Leopard Syndromes

Noonan syndrome, also known as the male Turner syndrome, is characterized as a wide spectrum of CHD, short stature, pterygium colli, thoracic and facial abnormalities, and also bleeding diathesis. Facial features include a broad forehead, hypertelorism, a high-arched palate, low-set and posteriorly rotated ears, and also down-slanting palpebral fissures. Cardiovascular involvement is present in up to 90 % of patients [9–12]. The anomaly has at least eight subtypes. Type 1 is caused by mutations in PTPN11, a gene encoding the protein tyrosine phosphatase SHP-2 located at chromosome 12q22-qter. It is the first disease gene identified for Noonan syndrome and accounts for 50 % of the cases. NS3 is caused by mutation in the KRAS gene; NS4, by mutation in the SOS1 gene; NS5, by mutation in the RAF1 gene; NS6, by mutation in the NRAS gene; NS7, by mutation in the BRAF gene; and NS8, by mutation in the RIT1 gene. Other different mutations in the same gene create Leopard syndrome, a genetic disorder with clinical findings overlapping those of Noonan syndrome and unique lentigines skin lesions and deafness too. In both syndromes, cardiac anomalies are common (about 60 % of cases), including pulmonary valve stenosis and also hypertrophic cardiomyopathy [11–17]. Noonan syndrome is more often associated with pulmonary valve stenosis with typically thickened leaflets classically unsuitable for interventional balloon dilation, thus needing surgical intervention [16–19].

Deletion in 22q11

This disorder becomes the second most common syndromic CHD after Down syndrome. The del22q11 syndrome (also known as velocardiofacial syndrome) is associated with a highly variable phenotype despite similar deletion sizes. Clinical features of 22q11 deletion also include cleft palate, facial dysmorphisms, and palatal abnormalities. Less frequent features included microcephaly, speech and learning disabilities, neonatal hypocalcaemia, short stature, immune deficiency, mental retardation, slender hands and digits, minor auricular anomalies, and also inguinal hernia.

The most common cardiac anomalies are ventricular septal defect, pulmonary atresia, and tetralogy of Fallot. Children with 22q11 deletion and tetralogy of Fallot present with extracardiac malformations like absent pulmonary valve and aortic arch abnormalities and aberrant left subclavian in 50 % of cases. The complex pulmonary arterial anatomy in these patients usually associated with additional surgical risk.

A routine screening for 22q11 deletion in all children with cleft palate is recommended.

Within the 22q11 interval, the TBX1 gene appears to be the most important determinant of the disease phenotypes, particularly the psychiatric diseases of this syndrome [20–22].

Turner Syndrome

Turner syndrome is created by the absence of an entire sex chromosome (Barr body), known as monosomy X, or less frequently by haploinsufficiency of specific genes on the X chromosome. It is part of the spectrum of short stature, idiopathic, X-linked syndrome. Clinical findings include CHD, gonadal dysgenesis, short stature, renal disorders, facial abnormalities, and pterygium colli. There is significant variability in cardiac defects, ranging from partial anomalous pulmonary venous connection, bicuspid aortic valve, and aortic coarctation to complex disorders of left-sided obstruction, i.e., hypoplastic left heart syndrome affecting up to 40 % of patients. CHD, especially aortic valve anomalies and aortic coarctation, appears to be more common in subjects with 45, X karyotype versus those with mosaicism (45, X/46, XY karyotype). In Turner syndrome patients with aortic coarctation, friability of the aortic wall with high risk of hemorrhages has been defined at surgery or after stent implantation [1, 2, 23, 24].

Early-onset aortic dilation, dissection, or rupture has been reported in subjects with a Turner syndrome with a frequency of 36/100,000 per year. The majority of Turner patients have either bicuspid aortic valve, aortic coarctation, or also systemic hypertension. However, aortic dissection caused by vasculopathy including intimal and medial layers of large arteries in the absence of CHD or systemic hypertension also occurs. Ascending aortic size index of 2.5 cm/m^2 or more is considered as significant risk factor for aortic dissection. Due to increased risk of cardiovascular disease in patients with Turner syndrome routine clinical and echocardiographic evaluations, including periodic monitoring of blood pressure is often recommended [23, 24].

Marfan Syndrome

Marfan syndrome is an autosomal dominant disorder in the connective tissue featuring musculoskeletal, ocular, and cardiovascular anomalies. The syndrome is caused by mutations in fibrillin 1 gene on chromosome 15. Fibrillin is the main and basic structural component of the elastin-related connective tissue microfibrils. Cardiovascular involvement is present in the 70–80 % of patients with Marfan syndrome, including aortic dilatation with the threat of aortic dissection and mitral valve leaflets prolapse with or without mitral valve regurgitation. Though pulmonary artery is also dilated in patients with Marfan syndrome, this anomaly seldom leads to clinical consequences. The aortic stiffness is described to be greater in patients with Marfan syndrome compared with patients with juvenile forms of ascending aortic dilation without this syndrome [25–29].

Ventricular tachyarrhythmia with increased left ventricular size and mitral valve leaflets prolapse can represent an additional risk factor for sudden cardiac death in these patients. Beta-blockers and angiotensin II receptor blockers are commonly used to delay the progression of aortic aneurysm and dissection in this syndrome [1–3, 29].

Loeys-Dietz Syndrome

The Loeys-Dietz syndrome (LDS) is another syndromic autosomal dominant aortic aneurysm disorder with multiple systemic involvements. The vascular phenotype is characterized by tortuous aneurysms. The extracardiac phenotypes include hypertelorism, a bifid uvula, or cleft palate. This syndrome consists of at least four subtypes. Patients with LDS type 1 have craniofacial involvement including craniosynostosis, hypertelorism, or cleft palate. Patients with LDS type 2 have only a bifid uvula and arterial aneurysms. LDS1 and LDS2 are caused by mutation in the TGFBR1 and TGFBR2 genes. Another form of Loeys-Dietz syndrome is associated with early-onset osteoarthritis and is created by mutations in the SMAD3 gene. LDS4 is caused by mutation in the TGFB2 gene [2, 27–29].

Williams Syndrome

Williams syndrome features CHD, mental retardation, typical facial anomalies, short stature, and also connective tissue abnormalities and is caused by a microscopic deletion of chromosome 7q11.23. More than 20 genes have been mapped inside the commonly deleted region. Many of the clinical features of Williams syndrome, including the cardiac defects, are caused by the deletion of the elastin gene. In vivo and in vitro studies have suggested that the abnormal elastin protein product induces arterial smooth muscle proliferation and intimal hyperplasia, particularly at the supravalvular aortic and pulmonary artery levels, leading to arterial stenosis. The disease also affects the mesenteric and renal arteries, predisposing the affected children to systemic hypertension. Supravalvular aortic stenosis is a progressive lesion, which can be discrete in the form of hourglass narrowing of the supravalvular region or diffuse extending into the aortic arch and into the origin of brachiocephalic arteries. Abnormalities of left ventricular myocardial mechanics have been described in children with Williams syndrome even in absence of supravalvular aortic stenosis or hypertension. Finally, coronary artery disease can happen in this syndrome even in patients without supravalvular aortic stenosis. Sudden cardiac death is rare and is restricted mainly to cardiac malformations with biventricular obstruction and/or to coronary artery stenosis [1, 2, 30].

CHAR Syndrome

Patent ductus arteriosus (PDA) is a common CHD that results when the ductus arteriosus, a muscular artery that connects the aorta to main pulmonary artery during fetal life, fails to completely close after birth. A syndromic form of this disease, Char syndrome, is an autosomal dominant disorder that features PDA, facial dysmorphology including broad forehead, saddle nose with a patulous tip, polydactyly, or fifth-finger clinodactyly. Only the small numbers of families have been reported with this syndrome. The disease is created by mutation in *TFAP2B*, the gene encoding a neural crest-derived transcription factor. Disease-causing mutations are missense and are both losses of function and dominant negative mutations [1–3, 31–33].

Holt-Oram Syndrome

This autosomal dominant disorder features thumb anomaly and atrial septal defect. Other cardiovascular anomalies may include hypoplastic left heart syndrome, ventricular septal defect, and PDA. The extracardiac features include absent pectoralis major muscle, thoracic scoliosis, and pectus excavatum or carinatum. The thumb may be absent, may have extracarpal bones or be triphalangeal, may appear as curved inward, or may appear as nonopposable, finger-like digit. The disease is caused by mutations in the T-box 5 gene [1, 34].

The gene is essential in cardiac development, as it associates with NKX2-5 and promotes cardiomyocyte differentiation. There is a strong genotype-phenotype association in this disorder with mutations in the highly conserved T-box sequences that interact with the major groove of target DNA causing significant cardiac anomalies but only minor skeletal deformities while mutations located in the T-box domain that bind to the minor groove of DNA causing extensive upper limb malformations but less significant cardiac abnormalities.

Loss of Tbx5 in the mouse ventricle results in a single chamber lacking distinct identity, indicating a requirement for Tbx5 in septation [34].

Other Syndromes

Trisomy 13 and trisomy 18 are responsible for CHD and carry an unfavorable short- to midterm prognosis per se. The related cardiac malformations like ventricular septal defects, tetralogy of Fallot, atrioventricular canal defects, and also aortic coarctation have been traditionally considered unsuitable for repair. Nonetheless, recent data suggests improvement of the overall prognosis [1–3, 32, 33].

Conclusion

Roughly 1/3 of all patients with cardiac defects have associated extracardiac malformations, giving rise to discrete syndromes that are often genetically determined. Presence of the extracardiac syndromic features should prompt clinicians to screen for associated cardiovascular anomalies. Genetic testing can help establish the diagnosis. These patients represent a management challenge not limited to their cardiovascular diseases but also due to extracardiac anomalies.

References

1. Eskedal L, et al. A population-based study of extra-cardiac anomalies in children with congenital cardiac malformations. Cardiol Young. 2004;14:600–7.
2. Marino B, Digilio MC. Congenital heart disease and genetic syndromes: specific correlation between cardiac phenotype and genotype. Cardiovasc Pathol. 2000;9:303–15.
3. Clementi M, et al. Apparent CHARGE association and chromosome anomaly: chance or contiguous gene syndrome. Am J Med Genet. 1991;41:246–50.
4. Tanaka M, Chen Z, Bartunkova S, Yamasaki N, Izumo S. The cardiac homeobox gene Csx/Nkx2.5 lies genetically upstream of multiple genes essential for heart development. Development. 1999;126:1269–80.
5. Atkins L, Bartsocas CS. Down's syndrome associated with two Robertsonian translocations, 45, XX,-15,-21, + t(15q21q) and 46, XX,-21, + t(21q21q). J Med Genet. 1974;11:306–9.
6. Tandon R, Edwards JE. Cardiac malformations associated with Down's syndrome. Circulation. 1973;47: 1349–55.
7. Schott JJ, et al. Congenital heart disease caused by mutations in the transcription factor NKX2-5. Science. 1998;281:108–11.
8. Laing CR, Harper WH. Rubinstein-Taybi syndrome: broad thumbs and toes, facial abnormalities and mental retardation. Ariz Med. 1967;24:536–40.

9. Park SC, Needles CF, Dimich I, Sussman L. Congenital heart disease in an infant with the Smith-Lemli-Opitz syndrome. J Pediatr. 1968;73:896–902.
10. Antonarakis SE, Adelsberger PA, Petersen MB, Binkert F, Schinzel AA. Analysis of DNA polymorphisms suggests that most de novo dup(21q) chromosomes in patients with Down syndrome are isochromosomes and not translocations. Am J Hum Genet. 1990;47:968–72.
11. Robinow M, Shaw A. The McKusick-Kaufman syndrome: recessively inherited vaginal atresia, hydrometrocolpos, uterovaginal duplications, anorectal anomalies, postaxial polydactyly, and congenital heart disease. J Pediatr. 1979;94:776–8.
12. Hook EB, Cross PK, Schreinemachers DM. Chromosomal abnormality rates at amniocentesis and in live-born infants. JAMA. 1983;249:2034–8.
13. Tartaglia M, et al. PTPN11 mutations in Noonan syndrome: molecular spectrum, genotype-phenotype correlation, and phenotypic heterogeneity. Am J Hum Genet. 2002;70:1555–63.
14. Schubbert S, et al. Germline KRAS mutations cause Noonan syndrome. Nat Genet. 2006;38:331–6.
15. Roberts AE, et al. Germline gain-of-function mutations in SOS1 cause Noonan syndrome. Nat Genet. 2007;39:70–4.
16. Razzaque MA, et al. Germline gain-of-function mutations in RAF1 cause Noonan syndrome. Nat Genet. 2007;39:1013–7.
17. Cirstea IC, et al. A restricted spectrum of NRAS mutations causes Noonan syndrome. Nat Genet. 2010;42:27–9.
18. Niihori T, et al. Germline KRAS and BRAF mutations in cardio-facio-cutaneous syndrome. Nat Genet. 2006;38:294–6.
19. Aoki Y, et al. Gain-of-function mutations in RIT1 cause Noonan syndrome, a RAS/MAPK pathway syndrome. Am J Hum Genet. 2013;93:173–80.
20. Mehraein Y, et al. Microdeletion 22q11 in complex cardiovascular malformations. Hum Genet. 1997;99: 433–42.
21. Wilson DI, et al. DiGeorge syndrome with isolated aortic coarctation and isolated ventricular septal defect in three sibs with a 22q11 deletion of maternal origin. Br Heart J. 1991;66:308–12.
22. Lindsay EA, et al. Tbx1 haploinsufficiency in the DiGeorge syndrome region causes aortic arch defects in mice. Nature. 2001;410:97–101.
23. Ellison JW, et al. PHOG, a candidate gene for involvement in the short stature of Turner syndrome. Hum Mol Genet. 1997;6:1341–7.
24. Prandstraller D, et al. Turner's syndrome: cardiologic profile according to the different chromosomal patterns and long-term clinical follow-Up of 136 nonpreselected patients. Pediatr Cardiol. 1999;20: 108–12.
25. Dietz HC, et al. Marfan syndrome caused by a recurrent de novo missense mutation in the fibrillin gene. Nature. 1991;352:337–9.
26. Keramati AR, Sadeghpour A, Farahani MM, Chandok G, Mani A. The non-syndromic familial thoracic aortic aneurysms and dissections maps to 15q21 locus. BMC Med Genet. 2010;11:143.
27. Loeys BL, et al. A syndrome of altered cardiovascular, craniofacial, neurocognitive and skeletal development caused by mutations in TGFBR1 or TGFBR2. Nat Genet. 2005;37:275–81.
28. van de Laar IM, et al. Mutations in SMAD3 cause a syndromic form of aortic aneurysms and dissections with early-onset osteoarthritis. Nat Genet. 2011;43: 121–6.
29. Boileau C, et al. TGFB2 mutations cause familial thoracic aortic aneurysms and dissections associated with mild systemic features of Marfan syndrome. Nat Genet. 2012;44:916–21.
30. Pober BR. Williams-Beuren syndrome. N Engl J Med. 2010;362:239–52.
31. Satoda M, et al. Mutations in TFAP2B cause Char syndrome, a familial form of patent ductus arteriosus. Nat Genet. 2000;25:42–6.
32. Wynne-Davies R. Genetics and malformations of the hand. Hand. 1971;3:184–92.
33. Mani A, et al. Syndromic patent ductus arteriosus: evidence for haploinsufficient TFAP2 mutations and identification of a linked sleep disorder. Proc Natl Acad Sci U S A. 2005;102:2975–9.
34. Terrett JA, et al. Holt-Oram syndrome is a genetically heterogeneous disease with one locus mapping to human chromosome 12q. Nat Genet. 1994;6:401–4.

Basic Principles and Systemic Segmental Approach to Congenital Heart Disease in Echocardiography

11

Anita Sadeghpour

Keywords
Adult congenital heart disease • Echocardiography • Segmental approach • Atrioventricular connection • Ventriculoarterial connection • Great arteries

Basic Principles of Echocardiography in Congenital Heart Disease

Patients with adult congenital heart disease (ACHD) have a range of heart conditions, varying from simple "holes in the heart" to complex single-ventricle anatomy. Some patients have undergone palliation or complete surgical repair, whereas others remain with their native heart condition. *In all of these situations, echocardiography remains the mainstay of diagnosis for patients with CHD.*

The following basic principles should be borne in mind in the imaging of patients with suspected CHD [1–5]:

1. *In all probability, the presence of one congenital abnormality denotes the existence of more.* Whether we seek to diagnose the most basic of communications between the atria or we endeavor to detect the most complex of malformations, the objective of the sequential segmental modality is to prove normality. That is why we subject a patient with an isolated atrial septal defect in the setting of a normally constructed heart to the same painstaking analysis as a patient with congenitally corrected transposition of the great arteries allied to multiple intracardiac defects.
2. A patient's history and/or written surgical report are to be meticulously perused even prior to meeting the patient. *The echocardiographer's thorough understanding of the particulars of the patient's earlier repairs affords a more clear-cut and efficient imaging investigation.*
3. Inspection of the patient's color, fingers, and chest would be helpful. Is the patient cyanotic with clubbed fingers? After all, *a cyanotic patient is more likely to have complex malformations.* The presence of the scars of sternotomy or lateral thoracotomy is proof of preceding surgical interventions.
4. The so-called rules of cardiac development and congenital abnormalities are not "gospel truth." The echocardiographer should, therefore,

A. Sadeghpour, MD, FACC, FASE
Echocardiography Lab, Department of Cardiology, Adult Congenital Heart Disease Clinic,
Rajaie Cardiovascular Medical and Research Center, Iran University of Medical Science, Tehran, Iran
e-mail: anita.sadeghpour@gmail.com, asadeghpour@rhc.ac.ir

A. Sadeghpour et al. (eds.), *Comprehensive Approach to Adult Congenital Heart Disease*,
DOI 10.1007/978-1-4471-6383-1_11, © Springer-Verlag London 2014

describe what is present, even if it does not chime in with the known conventional lesions.

5. *The philosophy of segmental analysis is based on the morphologic method. Accordingly, the recognition of the cardiac chambers should be on the basis of their morphology rather than their position.*
6. *Never hesitate to seek a second opinion if there is a complex anatomy.*
7. The sequential segmental approach is a systematic and standard approach for echocardiography in CHD. Generally, the sequential segmental approach consists of the following steps: cardiac position and orientation, visceroatrial situs, ventricular position (ventricular looping), and the great arteries position (looping). *Thereafter, the atrioventricular and ventriculoarterial connections are analyzed in terms of connections and relations.*
8. *The key to the echocardiography of CHD is an appreciation of the sequential segmental approach for the diagnosis of both simple and complex lesions.*
9. *In the evaluation of patients with CHD, the echocardiographic examination should be far more than a mere definition of the cardiac anatomy.* Not only does a comprehensive echocardiographic assessment define the cardiovascular anatomy but also it seeks to provide a description of the function of the myocardium, abnormalities of the valves, and overall hemodynamic status.
10. *Atrioventricular and semilunar valves have common abnormalities, even with normal segmentation.* Bicuspid aortic valves, Ebstein's anomaly of the tricuspid valve, and cleft mitral valves account for the most frequent findings.
11. Echocardiography is deemed a frontline diagnostic modality inasmuch as it can provide information on the anatomy of the heart, morphology of the cardiac chambers, function and size of the ventricles, communications between the atria and the ventricles, origins of the great arteries, and venous return.
12. There may be suboptimal echocardiography imaging in ACHD patients due to the larger body habitus and chest deformity. Consequently, off-axis and nonstandard views are frequently used to assess complex anatomy. Completion of echocardiographic data in these patients may necessitate other strategies such as transesophageal echocardiography (TEE), magnetic resonance imaging (MRI), computed tomography (CT) scanning, and even cardiac catheterization.

Sequential Segmental Approach

The following echocardiographic steps in the sequential segmental analysis [1–3, 5–8] are crucial in any patient with CHD:

Cardiac location: The term signifies the gross position of nearly all the heart in the thoracic cavity in connection with the midline. This definition is particularly useful radiographically; also it should *be determined by echocardiography from a standard subcostal view.*

Levoposition or left-sided heart: In this condition, most of the cardiac mass is positioned to the left of the midline (Fig. 11.1).

Dextroposition or right-sided heart: It is a condition where most of the cardiac mass is ositioned to the right of the midline (Fig. 11.2).

Mesoposition or midline heart: It is a condition where the heart is evenly distributed around the midline.

Cardiac Orientation (Base-to-Apex Axis)

Cardiac orientation (base-to-apex axis) should be determined, independent of cardiac location, from a standard subcostal view as leftward, midline, or rightward orientation (Figs. 11.3, 11.4 and 11.5).

A normal heart is a left-sided heart with a leftward-pointing apex. Cardiac location and orientation usually go together.

Visceral Situs or Sidedness

Embryological development sees all major organ systems starting with a bilaterally sym-

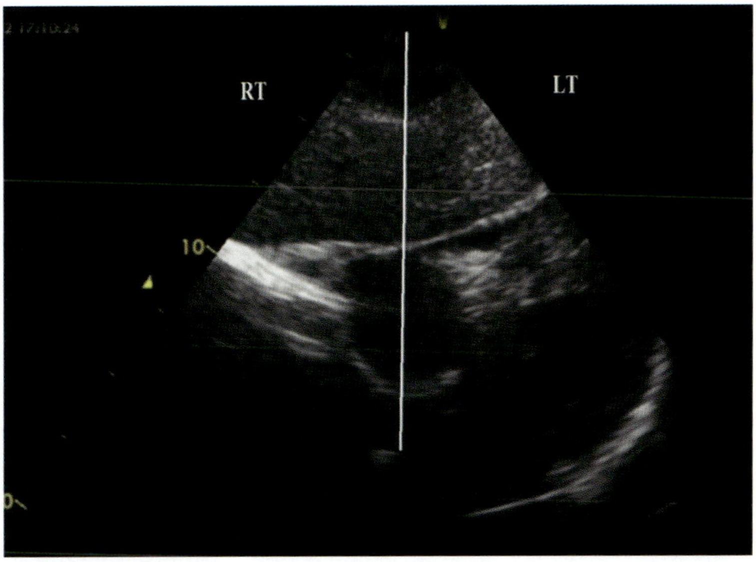

Fig. 11.1 Levoposition of the heart: most of the cardiac mass is positioned to the left of the midline in subcostal view. *RT* right, *LT* left

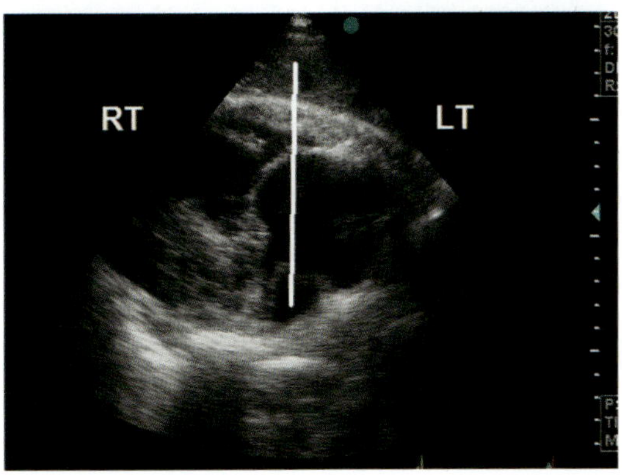

Fig. 11.2 Dextroposition of the heart: most of the cardiac mass is positioned to the right of the midline in subcostal view. *RT* right, *LT* left

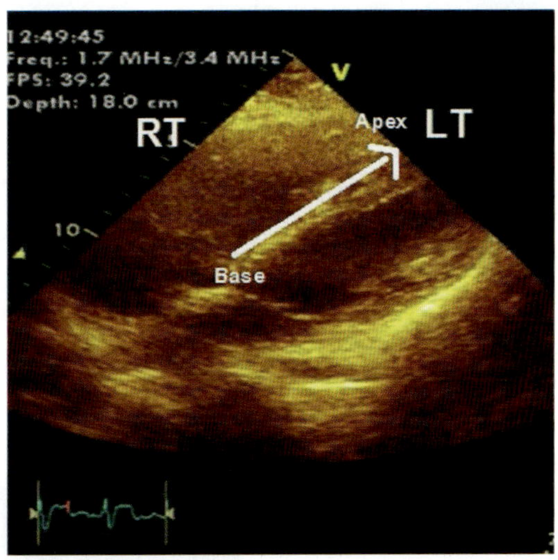

Fig. 11.3 Levoposition of the heart, with a leftward-pointing apex (levocardia) (*arrow*). *RT* right, *LT* left

metric midline orientation. The cardiovascular, respiratory, and digestive systems subsequently become asymmetric and are, thus, characterized by situs (sidedness or handedness).

Situs may be solitus (normal), inversus (mirror image), or ambiguus (isomeric or indeterminate).

Visceral situs describes the position of the organs in the abdomen that are not bilaterally symmetric. Visceral situs is determined by the position of the liver, stomach, and abdominal great vessels such as the aorta and the inferior vena cava (IVC) from a standard subcostal view, with the probe pointing at a right angle to the spine [1, 6, 9]. The echocardiographer can visualize the abdominal aorta together with the IVC and the spine posteriorly.

Abdominal situs solitus refers to a condition where the aorta and the IVC are positioned to the left and to the right of the spine, respectively (Figs. 11.6, 11.7 and 11.8). The spleen and pancreas are normally on the same side of the spine as the stomach.

Visceral situs solitus or normal sidedness refers to a condition where the liver is positioned to the right and the stomach and spleen to the left of the vertebral column. The term "situs inversus" means the reversal of the thoracic and abdominal viscera.

Atrial Situs

Cardiac situs is determined by the position of the atria in the chest. There are four types of atrial arrangements: (1) atrial situs solitus, denoting a right-sided right atrium; (2) atrial situs inversus, indicating a left-sided morphologic right atrium; (3) bilateral right atria, signifying right cardiac isomerism; and (4) bilateral left atria, representing left cardiac isomerism [4, 5, 10].

The right and left atria differ morphologically with regard to their appendages. A morphologic right atrium has a broad right atrial appendage (Fig. 11.9), whereas a morphologic left atrium has a narrow left atrial appendage (Fig. 11.10).

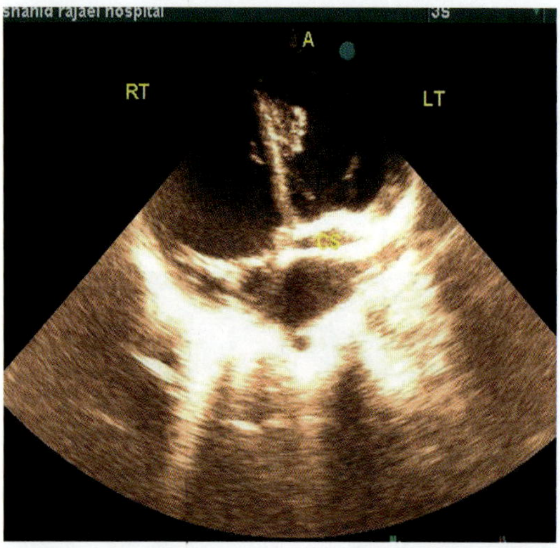

Fig. 11.4 Middle position of the heart, with a boxed-shaped apex (mesocardia). *RT* right, *LT* left

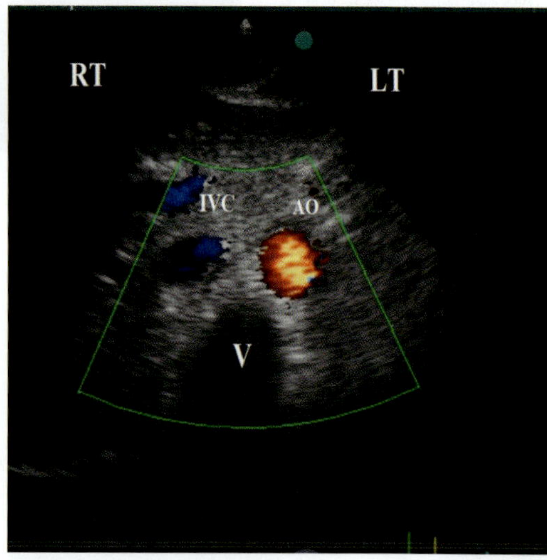

Fig. 11.6 Abdominal situs solitus, with the aorta to the left and the inferior vena cava to the right of the spine. *RT* right, *LT* left, *IVC* inferior vena cava, *AO* aorta, *V* vertebra

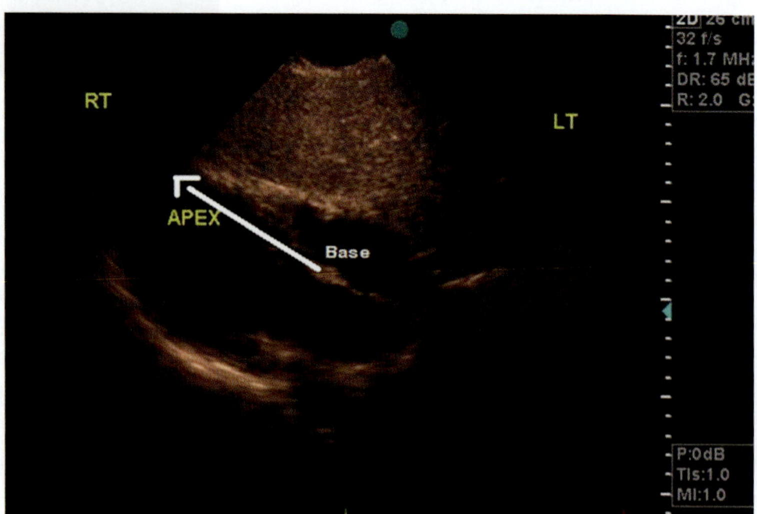

Fig. 11.5 Dextroposition of the heart, with a rightward base-to-apex axis (dextrocardia) (*arrow*). *RT* right, *LT* left

However, the atrial appendage is difficult to visualize by transthoracic echocardiography, and confident assignment of a morphologic left atrium and right atrium cannot be made by transthoracic echocardiography. Transesophageal echocardiography can assist with visualizing the atrium and determining the atrial situs. In about 70–80 % of the cases, atrial situs follows abdominal situs. When atrial and visceral situs is indeterminate, it is called situs ambiguus. If both the aorta and inferior vena cava are positioned to the left of the spine and the two morphologic atria are to the left (Fig. 11.11a, b), there is abdominal and atrial left isomerism.

Azygos venous return of the inferior vena cava is common in left isomerism (Figs. 11.12 and 11.13). When both the aorta and inferior vena cava are to the right of the spine and the two morphologic atria are to the right, there is abdominal and atrial right isomerism.

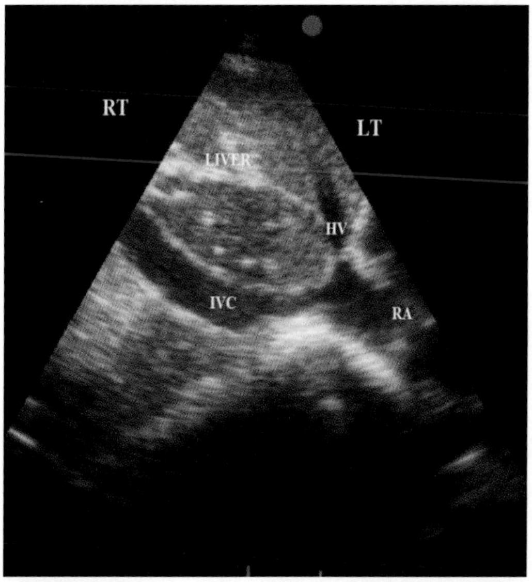

Fig. 11.7 Abdominal situs solitus, with the right-sided liver and inferior vena caval continuity to the right atrium. *RT* right, *LT* left, *IVC* inferior vena cava, *HV* hepatic vein, *RA* right atrium

Ventricular Situs (Ventricular Looping)

Once the visceroatrial situs is determined, the position and the morphology of the ventricles should be assessed. It is very important to define whether there is biventricular or univentricular anatomy. In biventricular anatomy, a D-loop ventricle indicates that the inflow portion of the morphologic right ventricle lies to the right of the morphologic left ventricle (Fig. 11.14) and an L-loop ventricle indicates that the inflow portion of the morphologic right ventricle lies to the left of the morphologic left ventricle (Fig. 11.15). As we mentioned before, chambers are recognized according to their morphology rather than their position [4–6].

The morphologic right ventricle has four characteristic features distinguishing it from the morphologic left ventricle: (1) heavy trabeculation, (2) moderate band, (3) septal attachment of the tricuspid valve and a coarse septal surface, and (4) apical insertion of the tricuspid valve.

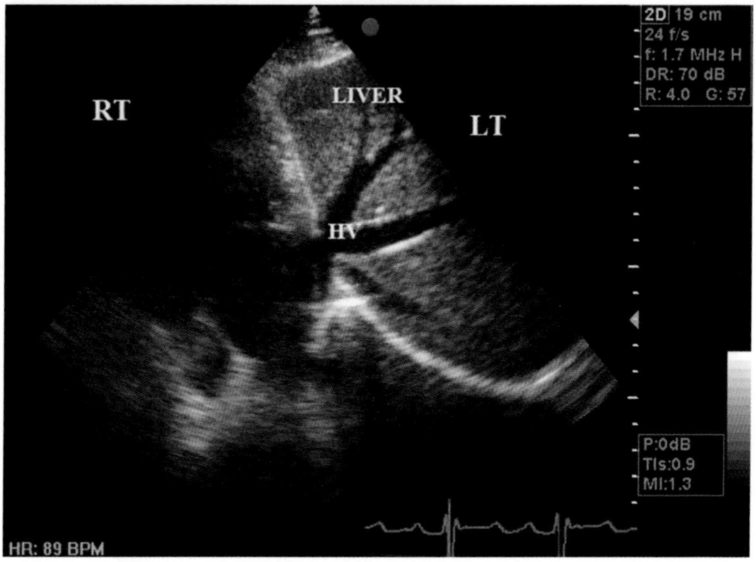

Fig. 11.8 Abdominal situs inversus, with a left-sided liver. *RT* right, *LT* left, *HV* hepatic vein

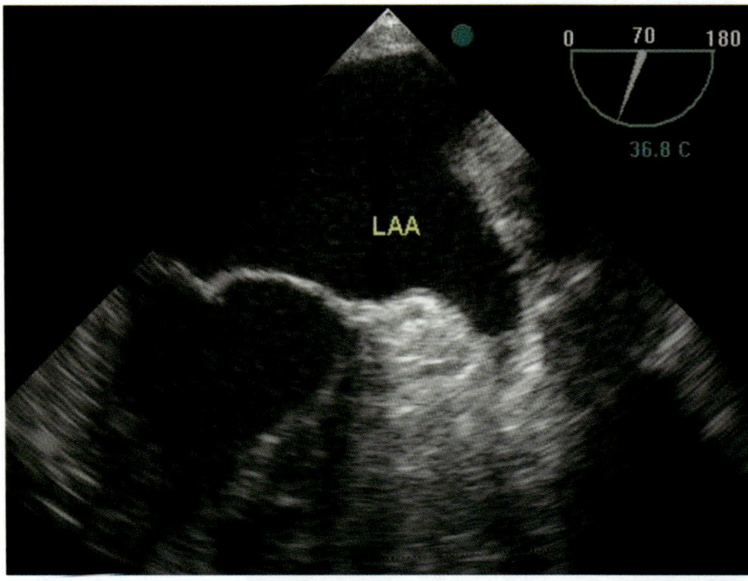

Fig. 11.9 Transesophageal echocardiography, showing a narrow and fingerlike. *LAA* left atrial appendage

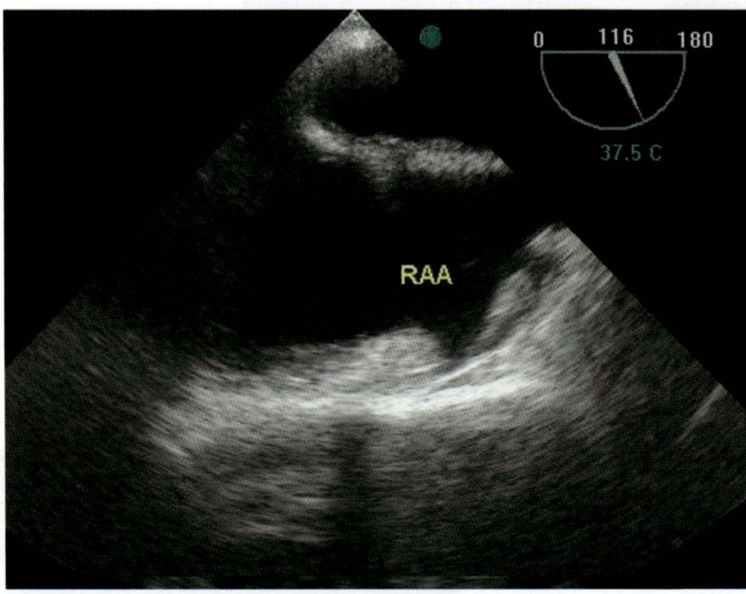

Fig. 11.10 Transesophageal echocardiography, showing a broad-based. *RAA* right atrial appendage

The asymmetric attachment of the two atrioventricular valves has been suggested as the most reliable feature for distinguishing the right ventricle from the left ventricle. If this landmark is unavailable, one can rely on the ventricular myocardial structure.

The tricuspid valve is always attached to the morphologic right ventricle as the mitral valve is attached to the morphologic left ventricle.

The morphologic left ventricle has these four characteristic features: (1) smooth apex and septal surface, (2) basal insertion of the mitral

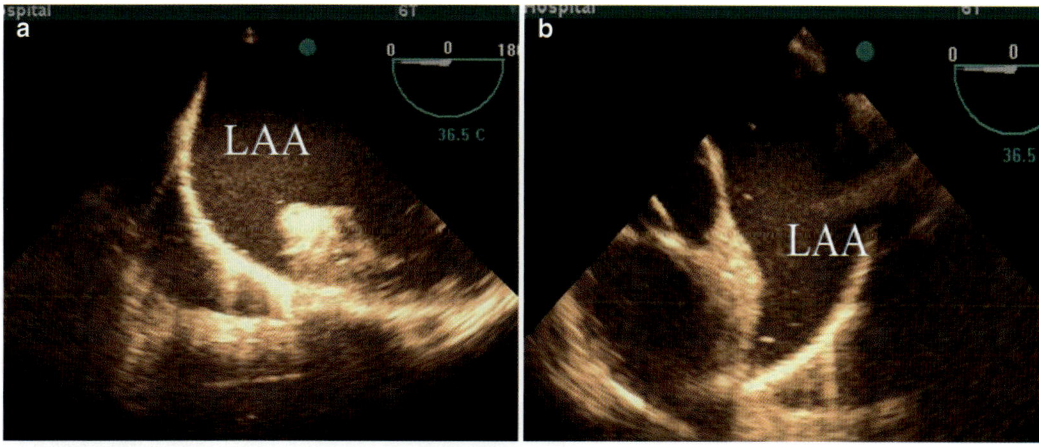

Fig. 11.11 (**a**, **b**) Transesophageal echocardiography, showing left isomerism with bilateral left atria. *LAA* left atrium appendage

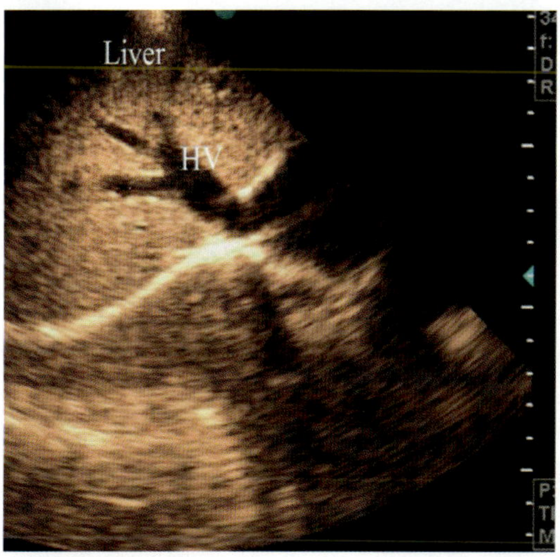

Fig. 11.12 Subcostal view, showing an interrupted inferior vena cava. *HV* hepatic vein

valve without septal attachment, (3) absence of the moderator band, and (4) mitral-aortic fibrous continuity.

Atrioventricular Connection

Once the position of the ventricles is established, the atrioventricular relationship should be determined. The atrioventricular valves connect the atria to the ventricles in either a normal (concordant) or abnormal (discordant) manner (Figs. 11.16 and 11.17).

In the normal biventricular heart with atrioventricular concordance, the morphologic right atrium via the tricuspid valve empties into the morphologic right ventricle and the morphologic left atrium empties into the morphologic left ventricle through the mitral valve. Atrioventricular discordance implies that the morphologic right atrium empties into the morphologic left ventricle and the morphologic left atrium drains into the morphologic right ventricle. When both atria predominantly connect to one ventricle (right or left), the atrioventricular connection is called "a double-inlet" ventricle (Fig. 11.18). For the assessment of atrioventricular and ventriculoarterial connections, the 50 % rule can be applied. An atrium is considered to connect to the ventricle into which greater than 50 % of the valve orifice drains [2, 3, 5, 6].

Ventriculoarterial Connection

Similar to the assessment of the atrioventricular connection, the position of the great arteries and associated valves in relation to the ventricles should be determined. Semilunar valves, which

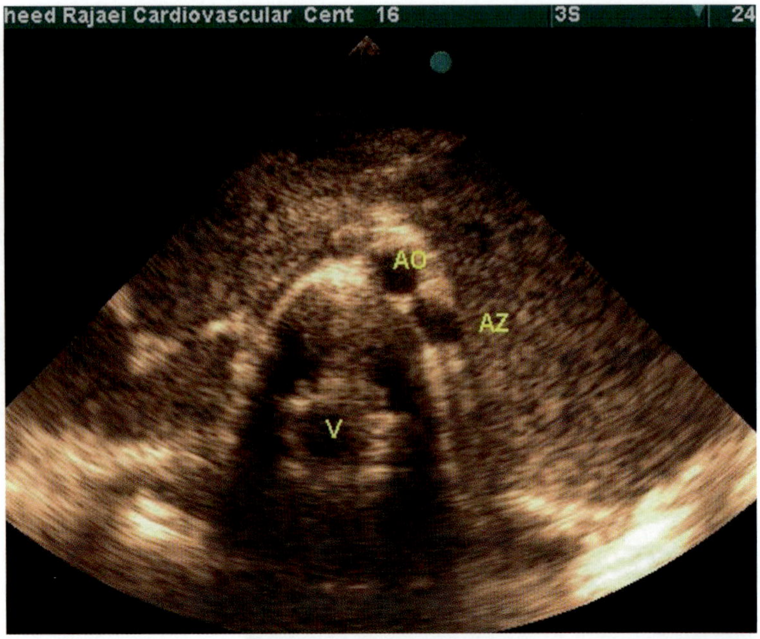

Fig. 11.13 Subcostal view, showing an interrupted inferior vena cava with azygos continuity. *AO* aorta, *AZ* azygos vein, *V* vertebra

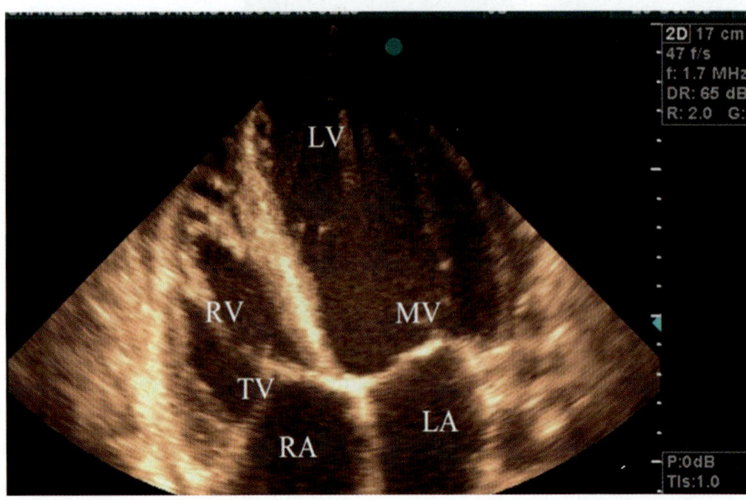

Fig. 11.14 Normal D-loop ventricle: the inflow portion of the morphologic right ventricle lies to the right of the morphologic left ventricle. *LV* left ventricle, *RV* right ventricle, *TV* tricuspid valve, *RA* right atrium, *MV* mitral valve, *LA* left atrium

serve to connect a ventricle to a great artery, encompass the aortic, pulmonary, and truncal valves. Interestingly, the aortic and pulmonary valves are anatomically identical and each of the semilunar valves is determined according to the artery into which it drains. Consequently, the aortic valve is always attached to the aorta and the pulmonic valve is attached to the pulmonary artery. The great arteries can be distinguished simply by their arterial branching. The pulmonary artery has its early branching into the left and right pulmonary arteries. Similarly, the aorta can be distinguished by the branching of its coronary and head and neck vessels. Generally, the position of the aorta is described in relation to the pulmonary artery. In the normal hearts, aorta lies in the right and posterior (Fig. 11.19).

Abnormalities in aortic position are important to assess because each generally occurs in only a limited number of conditions, and once

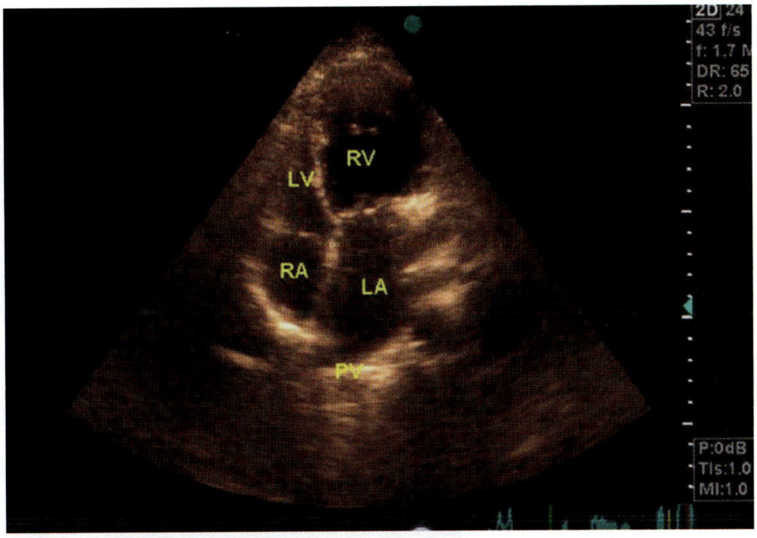

Fig. 11.15 L-loop ventricle, indicating which inflow portion of the morphologic right ventricle lies to the left of the morphologic left ventricle. *LV* left ventricle, *RV* right ventricle, *RA* right atrium, *LA* left atrium, *PV* pulmonary vein

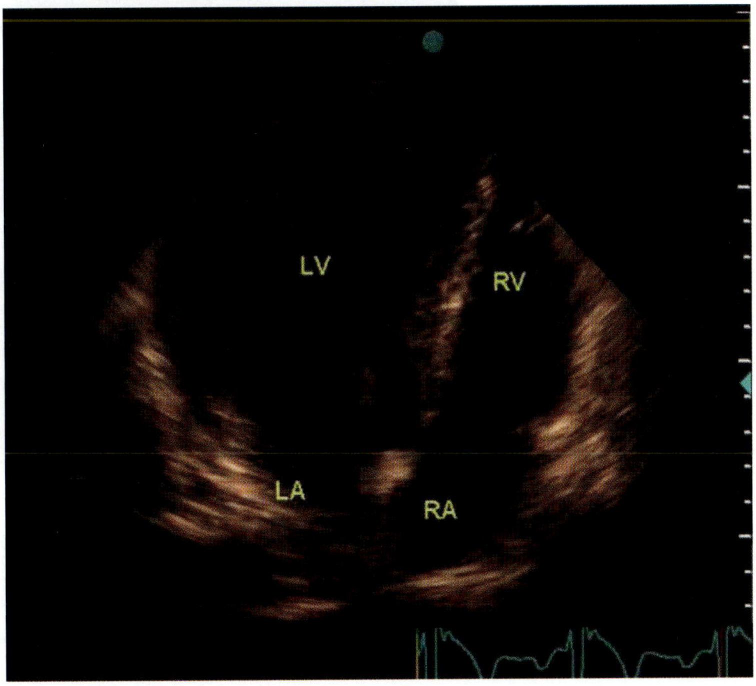

Fig. 11.16 Transthoracic echocardiography in four-chamber view, showing an L-loop ventricle and a concordant atrioventricular connection. *LV* left ventricle, *RV* right ventricle, *RA* right atrium, *LA* left atrium

the position of the semilunar and great arteries is established, the ventriculoarterial relationship should be determined. When the morphologic right ventricle gives rise to the pulmonary artery and the morphologic left ventricle empties into the aorta, there is ventriculoarterial concordance. When the morphologic right ventricle gives rise to the aorta and the morphologic left ventricle drains into the pulmonary artery, there is ventriculoarterial discordance (Fig. 11.20). By applying the 50 % rule, the condition where more than 50 % of both great arteries exit from one ventricle (right or left) is called "a double-outlet" (right or left) ventricle [2–5]. The completion of segmental analysis should be followed by an evaluation of myocardial function, valvular abnormality,

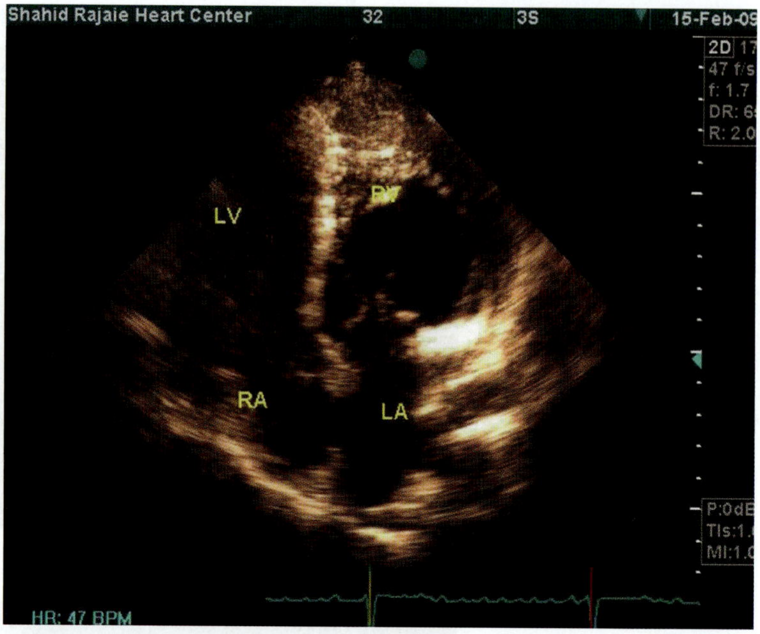

Fig. 11.17 Transthoracic echocardiography in four-chamber view, showing an L-loop ventricle and a discordant atrioventricular connection. *LV* left ventricle, *RV* right ventricle, *RA* right atrium, *LA* left atrium

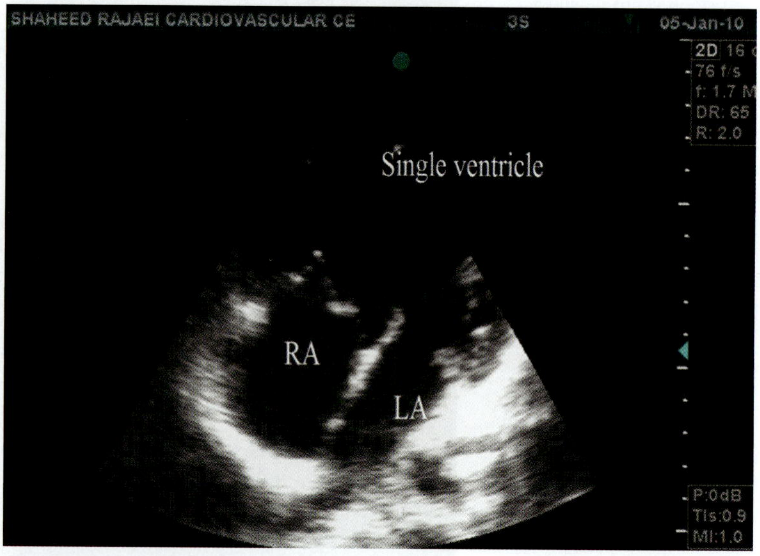

Fig. 11.18 Transthoracic echocardiography in four-chamber view, showing a double-inlet left ventricle (DILV). *RA* right atrium, *LA* left atrium

and lesion-specific approach with overall hemodynamic consequence.

In contrast to acquired heart disease, in the assessment of congenital heart disease, the right ventricle, if not more, is as important as the left ventricle. The comprehensive sequential segmental approach to the diagnosis of congenital heart disease via transthoracic echocardiography affords a noninvasive assessment of the cardiovascular structure and function in adults with congenital heart disease. Because of its widespread availability, user-friendliness, and speed of interpretation, transthoracic echocardiography has remained the technique of choice for the initial diagnosis and follow-up in most adults with congenital heart disease.

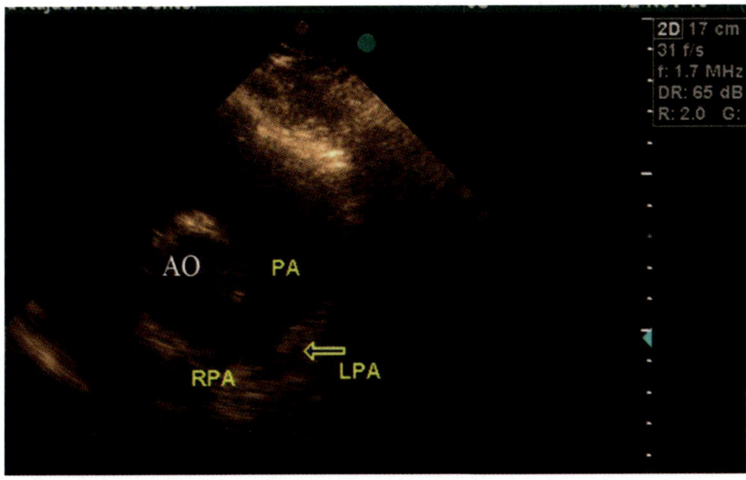

Fig. 11.19 Normally related great arteries: the aorta lies in the right and posterior of the pulmonary artery. *AO* aorta, *PA* pulmonary artery, *RPA* right pulmonary artery, *LPA* left pulmonary artery

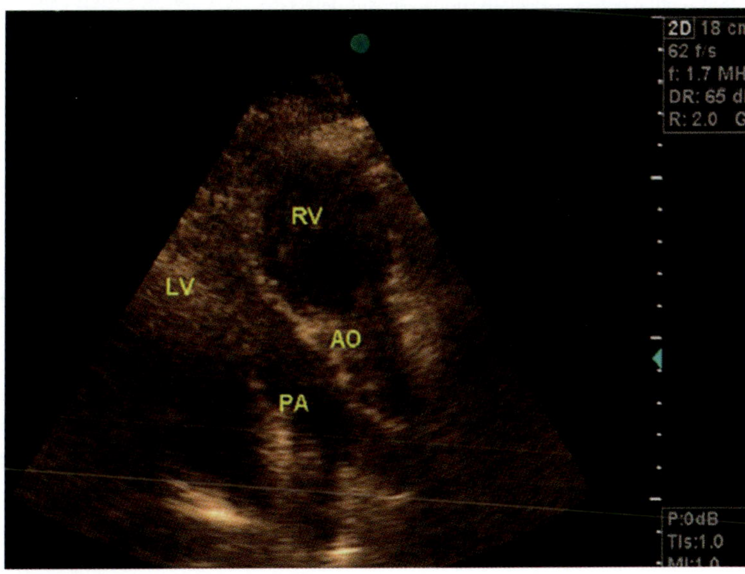

Fig. 11.20 Ventriculoarterial discordant connection: the morphologic right ventricle gives rise to the aorta and the morphologic left ventricle drains into the pulmonary artery. *AO* aorta, *PA* pulmonary artery, *RV* right ventricle, *LV* left ventricle

Shunt Study

Cardiac shunts are best visualized by two-dimensional echocardiography and color flow imaging. The severity of a shunt can be evaluated through the physiological consequences of the shunt and chronic volume overload on the receiving chambers as well as the QP:QS calculation by Doppler study. The stroke volume of the systemic circulations is expressed as QS and the stroke volume of the pulmonary circulation as QP. Shunt severity can be estimated based on the measurement of the stroke volume via Doppler echocardiography (Table 11.1). The stroke volume of the systemic and pulmonary circulation is a product of the time velocity integral of the blood flow through a given cross-sectional area. The sites of measurements are demonstrated in (Table 11.1). It is noteworthy that clinical decisions are not derived from Doppler-based QP:QS shunt study calculation alone. Instead, shunt severity estimation and clinical decision-making should be based on the patient's volume-loaded chamber as well as his symptoms, physical examination, electrocardiogram, and chest radiograph.

Table 11.1 Sites for the Doppler-based measurements of systemic and pulmonary stroke volumes, QP and QS, for the determination of shunt severity

Atrial septal defects
Pulmonary outflow or tricuspid inflow = QP
Aortic outflow or mitral inflow = QS
Ventricular septal defects
Pulmonary outflow or mitral inflow = QP
Aortic outflow or tricuspid inflow = QS
Patent ductus arteriosus
Aortic outflow or mitral inflow = QP
Pulmonary outflow or tricuspid inflow = QS

Table 11.2 Advantages of transesophageal echocardiography over transthoracic echocardiography in adults with congenital heart disease

Atrial septum defect, especially sinus venosus defects and pulmonary veins
Atrial baffle and Fontan circuit
Superior vena caval anatomy and Glenn shunts
Prosthetic valves
Evaluation of mitral valve leaflet morphology and suitability for mitral valve repair
Ventricular outflow tracts
Aorta and aortopulmonary shunts
Before cardioversion
Guiding transcatheter or surgical procedure

It has been suggested that in an isolated and uncomplicated secundum-type atrial septal defect in adults, a jet diameter >1 cm in color Doppler imaging in transesophageal echocardiography is associated with a clinically significant left-to-right shunt and a jet width ≤15 mm is correlated with a QP:QS <2:1 [3, 9, 11, 12].

Transesophageal Echocardiography

Transesophageal echocardiography plays an important role in the evaluation of posterior regions of the heart such as the left atrium, pulmonary veins, interatrial septum, thoracic aorta, ventricular outflow tracts, and valved conduits (Table 11.2).

In adult patients with congenital heart disease, transesophageal echocardiography offers a better two-dimensional resolution in patients with multiple previous cardiac operations and inadequate transthoracic windows.

Transesophageal echocardiography should be considered in the following situations:

1. When transthoracic echocardiography does not provide adequate data or when there is a complex congenital heart anatomy.
2. When we need to monitor therapeutic interventions in the cardiac catheterization laboratory, especially at the time of transcatheter atrial septal defect closure [13–15].
3. When we evaluate the mitral valve leaflet morphology and suitability for mitral valve repair versus replacement [16].
4. When we assess intraoperative and postoperative surgical repair. This imaging modality plays a significant role in the intraoperative assessment of the adequacy of valve repair and congenital cardiac surgery. Furthermore, intraoperative transesophageal echocardiography by an expert echocardiologist is an essential requirement for adult congenital heart disease centers performing adult congenital cardiac surgery [2, 11, 17].
5. When we study infective endocarditis and its related complications, transesophageal echocardiography may be more sensitive and specific than transthoracic echocardiography in adult congenital heart disease patients with possible infective endocarditis [18–22].

Three-Dimensional Echocardiography

One of the momentous developments in the ultrasound imaging of the heart has been the evolution of three-dimensional imaging from slow and offline reconstruction to real-time volumetric imaging. Currently, many echo labs perform full two-dimensional (2D) echocardiographic examinations, followed by focused three-dimensional (3D) echocardiographic studies. The reason for this is that the quality of a two-dimensional image obtained with three-dimensional transthoracic echocardiography probes is inferior to that of dedicated 2D transthoracic echocardiography probes. 3D transesophageal echocardiography affords precise anatomic detail of the atrial septal defect morphology, size, and surrounding rims and thus assists with stretched balloon sizing and device deployment (Fig. 11.21).

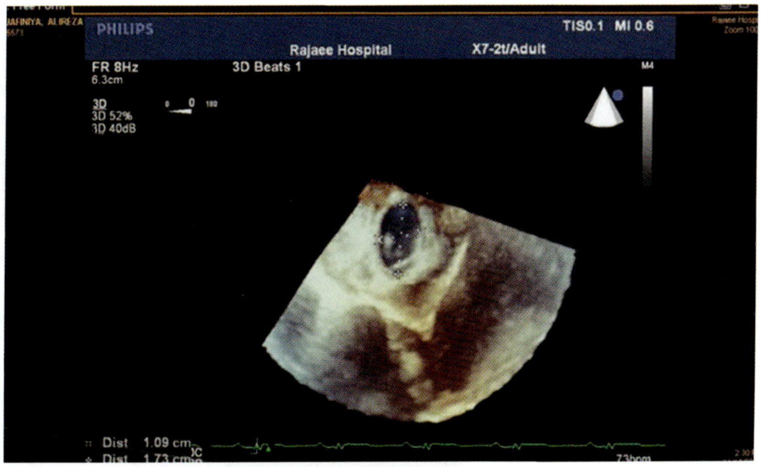

Fig. 11.21 Three-dimensional transesophageal echocardiography, showing precise anatomic detail of an atrial septal defect

The assessment of the RV size and function is not only an issue of great significance but also a very challenging issue in adult patients with congenital heart disease. Given the complexity of the right ventricular anatomy, a precise evaluation of the right ventricular size and function by 2D echocardiography is nearly impossible. The foreshortening of 2D echocardiography can be swiftly remedied via 3D echocardiography-gated wide-angle acquisition inasmuch as it affords a thorough evaluation of RV geometry, volumes, and ejection fraction. The volumetric quantification of the right ventricular volume can be performed by cardiac magnetic resonance imaging, cardiac computed tomography, and real-time three-dimensional echocardiographic images. Cardiac magnetic resonance imaging is deemed the best standard method for the evaluation of the right ventricular size and function; nevertheless, issues concerning claustrophobia, cost, or the presence of pacemakers or defibrillators can render this imaging modality prohibitive.

Several clinical studies have reported a good correlation between cardiac magnetic resonance imaging and 3D echocardiography volumes and ejection fraction of the right ventricle in selected populations, with the majority of these studies demonstrating a slight underestimation of the volumes compared with the reference technique.

Adults with chronic severe pulmonary regurgitation secondary to previous total repair of tetralogy of Fallot or pulmonary valvotomy require regular right ventricular assessment because they are at risk of progressive right ventricular dilation and dysfunction, arrhythmias, and sudden cardiac death unless there is a timely replacement of the pulmonary valve. In a recent study by Sugeng et al. [26], volumetric quantification of the right ventricular volume was performed by cardiac magnetic resonance imaging, cardiac computed tomography, and real-time three-dimensional echocardiography. The measurements obtained with cardiac computed tomography and real-time three-dimensional echocardiography correlated highly with the cardiac magnetic resonance imaging reference (r 0.79–0.89): the cardiac computed tomography measurements showed a slight (4 %) but consistent overestimation and the real-time three-dimensional echocardiography measurements demonstrated a small underestimation.

The advantages of 3D echocardiography (transthoracic and transesophageal) over 2D echocardiography have been suggested in the following situations [23–28]:

1. Assessment of the left ventricular volumes and ejection fraction; 3D echocardiography has been clearly demonstrated to yield more accurate and reproducible measurements.
2. Assessment of the mitral valve pathology should be integrated into routine clinical practice in that three-dimensional

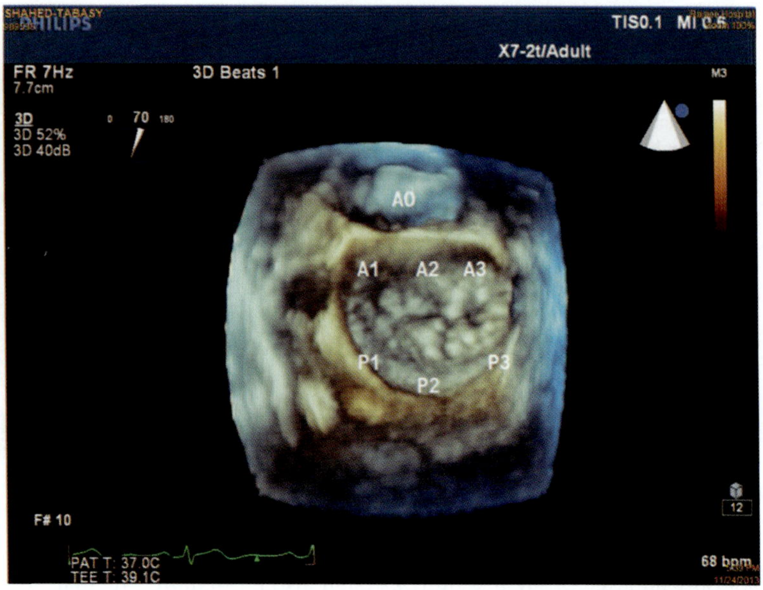

Fig. 11.22 Three-dimensional transesophageal echocardiography, yielding the best morphological information regarding the mitral valve scallops (P2 and P3 scallops prolapse). *Ao* aorta, *A1* anterolateral scallop, *A2* anteromiddle scallop, *A3* anteromedial scallop, *P1* posterolateral scallop, *P2* posteromiddle scallop, *P3* posteromedial scallop

Table 11.3 Indications for three-dimensional echocardiography in clinical practice

	Recommended for clinical practice	Promising clinical studies
Left ventricle functional assessment		
Volume	✓	
Ejection fraction	✓	
Left ventricle functional assessment		
Volume		✓
Ejection fraction		✓
Mitral valve assessment		
Anatomy	✓	
Stenosis	✓	
Guidance of transcatheter procedures[a]	✓	

[a]Mitral clips, mitral valvuloplasty, transcatheter aortic valve implantation, paravalvular leak closure, atrial septal defect closure, ventricular septal defect closure, and left atrial appendage closure

echocardiography affords the best physiological and morphological information regarding the mitral valve (Fig. 11.22).

3. Guidance of interventional mitral valve procedures (three-dimensional transesophageal echocardiography).

It is worthy of note, however, that the three-dimensional evaluation of the tricuspid valve, pulmonic valve, and prosthetic valves has yet to be fully investigated.

Indications for three-dimensional echocardiography in clinical practice are summarized in Table 11.3.

References

1. Bonow RO, Mann DL, Zipes DP, Libby P. (eds.) Braunwald's heart disease: a textbook of cardiovascular medicine. 9th ed. Philadelphia: Saunders Elsevier; 2011.
2. Otto CM. The practice of clinical echocardiography. 3rd ed. Philadelphia: Saunders Elsevier; 2007.
3. Eidem BW, Cetta F, Oleary P. Echocardiography in pediatric and adult congenital heart disease. Philadelphia: Lippincott Williams & Wilkins; 2010.
4. Allen HD, Driscoll DJ, Shaddy RE. Moss and Adams' heart disease in infants, children, and adolescents: including the fetus and young adults. 7th ed. Philadelphia: Lippincott Williams & Wilkins; 2008.
5. Snider AR, Serwer GA, Ritter SB. Echocardiography in pediatric heart disease. 2nd ed. St. Louis: Mosby; 1997.
6. Perloff J, Marelu A. Perloff's clinical recognition of congenital heart disease. 6th ed. Philadelphia: WB Saunders; 2013.
7. Warnes C, Williams RG, Bashore TM, et al. ACC/AHA, guidelines for the management of adults with congenital heart disease. JACC. 2008;52(23):2008.
8. Baumgartner H, Bonhoeffer P, De Groot NM, et al. ESC Committee for Practice Guidelines (CPG). ESC Guidelines for the management of grown-up congenital heart disease (new version 2010). Eur Heart J. 2010;31:2915–57.

9. Perloff JK, Child JS, Aboulhosn J. Congenital heart disease in adults. 3rd ed. Philadelphia: Saunders Elsevier; 2009.
10. Saremi F, Achenbach S, Arbustini E. Revisiting cardiac anatomy, a computed-tomography-based atlas and reference. Chichester: Wiley-Blackwell; 2011.
11. Lewim MB, Stout K. Echocardiography in congenital heart disease. Philadelphia: Saunders/Elsevier; 2012.
12. Oh JK, Seward JB, Tajik AJ, editors. The echo manual. 3rd ed. Philadelphia: Lippincott Williams & Wilkins; 2007.
13. Awad SM, Cao QL, Hijazi ZM. Intracardiac echocardiography for the guidance of percutaneous procedures. Curr Cardiol Rep. 2009;11:210.
14. Suematsu Y, Kiaii B, Bainbridge DT, et al. Robotic-assisted closure of atrial septal defect under real-time three-dimensional echo guide: in vitro study. Eur J Cardiothorac Surg. 2007;32:573.
15. Stephens DN, O'Donnell M, Thomenius K, et al. Experimental studies with a 9F forward-looking intracardiac imaging and ablation catheter. J Ultrasound Med. 2009;28:207.
16. Baharestani B, Sadeghpour A, Ghaffari Nejad MH. The principles of the mitral valve repair associated with echocardiographic evaluation. 1st ed. Iran: Omran publication; 2011.
17. Shanewise S, Cheung A, Aronson S, et al. ASE/SCA guidelines for performing a comprehensive intraoperative multiplane transesophageal echocardiograph examination: Recommendations of the American Society of Echocardiography Council for Intraoperative Echocardiography and the Society of Cardiovascular Anesthesiologists Task Force for Certification in Perioperative Transesophageal Echocardiography. Anesth Analg. 1999;89:870–84.
18. Child JS, Perloff JK, Kubak B. Infective endocarditis: risks and prophylaxis. In: Perloff JK, Child JS, editors. Congenital heart disease in adults. Philadelphia: W.B. Saunders; 1998. p. 129.
19. Bayer AS, Bolger AF, Taubert KA, et al. Diagnosis and management of infective endocarditis and its complications. Circulation. 1998;98:2936–48.
20. Fowler VG, Durack DT. Infective endocarditis. Curr Opin Cardiol. 1994;9:389–400.
21. Horstkotte D, Follath F, Gutschik E, et al. Guidelines on prevention, diagnosis and treatment of infective endocarditis executive summary; the task force on infective endocarditis of the European Society of Cardiology. Eur Heart J. 2004;25:267–76.
22. Krivokapich J, Child JS. Role of transthoracic and transesophageal echocardiography in diagnosis and management of infective endocarditis. Cardiol Clin. 1996;14:363–82.
23. den Ven AE, Robbers-Visser D, Krenning BJ, et al. Real-time transthoracic three-dimensional echocardiographic assessment of left ventricular volume and ejection fraction in congenital heart disease. J Am Soc Echocardiogr. 2006;19:1.
24. Lang RM, et al. EAE/ASE recommendations for image acquisition and display using three-dimensional echocardiography. J Am Soc Echocardiogr. 2012;25:3–46.
25. Grewal J, Majdalany D, Syed I. Three-dimensional ultrasound was comparable with MRI in determining RV size and function in most patients with complex congenital heart disease. J Am Soc Echocardiogr. 2010;23:127–33.
26. Sugeng L, Mor-Avi V, Weinert L, et al. Multimodality comparison of quantitative volumetric analysis of the right ventricle. J Am Coll Cardiol Img. 2010;3:10-8.
27. Schindera ST, Mehwald P, Sahn D, et al. Accuracy of real-time three-dimensional echocardiography for quantifying right ventricular volume static and pulsatile flow studies in an anatomic in vitro model. J Ultrasound Med. 2002;21(10):1069–75.
28. Iriart X, Montaudon M, Lafitte S, et al. Right ventricle three-dimensional echography in corrected tetralogy of fallot: accuracy and variability. Eur J Echocardiogr. 2009;10(6):784–92.

Cardiovascular Magnetic Resonance Imaging in Adult Congenital Heart Disease

12

Majid Kyavar and Anita Sadeghpour

Keywords

Adult congenital heart disease • Cardiovascular magnetic resonance imaging (CMR) • Segmental approach • Atrioventricular connection • Ventriculoarterial connection • Great arteries

Cardiac Imaging Modalities in Adult Congenital Heart Disease

In the past half century, there has been a remarkable improvement in the survival of patients with congenital heart disease (CHD). We are now faced with a growing population of adult patients with a broad spectrum of simple to complex CHD [1–3]. On the other hand, there have been major advances in the field of diagnostic cardiac imaging.

Echocardiography, cardiovascular magnetic resonance imaging (CMR), and cardiac computed tomography (CT) are the basic imaging modalities for the evaluation of patients with CHD, and nuclear cardiac imaging is used in special situations. Of all noninvasive cardiac imaging modalities, cardiac nuclear imaging and cardiac CT have the disadvantage of ionizing radiation exposure [4, 5], not least in patients with multiple follow-up imaging studies. Children and young adults are more sensitive to ionizing radiation than adults [6–8]. Echocardiography remains the basic imaging modality for the initial evaluation, diagnosis, and follow-up of CHD patients, and CMR and cardiac CT play a complementary role [9, 10] and are usually required based on the clinical question. However, in the diagnostic field of cardiac imaging, echocardiography has a limited acoustic window in adult CHD patients, particularly in those with prior cardiac surgery.

Among noninvasive cardiac imaging modalities, CMR has an increasing role in the evaluation of adolescents and adults with CHD [1]. CMR provides an unrestricted access to almost all components of the cardiovascular system; this is a utility often desired in patients with adult CHD, especially in those with complex lesions necessitating thorough assessment of the heart, and arterial/venous great vessels simultaneously. Some of the well-established clinical applications of CMR in adult CHD are presented in Table 12.1.

M. Kyavar, MD, FACC
Cardiovascular Imaging Ward, Department of Cardiology, Adult Congenital Heart Disease Clinic, Rajaie Cardiovascular Medical and Research Center, Iran University of Medical Science, Tehran, Iran
e-mail: kiavar0049@gmail.com, kiavar@rhc.ac.ir

A. Sadeghpour, MD, FACC, FASE (✉)
Echocardiography Lab, Department of Cardiology, Adult Congenital Heart Disease Clinic, Rajaie Cardiovascular Medical and Research Center, Iran University of Medical Science, Tehran, Iran
e-mail: anita.sadeghpour@gmail.com, asadeghpour@rhc.ac.ir

A. Sadeghpour et al. (eds.), *Comprehensive Approach to Adult Congenital Heart Disease*,
DOI 10.1007/978-1-4471-6383-1_12, © Springer-Verlag London 2014

Table 12.1 Clinical application of cardiovascular magnetic resonance imaging in adult congenital heart disease

Anatomic delineation of cardiac and extracardiac anomalies before and after surgery
Quantification of biventricular function and mass
Assessment of coronary arteries [magnetic resonance angiography (MRA)]
Measurement of systemic and pulmonary blood flow
Quantification of valvular regurgitation
Detection and quantification of myocardial ischemia and fibrosis
Assessment of myocardial viability
Tissue characterization (such as fibrosis, fat, and iron)

CMR offers a number of advantages over other cardiac imaging modalities such as echocardiography, CT, and invasive catheterization. Most notably, CMR is a noninvasive technique which provides not only angiographic (magnetic resonance angiography) and anatomical delineation of the cardiovascular system and extracardiac structures but also functional assessment of both ventricles and flow measurements. Furthermore, CMR evaluates myocardial viability, which is a feature that cannot be achieved by CT. CMR is also able to measure ventricular volumes, ejection fraction, and relative distribution of the blood flow in the lungs [4, 5, 11, 12].

The absence of ionizing radiation and the use of iodinated contrast are important considerations in children and young adults with CHD. Children are more susceptible to the potentially harmful effects of these agents because of higher cell proliferation and increased lifetime risk per unit dose. In addition, the need for sequential studies in CHD patients gradually builds up irradiation exposure [4, 6–8].

CMR is also superior to echocardiographic examination in patients with CHD. This superiority is highlighted in adolescents and adults, whose more complex anatomy and scar tissue which resulted from previous palliative or reparative surgeries, interposition of the lungs, and the higher distance of the heart from the chest wall render the penetration of echocardiography ultrasound waves to all cardiac structures somewhat limited. Moreover, CMR is less operator dependent than echocardiography, although a thorough understanding of the anatomic and functional principles of CHD is a prerequisite to a reliable imaging study. The other advantage of CMR over transthoracic echocardiography is that whereas echocardiography can only visualize structures accessible through echocardiographic windows, CMR with its three-dimensional contiguous data sets affords a complete depiction of the heart and extracardiac anatomy such as the venoatrial and ventriculoarterial connections [4, 5, 11, 12].

The clinical utility of CMR is highly dependent on the age of the patient. Infants and children are less cooperative and as such require sedation [13]. Thus, CMR is usually performed as a second method and as an adjunct to transthoracic echocardiography in infants and young children. In contrast, CMR has become the first imaging technique of choice in adolescents and adults, in those with more complex anatomy, or in postoperative patients irrespective of their age on the grounds that surgery sequels make their echocardiographic examination more difficult.

Echocardiography is preferable in the detection of patent foramen ovale, structural abnormalities of the valve leaflets, small and mobile masses such as vegetations in infective endocarditis, and estimation of gradient and pulmonary artery pressure.

CMR prior to diagnostic catheterization can minimize the duration and potential risks of diagnostic catheterization and even its necessity. A precise depiction of the cardiac and great-vessel anatomy using CMR should decrease the duration of catheterization and the radiation dose, which is associated with more efficient diagnosis and more interventional procedures during a single anesthesia session. As a result, CMR makes diagnostic catheterization and simultaneous interventional procedures more likely to become a one-stage process.

Given all the advantages and disadvantages of CMR reported thus far in the literature (Table 12.2) [11, 12, 14, 15], CMR is highly recommended in centers specialized in the care of patients with adult CHD. CMR in adult CHD patients should be interpreted by expert specialists with long-term collaboration with level 2 or level 3 adult CHD specialists and cardiac surgeons involved in management of these patients [3, 11].

Table 12.2 Advantages and disadvantages of cardiovascular magnetic resonance imaging (CMR) in adult congenital heart disease (CHD)

CMR advantages	CMR disadvantages
It is safe insofar as it does not require ionizing radiation and iodinated contrast	There is a possibility of claustrophobia (albeit seen in only a small percentage of patients)
It is applicable in pregnant women with CHD (usually without contrast agent)	It is relatively expensive and its interpretation needs expertise
It is free of acoustic window, with unrestricted access to almost all the components of the cardiovascular system	It is not portable and is unable to provide real-time imaging during open heart surgery (although interventional CMR is under investigation)
It offers comprehensive anatomic, functional, and hemodynamic assessment	It has relative contraindications in the presence of pacemakers, internal defibrillators, or cerebral aneurysm clips (based on the type of these devices)
It is the method of choice for the quantification of the ventricular size and function with good reproducibility	Sedation is usually needed in infants and uncooperative children

Table 12.3 When we recommend cardiovascular magnetic resonance imaging (CMR) as an adjunct to echocardiography

In patients with suboptimal echocardiographic images and inadequate data
In patients with borderline echocardiographic measurements when these values are important for clinical decision-making
For further evaluation of the pulmonary and systemic veins (connection and obstruction)
For quantification of the ventricular volume, mass, and function (e.g., quantification of the right ventricular volume in patients with repaired tetralogy of Fallot)
For quantification of valve regurgitation (pulmonary regurgitation) and shunt severity
For evaluation of the major aortopulmonary collaterals
For better evaluation of the conduit between the right ventricular outflow tract to pulmonary artery and the stenosis in the pulmonary artery branches (Echocardiography is superior for pulmonary artery pressure and gradient measurement.)
For better evaluation of the aorta in coarctation, Marfan syndrome, and aneurysm
In coronary artery anomalies and assessment of myocardial fibrosis and viability
For evaluation of the intra- and extracardiac masses

Clinical Application of Cardiovascular Magnetic Resonance Imaging in Adult Congenital Heart Disease

Indubitably, echocardiography constitutes the bedrock of noninvasive cardiovascular imaging modalities in patients with adult CHD. However, the selection of the best imaging technique for an adult CHD patient requires a thorough understanding of the strengths and weaknesses of the available modalities [4, 11]. Based on the European Society of Cardiology (ESC) publication, CMR is recommended in grown-up congenital heart disease (GUCH) patients in the following specific situations (Table 12.3):

Basic Principles of CMR in ACHD [11, 12, 14]

When assessing the patient with CHD, the following points should be considered:

Many patients with ACHD will benefit from one baseline CMR study as a reference point for future study and detecting unexpected abnormalities.

Generally, the patients with CHD are followed by echocardiography but serial CMR may be needed in some patients. The 3-year intervals have been suggested in most of these patients except for rare cases who may need earlier studies.

In the first-time CMR study, the exam should be monitored by the CMR physician as the proto-

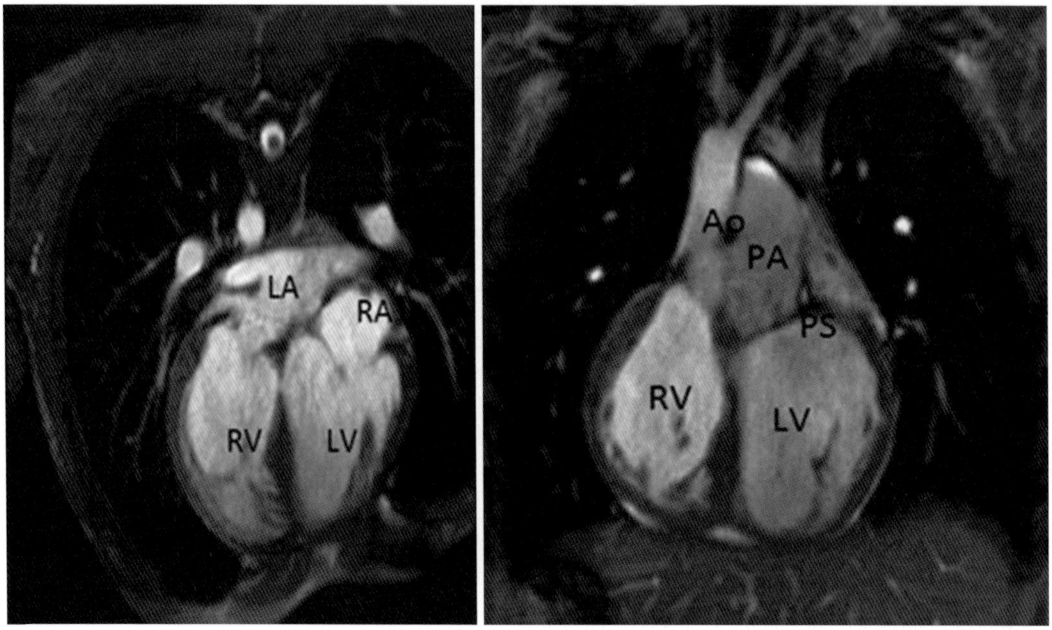

Fig. 12.1 *Patient with dextrocardia,* atrioventricular and ventriculoarterial *discordance suggestive of inverse congenitally corrected TGA. LA* left atrium, *RA* right atrium, *RV* right ventricle, *LV* left ventricle, *Ao* aorta, *PA* pulmonary artery, *PS* pulmonary stenosis

col may be needed to change based on the unexpected findings.

Most of the research in ACHD patients has been done with CMR 1.5 T. The superiority of CMR 3T needs to be confirmed.

In patients with CHD a comprehensive CMR study with a transaxial thin slice contiguous stacks for a complete coverage of mediastinal, cardiac, and upper abdomen is recommended. The CMR study will delineate the anomalous vessels, abdominal situs (including asplenia and polysplenia), cardiac location, atrial situs, ventricular and great arteries looping, atrioventricular and ventriculoarterial connections and positions (Figs. 12.1–12.3), and intracardiac and extracardiac shunts (Fig. 12.4).

In all CHD CMR study protocol, magnetic resonance angiography should be a part of the protocol.

CMR is the reference imaging modality for quantitative measurements of ventricular size and function with excellent LV assessment reproducibility and challenging RV measurements

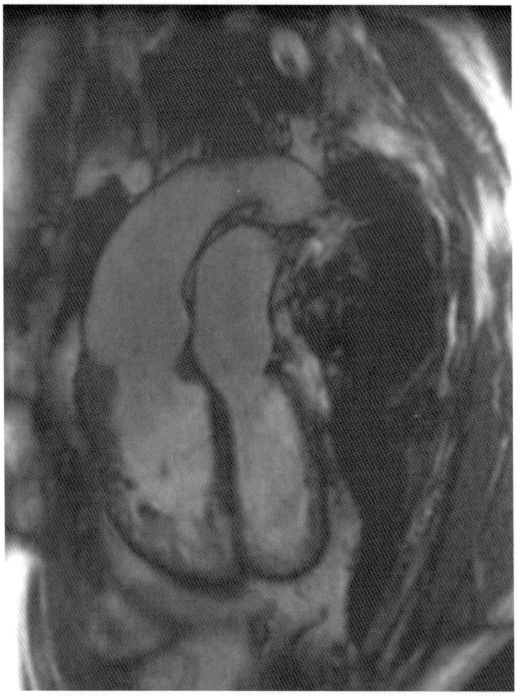

Fig. 12.2 Showing D-TGA with D-loop ventricle with hypertrophied RV which serve as a systemic subaortic ventricle and associated arterioventricular discordance

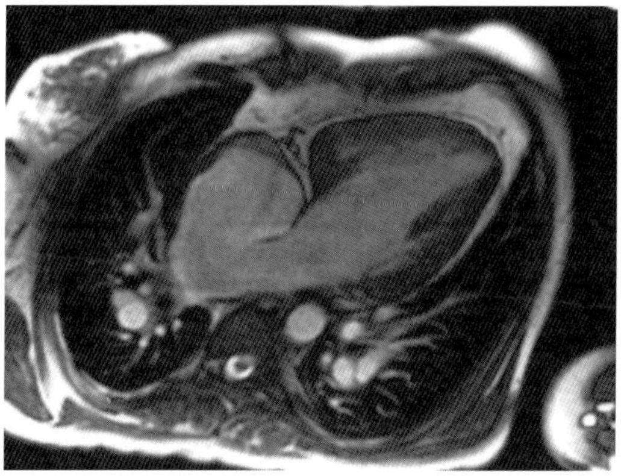

Fig. 12.3 Illustrating patient with levocardia and tricuspid atresia

[16–20]. RV assessment by CMR has a major role in clinical decision-making in patients with repaired tetralogy of Fallot and severe pulmonary regurgitation.

In the Following Specific CHD, CMR Has a Specific Role in Diagnosis, Clinical Decision-Making, and Follow Up [4, 5, 11, 12]

- Repaired tetralogy of Fallot
- Double-chambered right ventricle
- Major aortopulmonary collateral arteries
- Congenitally corrected transposition of the great arteries
- Fontan operations for functionally single ventricle
- Marfan syndrome and other connective tissue disorders
- Aortic coarctation
- Coronary artery anomalies
- Pulmonary hypertension
- Shunts: atrial septal defect, ventricular septal defect, or patent ductus arteriosus

Conclusion

CMR offers a number of advantages over other cardiac imaging modalities in patients with congenital heart disease. CMR allows comprehensive assessment of mediastinal and abdominal anatomy, ventricular size and function, valve regurgitation, shunt quantification tissue characterization, and viability.

CMR is particularly valuable in the evaluation and follow-up of the adult patients after repairs of tetralogy of Fallot, coarctation of aorta, and transposition of the great arteries and patients with history of Fontan operations.

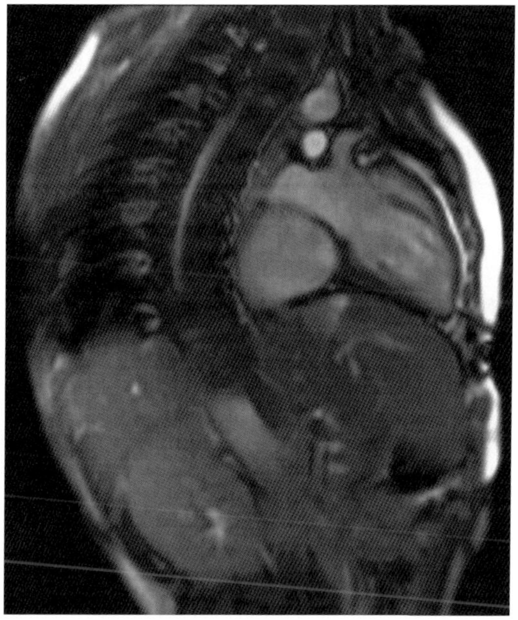

Fig. 12.4 Stagnant flow in the lateral tunnel of a patient with a past history of Fontan procedure

References

1. Warnes CA, Liberthson R, Danielson GK, et al. Task Force 1: the changing profile of congenital heart disease in adult life. J Am Coll Cardiol. 2001;37:1170–5.
2. Williams R, Pearson G, Barst R, et al. Report of the National Heart, Lung and Blood Institute Working Group on research in adult congenital heart disease. J Am Coll Cardiol. 2006;47:701–7.
3. Warnes C, Williams R, Bashore T, et al. ACC/AHA 2008 guidelines for the management of adults with congenital heart disease: a report of the American College of Cardiology/American Heart Association Task Force on Practice Guidelines. J Am Coll Cardiol. 2008;52(23):e143–263. doi:10.1016/j.jacc.2008.10.001.
4. Prakash A, Powell AJ, Geva T. Multimodality noninvasive imaging for assessment of congenital heart disease. Circ Cardiovasc Imaging. 2010;3:112–25.

5. Baumgartner H, Bonhoeffer P, De Groot NM, et al. ESC Guidelines for the management of grown-up congenital heart disease (new version 2010). Eur Heart J. 2010;31(23):2915–57.
6. Brenner DJ, Hall EJ. Computed tomography: an increasing source of radiation exposure. N Engl J Med. 2007;357:2277–84.
7. Brenner DJ, Doll R, Goodhead DT, et al. Cancer risks attributable to low doses of ionizing radiation: assessing what we really know. Proc Natl Acad Sci U S A. 2003;100:13761–6.
8. Coles DR, Smail MA, Negus IS. Comparison of radiation doses from multislice computed tomography coronary angiography and conventional diagnostic angiography. J Am Coll Cardiol. 2006;47:1840–5.
9. Tworetzky W, McElhinney DB, Brook MM, et al. Echocardiographic diagnosis alone for the complete repair of major congenital heart defects. J Am Coll Cardiol. 1999;33:228–33.
10. Dorfman AL, Levine JC, Colan SD, et al. Accuracy of echocardiography in low birth weight infants with congenital heart disease. Pediatrics. 2005;115:102–7.
11. Kilner PJ, Geva T, Kaemmerer H, et al. Recommendations for cardiovascular magnetic resonance in adults with congenital heart disease from the respective working groups of the European Society of Cardiology. Eur Heart J. 2010;31:794–805.
12. Gatzoulis M, Webb GD, Daubeney PEF. Diagnosis and management of adult congenital heart disease. 2nd ed. Philadelphia: Saunders/Elsevier; 2011.
13. Napoli KL, Ingall CG, Martin GR. Safety and efficacy of chloral hydrate sedation in children undergoing echocardiography. J Pediatr. 1996;129:287–91.
14. Plein S, Greenwood JP, Ridgway JP. Cardiovascular MR manual. London/New York: Springer; 2011.
15. Bellenger NG, Marcus NJ, Rajappan K, et al. Comparison of techniques for the measurement of left ventricular function following cardiac transplantation. J Cardiovasc Magn Reson. 2002;4:255–63.
16. Karamitsos T, Hudsmith L, Selvanayagama J, et al. Operator induced variability in left ventricular measurements with cardiovascular magnetic resonance is improved after training. J Cardiovasc Magn Reson. 2007;9:777–83.
17. Mooij CF, de Wit CJ, Graham DA, et al. Reproducibility of MRI measurements of right ventricular size and function in patients with normal and dilated ventricles. J Magn Reson Imaging. 2008;28:67–73.
18. Grothues F, Smith GC, Moon JC, et al. Comparison of interstudy reproducibility of cardiovascular magnetic resonance with two-dimensional echocardiography in normal subjects and in patients with heart failure or left ventricular hypertrophy. Am J Cardiol. 2002;90:29–34.
19. Van den Bosch AE, Robbers-Visser D, Krenning BJ, et al. Comparison of real-time three-dimensional echocardiography to magnetic resonance imaging for assessment of left ventricular mass. Am J Cardiol. 2006;97:113–7.
20. Mannaerts HF, Van Der Heide JA, Kamp O, et al. Quantification of left ventricular volumes and ejection fraction using freehand transthoracic three-dimensional echocardiography: comparison with magnetic resonance imaging. J Am Soc Echocardiogr. 2003;16:101–9.

Basic Principles in Cardiovascular Computed Tomography Imaging with Comprehensive Evaluation of Adult Congenital Heart Disease by Computed Tomography Imaging

13

Majid Kyavar and Anita Sadeghpour

Keywords
Congenital heart disease • Computed tomography • Cardiovascular imaging • Anatomy • Sequential segmental analysis

Computed Tomography in Congenital Heart Disease

Cardiac anatomy is the first important step in understanding congenital heart disease (CHD). In this chapter we will discuss about cardiac chambers, great arteries, and also cardiac anomalies.

Atria

The atrium is a thin-walled structure consisting of the atrium and the atrial auricle. Defining features of the morphologic right atrium (RA) and left atrium (LA) are based on their venous connections and their auricles and pectinate muscle morphology [1]. The suprahepatic portion of the inferior vena cava (IVC) connection to RA allows its definite identification.

Two atria are placed side by side on the base of the ventricles, and they are separated by the interatrial septum. The pectinate muscle is present in the atrial appendage, and its extent is the accurate anatomic determinant for atrial situs and thoracic situs: situs solitus, situs inversus, right isomerism, and left isomerism. The right atrial appendage is triangular and oriented anteriorly and superiorly, whereas the left atrial appendage is toe shaped and directed laterally (Fig. 13.1).

The normal superior vena cava (SVC) inserts into the right-sided morphologic right atrium, whereas the IVC inserts into the medial, posterior, and inferior portion of the right atrium. The hepatic veins communicate with the IVC. A left SVC may be present with or without a crossing brachiocephalic vein that connects to a right SVC. It is important to determine whether the left SVC empties into a coronary sinus that then drains to the RA or whether it empties directly into the LA.

These alterations include left SVC to an unroofed coronary sinus, and bilateral SVC, with the left SVC draining into the coronary sinus. We should remember that SVC is not an

M. Kyavar, MD, FACC
Cardiovascular Imaging Ward, Department of Cardiology, Adult Congenital Heart Disease Clinic, Rajaie Cardiovascular Medical and Research Center, Iran University of Medical Science, Tehran, Iran
e-mail: kiavar0049@gmail.com, kiavar@rhc.ac.ir

A. Sadeghpour, MD, FACC, FASE (✉)
Echocardiography Lab, Department of Cardiology, Adult Congenital Heart Disease Clinic, Rajaie Cardiovascular Medical and Research Center, Iran University of Medical Science, Tehran, Iran
e-mail: anita.sadeghpour@gmail.com, asadeghpour@rhc.ac.ir

A. Sadeghpour et al. (eds.), *Comprehensive Approach to Adult Congenital Heart Disease*, DOI 10.1007/978-1-4471-6383-1_13, © Springer-Verlag London 2014

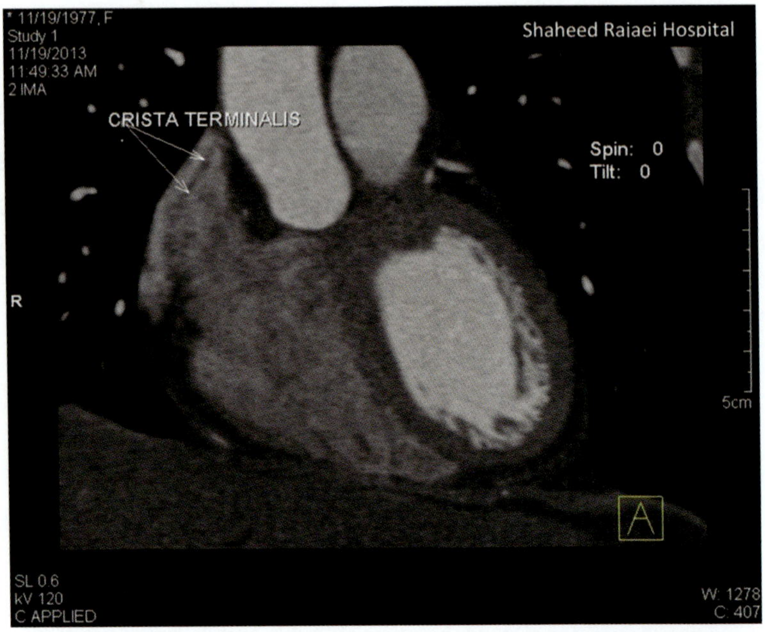

Fig. 13.1 Pectinate muscles in the right atrial appendage arise from crista terminalis

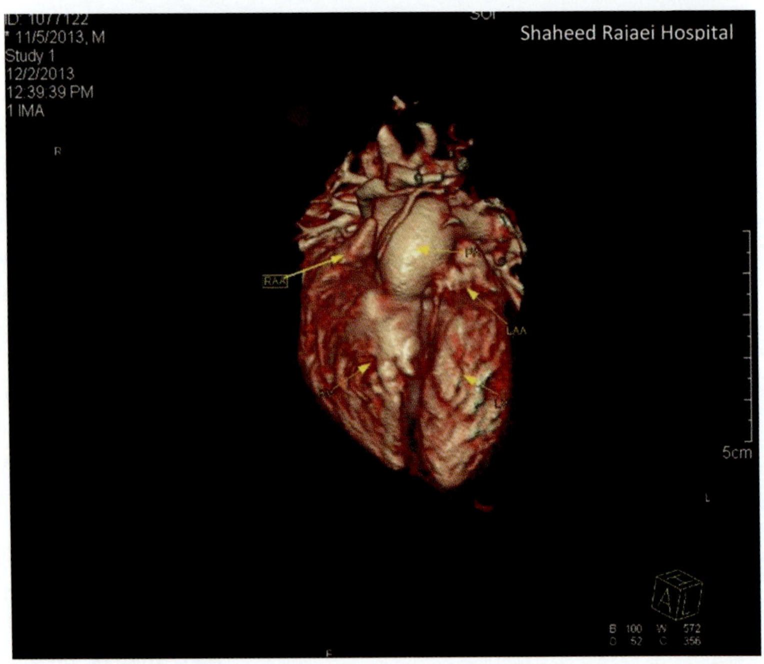

Fig. 13.2 The right atrial appendage has a broader opening and a triangular configuration. In addition, the pectinate muscles in the right atrial appendage reach the tricuspid valve annulus (*arrows*). The pulmonary valve is located anterior and left to the aortic valve. *PA* pulmonary artery, *RAA* right atrial appendix, *LAA* left atrial appendix, *LV* left ventricle, *RV* right ventricle

accurate criterion to the identification of morphologic right atrium. The pectinate muscles in the RA auricle extend to the tricuspid valve annulus. In the right atrial appendage, the comb-like pectinate muscles arise from the crista terminalis (Figs. 13.2, 13.3 and 13.4).

The morphologic LA is specified by a toe-shaped auricle and four pulmonary veins connecting to the morphologic LA. Pulmonary veins that drain anomalously should be identified—one, some, or all of the pulmonary veins may drain to the IVC, hepatic vein, SVC, or brachiocephalic vein. Total anomalous pulmonary venous connection occurs if all pulmonary veins drain abnormally together either through a common venous chamber or through mixed different locations. The most common association of a right upper or lower partial anomalous pulmonary vein

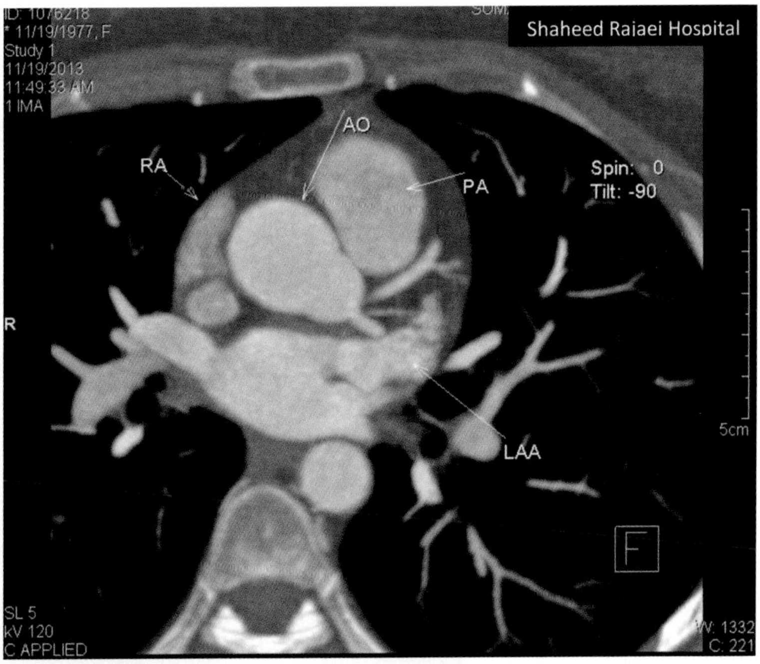

Fig. 13.3 Left atrium with toe-shaped auricle and four related veins. *PA* pulmonary artery, *LAA* left atrial appendix, *RA* right atrium, *AO* aorta

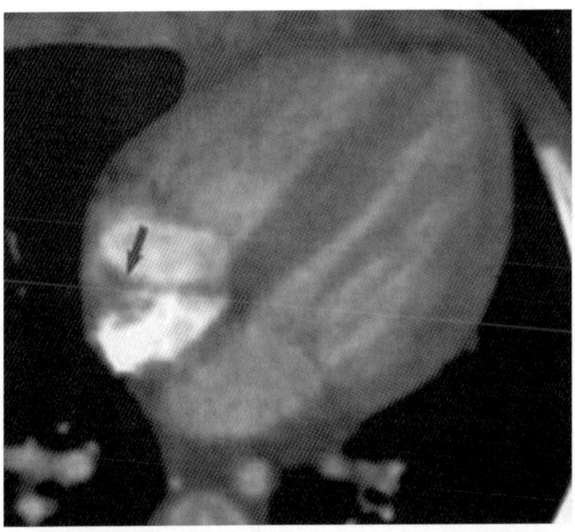

Fig. 13.4 Hypodense structure adjacent to the junction of the inferior vena cava and the right atrium that is the normal Chiari network (*arrow*)

on the right vein is the presence of a sinus venosus-type atrial septal defect (ASD) (Fig. 13.5).

Ventricles

Two ventricles are located side by side under the base of the atria, and they are separated by the atrioventricular septum and the interventricular septum. The apex of the heart is the most inferior external part of the heart that is normally formed by both ventricles and is normally on the left side of the thorax; the apex of the heart may be directed to the middle (mesocardia) or the right (dextrocardia) of the thorax. The right ventricle (RV) has three components:

1. The inlet
2. The apex
3. The outlet

Three prominent muscular bands divide the RV: the parietal, the septal, and the moderator band. The parietal band and the infundibular septum make up the crista supraventricularis, which separates the sinus and the conus regions. The tricuspid and pulmonary valves represent inlet and outlet portions, respectively. The moderator band is one of the determinant of morphologic RV.

Morphologic characteristics of the right ventricle include heavy trabeculations, coarse septal surface, moderator band, and the infundibulum (the crista supraventricularis); the infundibulum is identified as a muscular tissue that separates the atrioventricular valve from the semilunar valve and creates tricuspid-pulmonary discontinuity, and the septal attachment of the tricuspid valve is more apical than the mitral valve [2] (Figs. 13.6 and 13.7).

The anterior mitral valve leaflet forms part of the left ventricular (LV) outflow tract with

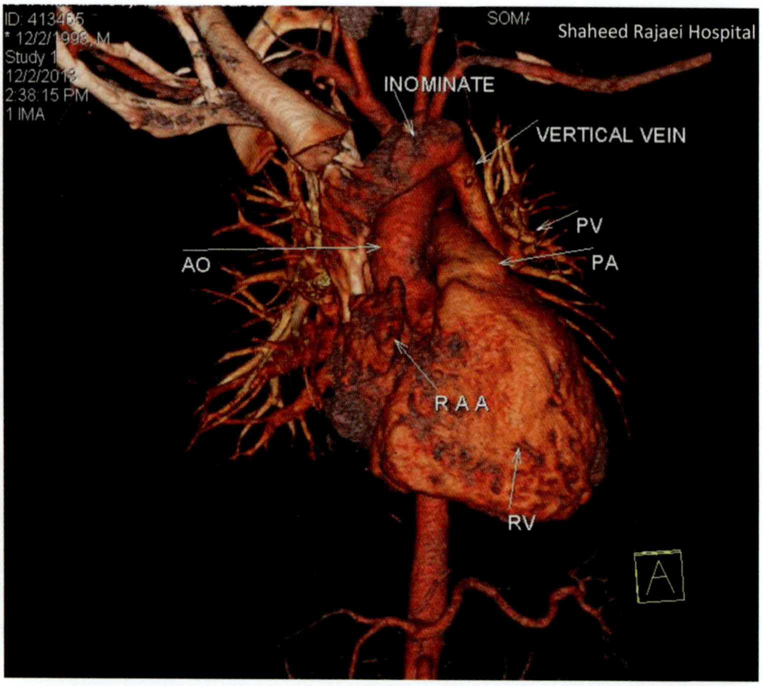

Fig. 13.5 Partial anomalous pulmonary veins drain into the innominate vein by vertical vein. *PA* pulmonary artery, *PV* pulmonary vein, *RV* right ventricle, *RAA* right atrial appendix, *AO* aorta

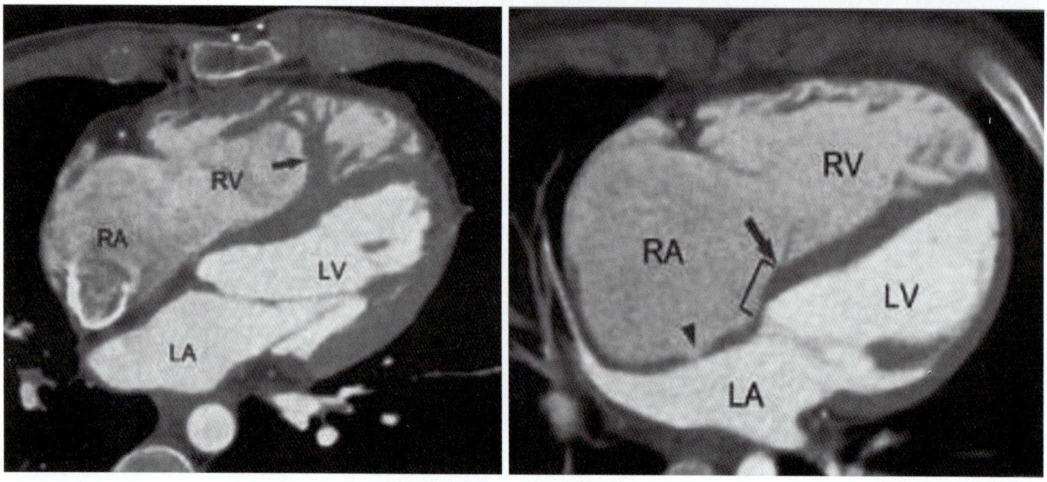

Fig. 13.6 The right ventricle has three, e.g., the anterior, posterior, and medial, papillary muscles for the tricuspid valve, while the left ventricle has two, e.g., the anterolateral and posteromedial, papillary muscles for the mitral valve. Some call the tricuspid valve as a septophilic valve, whereas the mitral valve is a septophobic valve. We should remember that neither the shape nor the degree of trabeculation is a reliable character of ventricular identification, because these markers are altered by pressor and volume load. *LA* left atrium, *RA* right atrium, *LV* left ventricle, *RV* right ventricle

marked thinning of the left ventricular myocardium at the apex. The left ventricle is morphologically specified by smooth trabeculations, smooth septal surface, and aortomitral fibrous continuity; septal attachment of the mitral valve of the LV is more cephalad than RV.

The atrioventricular valve is designated according to the ventricle morphology (e.g., the tricuspid valve for the morphologic RV, the mitral valve for the morphologic left ventricle). This means that atrioventricular valves follow the ventricle, rather than the atrium. The three leaflets of the tricuspid valve are named for their anatomic location: septal, anterosuperior, and inferior (posterior). Normal apical displacement of the tricuspid valve is characteristic.

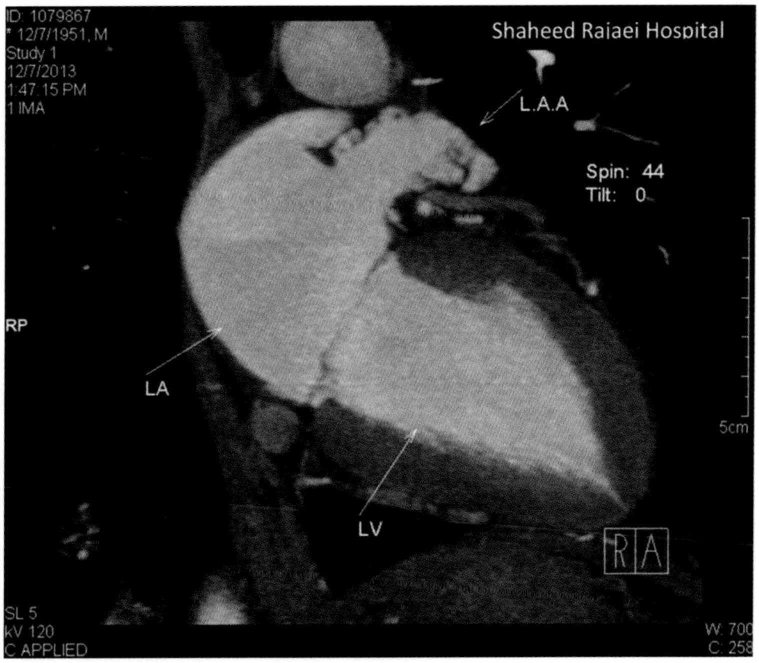

Fig. 13.7 LV and left atrium and left atrial auricle with apical thinning. *LA* left atrium, *LAA* left atrial appendix, *LV* left ventricle

The pulmonary infundibulum (conus) is a cone-shaped muscular structure that supports the leaflets of the pulmonary valve. Crista supraventricular separates the tricuspid and pulmonary valves. This is in contrast to what is seen in the LV where the aortic and mitral valves are in fibrous continuity. The apical trabecular component of the LV extends to the apex. It is characterized by fine trabeculations where the myocardium is surprisingly thin. The trabeculations of the LV including its septal wall are quite fine compared with those of the RV; this is the most useful characteristic in diagnosis of ventricular morphology in congenital heart disease. The two papillary muscles are termed posteromedial and anterolateral; arising from the posterior and lateral walls at midventricular level, the circumflex coronary artery and the coronary sinus run close to the posterior mitral annuls.

Great Arteries

The aorta gives branches to the body as well as the coronary arteries. Intercoronary segment of the aortic valve lies posterior and to the right of the pulmonary valve (Figs. 13.8 and 13.9).

Sequential Segmental Analysis

The heart can be considered in three segments: the atrial chambers, the ventricular mass, and the great arteries. By assessing the location of the component parts of the heart and their relationship, each case is described in a sequential manner. This approach was introduced by Van Praagh over 40 years ago [3, 4]. This approach is clinically useful and applicable to all imaging modality of congenital heart disease. This logical approach is determined by six steps:

(Step1) Visceroatrial situs
(Step 2) Ventricular loop
(Step 3) Great arterial spatial relationship
(Step 4) Atrioventricular and ventriculoatrial relationship
(Step 5) Cardiac position
(Step 6) Associated malformation

Our cardiac computed tomographic angiography study will follow these steps. All cardiac CT examinations were performed with a dual-source 256-slice CT scanner. The maximum dose of radiation was 2–3 mSv.

The first step of any segmental approach to the diagnosis of CHD is to establish the situs of the heart, namely, the atrial situs and the venous drainage.

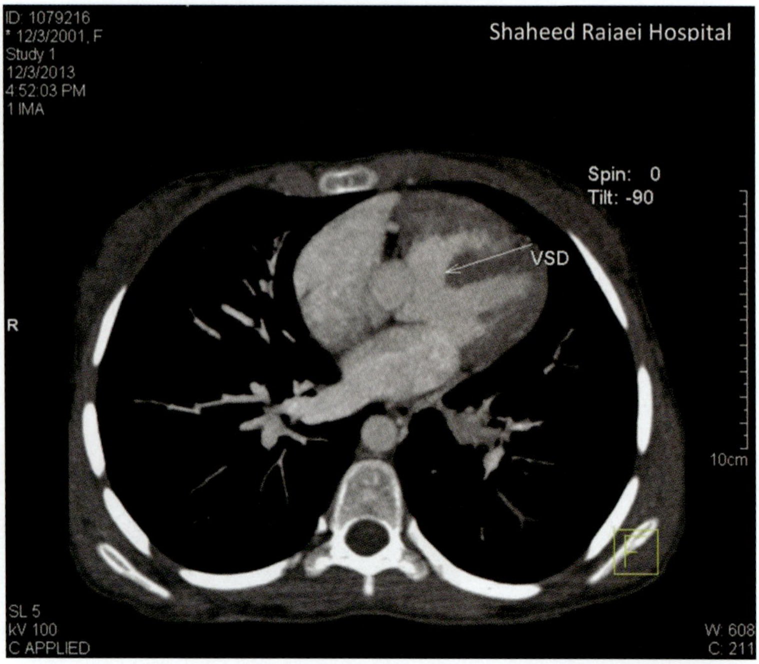

Fig. 13.8 A 12-year-old boy with subaortic VSD and atretic pulmonary artery with dilated aorta

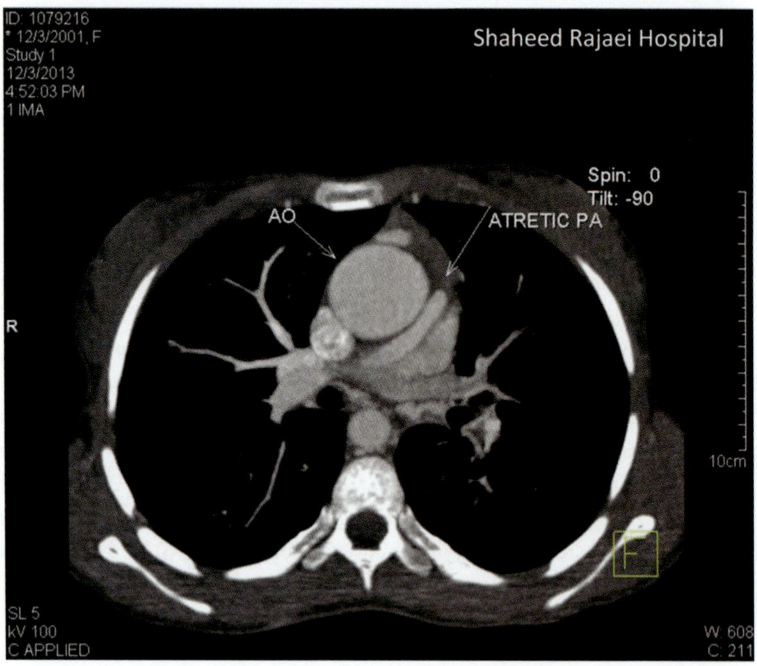

Fig. 13.9 Atretic pulmonary artery with dilated aorta. AO aorta

Situs Solitus

The morphologically right atrium is on the right side and the morphologically left atrium in the left side. The lungs and bronchi are concordant with such position, with a trilobed lung with short bronchus on the right side and bilobed lung and related long bronchus on the left side. The systemic veins (superior and inferior venae cavae) drain into the right atrium and the pulmonary veins into the left atrium [2].

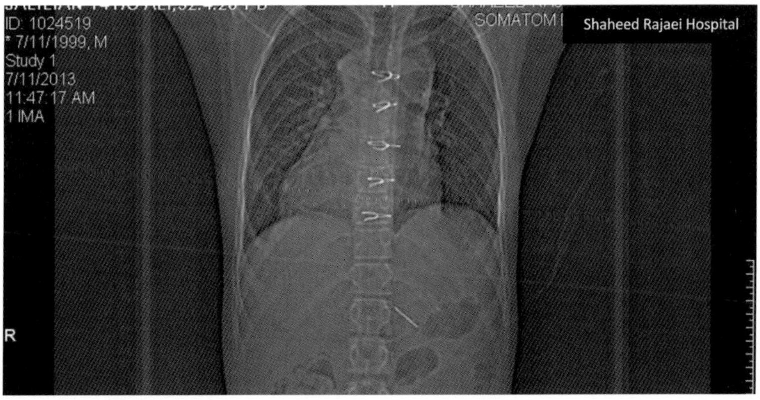

Fig. 13.10 Bilateral hyparterial bronchi with bilateral bilobed lungs in a 14-year-old boy with right Glenn shunt

Visceral situs solitus is characterized by the presence of a right-sided liver, left-sided spleen, and three-lobed right lung, and two-lobed left lung. The left bronchus is hyparterial and the right is eparterial.

Situs Inversus

With the reversed position of the atria and lungs, situs inversus is morphologically right on the left side and morphologically left on the right side.

In Situs Ambiguous

Both atria and lungs may exhibit right or left atrio-pulmonary isomerism [5]. This visceral symmetry is related to asplenia and polysplenia syndromes [6–13], with heterotaxia of subdiaphragmatic organs. Both atria and lungs may show right or left atrio-pulmonary isomerism. The key point is that the atrial situs almost always follows the thoracic and visceral situs, and bronchial morphology is a reliable predictor of atrial situs. A morphologic right bronchus is short and straight with early branching, whereas a morphologic left bronchus is relatively long and curved.

Polysplenia Syndrome Type of Heterotaxy

Polysplenia syndrome type of heterotaxy is characterized by polysplenia; anomalous pulmonary venous drainage, most often is partial; bilateral superior vena cava (SVC); left isomerism of the atrial appendages; bilateral hyparterial bronchi with bilateral bilobed lungs; and azygous continuation of the IVC. The hepatic to renal segment of IVC is absent (Fig. 13.10).

Asplenia Syndrome Type of Heterotaxy

Right isomerism of the atrial appendages consists of a bilateral SVC, bilateral right-sided bronchial branching, and anomalous pulmonary venous connections with complex congenital heart disease. Asplenia includes bilateral three-lobed lungs with transverse or symmetric liver. The spleen is absent.

The third type of heterotaxy syndrome was introduced by Van Praagh manifested by a single right-sided spleen with levocardia [3]. CT or MRI is required for evaluating the status of the liver and spleen.

Ventricular Loop

If morphologic RV lies to the right and anterior of the morphologic LV, it is called d loop. If morphologic RV lies to the left and anterior of morphologic LV, it is called L loop [14].

Great Arterial Spatial Relationship

Normally, aortic annulus is posterior and to the right of the pulmonary artery. In situs inversus the aorta lies posterior and to the left of pulmonary valve. Any position of the aortopulmonary valve other than solitus or inversus is called malposition. In transposition of the great arteries, there is a discordant relation between the great arteries and ventricles.

Complete Transposition of the Great Vessels/Atrioventricular Concordance and Ventriculoarterial Discordance

In this anomaly, the pulmonary artery arises from the left ventricle, and the aorta arises from the right ventricle; however, the ventricles are in their normal position [15]. Therefore, the pulmonary and systemic circulations are in two separate circulations. So usually in a VSD or an ASD, PDA must be present for oxygenated blood to reach the systemic circulation. This condition is sometimes called "d-complete transposition" to distinguish it from corrected transposition or "L-transposition" since the aorta is usually anterior and to the right of the pulmonary artery [16].

Congenitally Corrected Transposition of the Great Arteries

When the morphologic ventricles are on the opposite side of the heart (L loop) but the atria are in the appropriate location (normal atrial situs) and the great vessels connect with the appropriate side of the heart (the inappropriate morphologic ventricles), it is called AV and ventriculoarterial discordance.

Double Outlet Right Ventricle (DORV)

When both great arteries arise primarily from one ventricle, it is called as double outlet ventricle. In double outlet right ventricle (DORV), both great arteries originate principally from the right ventricle, and the semilunar valves commonly have bilateral conus [17, 18].

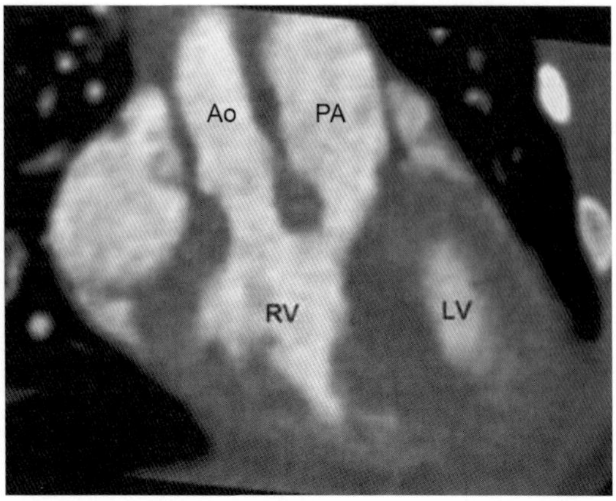

Fig. 13.11 DORV: both great arteries originate principally from the right ventricle, and the semilunar valves commonly have bilateral conus. *AO* aorta, *PA* pulmonary artery, *LV* left ventricle, *RV* right ventricle

A 50 % rule, in which more than a half of each great artery arises from the corresponding ventricle, should be used for this ventriculoarterial connection [19] (Fig. 13.11).

Malposition

The relationships of the great arteries are a wide spectrum. They are typically divided into three categories: normal, d-malposition, and l-malposition. In normal relationship, the pulmonary trunk is anterior and left to the ascending aorta. In contrast, the ascending aorta is anterior to the pulmonary trunk in malposition of the great arteries, either on the right (d-malposition, typical of complete TGA) or on the left (l-malposition, typical of congenitally corrected TGA). In malposition there is a concordant arterio-ventricular relationship.

Some Interesting Cases' Pictures (Figs. 13.12, 13.13, 13.14, 13.15 and 13.16)

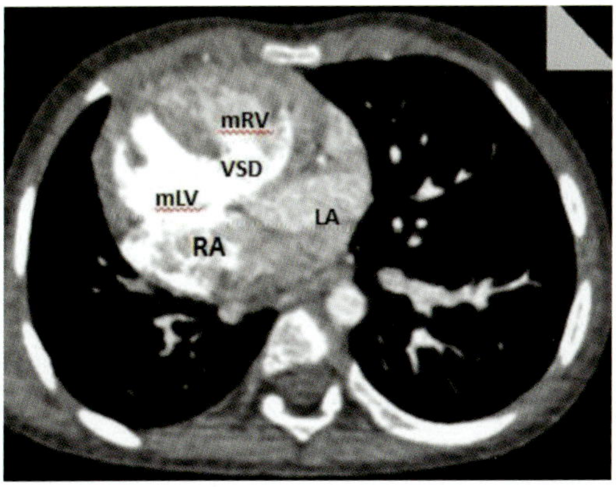

Fig. 13.12 Dextrocardia with morphologic trabeculated RV (*mRV*) located anteriorly and left-sided and morphologic LV (*mLV*) with atrioventricular discordance and large VSD. *LA* left atrium, *RA* right atrium

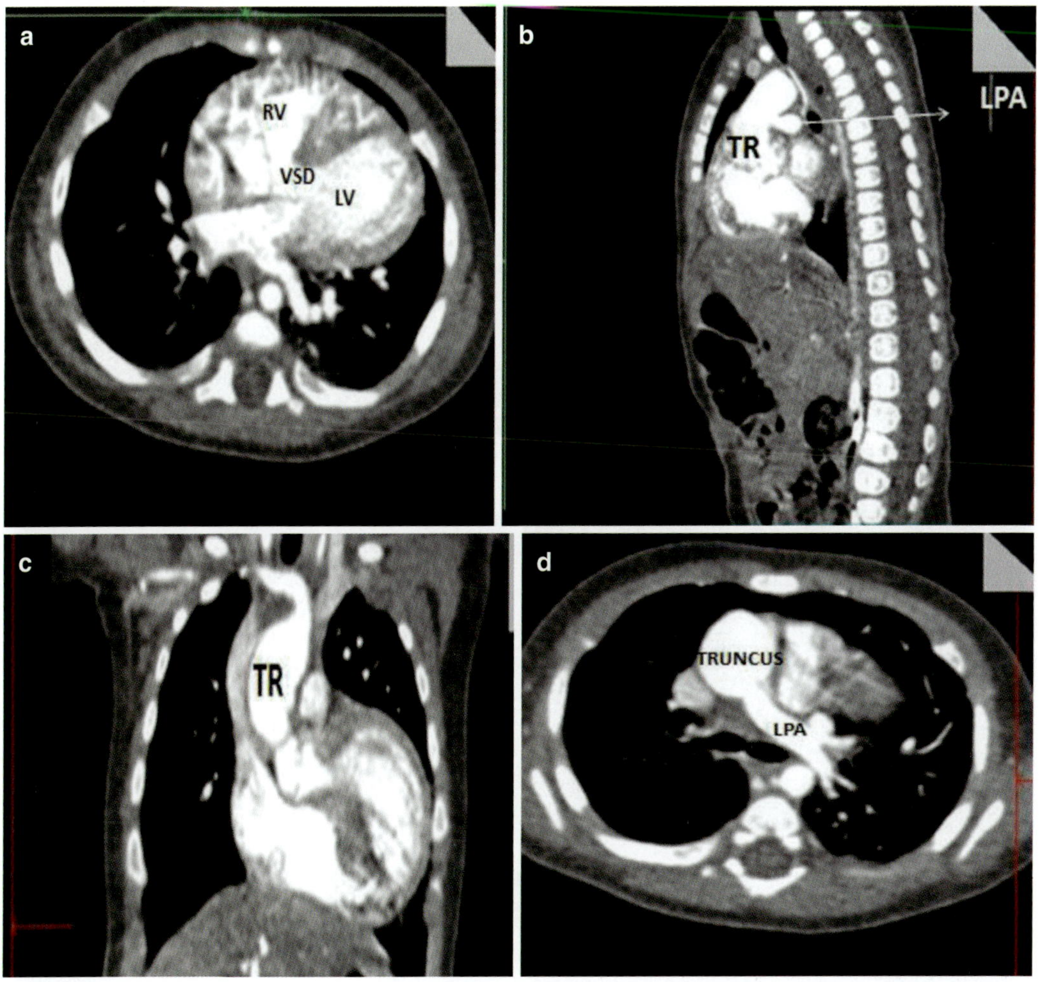

Fig. 13.13 (**a–d**) A case of truncus arteriosus, sub-truncus *VSD*; left pulmonary originates from truncus. *LPA* left pulmonary artery, *LV* left ventricle, *RV* right ventricle, *TR* truncus arteriosus, *VSD* ventricular septal defect

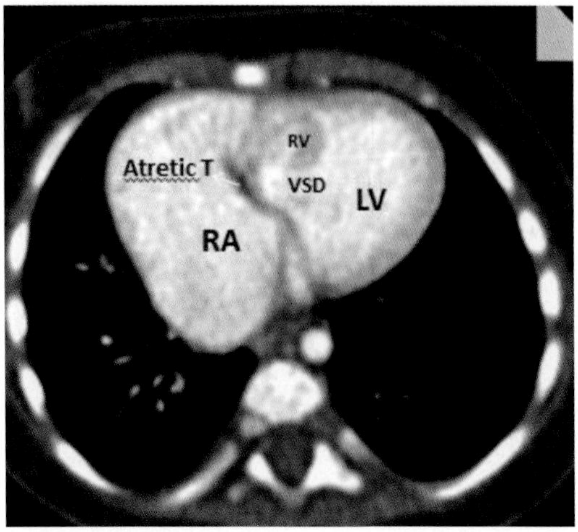

Fig. 13.14 A case of tricuspid atresia with diminutive RV. *LV* left ventricle, *RV* right ventricle, *RA* right atrium, *VSD* ventricular septal defect

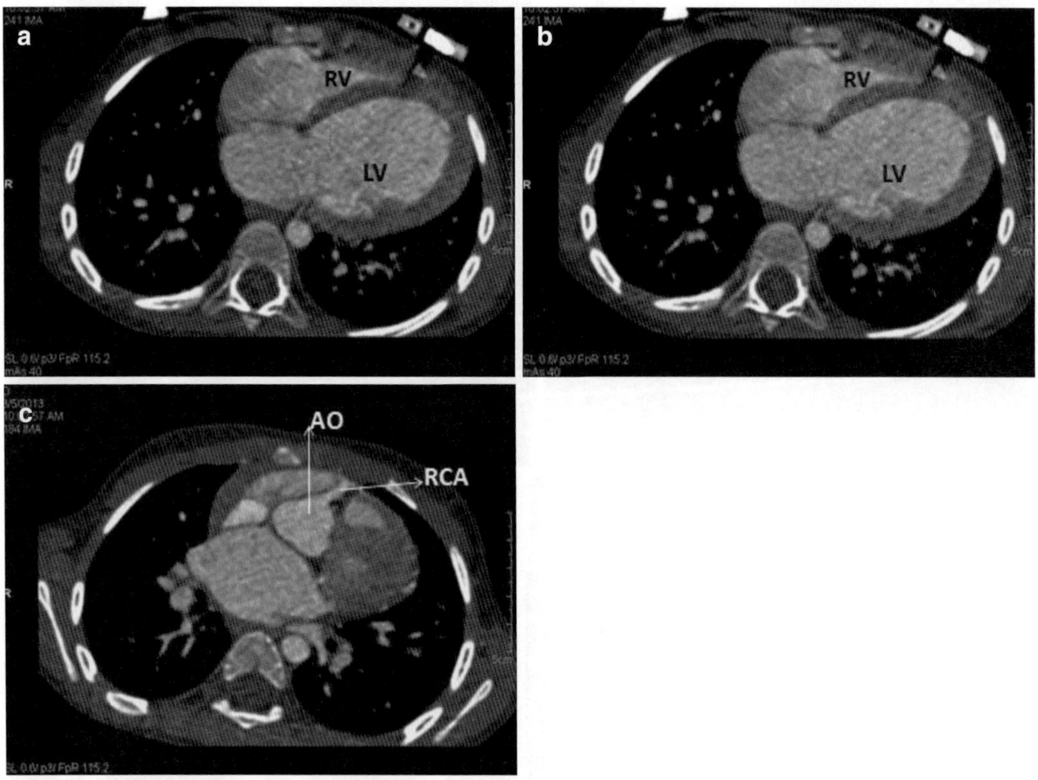

Fig. 13.15 (**a–c**) A case of ALCAPA (anomalous origin of LM from pulmonary artery). *LV* left ventricle, *RV* right ventricle, *AO* aorta, *RCA* right coronary artery

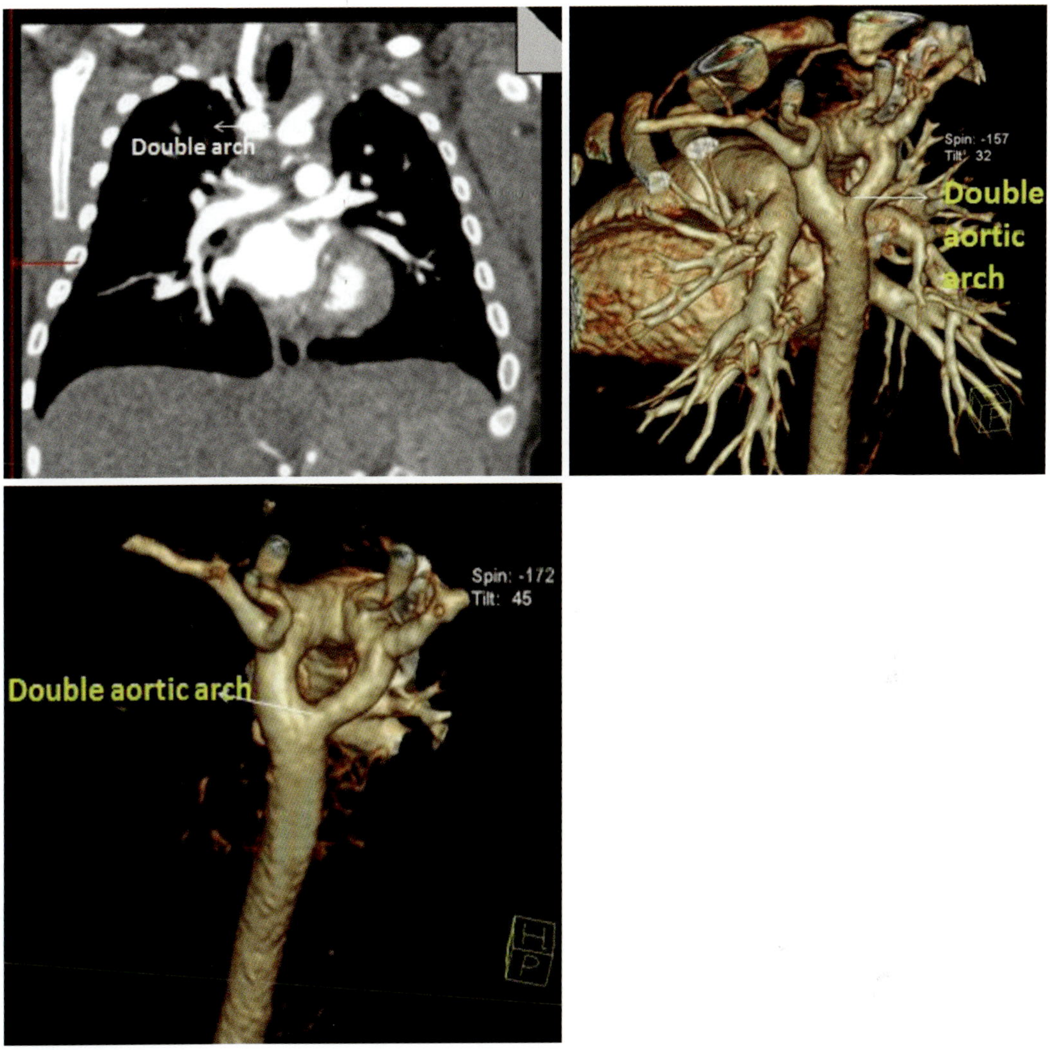

Fig. 13.16 A case of double aortic arch

References

1. Anderson RH, Brown NA. The anatomy of the heart revisited. Anat Rec. 1996;246:1–7.
2. Wilcox BR, Cook AC, Anderson RH. Surgical anatomy of the heart. Cambridge: Cambridge University Press. 2004. p. 11–82.
3. Van Praagh R. Terminology of congenital heart disease. Glossary and commentary. Circulation. 1977;56: 139–43.
4. Van Praagh R. The segmental approach to diagnosis in congenital heart disease. Birth Defects: Original Article Series 1972;8:4.
5. Van Mierop LHS, Gessner IH, Schiebler GL. Asplenia and polysplenia syndrome. Birth Defects: Original Article Series 1972;8:74.
6. Cotran RS, Kumar V, Robbins SL. Robbins pathologic basis of disease. 4th ed. Philadelphia: WB Saunders Co; 1989. p. 777.
7. Fraser RS, Muller NL, Colman NC, Pare PD. Fraser and Pare's diagnosis of diseases of the chest, vol. 3. 4th ed. Philadelphia: WB Saunders Co; 1999. p. 2281–3.
8. Gutgesell HP. Cardiac malposition and heterotaxy. In: Garson Jr AG, Fisher DJ, Neish SR, editors. Science and practice of pediatric cardiology, vol. 2. 2nd ed. Baltimore: Williams & Wilkins; 1998. p. 1539–61.
9. Hagler DJ, O'Leary PW. Cardiac malpositions and abnormalities of atrial and visceral situs. In: Emmanouilides GC, Riemenschneider TA, Allen HD, Gutgesell HP, editors. Moss and Adams' heart disease in infants, children, and adolescents: including the fetus and young adult, vol. 2. 5th ed. Baltimore: Williams & Wilkins; 1995. p. 1307–36.

10. Higgins CB. Essentials of cardiac radiology and imaging. Philadelphia: JB Lippincott Co; 1992. p. 283–331.
11. Jefferson K, Rees S. Clinical cardiac radiology. 2nd ed. London: Butterworths; 1980. p. 9–67.
12. Perloff JK. Clinical recognition of congenital heart disease. 4th ed. Philadelphia: WB Saunders Co; 1994.
13. Stanger P, Rudolph AM, Edwards JE. Cardiac malpositions: an overview based on study of 65 necropsy specimens. Circulation. 1977;56:159.
14. Van Praagh R, Ongley PA, Swan HJC. Anatomic types of single or common ventricle in man. Am J Cardiol. 1964;13:367.
15. Kirklin JW, Pacifico AD, Bargeron LM, Soto B. Cardiac repair in anatomically corrected malposition of the great arteries. Circulation. 1973;48:153.
16. Anderson RH, Ho HY, Becker AE. Anatomy of the human atrioventricular junctions revisited. Anat Rec. 2000;260:81–91.
17. Taussig HB, Bing RJ. Complete transposition of aorta and levoposition of pulmonary artery. Am Heart J. 1949;37:551.
18. Van Praagh R. What is the Taussig-Bing malformation? Circulation. 1966;38:445.
19. Anderson RH. Clinical anatomy of the aortic root. Heart. 2002;84:670–3.

Electrocardiography and Cardiac Arrhythmias in Adult Congenital Heart Disease

14

Abolfath Alizadeh Diz and Azin Alizadehasl

Keywords
Electrocardiography • Cardiac arrhythmias • Adult congenital Heart disease • Atrial fibrillation • Atrial flutter

Introduction

Arrhythmias make difficult the care of many adults with congenital heart disease (CHD). They are one of the leading causes of morbidity and also mortality in these patients. Their incidence and the trouble of management have made arrhythmia a reason of interest for physicians that are working in this area. In the USA, it is evaluated that there are about one million CHD patients, up to 20 % with severe disease, who need surgical intervention. The predisposing factors for arrhythmia in these patients may include aging, congenitally abnormal or displaced conduction system, abnormal hemodynamics, mechanical strain, hypoxia-induced stress, and residual or postoperative sequels. Indeed, the substrate of arrhythmia in adults with CHD is very complex. All arrhythmias that are prevalent in the normal population may also happen in CHD, and some other specific types are detected, for example, Wolff-Parkinson-White syndrome in Ebstein anomaly.

We, therefore, present the scope of the problem; clinical aspect of tachyarrhythmia and bradyarrhythmias, outlining therapeutic choices; conduction system abnormalities in CHD that are related with disease of the sinus node; and also AV conduction system. Also arrhythmias in common types of CHD are consequently discussed.

Congenital heart disease (CHD) is the most common type of birth lesion, with 1–2 % of moderate or severe forms [1, 2]. The spectrum of clinical consequences of arrhythmias in adult patients with CHD ranges from occult arrhythmia to sudden cardiac death. Recurrent or persistent arrhythmia may cause hemodynamic deterioration gradually, causing a vicious cycle of clinical decompensation. Thromboembolic events are also related to tachyarrhythmia [3]. Repeated hospitalization and the management of antiarrhythmic devices and also drugs create an important burden on quality of living. Cardiac arrhythmias in most patients with corrected surgery represent an acquired condition related to surgical scars and/or abnormal workload on the myocardium. In some patients, arrhythmias are related to the presence of intrinsic structural abnormalities, as is the case of accessory pathways in Ebstein anomaly.

The incidence of arrhythmias usually increases as the CHD patient ages. Really, by adulthood, arrhythmias are the main reason of morbidity and

A. Alizadeh Diz, MD
A. Alizadehasl, MD, FACC (✉)
Electrophysiology Lab, Department of Cardiology, Rajaie Cardiovascular Medical and Research Center, Iran University of Medical Science, Tehran, Iran
e-mail: alizadeasl@gmail.com, alizadeasl@rhc.ac.ir

A. Sadeghpour et al. (eds.), *Comprehensive Approach to Adult Congenital Heart Disease*,
DOI 10.1007/978-1-4471-6383-1_14, © Springer-Verlag London 2014

frequent hospital admissions, and sudden cardiac death with arrhythmic etiology is the most common source of mortality [4, 5].

The predisposing factors for arrhythmia in these patients may include aging, congenitally abnormal or displaced conduction system, abnormal hemodynamics, mechanical strain, hypoxia-induced stress, and residual or postoperative sequels. Indeed, the substrate of arrhythmia in adults with CHD is very complex [5, 6].

Physiopathological and Clinical Aspect

Bradyarrhythmias

Bradyarrhythmias may occur after sinus node dysfunction and/or block at the level of the atrioventricular (AV) node or His-Purkinje system.

Sinus Node Anatomical Location

Most patients with CHD have a normally placed sinus node in the epicardium at the junction of the superior vena cava (SVC) and right atrium (RA). Exceptions include:

1. Left juxtaposition of the atrial appendages
2. Situs inversus
3. Heterotaxy syndromes: RA isomerism (asplenia syndrome) or left atrial (LA) isomerism (polysplenia syndrome)

Sinus Node Dysfunction

Surgical procedures are the main causes of sick sinus syndrome in adult patients with CHD. The sinus node dysfunction occurs after the Mustard, Senning, and Fontan procedures. Patients with LA isomerism may also have congenital malformations in the sinus node independent of the special effects of their surgical techniques; in these patients sinus nodes are absent or hypoplastic and/or displaced posteroinferiorly. The patients with RA isomerism frequently have bilateral sinus nodes. The pacemaker may shift from one to the other. Paroxysmal atrial tachyarrhythmias and loss of sinus rhythm increase the risk of sudden cardiac death [7].

After Mustard procedure an electrophysiological study of patients identifies a variety of abnormalities such as prolonged sinus node recovery time (SNRT, Fig. 14.1), intra-atrial conduction times, and also atrial refractoriness. Direct surgical damage to the sinus node has been suggested as a cause of observed abnormalities of the sinus node's function. But the progressive loss of sinus rhythm observed over prolonged follow-up suggests further ongoing pathophysiological developments associated with chronic hemodynamic abnormality [8].

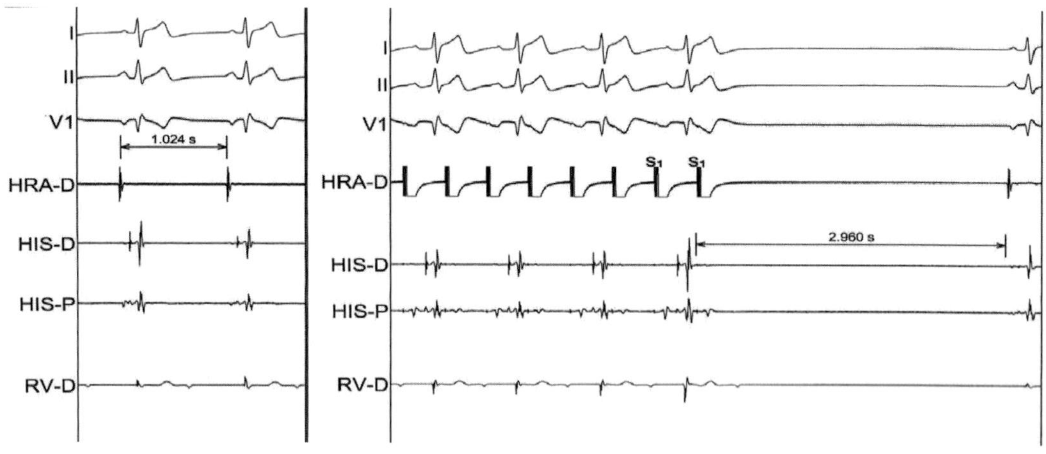

Fig. 14.1 Abnormal sinus node recovery time (SNRT) in a patient with sinus node dysfunction. Normal SNRT is lower than 1,500 ms

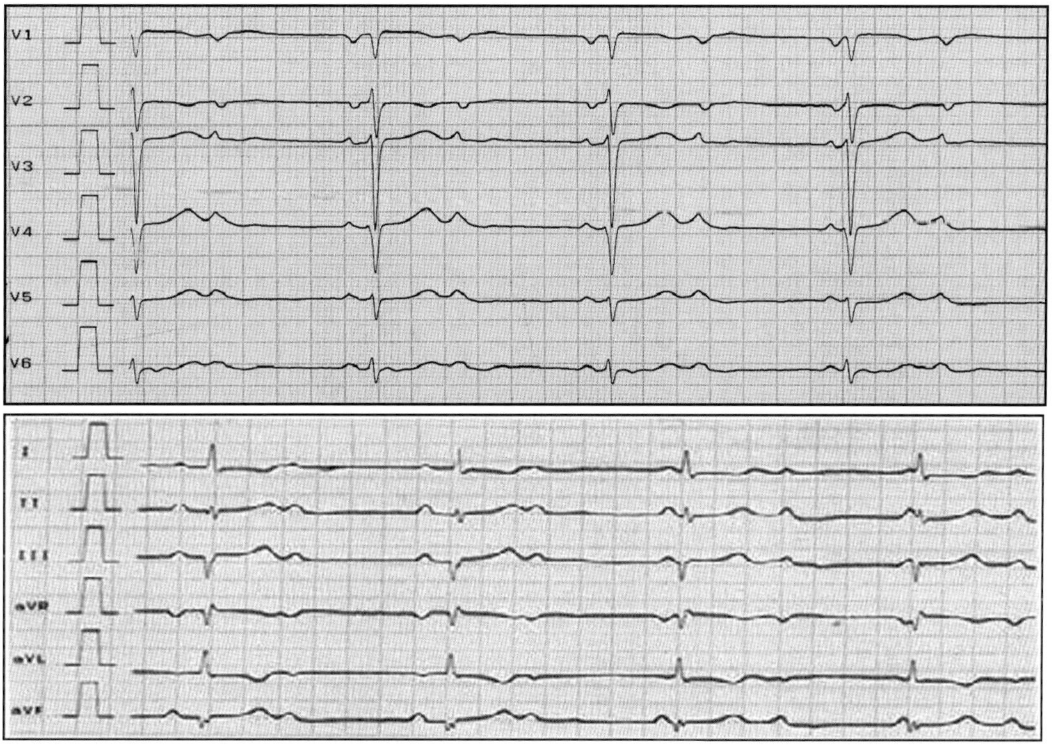

Fig. 14.2 CHB in a patient with complete TGA (d TGA)

AV Block

Complete heart block sometimes happens naturally in patients with specific structural heart disease, particularly endocardial cushion defects. This can be caused by abnormal anatomy of the AV node and His bundle, rendering them susceptible to injury. Though some of these patients are born with heart block, however, it can progress at any period of life.

Interventricular conduction delays, principally the right bundle branch block (RBBB), are very prevalent after any surgery for CHD. Complete postoperative heart block is formed either by direct surgical injury to the specialized conduction system or by indirect damage due to inflammation after surgery. It is characteristically related with surgical manipulation in the ventricular septum. Patients at uppermost risk are those experiencing surgery for left ventricular (LV) outflow tract obstructions and with L transposition of the great arteries (L TGA), but it is also common after ventricular septal defect (VSD) and tetralogy of Fallot (TOF) repair surgeries. Interestingly in patients with tricuspid atresia (TA), the AV node is typically found on the floor of the RA close to a small dent lined with endocardium. The His-Purkinje system's course is typically further leftward and away from the more anterior side of VSDs [9, 10] (Fig. 14.2).

A review of clinical consequences before cardiac pacing systems applicable for CHD patients who were accessible revealed that postoperative heart blocks had a high mortality rate [9, 10].

Tachyarrhythmias

Atrial Tachyarrhythmias

Supraventricular tachycardias are highly common and may be caused by accessory pathways (Figs. 14.3 and 14.4), dual AV nodal physiology (Fig. 14.5), twin AV nodes (e.g., in L-looped single left ventricles), automatic focus (Fig. 14.6), and macroreentrant circuits.

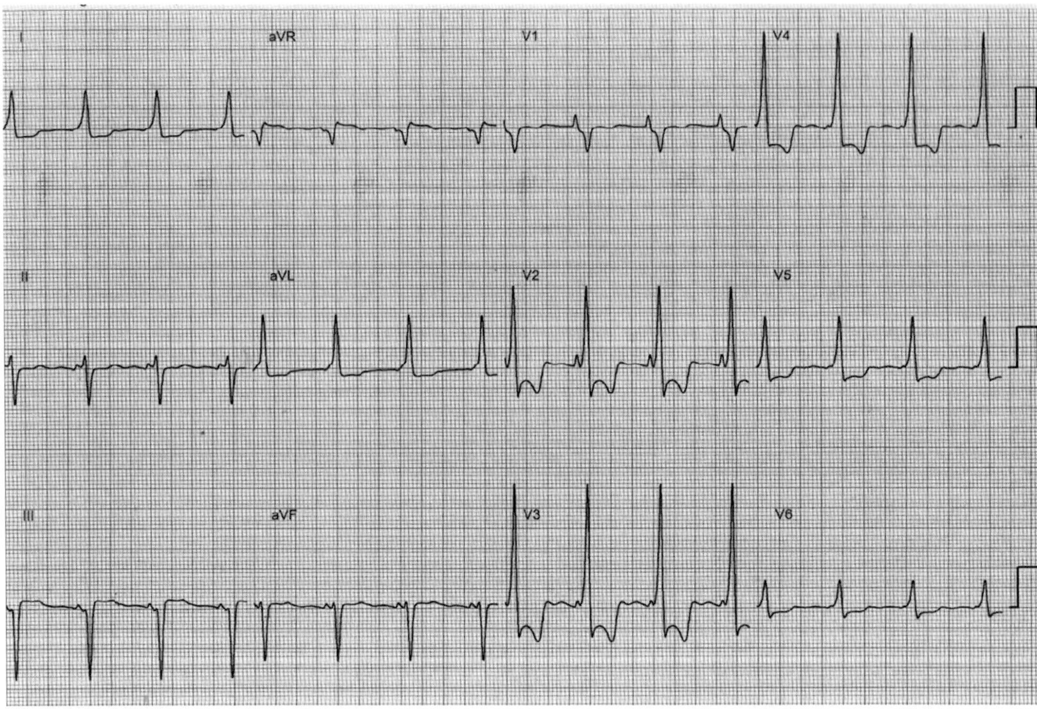

Fig. 14.3 Right posteroseptal accessory pathway in a patient with complex CHD (undergoing TCPC) presented with frequent episodes of drug-refractory SVT and WPW

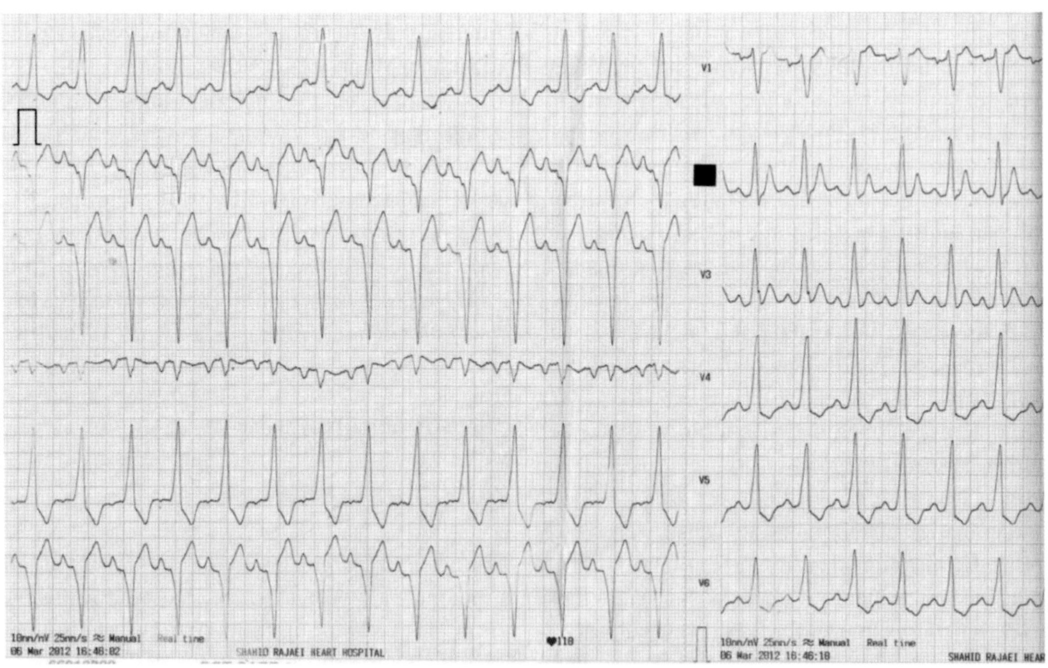

Fig. 14.4 WPW, right posteroseptal accessory pathway in a patient with Epstein's anomaly and frequent episodes of SVT

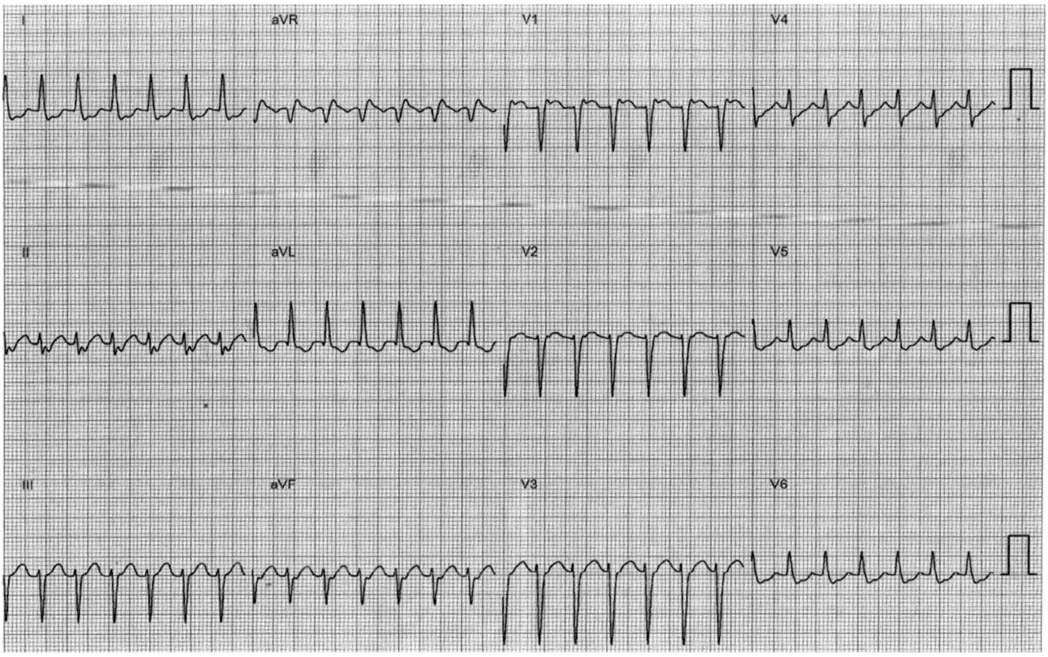

Fig. 14.5 Typical AVNRT in a patient with single ventricle physiology undergoing Fontan procedure and who presented with incessant SVT and dyspnea FC III

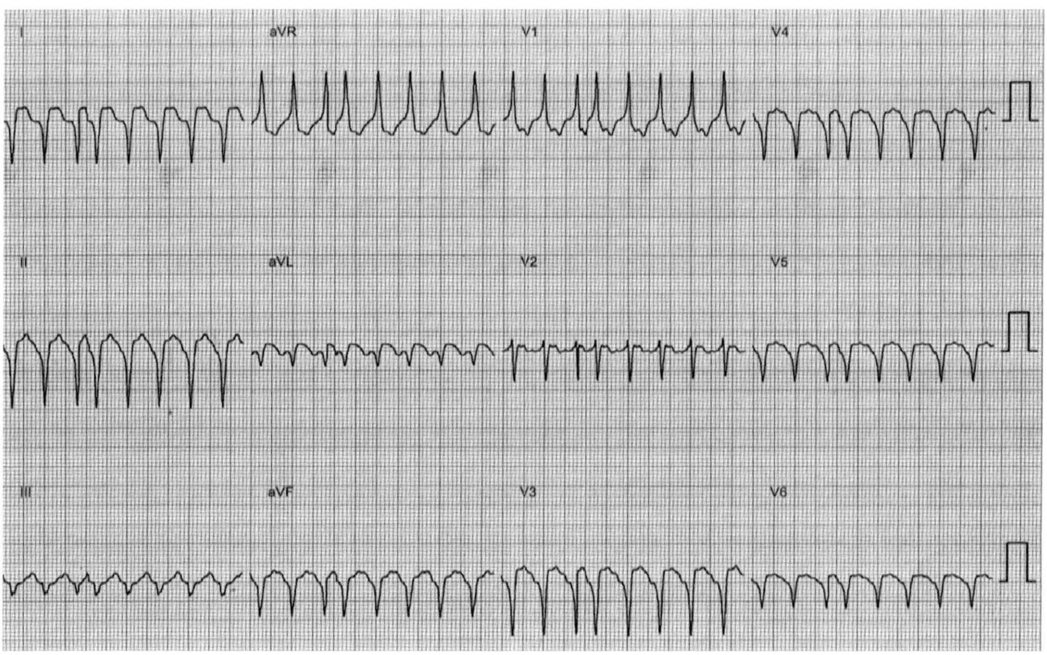

Fig. 14.6 Focal atrial tachycardia arising from anteroseptal area in a patient with complex CHD (abdominal and atrial situs inversus, mesocardia, atrioventricular discordance, ventriculo-arterial discordance, severe valvular and subvalvular PS, moderate secundum-type ASD, right-sided aortic arch, aorta in left and anterior side of PA, Ebstein-like anomaly of the tricuspid valve, right-sided RV (systemic ventricle) with EF=50 %, left-sided LV (subpulmonic) with EF=30 %). Atrial tachycardia was inducible with isoproterenol without response to atrial overdrive pacing or adenosine

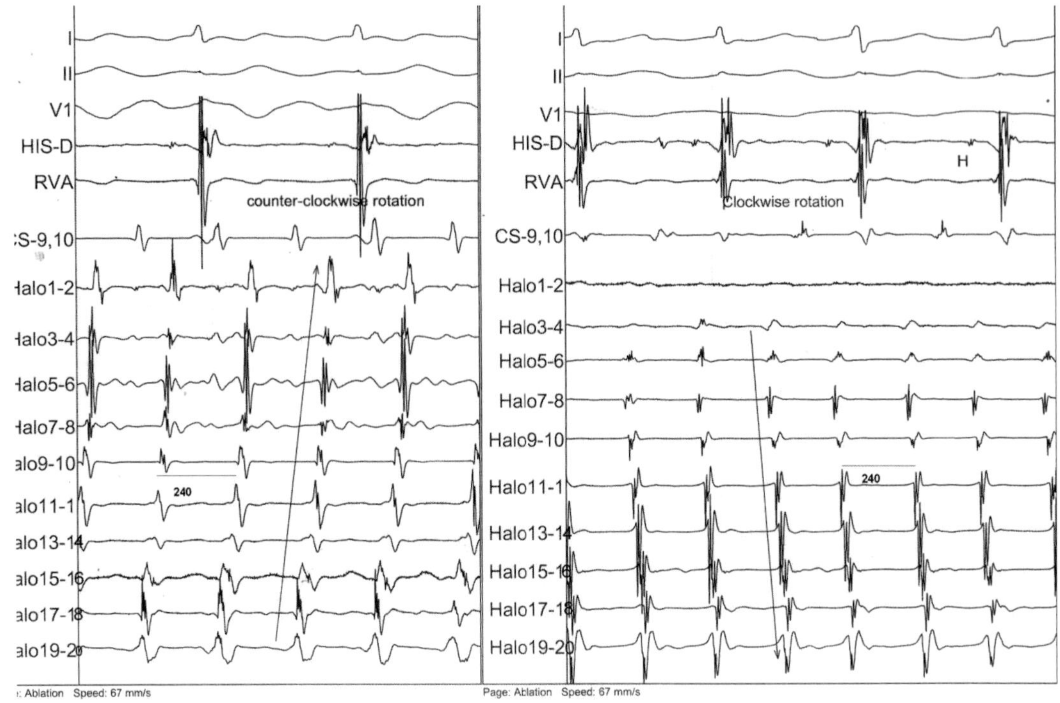

Fig. 14.7 Macroreentrant atrial tachycardia (typical cavo-tricuspid isthmus-dependent AFt in a patient with small ASD)

Reentrant tachycardia (RT) means macroreentrant atrial tachycardias other than cavo-tricuspid isthmus-dependent typical atrial flutter happening in the normal heart. This arrhythmia is a prevalent late complication in many types of CHD. Similar to typical atrial flutter (AFt), it has a stable cycle length and P wave morphology, suggesting that it is organized by a fixed and single substrate. Its prevalence has a particular dependence on surgical atrial damage (such as Mustard and Fontan surgeries) resulting in tachycardias like those observed clinically [11] (Fig. 14.7).

Atrial tachyarrhythmias are classified as focal or macroreentrant atrial tachycardia.

Atrial tachycardia:

1. Focal atrial tachycardia
2. Intra-atrial macroreentrant tachycardia or AFt
   Typical AFt (dependent to CTI)
   Atypical AFt (independent to CTI)

Focal atrial tachycardia (AT) was well defined as atrial activation starting rhythmically at a small area (focus) from which it spreads out centrifugally and also within endocardial activation over significant parts of the cycle length (Figs. 14.8 and 14.9).

In contrast, macroreentrant activation is traditionally defined as a circuit with a diameter of longer than 2 cm and often happens around a central obstacle (Fig. 14.10).

Frequently identified risk factors for intra-atrial reentrant tachycardia (AFt) include older age in operation time and longer follow-up period. Near half of those patients with old forms of Fontan surgery [12] and survivors of the Mustard and Senning surgeries are at risk for the development of sinus node dysfunction and reentrant tachycardia (RT). RT is more common in patients with repaired TOF (Fig. 14.9) than ventricular tachyarrhythmias (VT) [13]. AFt is common in repaired ASD (Figs. 14.11 and 14.12), and typical atrial flutter is more common than atypical atrial flutter.

Junctional tachyarrhythmias are prevalent, especially in young postoperative patients [14].

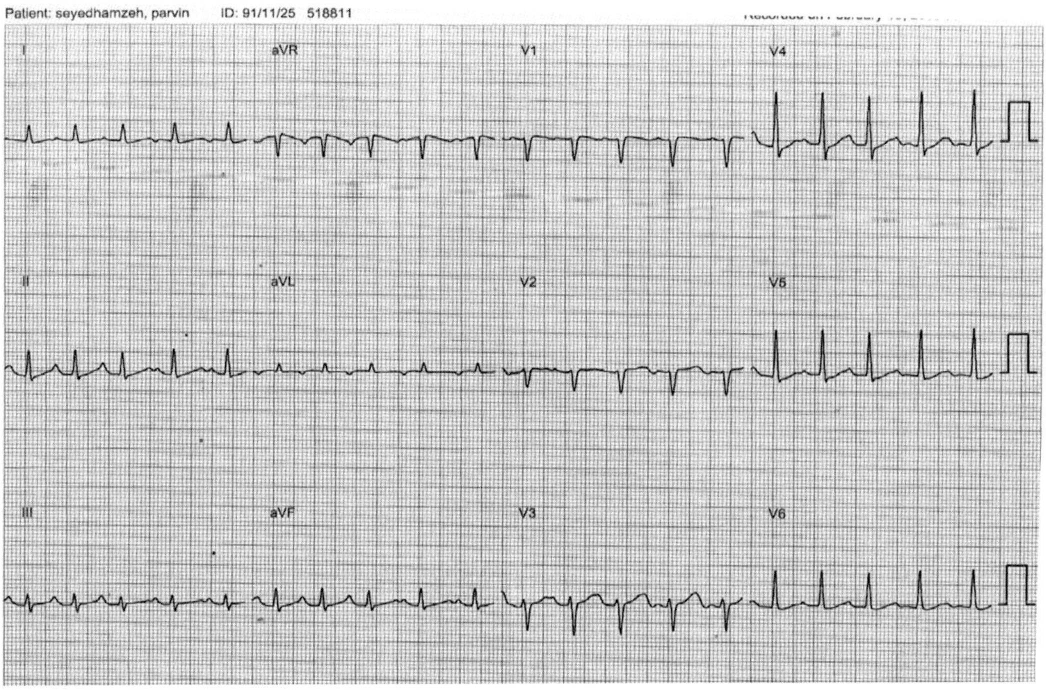

Fig. 14.8 Focal AT arising from left atrium

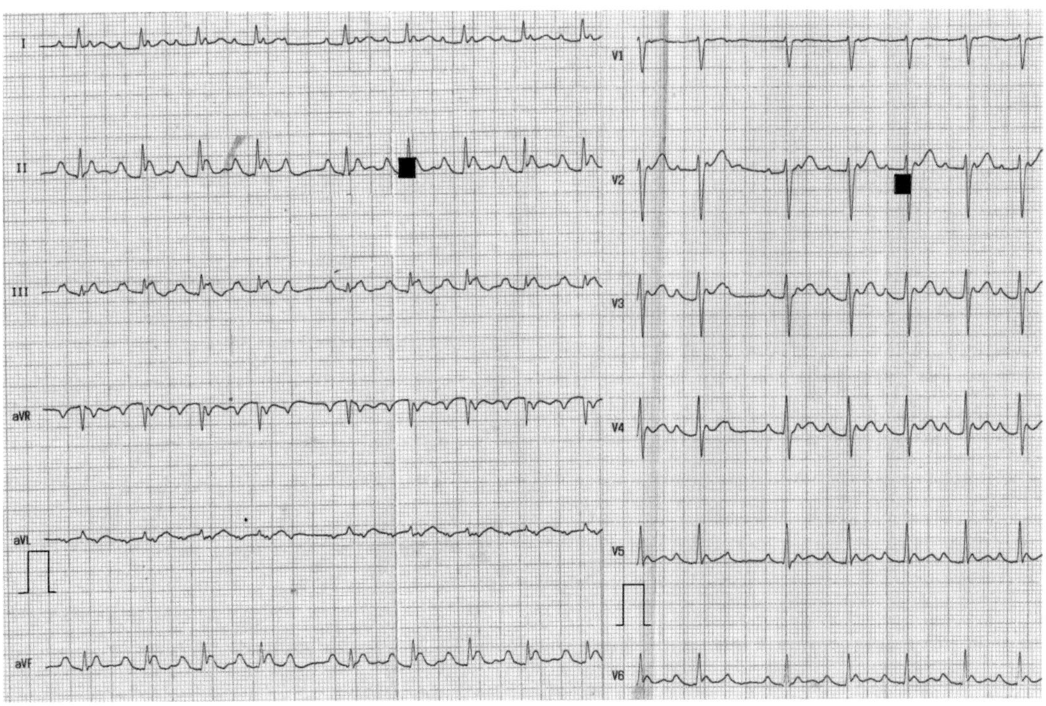

Fig. 14.9 Focal atrial tachycardia

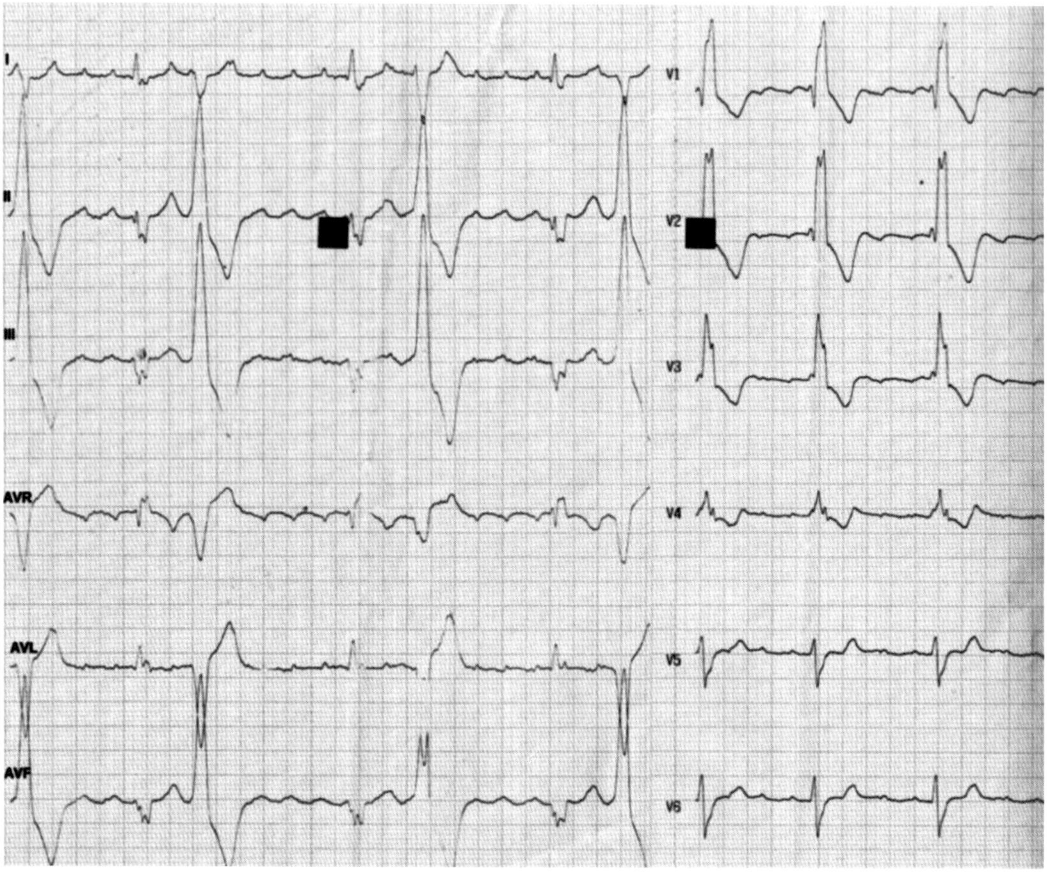

Fig. 14.10 Macroreentrant AT (typical AFt) in a patient with corrected TOF

Atrial Fibrillation

Atrial fibrillation (AF) is increasingly common in the aging population of adults with CHD. AF happens in as many as 25–30 % of patients with CHD and atrial tachyarrhythmias. The limited data available on these patients suggests that those with residual left-sided obstructive disease or unrepaired CHD are more prone to AF. The main beliefs of management are similar to the general adult population, containing anticoagulation and also rate control. The risk of thromboembolism is apparently high. Sinus rhythm is hemodynamically favored in CHD, and cardioversion, prophylactic antiarrhythmic drugs, and also sometimes atrial pacing are used to prevent establishing permanent AF if possible [1].

Ventricular Tachyarrhythmias

Large data are available on the natural history of ventricular arrhythmias and also clinical aspect outcomes in patients with TOF (Fig. 14.13). Mapping studies have revealed that, like intra-atrial RT, VT in TOF contains a macroreentrant circuit dependent on an anatomical problem, in this case the RV outflow tract patch and/or the conal septum [15].

Sudden cardiac death and VT happen with a frequency of 1–2 % over 5 years for young adults and an overall commonness of sudden death of 3–6 % [16]. Though the clinical presentation of TOF adult patients with sustained monomorphic VT is infrequent, such VT is inducible by programmed stimulation in 15–30 % of these patients, and half have recurrent and complex ventricular ectopy on ambulatory Holter ECGs

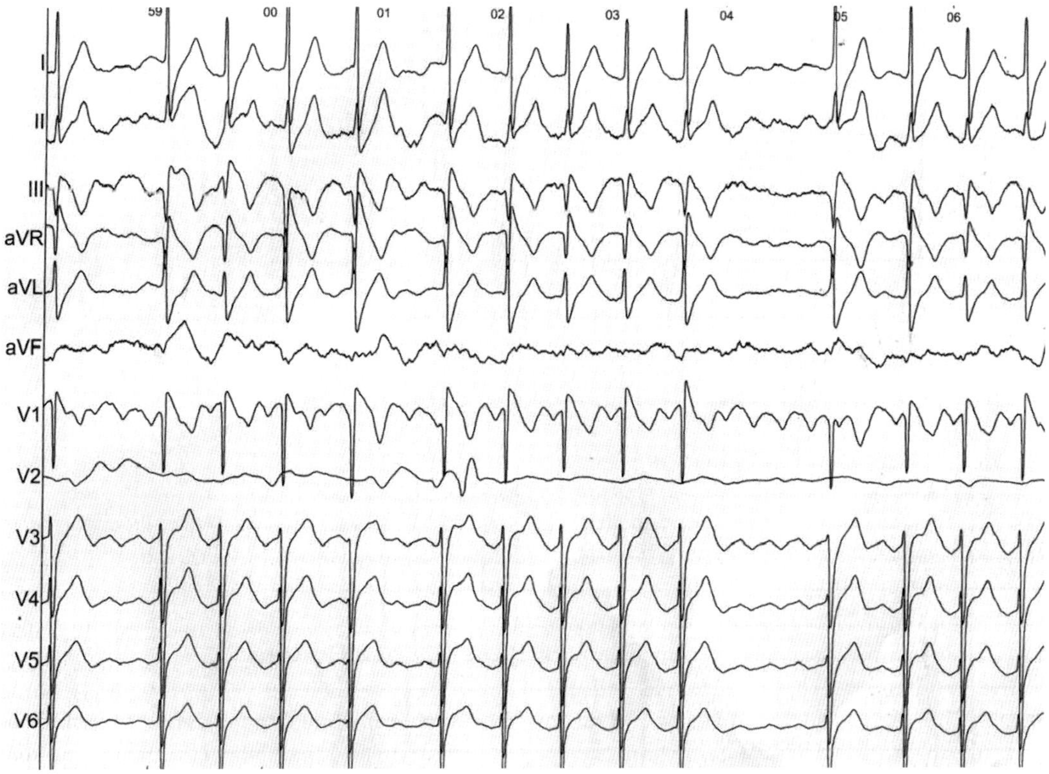

Fig. 14.11 Atypical AFt arising from lateral part of RA

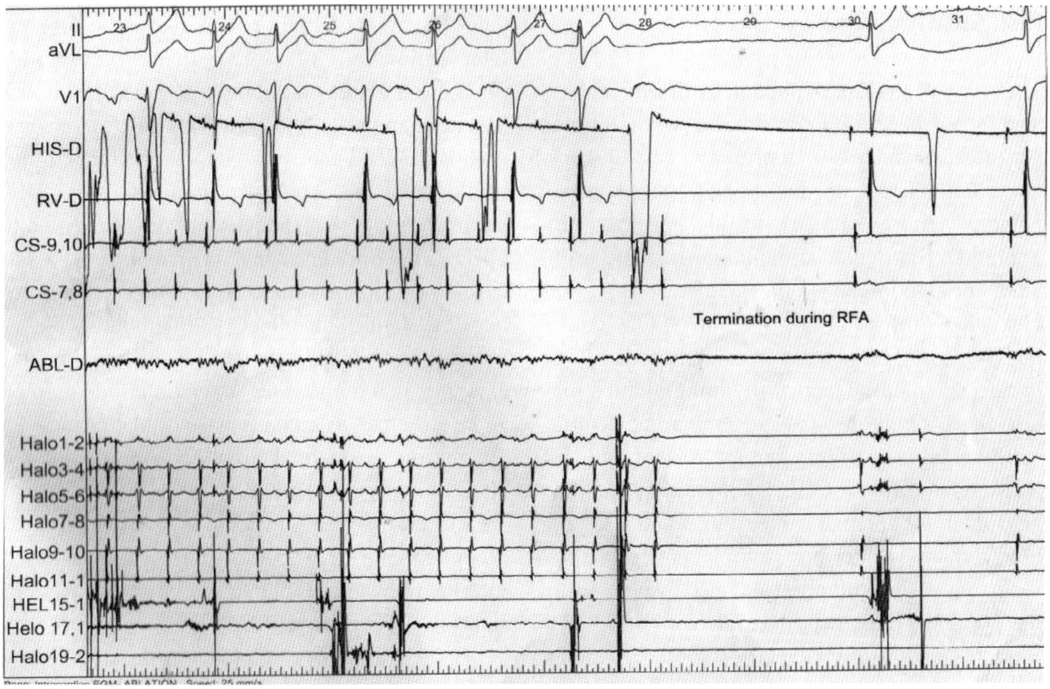

Fig. 14.12 Fragmented low amplitude potential recorded in the slow conduction zone in the lateral part of the right atrium. Atrial flutter was terminated during radiofrequency ablation in the mentioned area and extension to tricuspid isthmus

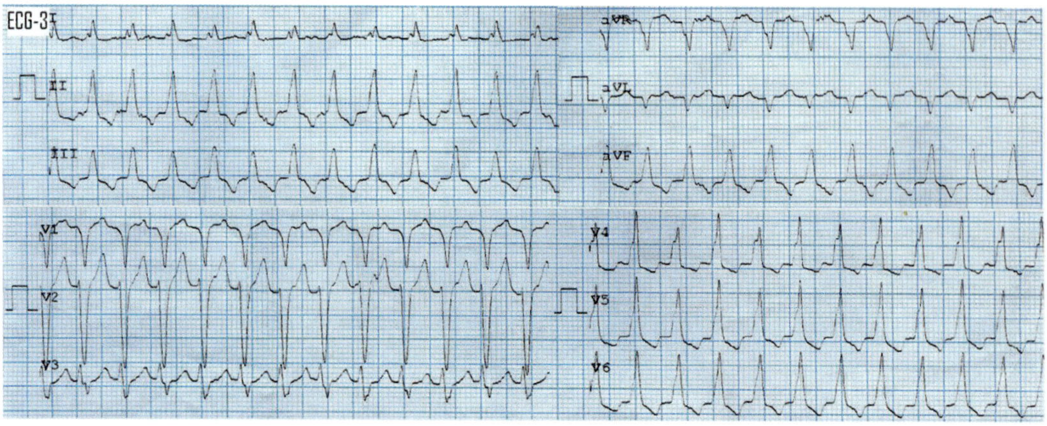

Fig. 14.13 RVOT VT in a patient with TOF

(Fig. 14.10). Sinus node dysfunction and also AFt happen in 20–30 % of patients with post-repair surgery for TOF and in up to 50 % of symptomatic patients mimicking VT symptoms and may cause wide complex tachycardias with underlying RBBB morphology. These issues make it challenging to apply standard diagnostic tools to screen patients with clinical arrhythmia symptoms for high risk of sudden cardiac death [17].

Risk Stratification

The study of the risk of sudden cardiac death created by VT needs an understanding of the limited prognostic standards of commonly used diagnostic examinations in this population. Through Holter, exercise tolerance testing and also programmed ventricular stimulation are very valuable for stimulating and also recording the clinically important arrhythmias. Of course the risk study is sometimes complicated by the occurrence of atrial tachyarrhythmias, which may also cause symptoms and sudden cardiac death.

Some clinical factors that are related with VT and sudden death in CHD adult patients are older age, older age at repair surgery time, and also poor hemodynamic status. For example, noticeable prolongation of QRS duration and also dispersions of the QT and JT segment intervals are related with mortality and also inducible VT in TOF patients. These findings identify a more arrhythmogenic myocardium and propose that both depolarization and depolarization are abnormal in TOF patients and the ambulatory ECG is frequently abnormal in high-risk patients with TOF [18, 19].

Therapeutic Options

Notably, arrhythmias can signal a change in hemodynamic outline and must ordinarily prompt a detailed study and workup. Care of the patient with CHD and concomitant arrhythmias may include drug therapy, implantable cardiac devices, catheter ablation, and also some surgical interventions.

There is a little data about the dosing and toxicity rate of antiarrhythmic drugs for the different age groups in CHD patients. Amiodarone-related thyroid dysfunction is prevalent in adults with CHD, particularly in women and those with cyanotic CHD [20]. Nowadays, there is much interest about class III of antiarrhythmic drugs with smaller number of systemic side effects and without increased mortality rate in the setting of LV dysfunction. For example, in a multicenter study, dofetilide seemed to be a helper to catheter-based ablation and an alternative in pharmacological management for atrial arrhythmias in adults with CHD [21].

Vascular access difficulties and anatomical complexities can complicate catheter-based interventions and implantation of pacemakers or ICDs in CHD patients [22, 23].

There are some challenges in device therapy in CHD patients including avoiding closed and obstructed vessels and conduits or baffles, identifying suitable candidates for cardiac resynchronization therapy, thromboembolic events risk in the presence of intracardiac shunts, and a high rate of inappropriate shocks, and also lead's complications [22, 24, 25]. Also some CHD patients may benefit from pacemakers having automated overdrive pacing systems to terminate the atrial tachyarrhythmias [26].

In specific circumstances, surgery for arrhythmia is frequently performed in combination with cardiac surgery for particular indications; of course it may complement fewer invasive choices. High recurrences and also the onset of any new arrhythmia continue to be challenging, principally in patients with a history of Fontan palliation.

References

1. Triedman JK. Arrhythmias in adults with congenital heart disease. Heart. 2002;87(4):383–9.
2. Hoffman JI, Kaplan S. The incidence of congenital heart disease. J Am Coll Cardiol. 2002;39:1890–900.
3. Feltes TF, Friedman RA. Transesophageal echocardiographic detection of atrial thrombi in patients with nonfibrillation atrial tachyarrhythmias and congenital heart disease. J Am Coll Cardiol. 1994;24:1365–70.
4. Khairy P, Dore A, Talajic M, Dubuc M, Poirier N, Roy D, Mercier LA. Arrhythmias in adult congenital heart disease. Expert Rev Cardiovasc Ther. 2006;4:83–95.
5. Oechslin EN, Harrison DA, Connelly MS, Webb GD, Siu SC. Mode of death in adults with congenital heart disease. Am J Cardiol. 2000;86:1111–6.
6. Kanter RJ, Garson Jr A. Atrial arrhythmias during chronic follow-up of surgery for complex congenital heart disease. Pacing Clin Electrophysiol. 1997;20:502–11.
7. Duster MC, Bink-Boelkens MT, Wampler D, et al. Long-term follow-up of dysrhythmias following the Mustard procedure. Am Heart J. 1985;109:1323–6.
8. Vetter VL, Tanner CS, Horowitz LN. Electrophysiologic consequences of the Mustard repair of d-transposition of the great arteries. J Am Coll Cardiol. 1987;10:1265–73.
9. Anderson RH, Becker AE, Arnold R, Wilkinson JL. The conducting tissues in congenitally corrected transposition. Circulation. 1974;50:911–23.
10. Bharati S, Lev M. The conduction system in tricuspid atresia with and without regular (d-) transposition. Circulation. 1977;56:423–9.
11. Garson Jr A, Bink-Boelkens MTE, Hesslein PS, et al. Atrial flutter in the young: a collaborative study in 380 cases. J Am Coll Cardiol. 1985;6:871–8.
12. Fishberger SB, Wernovsky G, Gentles TL, et al. Factors that influence the development of atrial flutter after the Fontan operation. J Thorac Cardiovasc Surg. 1997;113:80–6.
13. Roos-Hesselink J, Perlroth MG, McGhie J, et al. Atrial arrhythmias in adults after repair of tetralogy of Fallot. Correlations with clinical, exercise, and echocardiographic findings. Circulation. 1995;91:221413.
14. Khairy P, Balaji S. "Cardiac Arrhythmias In Congenital Heart Diseases" 312 early postoperative period. J Thorac Cardiovasc Surg. 2007;133:900–4.
15. Horton RP, Canby RC, Kessler DJ, et al. Ablation of ventricular tachycardia associated with tetralogy of Fallot: demonstration of bidirectional block. J Cardiovasc Electrophysiol. 1997;8:432–5.
16. Murphy JG, Gersh BJ, Mair DD, et al. Long-term outcome in patients undergoing surgical repair of tetralogy of Fallot. N Engl J Med. 1993;329:593–9.
17. Lucron H, Marcon F, Bosser G, et al. Induction of sustained ventricular tachycardia after surgical repair of tetralogy of Fallot. Am J Cardiol. 1999;83:1369–73.
18. Cullen S, Celermajer DS, Franklin RC, et al. Prognostic significance of ventricular arrhythmia after repair of tetralogy of Fallot: a 12-year prospective study. J Am Coll Cardiol. 1994;23:1151–5.
19. Gatzoulis MA, Till JA, Redington AN. Depolarization-repolarization inhomogeneity after repair of tetralogy of Fallot: the substrate for malignant ventricular tachycardia? Circulation. 1997;95:401–4.
20. Thorne SA, Barnes I, Cullinan P, Somerville J. Amiodarone-associated thyroid dysfunction: risk factors in adults with congenital heart disease. Circulation. 1999;100:149–54.
21. Wells R, Khairy P, Harris L, Anderson CC, Balaji S. Dofetilide for atrial arrhythmias in congenital heart disease: a multicenter study. Pacing Clin Electrophysiol. 2009;32:1313–8.
22. Stephenson EA, Batra AS, Knilans TK, Gow RM, Gradaus R, Balaji S, Dubin AM, Rhee EK, Ro PS, Thogersen AM, Cecchin F, Triedman JK, Walsh EP, Berul CI. A multicenter experience with novel implantable cardioverter defibrillator configurations in the pediatric and congenital heart disease population. J Cardiovasc Electrophysiol. 2006;17:41–6.
23. Batra AS, Balaji S. Pacing in adults with congenital heart disease. Expert Rev Cardiovasc Ther. 2006;4:663–70.
24. Khairy P, Landzberg MJ, Gatzoulis MA, Mercier LA, Fernandes SM, Cote JM, Lavoie JP, Fournier A, Guerra PG, Frogoudaki A, Walsh EP, Dore A. Transvenous pacing leads and systemic thromboemboli in patients with intracardiac shunts: a multicenter study. Circulation. 2006;113:2391–7.
25. Khairy P. Defibrillators and cardiac resynchronisation therapy in congenital heart disease. Exp Rev Med Devices. 2008;5:267–71.
26. Stephenson EA, Casavant D, Tuzi J, Alexander ME, Law I, Serwer G, Strieper M, Walsh EP, Berul CI. Efficacy of atrial antitachycardia pacing using the Medtronic AT500 pacemaker in patients with congenital heart disease. Am J Cardiol. 2003;92:871–6.

Pulmonary Hypertension Associated with Congenital Heart Disease, Eisenmenger Syndrome

15

Anita Sadeghpour and Azin Alizadehasl

Keywords
Pulmonary hypertension (PH) • Pulmonary arterial hypertension (PAH) • Eisenmenger syndrome • Pulmonary artery pressure (PAP) • Right heart catheterization (RHC)

Definition and Classification

Obviously, the proper management of every disease needs the proper definition and classification. Pulmonary hypertension (PH) which is a hemodynamic and pathophysiological condition has been defined as raised mean pulmonary arterial pressure ≥25 mmHg at rest that is confirmed by right heart catheterization (RHC). PH has been found in multiple different clinical conditions, and the American and European guidelines have been provided a clear classification based on the pathophysiological mechanisms, clinical presentations, and therapeutic approaches (Table 15.1).

We should be aware of the different definitions between PH and pulmonary arterial hypertension (PAH).

Table 15.1 Clinical classification of pulmonary artery hypertension

Group I. Pulmonary arterial hypertension (PAH)
Idiopathic PAH
Familial or heritable PAH
Drugs and toxins induced
Associated with risk factors and associated conditions
Connective tissue disease
Congenital heart disease
Portal hypertension
Associated with HIV
Chronic hemolytic anemia
Schistosomiasis
Associated with significant venous or capillary involvement
Persistent pulmonary hypertension of the newborn
Group II. Pulmonary hypertension associated with left heart disease
Group III. Pulmonary hypertension associated with lung disease and/or hypoxemia
Group IV. Pulmonary hypertension due to chronic thrombotic or embolic disease
Group V. Pulmonary hypertension with unclear or multifactorial mechanism

A. Sadeghpour, MD, FACC, FASE (✉)
Echocardiography Lab, Department of Cardiology, Adult Congenital Heart Disease Clinic, Rajaie Cardiovascular Medical and Research Center, Iran University of Medical Science, Tehran, Iran
e-mail: anita.sadeghpour@gmail.com, asadeghpour@rhc.ac.ir

A. Alizadehasl, MD, FACC
Echocardiography Lab, Department of Cardiology, Rajaie Cardiovascular Medical and Research Center, Iran University of Medical Science, Tehran, Iran
e-mail: alizadeasl@gmail.com, alizadeasl@rhc.ac.ir

A. Sadeghpour et al. (eds.), *Comprehensive Approach to Adult Congenital Heart Disease*,
DOI 10.1007/978-1-4471-6383-1_15, © Springer-Verlag London 2014

Table 15.2 Classification of pulmonary artery hypertension associated with congenital heart disease or CHD-related PAH (CHD-PAH) based on the ESC PH guidelines

1. *Eisenmenger's syndrome*
Large defects can lead to severe increase in PVR and consequently reversed (pulmonary-to-systemic) or bidirectional shunt
2. *Pulmonary arterial hypertension with systemic-to-pulmonary shunts*
Moderate to large-size defects associated with mild to moderate increase in PVR and still large systemic-to-pulmonary shunt with no cyanosis
3. *PAH with small defects*
Small defects (usually VSD less than 1 cm and ASD less than 2 cm of effective diameter when assessed by echocardiography) with similar clinical picture to idiopathic PAH
4. *PAH after corrective cardiac surgery*
PAH still present several months or years after total correction of congenital heart disease in the absence of significant residual defect

PAH has been classified as group I and hemodynamically is defined as a mean pulmonary artery pressure greater than 25 mmHg at rest, pulmonary capillary wedge pressure less than or equal to 15 mmHg, and PVR greater than 3 mmHg per L per min per m2. Normal mean PAP at rest is about 14+3 mmHg, with an upper limit of 20 mmHg.

Pulmonary arterial hypertension (PAH) of variable degrees is commonly associated with adult congenital heart disease (CHD). Approximately 5–10 % of CHD patients develop PAH of variable severity that affects quality of life, morbidity, and mortality [1, 2]. The dangerous manifestation of PAH in this setting, known as the Eisenmenger syndrome, has become the epitome of PAH associated with CHD [3, 4].

PAH in patients with CHD or CHD-related PAH (CHD-PAH) has been classified based on the ESC PH guidelines (Table 15.2) [5].

CHD-Related PAH

In patients with a large ventricular or arterial communication, shunt volume and direction are determined essentially by the difference in pressure between the systemic and pulmonary circulations. However, patients with a large atrial communication may have a right-to-left shunt not necessarily because of systemic or suprasystemic pulmonary pressures. In this group, a right-to-left shunt may rather reflect lower right ventricular compliance (e.g., a result of right ventricular hypertrophy). The natural sequence of patients with atrial communications is different. Although the penetrance of PAH is high and the onset of the Eisenmenger physiology is relatively early and is the rule in patients with large shunts at the ventricular or arterial level, the majority of patients with atrial septal defect (even large) do not develop the Eisenmenger physiology, and those who develop PAH often do so much later [6–13]. Accordingly, it is essential that additional information be collected when dealing with the Eisenmenger syndrome.

Pathophysiology

The vascular changes that occur in PAH allied to CHD are identical to those seen in idiopathic PAH. It is believed that endothelial cells release mediators that induce the development of pulmonary artery smooth muscle cells in response to changes in the pulmonary blood flow or pressure. Experimental data have recommended that medial hypertrophy can be converted to a neointimal pattern when pulmonary vascular injury is coupled with increased pulmonary blood flow. Early changes, characterized by the hypertrophy of the media and the intimal proliferation of the muscular pulmonary arteries and arterioles, are believed to be reversible. Advanced disease, characterized by the presence of concentric laminar fibrosis, with obliteration of many arterioles and small arteries, and plexiform lesions are considered irreversible [1, 2].

Clinical Findings

The clinical signs and symptoms of PAH are variable and depend on the underlying heart disease, patient's age, repair status, and degree, volume, and direction of shunting. General symptoms of PAH are nonspecific and include breathlessness, chest pain, palpitation, and syncope. In patients with the Eisenmenger syndrome, central cyanosis and clubbing are the most visible clinical consequences, and some may exhibit differential cyanosis. Patients with long-standing large left-to-right shunts who develop the Eisenmenger syndrome tend to have multisystem disorders.

Eisenmenger Syndrome

Definition

In 1897 Victor Eisenmenger, an Austrian physician (1864–1932), described a 32-year-old female cyanotic patient who had died due to hemoptysis (her autopsy showed a large ventricular septal defect (VSD) as well as right ventricular dilation, hypertrophy without evidence of pulmonary stenosis, pulmonary atherosclerosis, and pulmonary infarction) [6].

The Eisenmenger physiology or syndrome, as named later by Paul Wood is defined as pulmonary vascular disease resulting from any untreated large communications between the systemic and pulmonary circulation [8]. *When the pulmonary artery pressure reaches the systemic values, the direction of the blood flow reverses and a right-to-left or bidirectional shunt ensues.*

Traditionally, the Eisenmenger complex refers to the Eisenmenger physiology due to a VSD (as described originally by Eisenmenger) [14]. Left-to-right shunting leads to a rise in pulmonary artery vascular resistance and subsequently pulmonary artery pressure.

A number of congenital heart lesions can result in the Eisenmenger physiology, including unrepaired large systemic-to-pulmonary artery (left-to-right) shunts as in VSD, atrioventricular septal defect, and patent ductus arteriosus (PDA); aortopulmonary window; or more complex congenital heart diseases (CHD) such as partial or total anomalous pulmonary venous return, unrepaired or palliated conoventricular defects including truncus arteriosus, or transposition of the great arteries, and single-ventricle variants. Surgically created anastomoses (e.g., in the Pott and Waterson procedures) may also result in the Eisenmenger physiology.

Epidemiology

The Eisenmenger syndrome constitutes <5 % of patients in the adult congenital clinics. The incidence and prevalence of the Eisenmenger syndrome have been reported to decrease due to both earlier diagnosis and treatment of CHD.

Clinical Course

Initially, left-to-right shunting produces congestive heart failure due to an increased pulmonary blood flow. As pulmonary vascular resistance (PVR) increases, the symptoms of pulmonary congestion abate and the patient may improve symptomatically. Eventually, as pulmonary vascular resistance further increases, pulmonary pressure approaches the systemic circulation, and the converted direction of the blood flow (right to left) brings about the clinical manifestations of cyanosis.

Clinical Presentation

Clinical manifestation of the Eisenmenger syndrome in patients with PDA or VAD usually occurs during infancy or the first two years of age, while patients with the Eisenmenger syndrome due to ASD usually present during adulthood. Generally, the symptoms of the Eisenmenger syndrome are caused by either the inability to increase the pulmonary blood flow in response to physiologic stress due to pulmonary hypertension or the inability to provide sufficient pump action due to heart failure. Other symptoms are related to various multisystem complications associated with cyanotic CHD.

The most common symptoms of the Eisenmenger syndrome include:

- Dyspnea on exertion which is the most common presenting symptom of patients with Eisenmenger physiology.

  The average VO_2 in patients with the Eisenmenger physiology has been estimated as 12 ml/kg/min. More than 90 % of patients with the Eisenmenger syndrome are in the New York Heart Association (NYHA) functional class ≥II.

- Palpitation.
- Edema.
- Volume retention.
- Hemoptysis.
- Syncope.
- Progressive cyanosis.

Physical Examination

Cardiovascular findings in the Eisenmenger syndrome include:

- Central cyanosis (in patients with PDA, cyanosis may be more prominent in the lower extremities and sometimes in the left arm).
- Clubbing of the nail beds and digits.
- Jugular venous pulse wave may be A-wave dominant, and, in the presence of significant tricuspid regurgitation, the V wave may be prominent; central venous pressure may be elevated.
- Normal or diminished aortic pulses.
- Right parasternal heave and frequently a palpable pulmonary valve closure on precordial palpation.
- Pulmonary ejection click from a dilated main pulmonary artery.
- Loud pulmonic component of S_2.
- Right-sided fourth heart sound.
- Graham-steel murmur (high-pitched decrescendo murmur of pulmonic regurgitation).
- Holosystolic murmur of tricuspid regurgitation or mitral regurgitation.
- Murmurs related to VSD and PDA are usually not present.
- Abdominal tenderness/hepatic congestion.
- Peripheral edema.

Laboratory Investigation

Electrocardiography

Evidence of right atrial overload in association with right ventricular hypertrophy and right axis deviation is seen in patients with the Eisenmenger syndrome. Concomitant arrhythmias may also be seen.

Cardiovascular Imaging Modalities

Chest X-ray, echocardiography, multislice CT, and CMR have variable success in detecting the presence and severity of PH.

Chest X-ray

Chest radiographic examination reveals the following:

- Prominent dilated central pulmonary artery.
- *Decreased peripheral lung vascular markings (pruning).* Although in contrast to primary pulmonary hypertension, the attenuation of peripheral vascular markings is not common in these patients.
- Calcification of the central pulmonary artery may also be present due to long-lasting pulmonary hypertension.
- VSD or PDA usually has a normal or minimally increased cardiothoracic ratio.
- Right ventricular enlargement.
- ASD usually has cardiomegaly due to the dilatation of the right atrium and ventricle.
- PDA usually has an enlarged aorta (ductal calcification may also be present), while in patients with ASD, the aorta seems inconspicuous.

Echocardiography

Intracardiac communication and concomitant bidirectional shunting should be assessed in all patients with the Eisenmenger syndrome. Assessment of right ventricular function is mandatory for prognostic implications.

Echocardiography has been suggested as a pivotal screening test in PH evaluation. Doppler echocardiography can be used for estimation of systolic pulmonary arterial pressure (PAP), pulmonary artery (PA) diastolic pressure, mean PA pressure, and pulmonary vascular resistance (PVR). Echocardiographic estimation of systolic PAP is mainly based on the tricuspid regurgitation (TR) peak velocity.

Based on the European guidelines for PH assessment, echocardiographic assessment of the PH has been classified as [1]:

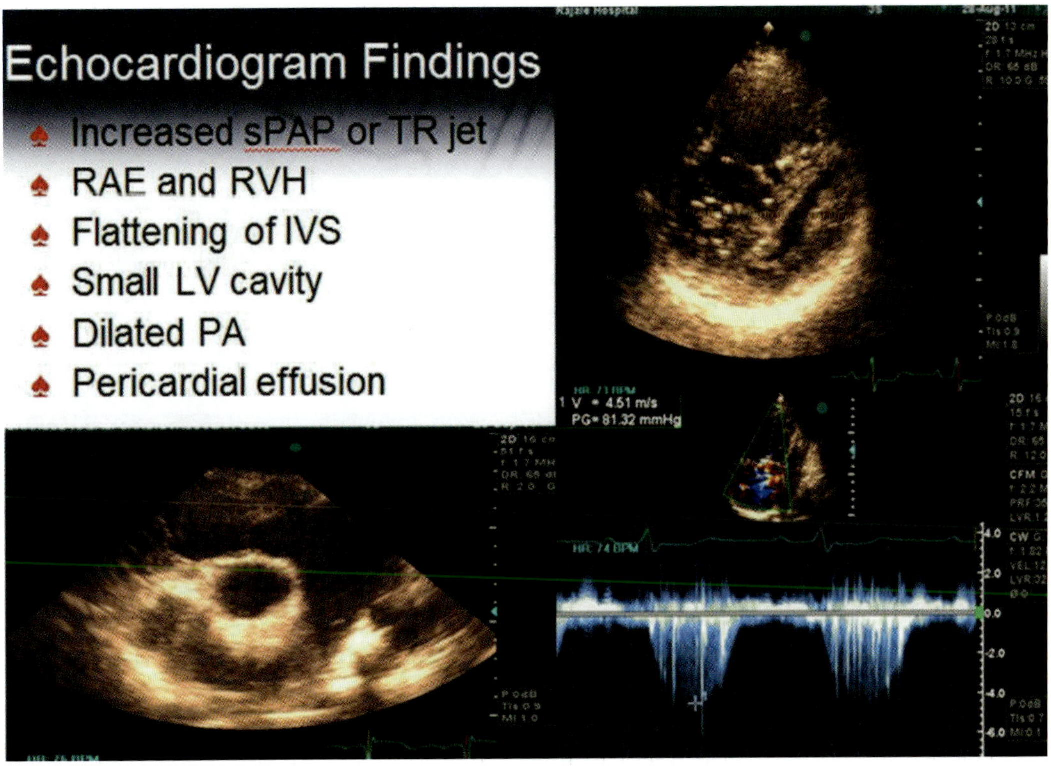

Fig. 15.1 Showing additional echocardiographic variables suggestive of PH

- PH unlikely when TR peak velocity is <2.8 m/s (assuming normal RAP about 5 mmHg) or (sPAP is <36 mmHg) with no additional variables suggestive for PH
- Possible PH when TR peak velocity is between 2.9 and 3.4 m/s (or sPAP is between 37 and 50 mmHg), with or without additional echocardiographic signs for suggestive of PH, or when TR peak velocity is <2.8 m/s (or sPAP is <36 mmHg) with additional variables suggestive for PH
- PH likely when TR peak velocity is >3.4 m/s (or sPAP is >50 mmHg), with or without additional echocardiographic variables suggestive for PH

However, there are additional variables (Figs. 15.1 and 15.2) that suggest PH although tend to occur late in the course of PAH as the following:

- Increased pulmonary regurgitant velocity
- RV hypertrophy (RVH) or dilation
- Short acceleration time of RV ejection
- Abnormal shape of inter ventricular septum (IVS)
- Dilated main PA

Janda et al. [15] in a meta-analysis of 29 studies showed 83 % (95 % CI 73–90) sensitivity and 72 % (95 % CI 53–85; $n=12$) specificity for echocardiographic diagnosis of pulmonary hypertension. They concluded that although echocardiography is a useful and noninvasive modality for initial assessment of PAP, but due to its limitations, RHC should be used for definite diagnosis and monitoring PAH.

Based on the guideline, echocardiographic parameters with established prognostic value are pericardial effusion and tricuspid annular plane systolic excursion (TAPSE) <1.5 cm [1].

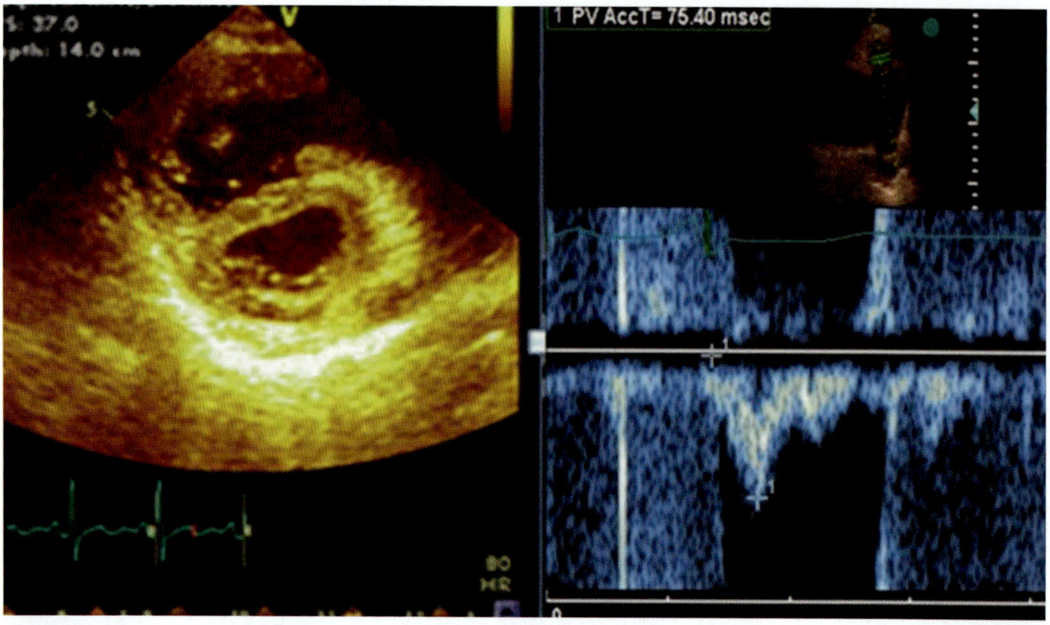

Fig. 15.2 Showing short acceleration time (AT) of RV ejection and abnormal IVS as systolic flattening of *IVS* interventricular septum

Cardiac Computed Tomography

Dilated main pulmonary artery exceeding the ascending aorta or main PA ≥ 29 mm at its widest point has been suggested accurate parameter for diagnosis of PH (with positive predictive value more than 95 % and a specificity of 89 %) [1].

Cardiac Magnetic Resonance (CMR)

CMR is not recommended for patients with pulmonary hypertension as a routine [1]. However, CMR is particularly useful in patient with PAH associated with CHD. CMR accurately, with a high degree of reproducibility assesses the RV size and function which has an important prognostic role in PAH.

Cardiac Catheterization

Cardiac catheterization allows the direct measurement of the pulmonary pressures, establishment of the diagnosis of pulmonary artery hypertension, and assessment of the severity of pulmonary vascular disease. It also could aid us in the future treatment planning through the assessment of the reactivity of the pulmonary vasculature to pulmonary arterial vasodilators. Right heart catheterization (RHC) is the gold standard for the definite diagnosis of PAH.

Open Lung Biopsy

Currently, open lung biopsy has a very limited role in the diagnosis or management of patients with the Eisenmenger physiology.

Complications

A summary of the complications seen in patients with the Eisenmenger physiology is depicted in Table 15.3.

Prognosis

Median age at death for patients with the Eisenmenger syndrome is 53 years (i.e., 20 years less than expected). However, patients with the Eisenmenger syndrome have a substantially better long-term prognosis than patients with primary pulmonary hypertension.

Table 15.3 Clinical complications of Eisenmenger syndrome

Cyanotic complications	Hematologic complications
	Thrombosis
	Bleeding
	Hyperviscosity
	Iron deficiency
	Central nervous system
	Rheumatologic complications
	Renal and gastrointestinal dysfunction
	Endocarditis
Non-cyanotic complications	Hemoptysis
	Pulmonary artery complications
	Aneurysms
	Thrombi
	Rupture
	Arrhythmias
	Atrial flutter
	Atrial fibrillation
	Ventricular tachycardia (rare)
	Progressive valvular disease
	Congestive heart failure
	Sudden death

Long-term survival of patients with the Eisenmenger syndrome usually depends on:

- The patient's age at the onset of pulmonary hypertension.
- Poor functional class [16].
- Syncope.
- Complex CHD.
- Arrhythmias.
- Worsened hypoxemia [16].
- Higher serum creatinine and uric acid levels.
- Right ventricular dysfunction.
- Left ventricular systemic dysfunction [16].
- Right ventricular hypertrophy.
- It has been suggested that voltage criteria for RVH, derived as the sum of the R-wave amplitude in V_1 and the maximum amplitude of the S wave in V_5 or V_6, may provide prognostic information in patients with the Eisenmenger physiology [16].
- QRS duration in the ECG.
- Down's syndrome.
- Reduced peak oxygen consumption and 6-min walk distance are associated with impaired prognosis in patients with pulmonary artery hypertension [17–19].
- Pulmonary vasoreactivity was recently shown to have prognostic value for adult patients with the Eisenmenger physiology [20].
- Right ventricular function affects survival predominantly.

The immediate causes of death in the Eisenmenger syndrome include pulmonary ventricular failure, severe hemoptysis from bronchial artery rupture or pulmonary infarction, complications during pregnancy, and cerebral vascular events including occlusive strokes, systemic paradoxical embolization, and brain abscesses [21–23]. Death also occurs during noncardiac surgeries.

Management Strategies

General Considerations

Patients with the Eisenmenger syndrome should avoid the following activities or exposures:

- Pregnancy.
- Dehydration.
- Moderate and severe strenuous exercise, particularly isometric exercise.
- Acute exposure to excessive heat (e.g., hot tub or sauna).
- Chronic high-altitude exposure (particularly at an elevation >5,000 feet above the sea level).
- Iron deficiency.
- Arrhythmias and infections should be promptly treated in patients with the Eisenmenger syndrome.

The principal medical treatment approaches in patients with the Eisenmenger physiology are primarily symptomatic and may include:

- Oxygen therapy.
- Therapeutic phlebotomy or erythropheresis should only be performed if the hemoglobin is >20 g per dL and the hematocrit is >65 % with associated symptoms of hyperviscosity and no evidence of dehydration.
- Iron replacement in patients with iron deficiency.

- Medical treatment of congestive heart failure.
- Antiarrhythmic for atrial arrhythmias.
- Pulmonary vasodilators such as endothelin receptor antagonists or phosphodiesterase inhibitors to improve the symptoms of pulmonary hypertension.

However, corrective surgeries or lung/heart-lung transplantation may also be considered in selected patients.

References

1. Galie N, Hoeper MM, Humbert M, et al. Guidelines for the diagnosis and treatment of pulmonary hypertension. Eur Respir J. 2009;34:1219–63.
2. Galiè N, Hoeper MM, Humbert M, et al. Guidelines for the diagnosis and treatment of pulmonary hypertension: the Task Force for the Diagnosis and Treatment of Pulmonary Hypertension of the European Society of Cardiology (ESC) and the European Respiratory Society (ERS), endorsed by the International Society of Heart and Lung Transplantation (ISHLT). Eur Heart J. 2009;30:2493–537.
3. McLaughlin V, Archer SL, Badesch DB, et al. Expert consensus document on pulmonary hypertension. J Am Coll Cardiol. 2009;53(17):1573–619.
4. Kidd L, Driscoll DJ, Gersony WM, et al. Second natural history study of congenital heart defects: results of treatment of patients with ventricular septal defects. Circulation. 1993;87:138–51.
5. Baumgartner H, Bonhoeffer P, De Groot NM, et al. ESC Guidelines for the management of grown-up congenital heart disease (new version 2010). Task Force on the Management of Grown-up Congenital Heart Disease of the European Society of Cardiology (ESC); Association for European Paediatric Cardiology (AEPC); ESC Committee for Practice Guidelines (CPG). Eur Heart J. 2010; 31(23):2915–57.
6. Eisenmenger V. Die angeborenen Defekte der Kammerscheidewände des Herzens. Zeitschr Klin Med. 1897;32:1–28.
7. Partin C. The evolution of Eisenmenger's eponymic enshrinement. Am J Cardiol. 2003;92:1187–91.
8. Wood P. The Eisenmenger syndrome or pulmonary hypertension with reversed central shunt. BMJ. 1958;46:755–62.
9. Oechslin EN, Harrison DA, Connelly MS, et al. Mode of death in adults with congenital heart disease. Am J Cardiol. 2000;86:1111–6.
10. Barst RJ, Mc Goon M, Torbicki A, et al. Diagnosis and differential assessment of pulmonary arterial hypertension. J Am Coll Cardiol. 2004;43(Suppl S): 40S–7.
11. Simonneau G, Galie N, Rubin LJ, et al. Clinical classification of pulmonary hypertension. J Am Coll Cardiol. 2004;43(suppl S):5S–12.
12. Farber HW, Loscalzo J. Pulmonary arterial hypertension. N Engl J Med. 2004;351:1655–65.
13. Ghofrani HA, Wiedemann R, Rose F, et al. Sildenafil for treatment of lung fibrosis and pulmonary hypertension: a randomized controlled trial. Lancet. 2002;360:895–900.
14. Hillis LD, Lange RA, Winniford MD, et al. Manual of clinical problems in cardiology, with annotated key references. Philadelphia: Lippincott Williams & Wilkins; 2003. ISBN 0781723817.
15. Janda S, Shahidi N, Gin K, Swiston J. Diagnostic accuracy of echocardiography for pulmonary hypertension: a systematic review and meta-analysis. Heart. 2011;97(8):612–22.
16. Cantor WJ, Harrison DA, Moussadji JS, et al. Determinants of survival and length of survival in adults with Eisenmenger syndrome. Am J Cardiol. 1999;84:677–81.
17. Wensel R, Opitz CF, Anker SD, Winkler J, Hoffken G, Kleber FX, Sharma R, Hummel M, Hetzer R, Ewert R. Assessment of survival in patients with primary pulmonary hypertension: importance of cardiopulmonary exercise testing. Circulation. 2002;106:319–24.
18. Miyamoto S, Nagaya N, Satoh T, Kyotani S, Sakamaki F, Fujita M, Nakanishi N, Miyatake K. Clinical correlates and prognostic significance of six-minute walk test in patients with primary pulmonary hypertension: comparison with cardiopulmonary exercise testing. Am J Respir Crit Care Med. 2000;161:487–92.
19. Paciocco G, Martinez FJ, Bossone E, Pielsticker E, Gillespie B, Rubenfire M. Oxygen desaturation on the six-minute walk test and mortality in untreated primary pulmonary hypertension. Eur Respir J. 2001;17:647–52.
20. Post MC, Janssens S, Van de Werf F, Budts W. Responsiveness to inhaled nitric oxide is a predictor for mid-term survival in adult patients with congenital heart defects and pulmonary arterial hypertension. Eur Heart J. 2004;25:1651–6.
21. Daliento L, Somerville J, Presbitero P, et al. Eisenmenger syndrome. Factors relating to deterioration and death. Eur Heart J. 1998;19:1845–55.
22. Saha A, Balakrishnan KG, Jaiswal PK, et al. Prognosis for patients with Eisenmenger syndrome of various aetiology. Int J Cardiol. 1994;45:199–207.
23. Vongpatanasin W, Brickner ME, Hillis LD, Lange RA. The Eisenmenger syndrome in adults. Ann Intern Med. 1998;128:745–55.

Cardiac Catheterization in Congenital Heart Disease

16

Shabnam Mohammadzadeh
and Mohammad Mahdavi

Keywords
Congenital heart disease (CHD) • Cardiac catheterization • Angiography • Pulmonary vascular resistance • Coronary anomalies

Cardiac Catheterization in Adult Congenital Heart Disease

The role of heart catheterization in patient management continues to evolve as anatomic and physiologic imaging with cardiac magnetic resonance imaging (CMR) and computed tomography (CT) improves and as the breadth of interventional catheter techniques dramatically widens [1, 2].

Indications for Cardiac Catheterization in Adult Congenital Heart Disease (ACHD)

Catheterization is the only gold standard method of pressure measurement in a vessel or a chamber. Pulmonary artery pressure and pulmonary vascular resistance, two values of utmost importance in patients with congenital heart disease (CHD), can be determined accurately by catheterization. There are a number of situations in which noninvasive imaging cannot provide the anatomic detail required for decision-making, and that is where the role of diagnostic catheterization becomes much more salient in CHD [1].

The three major indications for performing a diagnostic cardiac catheterization are as follows [3]:

1. A complete anatomic diagnosis or necessary hemodynamic information cannot be obtained by noninvasive methods.
2. Clinical signs and symptoms are not consistent with the patient's diagnosis.
3. The patient's clinical course is not progressing as expected.

Planning the Procedure

An exhaustive appraisal of the patient's clinic chart and paying due heed not only to the structural anatomy but also to the details of previous surgical repairs is of vital importance. Review of serial imaging and previous hemodynamic and angiocardiographic evaluations helps to consolidate an understanding of potential problems or issues requiring specific attention at the time of catheterization that may not be readily apparent.

S. Mohammadzadeh, MD (✉)
Department of cardiology,
Emam Khomeini General Hospital, Tehran, Iran
e-mail: dewsfar@yahoo.com

M. Mahdavi, MD
Pediatric Ward, Department of Pediatric Cardiology,
Rajaie Cardiovascular Medical and Research Center,
Iran University of Medical Science, Tehran, Iran

A. Sadeghpour et al. (eds.), *Comprehensive Approach to Adult Congenital Heart Disease*,
DOI 10.1007/978-1-4471-6383 1_16, © Springer-Verlag London 2014

The operator must have a thorough understanding of the anatomy and physiology of congenital cardiac defects and with the concomitant pathologies that might be present along with the primary disorder. Furthermore, the operator should be able to prioritize the information as to its level of importance. Information can be placed in the following categories:

1. Information that is absolutely essential to establish the diagnosis or plan the treatment
2. Information that is useful but not critical
3. Information that is already available from other imaging studies

Prioritization of such information and the resulting preparedness can significantly lessen the duration of the procedure and thus minimize exposure to radiation and the amount of contrast media. It is crucial to avoid unnecessary renal injury through the pointless utilization of large volumes of contrast agent to show an anatomy previously assessed through other imaging modalities.

Management choice normally necessitates the measurement of pulmonary artery pressure, pulmonary artery resistance, pulmonary vasculature reactivity, and shunt calculations. If access to the pulmonary artery is difficult, time invested here may be far more valuable than reevaluating other data already acquired from other diagnostic methods. Such information should be acquired in a steady state, and the occurrence of vagal reaction, administration of certain drugs such as atropine, and pain from the access site may lead to inaccuracy. An appropriate amount of sedation for most adults is mandatory; oversedation usually elevates pulmonary pressure, pulmonary resistance, and arterial hypoxemia [1, 4, 5].

To summarize, it is essential that the operator have the following checklist at the beginning of the procedure:

1. What constitutes critical hemodynamic information?
2. Which chamber(s) and great vessel(s) require angiography?
3. Must the coronary anatomy be determined?
4. What catheters will be most useful?
5. What constitutes the sequence to be followed throughout the procedure?

Catheter Course

The normal course of the catheter through the right side of the heart and into the pulmonary artery or through the arterial system into the left side of the heart should be easily recognizable, although there are some variations (Fig. 16.1) [6, 7].

The most common catheter positions in ACHD are depicted in anteroposterior and lateral projections in (Figs. 16.2, 16.3, 16.4, 16.5, 16.6, 16.7, 16.8, 16.9, 16.10, 16.11, 16.12, 16.13, 16.14, and 16.15).

Pressure Measurements

Waveforms

Right Atrial Pressure (RAP)

Normal waveform consists of two or three positive waves (a, c, and v) and three negative waves (x, x′, and y, respectively). The a wave denotes atrial contraction. The x decent follows the a wave and reflects atrial relaxation, followed by

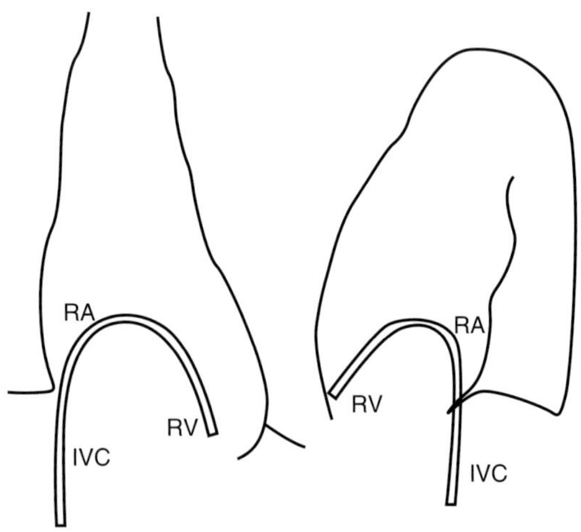

Fig. 16.1 Normal right heart catheter course: Catheter passes from inferior vena cava through right atrium anteriorly into right ventricle. *IVC* inferior vena cava, *RA* right atrium, *RV* right ventricle

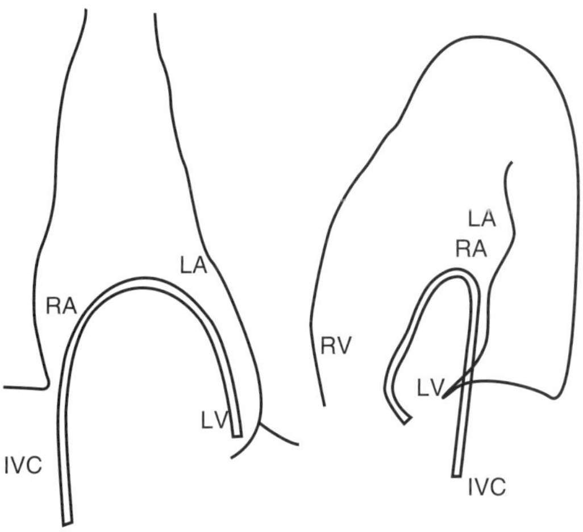

Fig. 16.2 Left ventricle: Catheter passes from inferior vena cava (*IVC*) across atrial septum, then inferiorly and posteriorly into left ventricle (*LV*), *LA* left atrium, *RA* right atrium, *RV* right ventricle

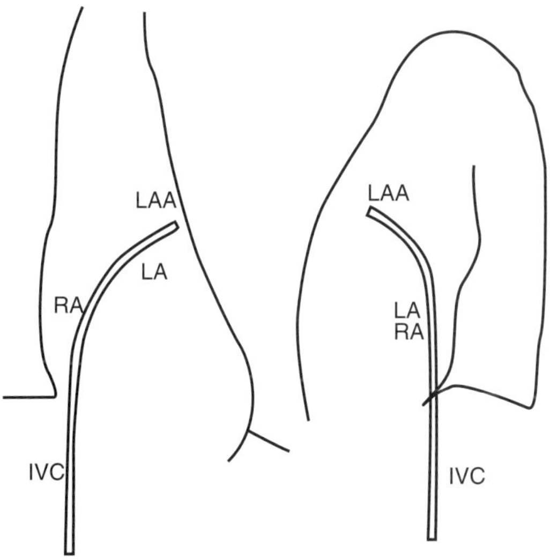

Fig. 16.3 Left atrial appendage: Catheter passes from inferior vena cava (*IVC*), through atrial septum, and superiorly and leftward into left atrial appendage (*LAA*). *RA* right atrium, *LA* left atrium

tricuspid valve closure. The c wave is sometimes evident and is due to ventricular systole as the closed tricuspid valve bulges into the atrium. The subsequent x′ decent results from the combined effects of continued atrial relaxation and descent of the tricuspid valve during continued ventricular contraction. The wave that follows is the v wave,

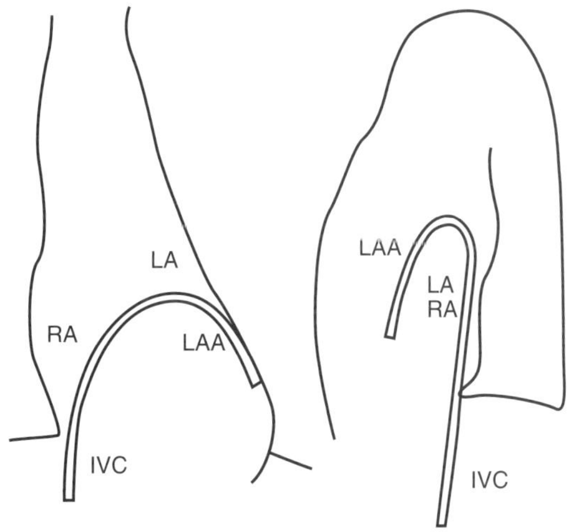

Fig. 16.4 Pericardial sac, through left atrial appendage: Catheter enters heart from inferior vena cava (*IVC*), passes from right atrium (*RA*) to left atrium (*LA*), and then follows cardiac border. This course may mimic passage into the left lower pulmonary vein (LLPV), but blood cannot be withdrawn, pressure is negative, and injection of a minute amount of contrast material confirms location. *LAA* left atrial appendix

which denoted atrial filling, while the atrioventricular valve (AVV) is still closed. The opening of the AVV, followed by atrial emptying, is represented by the y descent [3, 8–11].

Right Ventricular Pressure (RVP)

Normal (subpulmonary) right ventricular (RV) pressure also varies considerably with age, respiratory status, heart rhythm, structure, and function. Peak systolic pressure is typically 20–30 mmHg. End-diastolic pressure is typically equal or just slightly less than the right atrial a wave at 3–6 mmHg. RV waveform is marked by a rapid rise during isovolumetric contraction, followed by the peak systolic pressure before isovolumetric relaxation and a fall to minimum diastolic pressure (often near zero). There is a slow rise during diastolic filling, during which a small RV "a wave" inflection may be seen as a result of atrial contraction just prior to end-diastole and subsequent isovolumic contraction. This a wave is sometimes referred to as the atrial kick, with first-degree AV bock. Peak RV systolic pressure is elevated in the presence of any

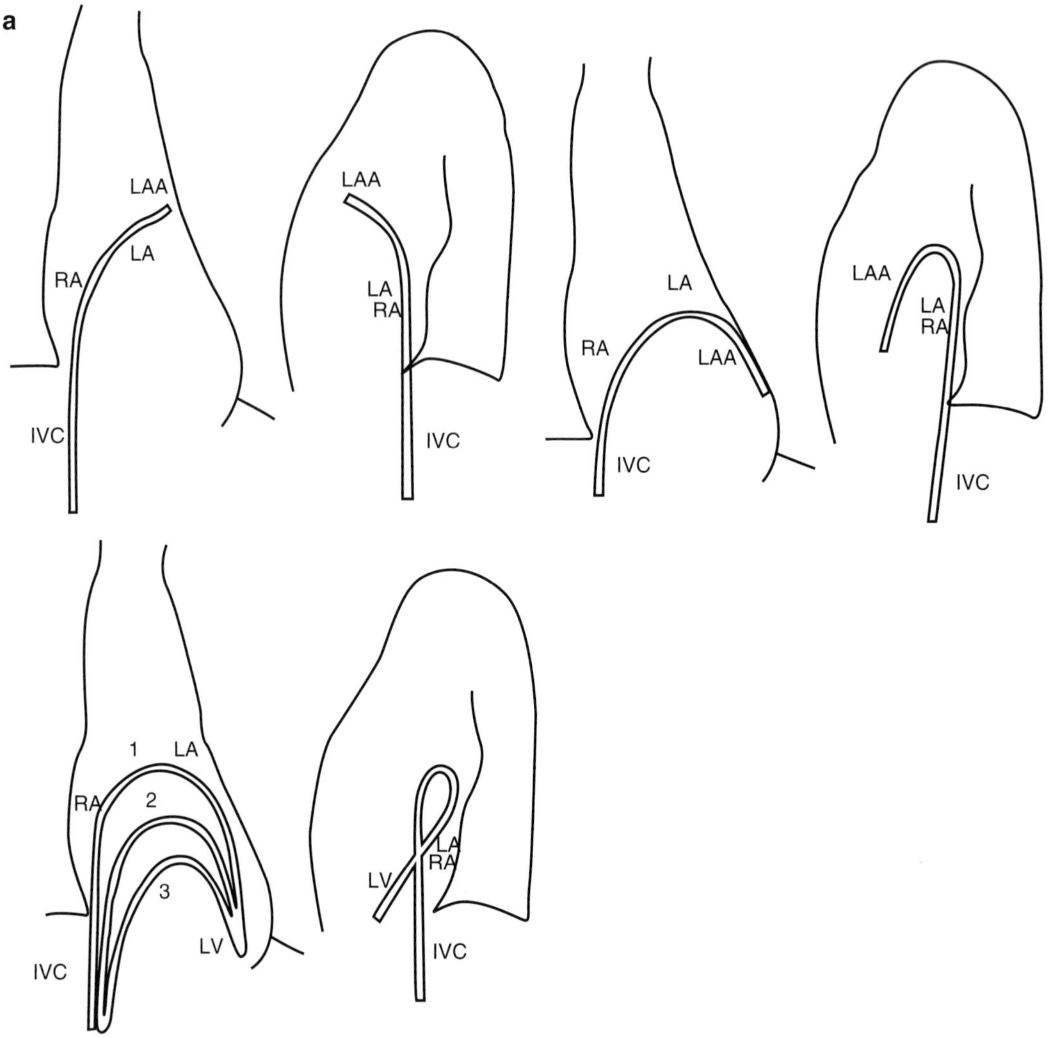

Fig. 16.5 (**a**) Atrial septal defects: Catheter passed from inferior vena cava (*IVC*), through various atrial defects. (*1*) The most superior catheter has passed through a sinus venosus. (*2*) The lower one through an ostium secundum. (*3*) The lowest through an ostium primum defect. (**b**) Left upper pulmonary vein (LUPV): Catheter enters heart from inferior vena cava (*IVC*), passes from right atrium (*RA*) to left atrium (*LA*), and leaves cardiac silhouette into left lung field. On lateral projection, however, it is located within cardiac shadow. (**c**) Left lower pulmonary vein (*LLPV*): Catheter passes from inferior vena cava (*IVC*) through right atrium (*RA*) and left atrium (*LA*) into LLPV. On lateral projection catheter is posteriorly in lung field. This course is more common with catheterization from the IVC because the catheter tip is guided by the limbus of the fossa ovalis. (**d**) Right upper pulmonary vein (*RUPV*): Catheter passes from inferior vena cava (IVC) through right atrium (RA) and ultimately to RUPV. Usually, this course is through a patent foramen ovale. Rarely, it indicates direct connection of pulmonary vein to right atrium. (**e**) Partial anomalous pulmonary venous connection (PAPVC) of right upper pulmonary vein (*RUPV*) to superior vena cava (*SVC*): Catheter passes from inferior vena cava (*IVC*) through right atrium (*RA*) and proximal superior vena cava into right upper lung field. *LA* left atrium, *RA* right atrium, *LV* left ventricle, *LAA* left atrial appendix

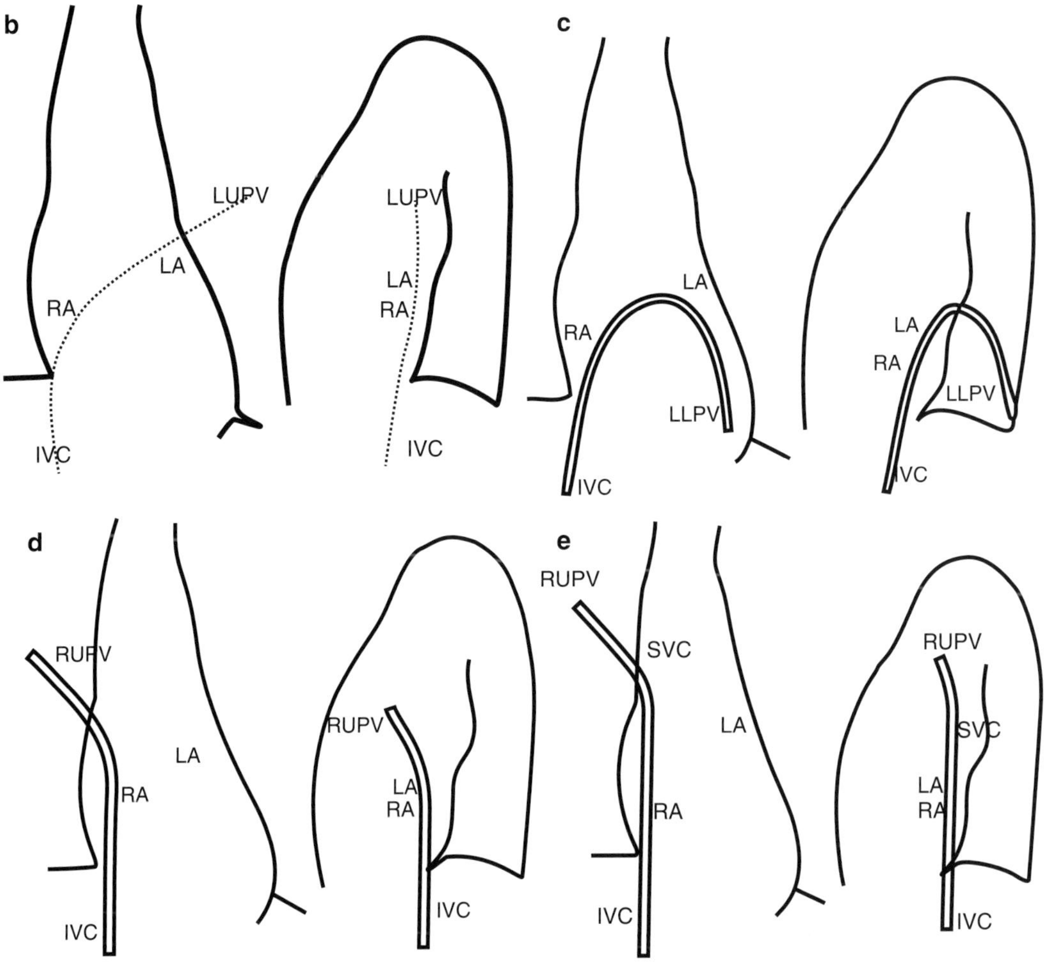

Fig. 16.5 (continued)

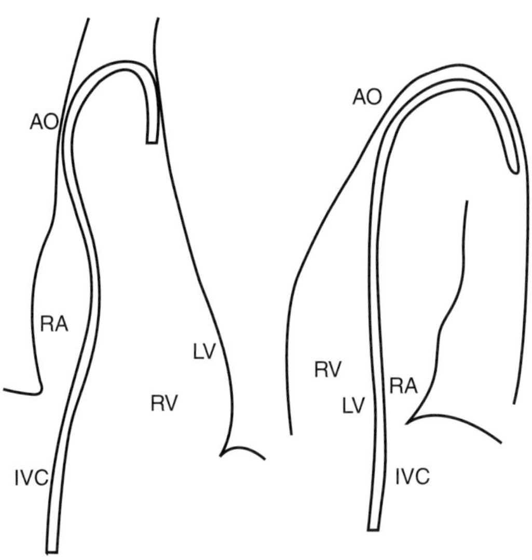

Fig. 16.6 Membranous ventricular septal defect (*VSD*): Catheter enters heart from inferior vena cava (*IVC*), passes through tricuspid valve following typical course close to spine, through ventricular septal defect, and into the aortic arch. *AO* aorta, *RA* right atrium, *RV* right ventricle, *LV* left ventricle

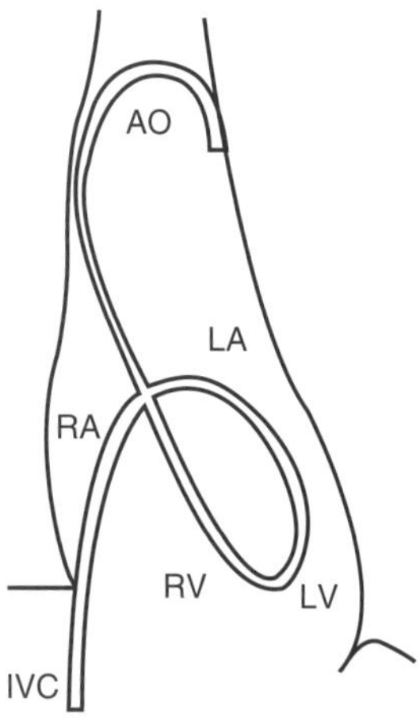

Fig. 16.7 Ascending aorta through patent foramen ovale: Catheter enters heart from inferior vena cava (*IVC*), passes from right atrium (*RA*) to left atrium (*LA*) through area of foramen ovale, and into left ventricle (*LV*), where it curves upon itself and then shows typical course through ascending aorta (*AO*) and aortic arch. *RV* right ventricle

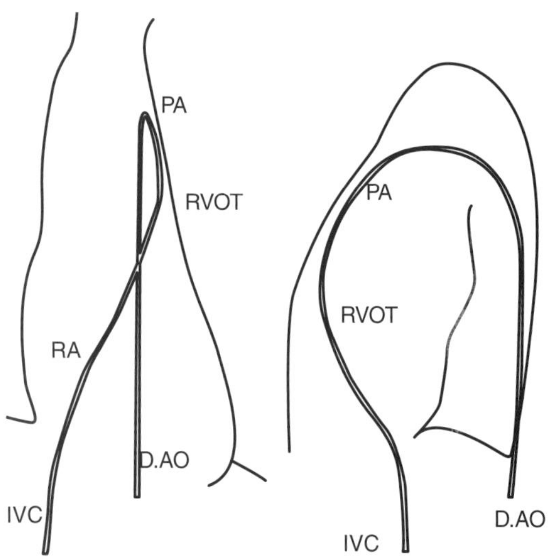

Fig. 16.8 Patent ductus arteriosus (PDA) or Potts anastomosis: Catheter passes from inferior vena cava (*IVC*) through right atrium (*RA*) and right ventricle (*RV*) into pulmonary trunk. On lateral projection, posterior direction of passage from pulmonary artery (*PA*) to aorta (*AO*) is evident. The catheter is then advanced below the diaphragm, confirming its location in the aorta. It is this important subdiaphragmatic location of the catheter which rules out the much more common passage into a left pulmonary artery

downstream obstruction, including RV outflow obstruction (subpulmonary stenosis or valvular pulmonary stenosis), main or branch pulmonary

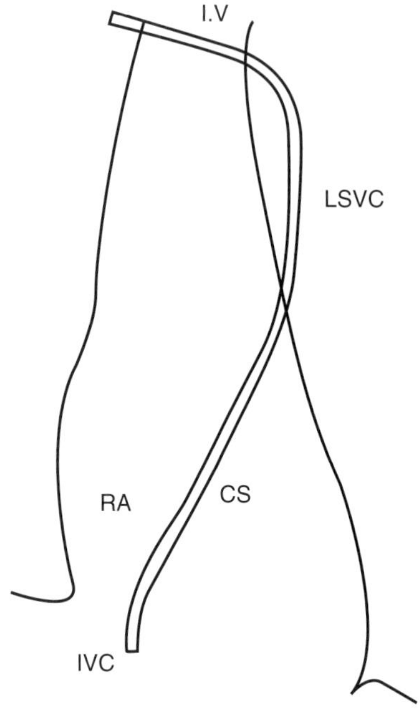

Fig. 16.9 Coronary sinus (*CS*) and left superior vena cava (*LSVC*): Catheter passes from superior vena cava (*SVC*) into right atrium (*RA*) and then posteriorly and into typical "reverse J" shape. On the anteroposterior projection, catheter position could be mistaken for right ventricle. Catheter can be advanced superiorly beyond cardiac contour into LSVC. *IVC* inferior vena cava

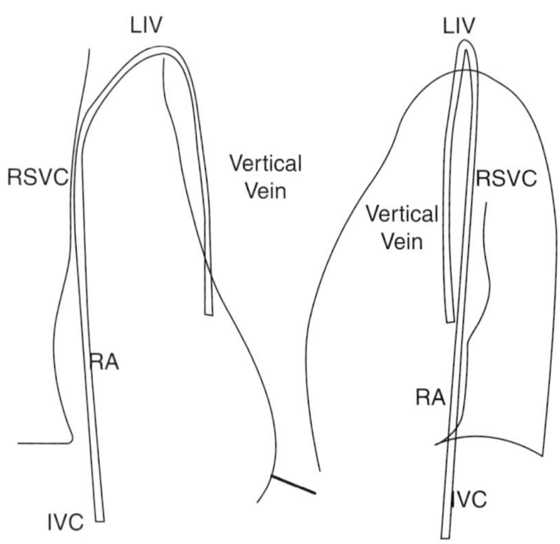

Fig. 16.10 Vertical vein in total anomalous pulmonary venous connection (TAPVC): Catheter passes from inferior vena cava (*IVC*) to right superior vena cava (*RSVC*). Left innominate vein (*LIV*) and vertical vein. If oxygen saturation is high, partial or total anomalous venous return must be considered. *RA* right atrium

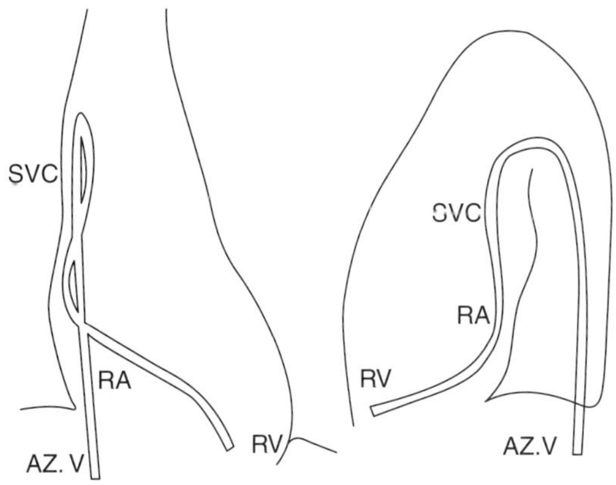

Fig. 16.11 Interruption of the inferior vena cava with azygos vein (*AZ.V*) continuation. On anteroposterior projection, leading portion of catheter appears within cardiac silhouette, but on lateral projection, it lies behind the heart in azygous vein and passes anteriorly into superior vena cava (*SVC*). Once there, it passes inferiorly into right atrium (*RA*) and, typically, into apex of right ventricle (*RV*)

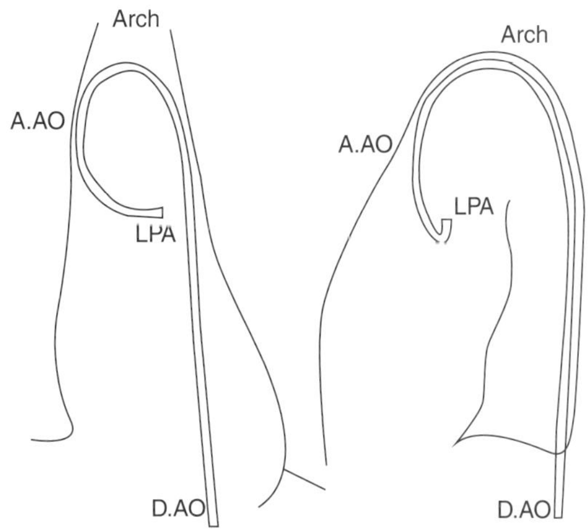

Fig. 16.13 Pots shunt: Catheter passes through aortic arch. Above aortic valve, catheter passes leftward into proximal left pulmonary artery (*LPA*). *D.AO* descending aorta, *A.AO* ascending aorta

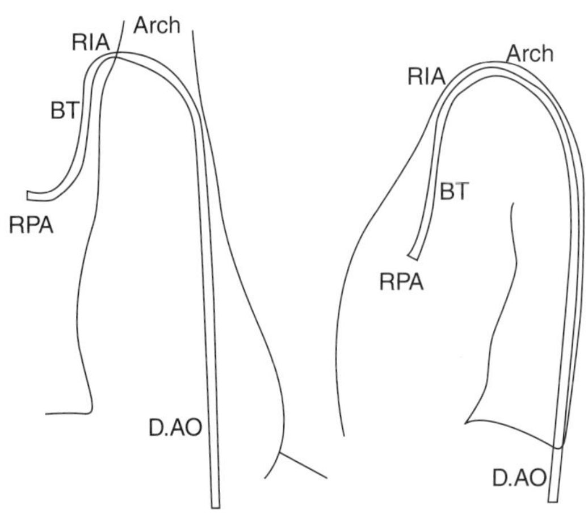

Fig. 16.12 Right Blalock-Taussig (*BT*) shunt: Catheter passes through aortic arch, into innominate artery (IA), and through shunt into right pulmonary artery (*RPA*). *RIA* right innominate artery, *D.AO* descending aorta

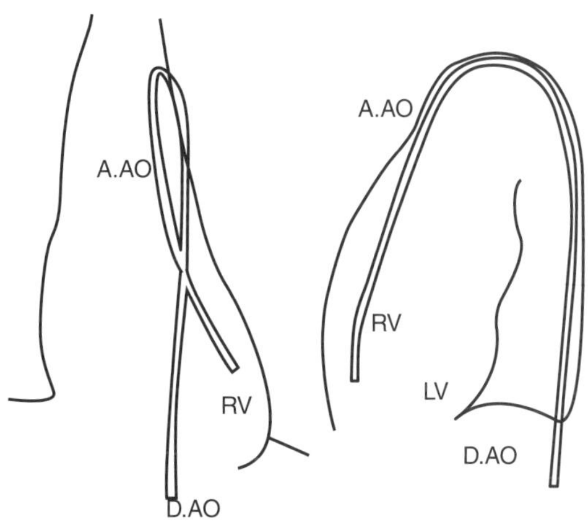

Fig. 16.14 Congenitally corrected transposition (arterial approach): Catheter passes through descending aorta (*D. O*) and aortic arch. The ascending aorta (*A.AO*) is located anteriorly and to the left. The catheter enters the systemic ventricle, located anteriorly and to the left (*RV*). *LV* left ventricle

artery stenosis, elevated pulmonary vascular resistance (PVR) (pulmonary hypertension), or any lesion causing significant pulmonary venous or left atrial hypertension [3, 8–11].

Pulmonary Artery Pressure (PAP)

The mean pulmonary artery pressure (PAP) is usually less than 20 mmHg, with a systolic peak equal to or slightly less than that of RVP. The pressure pulse is characterized by a relatively slow upstroke, peak systolic pressure, small dicrotic notch, and slow fall to end-diastole. The PAP tracing provides, in a single waveform, a significant insight into both right and left heart hemodynamics. If the operators arrive at PA through the right atrium and ventricle, a peak systolic pressure significantly lower (>10 mmHg) than RVP denotes RV outflow tract obstruction, which deserves further characterization to distinguish subvalvular,

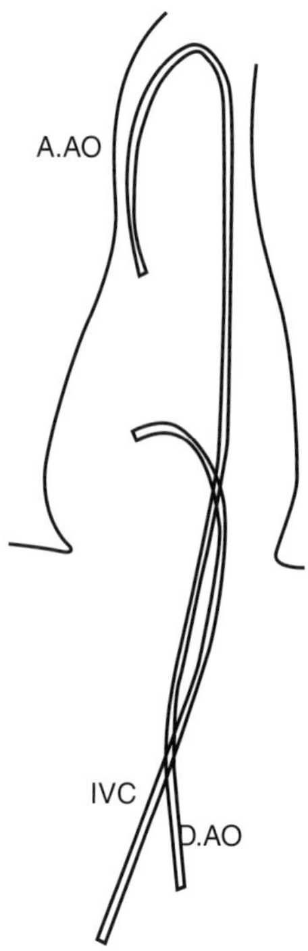

Fig. 16.15 Situs ambiguous (abdominal heterotaxia): Both venous and arterial catheters are to the left of the spine and cross in abdomen, indicating an indeterminate (ambiguous) situs. *D.AO* descending aorta, *A.AO* ascending aorta, *IVC* inferior vena cava

valvular, or supravalvular stenosis. Normally, there is a demonstrable diastolic pressure gradient between PA and RV, the absence of which suggests truly "free" pulmonary regurgitation. Otherwise, PA diastolic pressure more typically approaches LA pressure. Elevated PAP can occur with either increased flow (e.g., ventricular septal defect [VSD]), increased resistance (e.g., pulmonary vascular occlusive disease [PVOD]), or downstream obstruction (e.g., left atrial hypertension). As such, it is important to use precise and unambiguous terminology. Remember that PA hypertension, that is, high PAP, is not synonymous with high pulmonary vascular resistance. For example, elevated PAP can occur with an unrestrictive VSD and normal pulmonary resistance. Full hemodynamic assessment is critical to distinguish between these inasmuch as important management decisions are based on the ability to manipulate the underlying process (e.g., the operator can replace/dilate a stenotic mitral valve, but he/she cannot as easily replace end-stage PVOD-affected lungs) [3, 8–11].

Pulmonary Capillary Wedge Pressure (PCWP)

A good pulmonary capillary wedge pressure (PCWP) resembles left atrial pressure and waveform with a time delay of somewhere between 0.02 and 0.08 s unless there are significant collaterals or pulmonary vein stenosis. As such, this waveform should have interpretable a and v waves and normal respiratory variation. An underwedged tracing usually has exaggerated systolic peaks as PAP is transmitted around the catheter. An overwedged PCWP typically lacks identifiable waveform morphology with a high drifting mean pressure [3, 8–11].

Left Atrial Pressure (LAP)

In the normal heart, left atrial pressure (LAP) is higher than right atrial pressure, with mean pressures in the range of 6–9 mmHg. Even with respiratory variation, LAP is never normally below atmospheric pressure. The right and left atrial pressure waveforms are similar, but the v wave is usually dominant in the LA, presumably because of pulmonary venous contraction (e.g., the left atrial a wave is dominant in total anomalous pulmonary venous connection [TAPVC]). Increased a waves may be seen in mitral stenosis or in situations of poor LV compliance. Prosthetic mitral valves in the supra-annular position characteristically result in an increased v wave, probably due to the combined effects of a small, noncompliant LA and pulmonary venous contraction. However, increased v waves are more classically seen in mitral regurgitation. Overall, an increased LAP can result from any of the above situations, significant left-to-right shunts, or LV dysfunction [3, 8–11].

Pulmonary Vein Wedge Pressure (PVWP)

Pulmonary venous wedge pressure (PVWP) operates under the same principle as PCWP, but in the opposite direction, and provides a reasonable estimate of PAP (albeit often slightly underestimating), when the mean pressure obtained is less than 15 mmHg. (Above this, it is imprecise.) When PAP is a major reason for catheterization and the patient is potentially unstable or access to the PAs may make him so, this can provide a quick estimate in case things go awry [3, 8–11].

Left Ventricular Pressure (LVP)

Left ventricular pressure (LVP) varies with age and a host of structural and hemodynamic factors. Peak systolic pressure should equal ascending aortic pressure, failing which there must be is subvalvular, valvular, or supravalvular obstruction that warrants further characterization. LV end-diastolic pressure (LVEDP) is a crude but valuable marker for LV diastolic health, in that elevated LVEDP (>10–12 mmHg in children) suggests poor diastolic ventricular properties and/or LV failure. Similarly, a steep slope of the diastolic portion of the LV waveform suggests poor ventricular compliance. "Normal" pressures vary according to age, with a progressive increase in the average LVEDP as patients progress to old age [3, 8–11].

Aortic Pressure

The aortic pressure pulse varies uniquely in morphology in health and disease, much of which is due to the timing and magnitude of the reflected waves. Generally, there is systolic rise, peak aortic pressure, and a variable dicrotic notch on the downstroke. The pulse pressure in the ascending aorta is usually 25–50 mmHg or <50 % of peak systolic aortic pressure. A widened pulse pressure (systolic minus diastolic pressure) is characteristic of "runoff" lesions, including significant aortic (or neoaortic) regurgitation, patent ductus arteriosus (PDA), surgical shunts or significant aortopulmonary collaterals, truncus arteriosus, systemic AV fistula, and ruptured sinus of Valsalva. More commonly in adults than children, a widened pulse pressure may be seen in the setting of arterial stiffening and bradycardia. In contrast, a decreased or "narrow" pulse pressure may be seen in low cardiac output states and/or tamponade. A gradient between the ascending and descending aorta suggests coarctation of the aorta [3, 8–11].

Flows and Shunts

Sample Run

Oxygen saturation data play a significant role in the decision-making process for an ACHD patient. The first saturation sample should be obtained from systemic blood. Arterial desaturation may be in consequence of right-to-left shunting or ventilation/perfusion mismatch. In the adult catheterization laboratory, arterial desaturation often tends to be the result of hypoventilation following sedation. In the sedated patient, a rise in CO_2 is likely to significantly influence pulmonary pressures and oximetry. Systemic venous saturation lower than 50 % requires that low cardiac output be taken into account and high saturation could signify either a high-output state or a left-to-right shunt. Calculation of shunts, cardiac output, and resistances are conditional on an accurate determination of oxygen saturation. Of all physiologic data obtained in the adult catheterization laboratory, the least sensitive and most prone to error is oxygen saturation information.

When using oxygen as an indicator, the following points should be considered:

1. A steady-state blood flow is vitally important for all measurements.
2. A minimum of two samples should be taken from no fewer than three sites in rapid succession. This can be a tall order in a patient with complex congenital heart lesions. The estimation of oxygen consumption in the majority of adult catheterization laboratories is on the basis of the body surface area and is, as such, prone to significant errors (up to 30 %).

If the patient has low mixed venous saturation, the addition of even a small amount of fully saturated blood to the mixed venous blood can significantly intensify the downstream saturation.

If the patient has a high cardiac output and high mixed venous saturation, the addition of a small amount of fully saturated blood does not result in a quantifiable rise in the downstream mixed venous saturation. In the presence of multiple levels of shunting, the exact significance of each level is not based on oxygen saturation study at a particular chamber, and the most significant level or location of shunting is documented more optimally with other data (angiograms, pressure data, indicator curves, etc.) [1, 3–5].

Mixed Venous Saturation

Mixed venous blood saturation has three variable sources: the superior vena cava (SVC), inferior vena cava (IVC), and coronary sinus (CS). Due to these different sources, SVC oxygen saturation is liable to vary by 10 %. (There is lower saturation in the jugular vein by comparison with the subclavian and azygos veins.) Accordingly, no fewer than two separate samples should be obtained from these different sites. When the saturation levels of two separate samples do not fall within one or two percent of each other, we need a third sample from the SVC (from the mid SVC level) so as to ascertain which of the first two samples is more representative.

Oxygen saturation levels in the IVC are varied, with the flow varying by 10–20 %. The sample from the IVC is generally 5–10 % more saturated than that from the SVC. The very low saturation of the coronary sinus (25–45 %), despite the fact that it is responsible for 5–7% of the total venous return, can impact total mixed saturation. In the absence of shunts, a sample from the SVC (unless the patient has a low cardiac output) and the right atrium can provide a mixed venous sample. Some cardiologists use a weighted average of SVC and IVC blood as a mixed venous sample. If there is a shunt lesion, several samples should be obtained in rapid succession. A pulmonary vein sample may be 50–100 % disparate from a true mixed pulmonary venous sample. In the absence of a right-to-left shunt, it is advisable to use LV or aorta saturation as opposed to single pulmonary vein saturation. A pulmonary venous sample constitutes an integral part of the evaluation of the cause of arterial desaturation in acquired disease when a right-to-left shunt is in doubt through a patent foramen ovale (PFO) as a cause [1, 8].

Sampling

Samples should be drawn in rapid succession, i.e., no more than 1–2 min for the sampling run. Duplicate samples should be obtained if possible and should not differ by more than 1 or 2 %. The operator must be aware of the following sources of error:

1. Potential equipment malfunction (e.g., a very high hemoglobin level (>200 g/L) can lead to a false reading).
2. The operator should clear the flush solution and blood from the catheter after having drawn a sample and subsequently fill the catheter with the next sample blood.
3. The blood sample may contain microbubbles and this can lead to oxygenation.
4. The operator must avoid obtaining samples from the side arm of a bleed-back tap because it has a compartment in which there is a possibility of the contamination of the sample.

A rise in O_2 saturation in the downstream chamber is also referred to as "step-up." Step-up is of significance when it exceeds 9 % in the atrial level and 6 % in the ventricular level and pulmonary level [1–3, 12–16]. Various reasons for step-up in the different sides of the heart are listed in the table below (Table 16.1). The following points should be taken into account: [3]

1. The absence of a significant step-up in the right atrium does not completely rule out a left-to-right shunt.
2. If the aortic saturation is below 92 % (sea level, normal ventilation) or if there is a greater than 3 % drop in oxygen saturation on the left side of the heart, a right-to-left shunt may be present.
3. Administration of 100 % oxygen raises pulmonary vein and systemic artery saturation, making it possible to distinguish between pulmonary parenchymal disease and a right-to-left shunt. Pulmonary vein desaturation that does not resolve with the administration of 100 % oxygen suggests an intrapulmonary

Table 16.1 Various reasons for step-up in different side of the heart

A step-up of >9 % at atrial level	1. Left-to-right shunt from an atrial septal defect 2. Anomalous pulmonary venous connection 3. Left ventricle-to-right atrium shunt 4. Ventricular septal defect with tricuspid insufficiency 5. Shunt from the aorta (ruptured sinus of Valsalva aneurysm, coronary artery fistula)
A step-up of >6 % at ventricular level	1. Low atrial septal defect 2. Ventricular septal defect 3. Ruptured sinus of Valsalva aneurysm 4. Coronary atrioventricular fistula draining into the right ventricle 5. Left-to-right shunt at the great vessel level with significant pulmonary valve insufficiency
A step-up of >6 % at the pulmonary artery	1. High outlet ventricular septal defect 2. Patent ductus arteriosus 3. Aortopulmonary window 4. Coronary artery fistula into the pulmonary artery 5. Anomalous origin of the coronary artery from the pulmonary artery also with fistula 6. Surgical aortopulmonary communication

shunt (e.g., from a pulmonary arteriovenous malformation).

Reason for left heart side desaturation are listed in Table 16.2

Clinical Applications

In patients with CHD, a communication between the two sides of the heart or between the pulmonary artery and the aorta allows a shunt to exist. In such cases, the following calculations can be made [1]:

1. The magnitude of a left-to-right shunt and a right-to-left shunt
2. Pulmonary blood flow
3. Pulmonary-to-systemic flow ratio (QP/QS)

QP/QS is the most useful measurement of all in that it yields a reliable estimate of the rise or drop in the pulmonary blood flow. Calculation of QP/QS is also very simple because it only requires the oxygen saturation data from systemic arterial blood, left atrial or pulmonary venous blood, pulmonary artery, and vena cava and right-sided heart samples. The operator must obtain the samples in room air or a gas mixture containing a maximum of 30 % oxygen, or else, the saturation data may not provide accurate information on the pulmonary blood flow. Under such circumstances, the pulmonary blood flow is usually overestimated, resulting in the exaggeration of the Qp:Qs ratio.

Calculation of the Flow

The most used method for the calculation of the flow is the Fick method.

The Fick Method

Oxygen content (mL O_2/dL plasma): O_2 bound to the hemoglobin + dissolved O_2

Oxygen content:

$$(\mathrm{mLO_2/L}) = [(\text{Oxygen capacity} \times \mathrm{SpO_2}) + (\mathrm{pO_2} \times 0.003\,\mathrm{mL/mm\,Hg/dL})] \times 10\,\mathrm{dL/L}$$

Qs = VO_2/[hemoglobin × 1.36 × 10 × (Aorta saturation – MVO_2 sat)]

Qp = VO_2/[hemoglobin × 1.36 × 10 × (Pulmonary vein sat – Pulmonary arterial sat)]

Qep = VO_2/[hemoglobin × 1.36 × 10 × (Pulmonary vein sat – MVO_2 sat)]

where MVO2 = mixed venous saturation, Qs = systemic flow, Qp = pulmonary flow, and Qep = effective pulmonary flow [1].

Table 16.2 Reason for left heart side desaturation

Pulmonary vein desaturation	Hypoventilation(sedation)
	Pulmonary parenchymal disease
	Pulmonary edema
	Pulmonary atrioventricular malformation
Left atrial desaturation	Desaturated pulmonary vein
	Markedly decreases right ventricular compliance or right ventricular failure
	With normal pulmonary vein saturation, usually resulting from a right-to-left shunt through an atrial septal defect or patent foramen ovale
	Platypnea-orthodeoxia syndrome
	Persistent left superior vena cava to the left atrium
Left ventricular desaturation	Any lesion that produces desaturation in the pulmonary veins or left atrium
	Right-to-left shunting at the ventricular level occurs with right ventricular systolic pressure is equal to or greater than left ventricular systolic pressure
Aortic desaturation (step-down in aorta)	Patent ductus arteriosus with pulmonary hypertension or peripheral pulmonary stenosis
	Aortopulmonary window with pulmonary hypertension or peripheral pulmonary stenosis
Step-down between ascending and descending aorta	Combination of a patent ductus arteriosus and coarctation of the aorta with pulmonary hypertension

Pulmonary-to-Systemic Blood Flow Ratio

This calculation is based on the Fick principle. In other words, factors such as oxygen-carrying capacity and oxygen consumption employed for each single flow calculation nullify each other when we are estimating only the ratio of the two flows: [1, 4–13, 17]

$$Qp / Qs : (\text{Sat Ao} - \text{Sat MV}) / (\text{Sat PV} - \text{Sat PA})$$

where Sat Ao = aortic saturation, Sat MV = mixed venous saturation, Sat PV = pulmonary vein saturation, and Sat PA = pulmonary artery saturation.

If a pulmonary vein has not been entered, a value of 96 % can be assumed. Similarly, LV or aortic saturation may be used instead of left atrial saturation on condition that there is no right-to-left shunt. For mixed venous saturation, the pulmonary artery sample may be used unless there is a shunt at the atrial or ventricular level. Mixed venous saturation is more similar to that of the SVC rather than the IVC. The following formula is often used:

$$\text{Mixed venous saturation} : (3\text{SVC} + 1\text{IVC}) / 4$$

In the presence of a large left-to-right shunt, the Q/Qs is merely reported as "greater than 3:1. [1–4]."

Right-to-Left Shunting [1–8]

If the patient has no left-to-right shunt, mixed venous saturation and pulmonary artery saturation are the same, and all of the pulmonary blood flow is "effective," that is, Qp = Qep′. For all patients in a steady hemodynamic state, we have Qep′ = Qes. When there is a left-to-right shunt, some oxygenated blood recirculates through the lungs; thus, the volume of a left-to-right shunt is the difference between the total pulmonary flow (Qp) and the effective pulmonary flow (Qep):

$$Q_{L-R} = Qp - Qep$$

Similarly, when there is a right-to-left shunt, some of the deoxygenated "blue" blood bypasses the lungs and recirculates through the body; thus, Qs > Qes. The volume of a right-to-left shunt is the difference between the total systemic flow (Qs) and the effective systemic flow (Qes):

$$Q_{R-L} = Qs - Qes(Qep)$$

The volume of the left-to-right shunt = QP -QEP l/min/m2

The volume of the right-to-left shunt = QS -QEP l/min/m2

Usefulness of the Shunt Ratio in Practice

In an atrial defect, if there is evidence of a significant shunt according to clinical and noninvasive testing, the shunt ratio should not be included in the decision-making process about treatment because atrial shunts depend on the compliance of the ventricles. It is not exceptional for a measured shunt to be small (e.g., <1.5:1) in spite of other evidence of a significant defect [1].

Resistance Calculations

Resistance: Delta Pressure/Flow [1–11, 17]

Therefore, PVR (pulmonary vascular resistance) = (mean PAP- mean LAP)/QP.

PVR is usually indexed and expressed as indexed Wood units (mmHg/L/min/m^2). Normal PVR is less than 2 indexed Wood units (WU).

SVR: (mean Aop- mean RAp)/QS: normal SVR 15 – 20WU

Assessment of PVR is particularly important in the following situations [12–17]:

1. Prior to Glenn and total cavopulmonary anastomoses (the risk of postoperative complications is higher in patients with PVR > 3WU)
2. For risk stratification before cardiac transplantation (the risk of postoperative right heart failure is higher in patients with PVR > 6WU)
3. For the evaluation of responsiveness to medical therapy in patients with pulmonary hypertension

Oxygen and Nitric Oxide Inhalation Studies

For patients with pulmonary hypertension, it is important to calculate PVR and also to identify responsiveness to certain pharmacologic interventions. After measurement of PVR in the adult cardiac catheterization laboratory, patients with elevated pulmonary arterial hypertension and PVR are given 100 % inhaled oxygen or nitric oxide (usually 20–80 ppm). After 10 min of 100 % O_2, everything should be measured once more and PVR should be calculated. (Dissolved O_2 should also be included.) In those with fixed elevated pulmonary vascular resistance, there may be no significant rise in left-to-right shunting (QP/QS) or significant drop in PVR following the administration of oxygen or nitric oxide. Conversely, patients with pulmonary hypertension, which is reactive, tend to exhibit a significant drop in the PVR index and PVR/SVR [3–18].

Coronary Angiography

Coronary anomalies are quite frequent in CHD. In such patients, if a catheter with a usual shape fails to identify the origin swiftly, the operator should try other catheters. If the left Judkins catheter cannot find the left coronary artery in the left coronary sinus, or if the left coronary artery or the circumflex is "missing," the next step is to approach the right coronary artery. In this way, the "missing" artery can be identified arising from the right coronary trunk. If the right coronary artery cannot be found, a review of the LV or aortic angiogram normally identifies the anomalous origin. At this juncture, the operator must select a catheter from a wide array of other catheter shapes. The Amplatz and multipurpose catheters are normally the operator's first choice for the identification of the anomalous origin. If the origin of the coronary artery is abnormal, the operator should seek to define the course of the coronary artery as well. In an experienced center, cardiac CT may prove more valuable than angiography [1, 19, 20].

Chamber Angiography

The majority of adult catheterization laboratories are not equipped with biplane configurations. Consequently, a thorough understanding of

Table 16.3 Projection angles in single-plane projection

Conventional RAO	40° RAO
Cranially tilted RAO	30° RAO + 30° cranial
Frontal (AP)	0°
Shallow LAO	1–30°
Straight LAO	31–60°
Steep LAO	61–89°
Cranially tilted shallow LAO	25° LAO + 30° cranial
Cranially tilted mid LAO (long-axis oblique)	60° LAO + 20–30° cranial
Cranially tilted steep LAO (hepatoclavicular view)	45–70° LAO + 30°cranial
Left lateral	90° left
Cranially tilted frontal (sitting up view)	30° or 45° cranial

LAO left anterior oblique, *LPA* left pulmonary artery, *MPA* main pulmonary artery, *PA* pulmonary artery, *RAO* right anterior oblique, *RVOT* right ventricular outflow tract

Table 16.4 Biplane combinations: A plane B plane

Anteroposterior and lateral	0° + left lateral
Long-axis oblique	30° RAO 60° LAO + 20° to 30°cranial
Hepatoclavicular view	45° LAO + 30° cranial 120° LAO + 15° cranial

RAO right anterior oblique, *LAO* left anterior oblique

Table 16.5 Angiographic projections with specific interest

Specific side or lesion	Angiographic projections
RVOT-MPA	(Sitting up) 10° LAO + 40° cranial Left lateral RAO
Pulmonary valve	Left lateral
Main PA and branches	45°straight cranial 30° caudal + 10° RAO 20° caudal
LPA long axis	(Single plane) 60° LAO + 20° cranial (Biplane) 30° RAO 60° LAO + 30° cranial
RPA	Frontal Shallow RAO (junction of RPA to MPA) RAO cranial 35° cranial and 45° RAO (distal RPA)
ASD	30–45° LAO + 30–45° cranial
ASD with right-to-left shunt PFO for valve and tunnel	Left lateral
ASD device after insertion	RAO, caudal (30° RAO and 30° caudal) LAO, caudal (*30° LAO and 30° caudal*) RAO, cranial
Perimembranous VSD	LAO, with cranial angulation
Outlet extension of perimembranous VSD Anterior muscular VSD Apical VSD	Steep LAO with cranial angulation
Inlet-type VSD	Shallow LAO with cranial angulation
Posterior VSD	45° cranial, 30–45° LAO
High outlet VSD	Left lateral
Most VSDs with high RV pressure (injection in RV)	Left lateral
Aortic arch	LAO

Table 16.5 (continued)

Specific side or lesion	Angiographic projections
LV outflow tract	45° cranial, 30° LAO
Coarctation of aorta	LAO
PDA	LAO Left lateral RAO
Bifurcation of the left coronary artery	LAO
Common AV valve	45° cranial + 45°LAO
Goose neck deformity in AVSD	Frontal
Left ventricular to right atrial shunting	45° cranial + 45°LAO
Peripheral systemic venous system	Frontal
IVC, SVC	Frontal
Entrance of SVC and IVC and hepatic vein to the RA	Left lateral
RA	Frontal
RV	Frontal
Pulmonary veins to LA	Frontal
Course of abnormal pulmonary vein	Frontal
LA, LAA	Frontal
BT shunts	Frontal
Aortopulmonary collaterals	Frontal Left lateral RAO
Aortopulmonary relationship	Frontal Left lateral
Outlet of single ventricle	Frontal
Right and left PA in truncus arteriosus	Frontal
Coronary sinus	Left lateral
Course of azygos and hemiazygos veins	Left lateral
Entrance of LSVC to the LA or CS	Left lateral
Mitral valve	RAO RAO, caudal (*30° RAO and 30° caudal*)
Tricuspid valve	RAO RAO, caudal 30° RAO and 30° caudal
Separation of MV with LVOT	*30° RAO and 30° caudal*
Devices on the atrial septum	RAO

LAO left anterior oblique, *LPA* left pulmonary artery, *MPA* main pulmonary artery, *PA* pulmonary artery, *RAO* right anterior oblique, *RVOT* right ventricular outflow tract, *ASD* atrial septal defect, *VSD* ventricular septal defect, *LSVC* left superior vena cava, *CS* coronary sinus, *RV* right ventricle, *LV* left ventricle, *LVOT* left ventricle outflow tract

the anatomy and the goals of the interventional procedure becomes essential to a successful procedure.

Angiographic Projections

Mostly used projections are listed in Tables 16.3 and 16.4; also, views with specific interest are listed in Table 16.5.

References

1. Gatzoulis MA, Webb GD, Daubeney P. Diagnosis and management of adult congenital heart disease. 2nd ed. Philadelphia: Elsevier Saunders; 2011. p. 68–85.
2. Deanfield J, Thaulow E, Warnes C, et al. Management of grown up congenital heart disease. The Task Force on the Management of Grown up Congenital Heart Disease of the European Society of Cardiology. Eur Heart J. 2003;24: 1035–84.

3. Allen HD, Driscoll DJ, Shaddy RE, et al. Moss and Adams' heart disease in infants, children, and adolescents including the fetus and young adult. 7th ed. Philadelphia: Lippincott Williams & Wilkins; 2008. p. 208–39.
4. Freedom RM, Mawson JB, Yoo SJ, et al. Congenital heart disease textbook of angiocardiography. Armonk: Futura Publishing; 1997. p. 39–93.
5. Freedom RM, Mawson JB, Yoo SJ, et al. Congenital heart disease textbook of angiocardiography. Armonk: Futura Publishing; 1997. p. 189–218.
6. Amplatz K, Moller JH, Castaneda-Zuniga W, Finch ME. Radiology of congenital heart disease. 1st ed. New York: Theime Medical Publisher; 1986. p. 131–9.
7. Mullins CE. Transseptal left heart catheterization: experience with a new technique in 520 pediatric and adult patients. Pediatr Cardiol. 1983;4:239–46.
8. Bergersen L, Forster S, Marshall AC, Meadows J. Congenital heart disease, the catheterization manual. 1st ed. New York: Springer; 2009. p. 4–8.
9. Ganz W, Donoso R, Marcus HS, et al. A new technique for measurement of cardiac output by thermodilution in man. Am J Cardiol. 1971;27:392–6.
10. Vargo TA, et al. Cardiac catheterization: hemodynamic measurements. In: Garson A et al., editors. The science and practice of pediatric cardiology. 2nd ed. Baltimore: Williams & Wilkins; 1998. p. 961–93.
11. Brown LK, et al. Anatomic landmarks for use when measuring intracardiac pressure with fluid-filled catheters. Am J Cardiol. 2000;86(1):121–4.
12. Freed MD, Miettinen OS, Nadas AS. Oximetric detection of intracardiac left-to-right shunts. Br Heart J. 1979;42:690–4.
13. Lister G, Hoffman JI, Rudolph AM. Oxygen uptake in infants and children: a simple method for measurement. Pediatrics. 1974;53(5):656–62.
14. LaFarge CG, Miettinen OS. The estimation of oxygen consumption. Cardiovasc Res. 1970;4(1):23–30.
15. Gutgesell HP, Williams RL. Caval samples as indicators of mixed venous oxygen saturation: implications in atrial septal defect. Cardiovasc Dis. 1974;1(3):160–4.
16. Krouskop RW, et al. Accuracy and clinical utility of an oxygen saturation catheter. Crit Care Med. 1983;11(9):744–9.
17. Mullins CE. Cardiac catheterization in congenital heart disease: pediatric and adult. Malden: Blackwell; 2006. p. 289–324.
18. Hill KD, Lim DS, Everett AD, et al. Assessment of pulmonary hypertension in the pediatric catheterization laboratory: current insights from the Magic registry. Catheter Cardiovasc Interv. 2010;76:865–73.
19. Greenberg MA, Fish BG, Spindola-Franco H. Congenital anomalies of the coronary arteries. Radiol Clin North Am. 1989;27:1127–46.
20. Ishikawa T, Brandt PWT. Anomalous origin of the left main coronary artery from the right anterior aortic sinus: angiographic definition of anomalous course. Am J Cardiol. 1985;55:770–6.

Anesthesia in Adults with Congenital Heart Disease

17

Rasoul Azarfarin

Keywords
Anesthetic management • Cardiac anesthesia • Adult • Congenital heart disease

Introduction

Nowadays, advances in prenatal diagnosis, interventional cardiological procedures, and pediatric cardiac anesthesia as well as improvements in complex surgical techniques and apparatus, postoperative critical care, and efficacy of cardiovascular pharmacologic agents have resulted in an overall increase in post-repair survival rates and have led to a growing number of adult patients with congenital heart disease (ACHD). The majority of these patients will require cardiac or noncardiac surgery; this constitutes a new challenge for anesthesiologists. What is more, these patients experience an increased rate of perioperative morbidity and mortality [1].

All the below-mentioned pre-, intra-, and postoperative recommendations for the anesthetic management of patients with ACHD are generalizable to both cardiac and noncardiac procedures, so the complexity of CHD and the extent of the operative procedure (either cardiac or noncardiac) mostly determine the early and late outcome of these patients. *Thus, it is strongly recommended that all surgical procedures (except for those with absolute emergency) be performed in a referral center specifying in congenital cardiology, with skilled surgeons and cardiac anesthesiologists.* Even minor noncardiac surgery may carry a high risk in ACHD patients, so consultation with ACHD experts and a cardiac anesthesiologist for the assessment of risk and for moderate- and high-risk patients, respectively, is recommended in patients with ACHD scheduled to undergo noncardiac surgery [2, 3].

Individualized management of these fragile and sophisticated patients with complex ACHD should be accomplished with a deep and extensive knowledge of the pathophysiology of various congenital heart anomalies (cyanotic or non-cyanotic, obstructive or regurgitant, etc.) and of the effect of these chronic pathologic changes, until adulthood, on other organ systems (pulmonary, cerebrovascular, hematologic, and coagulation systems). Suitable perioperative care of such a patient requires a cardiac anesthesiologist with a keen understanding of the patient's underlying cardiac anomaly and coexisting diseases [4]. To

R. Azarfarin, MD, FACC
Professor of Anesthesiology Fellowship of Cardiac Anesthesia, Cardiac Anesthesiology Ward, Department of Anesthesiology,
Rajaie Cardiovascular Medical and Research Center, Iran University of Medical Science, Tehran, Iran
e-mail: razarfarin@yahoo.com, razarfarin@rhc.ac.ir

A. Sadeghpour et al. (eds.), *Comprehensive Approach to Adult Congenital Heart Disease*,
DOI 10.1007/978-1-4471-6383-1_17, © Springer-Verlag London 2014

achieve this goal, a comprehensive preoperative (noninvasive or invasive) cardiac imaging study, consisting of transthoracic echocardiography (TTE) or transesophageal echocardiography (TEE), cardiac magnetic resonance imaging (CMRI), and CT angiography or cardiac catheterization, should be done for accurate diagnosis of the current complex CHD and associated pulmonary and peripheral vascular disease status [4].

Preoperative Evaluation

There are three types of ACHD patients expected to come for evaluation: (1) patients with uncorrected cardiac defects, (2) patients with previous palliative surgery for example tetralogy of Fallot (TOF) with a Blalock–Taussig shunt or patients with transposition of the great arteries with a history of atrial septostomy or septectomy, and (3) patients with ACHD who, despite having previously had total correction, may have residual defects or may develop a new abnormal finding requiring further procedures.

Preoperative assessment should contain comprehensive information about cardiac lesions and altered physiology and the consequences thereof. Proper perioperative management of ACHD patients requires a careful assessment of their general condition such as fatigue, headache, and dyspnea on exertion as well as their nutritional status (the degree of malnutrition or in severe cases cardiac cachexia), lean body mass, mental status, and extent of probable neurobehavioral changes. Especially in cyanotic ACHD, polycythemia could lead to some neurological symptoms such as visual disturbances, depressed mentation, and limb paresthesia.

Examining of ACHD patients for likely infection sources, including the upper or lower respiratory and genitourinary systems, or endocarditis in complex cardiac lesions is essential. These preoperative findings may, therefore, have extensive detrimental effects on the postoperative course in these fragile and high-risk patients. *The function of most organ systems (immune, endocrine, hematologic, coagulation, respiratory, etc.) must be optimized by proper consultation with relevant experts, and any significant coexisting problems should be resolved before admitting these patients for any major cardiac or noncardiac surgical procedures.*

There are some inquiries which should be conducted during the preoperative visit of ACHD patients such as comprehensive understanding of the anatomic changes due to cardiac defects or palliative or corrective procedures, direction and extent of an existing shunt, the presence of a low or high pulmonary flow and severity of pulmonary artery hypertension, extent of hypoxemia, and coexisting polycythemia. An anesthesiologist should also consider any possible abnormalities in platelet function and coagulation.

A prolonged high pulmonary flow leads to pulmonary congestion and even edema, causing repeated pulmonary infectious disease. Right-sided heart failure may give rise to fatigue, tachycardia, tachypnea, cardiomegaly, and hepatosplenomegaly and as such reduce the patient's desire for food or drink and eventually lead to malnutrition. Attempts should be made to avoid dehydration in all and especially cyanotic ACHD patients by permitting them to intake clear liquids 2 h prior to surgery. If the timing of surgery has not been determined, the anesthesiologist can start an intravenous line and give glucose-containing solutions.

Polycythemia is very common in cyanotic ACHD patients; it raises blood viscosity and results to cerebral, pulmonary, and renal vessel thrombosis and infarction. Also, coagulation abnormalities happen owing to hypofibrinogenemia and factor deficits. Platelet count, prothrombin time (PT), and partial thromboplastin time (PTT) must be measured in all patients scheduled for a surgical procedure. Preoperative phlebotomy can be done in those with symptomatic hyperviscosity and hematocrit more than 65 % [2].

Electrolyte disturbances are frequently observed in ACHD patients who take diuretics and also parenteral nutrition. Hypocalcaemia is usually seen in patients with the DiGeorge syndrome. The electrocardiogram (ECG) may show ventricular strain or hypertrophy patterns and axis deviation. Chest X-ray should be obtained to investigate the heart's position (levocardia, mesocardia, or dextrocardia) and size, lung atelectasis, pulmonary infection, vascular markings, and level of hemidiaphragm. An increased pulmonary blood flow raises pulmonary marking, whereas a decreased flow causes oligemic lung fields.

Echocardiography is an essential diagnostic tool and is usually sufficient for planning a correct surgical procedure. Echocardiographic 2D or 3D studies, accompanied by Doppler and color flow mapping, provide comprehensive reports on ACHD patients' cardiovascular anatomic and physiological abnormalities, while catheterization yields precise information on pressures in the heart's chambers, extent of shunt, and coronary anatomy. More specific cardiac imaging modalities such as cardiac MRI or CT angiography in sophisticated congenital lesions may be needed. Neurological assessment and brain MRI may also be required in patients with neurological symptoms because these findings could affect anesthetic management in such patients.

Intraoperative Considerations

The presence of CHD in adult patients poses a formidable challenge for the anesthesiologist as morbidity and mortality of surgical procedures are reasonably high. Anesthetic considerations in ACHD patients are directly affected by the patient's cardiac status (repaired or unrepaired lesions), degree of heart failure, and New York Heart Association (NYHA) class as well as by the length and extent of the cardiac or noncardiac surgical procedure and the majority of hemodynamic fluctuations and fluid exchanges.

Considering the relatively higher incidence of anatomic airway anomalies and craniofacial syndromes in patients with CHD and also reduced cardiopulmonary reserve, airway management in these patients could be challenging for the anesthesiologist. Compression of the airway is not uncommon and is a frequently undiagnosed consequence of congenital cardiac and aortic arch disease. Airway obstruction may be caused by the anomalies of the tracheobronchial tree and grate vessels such as dilated aortic arch and pulmonary arteries or left atrial enlargement and massive cardiomegaly. A high degree of suspicion of airway compression should be preserved in patients who present with repeated respiratory problems, stridor, wheezing, and dysphagia unexplained by other reasons. MRI can be a good diagnostic tool for depicting all anatomic elements around the airway and allowing for accurate anatomic description and better airway management [5]. Regarding growth retardation in the majority of adolescent and adult patients with CHD, choosing the proper size of the cuffed endotracheal tube according to the patient's body size may be challenging [6].

A confident intravenous (IV) line should be positioned in all ACHD patients even for minor procedures. *All IV tubing must be free of even small air bubble because of the probability of systemic air emboli through right-to-left shunts. Polycythemic patients must be adequately hydrated before induction of anesthesia via IV or orally*. Sevoflurane is favored over halothane owing to the superior hemodynamic stability in ACHD patients and much lower risk of hepatotoxicity. The majority of ACHD patients tolerate induction with IV drugs. On the other hand, in those with poor cardiac function, induction drugs such as hypnotics and opioids must be administered as titrated dosing while continuously monitoring the blood pressure. Various types of inotropes and vasopressors must be immediately available and should be used as needed. Especially in ACHD with stenotic lesions such as subvalvular, valvular, or supravalvular aortic stenosis or pulmonary stenosis, because of the fixed cardiac output, the anesthesiologist must provide adequate preload before induction and avoid profound reduction in afterload. Cardiopulmonary resuscitation has a very poor outcome in patients with stenotic lesions, and any severe arrhythmia or hypotension during the induction or maintenance of anesthesia in such patients could be fatal [7].

Monitoring

In patients with complex cardiac anomalies and underlying (right- or left-sided) heart failure scheduled to undergo major surgery, in addition to standard monitoring [ECG, peripheral oxygen saturation (SpO_2), and end-tidal CO_2 ($ETCO_2$)], what needs to be established is an extensive monitoring system encompassing invasive arterial and central venous pressure (CVP) measurements, TEE, cerebral oximeter, and advanced coagulation and blood glucose monitoring (activated clotting time and thromboelastography).

Although the ECG can be useful in the recognition of ST alterations, it is mainly utilized for arrhythmia recognition in ACHD patients. Even arrhythmia finding might be difficult if there is baseline tachycardia. A 3- or 5-lead system is commonly used.

Invasive BP monitoring not only delivers continuous beat-to-beat blood pressure measurement but also delivers an easy route for arterial blood sampling for gas analyses and other additional laboratory tests such as blood sugar, lactate, and electrolytes. *Pressure monitoring stopcocks and tubing must be de-aired to prevent air emboli and also damping of the system.* Dextrose solution can be used; however, commonly heparinized normal saline is the flushing fluid because bacterial growth is less possible.

Central venous access is useful in the monitoring of the CVP and also delivers a confident way for drugs, fluids, and blood. The right internal jugular vein is usually used because of its straight course to the right atrium. The subclavian and femoral veins can also be used, alternatively.

The pulse oximeter consists of two light-emitting diodes (LED) and one photodiode for the recognition of red and infrared lights. The accuracy of the pulse oximeter is distributed by some factors, including hypothermia, hypotension, and electrocautery. Also, thick skin, bright external light, dark color, or the presence of dyes such as methylene blue and indocyanine green and unusual hemoglobins such as methemoglobin and carboxyhemoglobin can cause artifacts [8].

Cerebral oximetry via transcranial near-infrared spectroscopy (NIRS) provides sensitive monitoring of regional hypoperfusion. It is valuable in cardiopulmonary bypass (CPB) and total circulatory arrest. The cerebral oximeter detects the intravascular (mostly venous and some arterial) hemoglobin oxygen saturation of the frontal cerebral cortex, over which the oximetry leads are placed.

Intraoperative TEE plays an essential role in betterment of surgical outcome in all cardiac surgeries, including ACHD surgical procedures, by approving diagnosis and recognizing residual defects. It is also useful in interventional procedures in the catheterization laboratory. Multiplane TEE probes and 3D technologies are novel developments in the echocardiography field. Intraoperative epicardial echocardiography is an alternate choice in centers where smaller TEE probes are not available. Adult TEE probes can be placed in patients with body weight >20 kg [8].

Anesthetic Management of Altered Circulation Physiology in Adult Congenital Heart Disease

Anesthetic management in ACHD is to some extent influenced by the presence or absence of shunts, direction of the shunt flow, pulmonary artery hypertension, severity of hypoxemia, left or right ventricular dysfunction and also pulmonary blood flow, and arrhythmia.

Shunting through congenital heart defects depends upon the diameter of the defect and the balance between systemic and pulmonary vascular resistance. *Balance between systemic vascular resistance and pulmonary vascular resistance is crucial in the anesthetic management of patients with shunts.* In a normal pulmonary blood flow, the systemic ratio (Qp:Qs ratio) is 1:1, which demonstrates either no shunting or a bidirectional shunt of equal amount. In the catheterization lab, this ratio is assessed by oxygen saturation measurement by sampling from the pulmonary artery and venous, arterial, and also mixed venous blood. Heart defects with left-to-right shunts (Qp:Qs ratio ≥2:1) consist of atrial septal defect (ASD), ventricular septal defect (VSD), patent ductus arteriosus (PDA), atrioventricular canal defects, and complete or partial anomalous venous return and also surgically created Blalock–Taussig shunts [7, 8].

In anesthetized patients, the left-to-right shunt decreases significantly with a fall in systemic vascular resistance (SVR) or a rise in pulmonary vascular resistance (PVR). A left-to-right shunt increases the pulmonary blood flow and eventually leads to pulmonary artery hypertension and right-sided heart failure, if left untreated. These patients are usually acyanotic, but worsening in gas exchange may occur due to pulmonary congestion. Applying 100 % oxygen and hyperventilation in these patients must be avoided. Patients with large patent ductus arteriosus are susceptible to coronary ischemia due to partial pulmonary runoff during diastole. Thus, diastolic blood pressure (BP) must be monitored throughout anesthesia in cases with patent ductus arteriosus. The blood pressure of the arm could be lower in patients with Blalock–Taussig shunt, so the opposite arm should be used. In patients with pulmonary atresia, the presence of major aortopulmonary collateral arteries may create significant left-to-right shunts.

Right-to-left (Qp:Qs ratio <1:1 ratio) shunts tend to prolong the inhalation induction. Such shunts are likely to occur in TOF. Shunt reversal happens when systemic vascular resistance falls or pulmonary vascular resistance rises. *A hypercyanotic spell during anesthesia will respond to fluid administration and increase systemic vascular resistance with alpha-agonist agents such as phenylephrine.* The inappropriate administration of beta-agonists such as ephedrine, dopamine, and dobutamine in patients with TOF anatomy and physiology leads to dynamic right ventricular outlet obstruction and severe desaturation and eventually systemic hypotension.

In cyanotic ACHD patients, blood desaturation and eventually ischemia result from an insufficient pulmonary blood flow and/or mixing of oxygenated with deoxygenated blood in the systemic circulation. Also, pulmonary congestion and poor exchange of O_2 can cause hypoxemia. Persistent hypoxemia leads to slightly increased heart rate, hyperventilation, erythrocytosis, and decreased chemoreceptor response to hypoxemia. In these patients, the CNS and myocardial oxygenation is maintained (although myocardial ischemia and dysfunction in some cases ensue) and splanchnic and muscular oxygenation is decreased. Moreover, the majority of these patients have growth retardation. The anesthetic management in cyanotic ACHD includes sufficient hydration, maintenance of systemic vascular resistance, reduction of further resistance to pulmonary blood flow, and prevention of an abrupt rise in oxygen demand (pain, agitation, and light anesthesia).

Pulmonary artery hypertension in early stages is reactive and reacts with pain, hypothermia, stress, metabolic acidosis, high $PaCO_2$, hypoxia, and elevated intrathoracic pressure, whereas advanced pulmonary artery hypertension becomes fixed. In this end stage, where pulmonary vascular resistance (PVR) exceeds systemic vascular resistance (SVR) and symptoms of a right-to-left shunt appear, the Eisenmenger syndrome occurs. The risk of anesthesia is very high, consisting of RV failure, bronchospasm, PAH crisis, and eventually cardiac arrest. *The emphasis in the management of anesthesia in the Eisenmenger syndrome is on avoiding a further rise in the right-to-left shunt by maintaining SVR higher and PVR lower, keeping adequate myocardial contractility, and avoiding any arrhythmia and volume depletion.*

Most ACHD patients experience some degrees of ventricular (left- or right-sided or biventricular) dysfunction due to long-lasting volume (excessive shunts or valvular insufficiency) or pressure (obstructive lesions) overload and cardiomyopathies. Arterial blood gas analyses and X-ray may demonstrate metabolic acidosis and pulmonary congestion, respectively. Patients are commonly on digoxin, diuretics, and inotropes.

Generally, the principle of anesthesia in patients with a poor ventricular function is based on opioid anesthesia. Etomidate and fentanyl maintain good cardiovascular stability during anesthesia induction. The anesthesiologists must avoid or minimize the use of inhalation anesthetics because of related myocardial depression. The patient's normal sinus rhythm, preload, and afterload should be maintained within an acceptable physiological limit [7, 8].

Neurological Sequels in Patients with Adult Congenital Heart Disease

There is increasing concern over quality of life and neurobehavioral outcomes in ACHD patients owing to the prolonged survival of these patients. About one-third to half of these patients may experience neurological deficiency and damage due to long-lasting hypoxemia, thromboembolic accidents due to hyperviscosity syndrome, and hemodynamic and inflammatory consequents of CPB (ischemia/reperfusion injury).

Coagulation Abnormalities

Coagulation defects are very prevalent in ACHD patients, especially in cyanotic lesions and those that are polycythemic. Coagulation abnormalities allied to high hemoglobin concentrations consist of low platelet count and performance, fibrinolysis, and compromised coagulation factor construction. The coagulopathy use of blood products is common during cardiac operations, not least those with CPB; as a result, various blood conservation protocols have been established to lower transfusion problems. Preoperative administration of 20 ml/kg fresh frozen plasma (FFP) to replace the same amount of blood is a reliable manner to prevent coagulopathy. Antifibrinolytic agents such as aprotinin and tranexamic acid have been used to reduce postoperative bleeding. Tranexamic acid is administered as a bolus dose of 100 mg/kg and then by 10 mg/kg/h infusion. Transfusion of whole blood is very effective in these patients. Although there is some warning about aprotinin usage, there are reports of using low doses or even ultra-low doses of this drug in cardiac surgical patients [9].

Postoperative Pain Management

Intraoperative use of high-dose opioids in adult congenital heart surgery is useful for continuing the analgesic effect until the postoperative period. *Appropriate intraoperative and postoperative analgesia is correlated with improvement in the surgical outcome*. Morphine in the dose of 25 μ/kg/h will deliver acceptable analgesia and moderate sedation in the postoperative period. Continuous infusions of 1–5 μ/kg/h of fentanyl will provide adequate analgesia along with minor sedation in the postoperative period. In moderate pain levels, non-opioid agents such as ketamine and paracetamol could also be employed in these patients [10].

Anesthesia in ACHD Undergoing Noncardiac Surgery

ACHD patients who undergo any noncardiac surgeries are at a greater risk of morbidity and mortality than matched control cohort patients [11]. Any adult with ACHD may require surgical procedure in any part of body in their life; however, some specific subgroups such as cyanotic patients may need certain procedures (i.e., operation for gallstones, cerebral abscess, or scoliosis). *The risk of noncardiac surgery is mostly influenced by the complexity of the underlying CHD and the extent and urgency of the procedure*. The patients at highest risk are those with a functional single ventricle (prior Fontan operation), suprasystemic PAH, dilated cardiomyopathy, LV outflow tract obstruction, complex CHD, or cyanotic CHD with residua such as cardiac failure [12]. Also those before stage II palliative surgery, undergoing major operations and getting inotropes, digoxin, and ACE inhibitors, seem to be at risk for hemodynamic abnormality during operation [13]. *Even for noncardiac operation, it is recommended that the preoperative assessment and surgery be done in an ACHD center by skilled surgeons and cardiac anesthesiologists.*

Preoperative phlebotomy can decrease the risk of bleeding when hematocrit >65 %. Prolonged surgeries accompanying with hemodynamic variability and large-volume fluid shift are related with higher perioperative death. Fluid balance is crucial in cyanotic and single ventricle lesions and those with CHF. Patients with CHD may need ICU monitoring services even after relatively minor procedures. Even for noncardiac surgery, special considerations should be planned that include endocarditis and deep venous thrombosis prophylaxis, perioperative anticoagulation, filters for IV lines in cyanotic patients, monitoring of renal function, and the decreased arm BP in patients with previous Blalock–Taussig shunt [3, 8].

References

1. Cannesson M, Collange V, Lehot JJ. Anesthesia in adult patients with congenital heart disease. Curr Opin Anaesthesiol. 2009;22(1):88–94.
2. Baumgartner H, Bonhoeffer P, De Groot N, et al. ESC guidelines for the management of grown-up congenital heart disease (new version 2010). Eur Heart J. 2010;31(23):2915–57. PMID: 20801927.
3. Warnes CA, Williams RG, Bashore TM, et al. ACC/AHA 2008 Guidelines for the Management of Adults With Congenital Heart Disease: a report of the American College of Cardiology/American Heart Association Task Force on Practice Guidelines (Writing Committee to Develop Guidelines on the Management of Adults With Congenital Heart Disease). Developed in Collaboration With the American Society of Echocardiography, Heart Rhythm Society, International Society for Adult Congenital Heart Disease, Society for Cardiovascular Angiography and Interventions, and Society of Thoracic Surgeons. J Am Coll Cardiol. 2008;52(23):e143–263.
4. Cosgrove MS. Anesthesia for the adult patient with an unrepaired congenital cyanotic heart defect: a case report. AANA J. 2012;80(3):197–203.
5. Kussman BD, Geva T, McGowan FX. Cardiovascular causes of airway compression. Paediatr Anaesth. 2004;14(1):60–74.
6. Azarfarin R, Seyedhejazi M, Bilehjani E, et al. Do pediatric patients undergoing cardiac surgeries require larger-size cuffed endotracheal tubes? A prospective study. Paediatr Anaesth. 2013;23(3):228–32.
7. Hamid M. Anaesthetic considerations for congenital heart disease patient. Aga Khan University, Pakistan. 2013. Available in URL 2: http://cdn.intechopen.com/pdfs/30197/InTech-Anaesthetic_considerations_for_congenital_heart_disease_patient.pdf
8. Lovell AT. Anaesthetic implications of grown-up congenital heart disease. Br J Anaesth. 2004;93(1):129–39.
9. Parvizi R, Azarfarin R, Hasanzadeh S. Ultra-low dose aprotinin effects on reducing the need for blood transfusion in cardiac surgery. Saudi Med J. 2007;28(1):49–53.
10. Brown ML, Dearani JA, Burkhart HM. The adult with congenital heart disease: medical and surgical considerations for management. Curr Opin Pediatr. 2009;21(5):561–4.
11. Maxwell BG, Wong JK, Kin C, et al. Perioperative outcomes of major noncardiac surgery in adults with congenital heart disease. Anesthesiology. 2013;119(4):762–9.
12. Gottlieb EA, Andropoulos DB. Anesthesia for the patient with congenital heart disease presenting for noncardiac surgery. Curr Opin Anaesthesiol. 2013;26(3):318–26.
13. Watkins SC, McNew BS, Donahue BS. Risks of noncardiac operations and other procedures in children with complex congenital heart disease. Ann Thorac Surg. 2013;95(1):204–11.

Surgical Management of Adults with Congenital Heart Disease

18

Alireza Alizadeh Ghavidel and Mitra Chitsazan

Keywords
Adult congenital heart disease (ACHD) • Surgery • Surgical techniques • Surgical approach • Median sternotomy • Re-sternotomy

Introduction

Over the past decades, due to tremendous improvement in cardiothoracic surgery, 95 % of newborns with congenital heart disease survive into adulthood in the current era. Although most of adult patients with congenital heart disease (CHD) have undergone surgical intervention during childhood and also there have been recently remarkable advances in percutaneous techniques to treat adult congenital heart disease (ACHD), a significant proportion of these patients will have to undergo cardiovascular surgery at some point in adulthood.

Surgeries may be considered in a number of patients with ACHD. These patients include those with prior palliative operations or residual defects. Patients with associated cardiac lesions who have not been operated due to missed diagnosis or lack of sever lesions may also need the surgery in adulthood. Underlying medical disorders, previous cardiac surgeries, and anatomic variations lead to a more complex operation. Despite the recent improvement in minimally invasive surgeries, the standard median sternotomy provides better surgical exposure to evaluate the various and even unexpected cardiac anomalies, safe cannulation and decannulation, de-airing, and cardioplegia administration. *History of multiple cardiac surgeries, previous mediastinitis, aneurysmal dilatations of the LVOT and RVOT, calcified arterial conduits, close adherence of the aorta, or right-sided heart chambers to the sternum are the main risk factors for tissue injuries during re-sternotomy.* Peripheral cannulation and pre-sternotomy establishment of the cardiopulmonary bypass may reduce the incidence of cardiac rupture in this high-risk group of patients with ACHD.

The detailed treatment strategies in adults with various CHD have been discussed in the related chapters, and the following section provides an overview on surgery in ACHD.

Progressive improvement in surgical techniques and medical care has led to a rise in the number of adults with congenital heart disease (CHD). Although most newborns with CHD sur-

A. Alizadeh Ghavidel, MD (✉)
Cardiac Surgery Ward, Department of Cardiac Surgery, Rajaie Cardiovascular Medical and Research Center, Iran University of Medical Science, Tehran, Iran
e-mail: aaghavidel@gmail.com, aghavidel@rhc.ac.ir

M. Chitsazan, MD
Rajaie Cardiovascular Medical and Research Center, Tehran, Iran

A. Sadeghpour et al. (eds.), *Comprehensive Approach to Adult Congenital Heart Disease*,
DOI 10.1007/978-1-4471-6383-1_18,

vive to adulthood, their life is fraught with long-term complications, residual defects, or progressive disease. A significant number of corrective surgical procedures are performed in CHD patients without important hemodynamic effects during the early years of life. *About 30–40 % of these patients have previous reconstructive cardiac surgery and need repetitive surgical re-interventions* [1, 2]. Adult patients with a history of tetralogy of Fallot repair form the largest group of the patients requiring redo operations [1].

Usually cardiac surgery in adult patients with CHD is more complex owing to concomitant diseases, coagulopathy, and need for re-sternotomy. Therefore, a multidisciplinary approach may play an important role in the achievement of favorable surgical results and better quality of life. A team approach and close follow-up are also important during the transition between childhood and adulthood.

Despite the remarkable advances in percutaneous intervention in some forms of CHD such as atrial septal defect (ASD), patent ductus arteriosus (PDA), ventricular septal defect (VSD), and coarctation of aorta, surgery remains the gold standard for most patients, especially in complex or recurrent diseases. Because of anatomic variations, previous surgical procedures, and unanticipated surgical findings, the surgery of complex congenital disorders should be done by trained cardiac surgeons in CHD and redo surgeries.

Surgical Approaches

Different surgical approaches have been described for the repair of CHD. Median sternotomy, however, remains the standard incision for adult patients with CHD. *Median sternotomy provides good surgical exposure not only for the evaluation of various and even unexpected cardiac anomalies but also for safe cannulation and decannulation, de-airing, and cardioplegia administration via different routes.* On the other hand, median sternotomy can cause unnecessary trauma to the collateral arteries. Although median sternotomy is the standard approach for redo operations, right anterolateral thoracotomy can be used for selected redo cases with mitral or tricuspid valve disease. The length of the incision and the higher chance of hypertrophic scar formation are two cosmetic disadvantages of median sternotomy. T-shaped or J-shaped mini-sternotomy can provide better cosmetic results for first-time operations in selected patients with isolated aortic valve disease, isolated subaortic stenosis [3, 4], or even hypertrophic obstructive cardiomyopathy.

Robotic and minimally invasive surgeries have been recently employed for the correction of defects in simple cardiac anomalies such as isolated primary or secondary ASD and PDA as well as isolated congenital mitral valve disease. Better cosmetic results, less pain, shorter intubation time, and shorter postoperative hospital stay are the main advantages of the right mini-thoracotomy approach in these patients. The major disadvantages of minimally invasive surgeries include the longer cardiopulmonary bypass (CPB) and aortic cross-clamping time, need for peripheral cannulation, and more complex surgical process [5]. Right anterior thoracotomy and central cannulation are also recommended for nonobese patients with isolated ASD or sinus venosus-type ASD.

Special Considerations in Re-sternotomy

As was mentioned before, reoperations are not uncommon in patients with CHD. Residual defects, progressive disorders, and conduit complications constitute the principal causes of redo surgeries in these patients. Heart failure and enlarged cardiac chambers (especially right atrium and right ventricle), degenerative and calcified conduit, aneurysm or pseudoaneurysm of the aortic root, aneurysmal transannular patch, collateral small arteries, baseline coagulopathies, and history of deep mediastinal wound infection are the risk factors for reentry injury. History of multiple cardiac operations and evidence of severe adhesion of the right ventricle, arterial conduit, or ascending aorta to the inner table of the sternum in chest computed tomography are the other risk factors for tissue injury during re-sternotomy [6, 7].

Re-sternotomy in Low-Risk Patients

Femoral vessel exploration and peripheral cannulation are not used routinely in low-risk cases. Usually, direct re-sternotomy with an oscillating saw after the excision of the previous scar tissue and removing the sternal wire is utilized to divide the sternum. To reduce the risk of soft tissue injury, we recommend pulling up the sternum during sawing using two towel clips from both sides of the sternum. Small bleeding from the soft tissue injury of the right ventricle can be usually stopped with a transient local pack. When major bleeding occurs immediately after sternotomy, the patient's position should be changed to Trendelenburg without delay. The bleeding site between the two segments of the sternum should be packed with sponge, and the two separate segments of the sternum should be closed together by the surgeon's assistant. The femoral vessels should be explored and cannulated by the senior surgeon as soon as possible. Rarely, when the femoral artery is not deemed suitable for cannulation based on the preoperative or intraoperative findings, the surgeon should extend the incision toward the neck to explore the innominate or the right carotid artery. Right axillary artery cannulation is usually time-consuming and is not recommended in emergent condition. After peripheral cannulation and establishment of CPB, the sternum should be opened carefully and tissue dissection in the surgical plane should be continued. The position of the venous cannula in the inferior vena cava should be checked by transesophageal echocardiography (TEE) guidance, and the superior vena cava should be cannulated if necessary.

Re-sternotomy in High-Risk Patients

We recommend the liberal use of peripheral cannulation for high-risk cases, not least in patients with aneurysmal or calcified biological conduits and aneurysmal dilatation of the transannular patch. A more conservative approach can be adopted for selected cases. The femoral vessels should be explored and controlled before sternotomy in these patients. If re-sternotomy is carried out uneventfully, central standard cannulation is performed. Emergent peripheral cannulation and CPB are employed when significant mediastinal bleeding occurs during re-sternotomy. *Usually trying to suture and control the severe mediastinal bleeding from the aorta, right ventricle, or right atrium before the establishment of CPB and decompression of the heart chambers is unsuccessful.* It is recommended to control the bleeding after cardiac decompression and adequate division of the two sides of the sternum. The Trendelenburg position helps reduce the risk of air emboli.

Axillary artery cannulation is recommended for patients with a dilated calcified homograft in the aortic position. This approach facilitates reentering and controlling the aorta and also facilitates inducing the hypothermic circulatory arrest with antegrade cerebral perfusion when needed. The same approach is appropriate for Marfan patients with aneurysm of the ascending aorta and the aortic arch and also for patients with large pseudoaneurysms of the aortic root. In complex surgeries for patients with frank heart failure, it is advisable to use peripheral cannulation and CPB before re-sternotomy. These patients are transiently weaned from CPB during the division of the sternum from the heart and control of the aorta to reduce the CPB time. CPB can be reestablished right before cross-clamping the aorta.

Atrial Septal Defect

Surgical closure has been considered the "gold standard" treatment for patients with atrial septal defect (ASD) [8]. Surgical closure of secundum ASD may be performed during a concomitant surgical repair/replacement of the tricuspid valve. Since a primum ASD or partial anomalous pulmonary venous drainage may be found unexpectedly during operation and pose additional challenges, surgical repair of this type of ASD should be performed by experienced surgeons in adult congenital heart disease. In such cases, anomalous pulmonary venous drainage should be repaired by creating a baffle with autologous pericardium or synthetic patches to divert the blood flow to the left atrium.

In patients that the anomalous pulmonary venous drainage connects to the mid- or upper superior vena cava, the incision of the right atrium (RA) should be extended toward the lateral side of the superior vena cava (SVC), and the defect should be repaired with a patch. The RA and SVC incision should be repaired by another pericardial patch or V-Y plasty of the right atrial appendage (RAA) to prevent the SVC stenosis. The Warden procedure may be an alternative method to a sinus venosus-type ASD [8]. In this technique, the azygous vein is ligated, and SVC is transected above the orifice of the anomalous pulmonary vein and is anastomosed to the RAA. Then SVC-RA junction is closed with a patch, and the superior vena cava with the anomalous draining pulmonary veins remains draining to the left atrium via the sinus venosus ASD.

Moreover, surgical closure of ASD may be preferred to percutaneous intervention for patients in whom the anatomic characteristics of the defect preclude the use of a percutaneous closure device. *Ideally, some types of ASD such as sinus venosus, coronary sinus, or primum ASD should be closed surgically rather than by percutaneous intervention.* However, it should be noted that ASD closure is contraindicated in patients with severe irreversible PAH and Eisenmenger physiology (class III, *level of evidence: B*) [8].

Depending on the size of the ASD, it can be closed primarily with continuous suture or using a patch by either right thoracotomy or sternotomy approaches. Concomitant tricuspid valve repair should be performed in the presence of significant tricuspid regurgitation (TR). *In adult patients who suffer from intermittent or chronic atrial tachyarrhythmia, a concomitant Maze procedure may also be considered during ASD closure which reduces the incidence of atrial fibrillation/flutter* (class IIb, *level of evidence: C)* [8]. However, atrial arrhythmias may develop after repair. Although SVC or pulmonary vein stenosis may necessitate reoperation following closure of sinus venosus-type ASDs, residual/recurrent ASD is an uncommon cause of reoperation in ASD patients.

Ventricular Septal Defect

Isolated VSD is usually repaired via trans-atrial approach using patch closure with a synthetic material or autologous pericardium. Primary closure is rarely used in isolated VSDs [8]. In the presence of multiple VSDs, shunting from the associated defects might only develop following closure of the dominant VSD. As a result, transesophageal echocardiography is required intraoperatively to carefully visualize the muscular septum and identify these lesions. Concomitant cardiac lesions should also be addressed during surgical repair of VSD. Associated infundibular RVOT obstruction should be corrected by myocardial resection or patch enlargement technique. Aortic valve replacement may be required in significant aortic regurgitation. Subaortic stenosis is usually treated by resection of the subaortic membrane. *Rarely, the complex tunnel-shaped LVOT obstruction or small aortic root can be repaired by the Konno-Rastan procedure* [9].

Reoperation due to residual VSD is not common; however, late reoperation may be necessary for significant tricuspid or aortic regurgitation.

Patent Ductus Arteriosus

Surgical closure of PDA in the adult is more challenging due to the fragile or calcified tissue of the ductus, aortic isthmus, and pulmonary artery. Moreover, device closure is usually feasible in patients with isolated PDA, and adults with PDA are usually preferred for percutaneous closure with either the occlusion device or coils [10]. A PDA in association with other concomitant lesions may be closed simultaneously at the time of cardiac operation. However, the preoperative device closure of the PDA may decrease the risk of cardiopulmonary bypass and should be undertaken in patients undergoing other cardiac surgeries such as coronary artery bypass grafting.

The primary surgical approach for PDA closure may be provided by either left thoracotomy or sternotomy, with or without cardiopulmonary bypass. It should be considered that in patients with a large PDA, severe reduction of the systemic arterial pressure occurs immediately after the establishment of the cardiopulmonary bypass (CPB), due to the large left to right shunt of the arterial blood flow. As a result, in these cases transient occlusion of the PDA orifice in PA side could be done by finger compression immediately before the CPB. The presence of ductal calcification may be associated with increased surgical risk. *Depending on the tissue characteristics and the size of the PDA, surgical strategies may include division and ligation or patch closure. Patch repair technique with cardiopulmonary bypass is recommended for larger or calcified PDA in adult patients*. More than 95 % of PDAs can be repaired surgically and recanalization is rare [8].

Coarctation of the Aorta

Although the appropriate management for native coarctation of the aorta (Co-A) in adults continues to be controversial, surgery should be considered in patients with previously repaired coarctation and long re-coarctation segment or concomitant hypoplasia of the aortic arch (which both affect the adjoining arch arterial branches). Since the unreliable tissue integrity of the paracoarctation region in young ladies in childbearing age, surgical repair with excision of the paracoarctation tissue may be the preferred method in these patients.

Reoperation is performed using sternotomy or posterolateral thoracotomy approaches, depending on the anatomic characteristics of coarctation in any given and associated lesions such as bicuspid aortic valve; dilated aortic root is required to be repaired concomitantly. *Single-stage extra-anatomic bypass of the coarctation segment and simultaneous aorta surgery by sternotomy approach under cardiopulmonary bypass can be performed in selected patients with Co-A and concomitant intracardiac congenital defects or aorta disease* [11]. In this technique, a tube graft was used to bypass the ascending aorta to the descending aorta in supradiaphragmatic region with two end-to-side anastomoses. Partial or full cardiopulmonary bypass may be needed to prevent spinal cord injuries. Preoperative administration of a beta-blocker may prevent or reduce the rebound hypertension which can be encountered early after repair.

Co-A repair with patch aortoplasty technique (especially with the use of a Dacron patch) or resection of coarctation shelf may be complicated by aneurysm formation at the site of repair. False or true aneurysms at the suture line or dissection in both sides of repair site may also develop later [12]. *Paraplegia secondary to the spinal cord injury is rare and more commonly seen in patients with poor collateral circulation.* Arm claudication or subclavian steal syndrome is also a rare complication; however, it may particularly be seen with the subclavian flap technique.

Tetralogy of Fallot

Usually, the residual defects and recurrent disease are the main causes of surgical intervention in adult patients with tetralogy of Fallot. The surgical technique of tetralogy of Fallot in adults (with or without history of palliative procedure) is the same as in children. VSD closure with synthetic or pericardial patch and relief of the RVOT obstruction are the main parts of the total correction of TF. Although simple resection of infundibular tissue may relieve the RVOT obstruction, RV outflow enlargement with limited infundibular patch or even transannular patch is necessary in patients with severe complex RVOT stenosis and small pulmonary annulus. Transannular patch increases the risk of subsequent pulmonary insufficiency and need for valve replacement due to disruption in the continuity of the pulmonary annulus and aneurysmal dilatation of the RVOT.

Infrequently, a homograft or other conduit must be used to relieve the RVOT obstruction in patients with an anomalous coronary artery across the RVOT.

To avoid interruption of this important coronary vessel, the AHA/ACC guideline recommends that the presence or absence of an anomalous anterior descending coronary artery across the RVOT should be determined prior surgery (class I, *level of evidence: C*) [8].

Valvotomy or resection of the pulmonary valve may also be required in the presence of pulmonary valve abnormalities, particularly when complete repair is performed in adulthood [13]. Pulmonary valve replacement is mandatory for severe pulmonary regurgitation in patients with related symptoms or in asymptomatic cases with decreased exercise tolerance and signs of progressive RV dysfunction or severe RV enlargement [8, 14]. A PFO, small ASD, or residual VSD is usually closed simultaneously.

Long-term survival after reparative surgery of tetralogy of Fallot is excellent and has been estimated as a 35-year survival of more than 85 % [15, 16]. *The most common complications encountered in the adulthood after the TF repair include pulmonary regurgitation, residual RVOTO, RV dilation and dysfunction with subsequent TR, residual VSD, aortic root dilation with AR, LV dysfunction, atrial/ventricular tachycardia, and rarely endocarditis* [14]. Sudden cardiac death (SCD) most commonly arises from VT/ventricular fibrillation (VF) due to progressive hemodynamic abnormalities and/or surgical scarring and has been reported in 1–6 % of cases. SCD also constitutes approximately one-third up to half of late deaths [17]. After the second decade of life, the need for pulmonary valve insertion increases the rate of re-interventions. RV-to-pulmonary artery conduit repairs may undergo conduit stenosis or regurgitation, necessitating further interventions. Moreover, in some patients aortic regurgitation deteriorates which requires surgical intervention.

Dextro-transposition of the Great Arteries

Dextro-transposition of the great arteries (d-TGA) generally presents with cyanosis in infancy, and admixture of blood is required for survival. Initial presentation in adulthood is extremely rare unless it has an appropriate admixture of blood. These patients usually have a VSD with pulmonary stenosis, or pulmonary vascular disease represents the TF physiology. As a result, most d-TGA adult patients who visited at adult congenital heart disease clinics have usually had 1 or more operations in infancy and childhood.

After Atrial Baffle Procedure (Mustard, Senning)

Baffle procedure (atrial switch) provides blood mixing and partial physiological correction in patients with complete TGA. This operation consists of anastomosis of the right pulmonary veins to the right atrium and of the inferior vena cava to the left atrium.

Patients with previous atrial switch may need the re-intervention due to the pulmonary venous pathway stenosis or SVC and IVC obstruction or severe subpulmonary stenosis. Pulmonary venous pathway stenosis is usually treated by patch augmentation technique under cardiopulmonary bypass. Superior and inferior vena cava baffle limb obstruction may manage by percutaneous interventions or surgical methods. Surgical options include the extra-anatomic conduit to connect the SVC to IVC, bidirectional cavopulmonary shunt, or patch augmentation technique.

Late subvalvular LVOT (pulmonary trunk) obstruction is usually managed by fibromuscular resection via transpulmonary approach.

After Arterial Switch Operation (Jatene Procedure)

This operation is used in complete TGA and consists of removal of the aorta from its attachment to the right ventricle and of the pulmonary artery from the left ventricle. The great arteries are reattached to the contralateral ventricles with reimplantation of the coronary arteries into the neoaorta. This operation provides the supporting of the systemic circulation by the left ventricle. A Lecompte procedure, translocation of the pulmonary artery confluence anterior to the ascending aorta, is often performed.

Surgery may be considered in patients after the arterial switch operation (ASO) if they had RVOT obstruction coronary artery stenosis with myocardial ischemia (not amenable to percutaneous intervention) and severe neoaortic valve problems.

In patients which have higher desired exercise level or concomitant severe pulmonary regurgitation or are planning for pregnancy lesser degrees of RVOT obstruction should conduct patients to reoperation after arterial switch [8, 18].

Severe RVOT obstruction can be treated surgically by fibromuscular resection, transannular patch, valvuloplasty, or valve replacement according to the type and level of the obstruction. Coronary artery stenosis is usually managed by standard coronary artery bypass grafting. Rarely coronary ostium reimplantation (with or without patch) may be considered in patients with coronary ostium stenosis.

Neoaortic root replacement or neoaorta surgery is usually more challenging because of previous Lecompte maneuver in arterial switch operation. Transection of the pulmonary trunk or its branches may be essential to facilitate the operation in these cases.

After Rastelli Procedure

Rastelli procedure is performed to repair a complete TGA in association with a large VSD and LVOT obstruction. In this operation, a communication is made between the left ventricle and the aorta through VSD closure with a baffle within the right ventricle. The right ventricle is then linked to the pulmonary artery via a valved conduit, and the left ventricle-to-pulmonary artery communication is blocked. The result is the left ventricular support for the systemic circulation.

Patients after Rastelli repair of d-TGA may need reoperation for conduit and/or valve replacement because of conduit stenosis, pulmonary artery branch stenosis, subaortic stenosis, and residual VSD severe aortic valve insufficiency (see Chap. 13).

Intermittent or chronic atrial tachyarrhythmia in adults with d-TGA can be treated effectively with a concomitant Maze procedure during reoperation for any reason [8, 14].

Ebstein's Anomaly

The primary operation in this anomaly generally includes closure of any interatrial communications; antiarrhythmia procedures such as surgical division of accessory conduction pathways, cryoablation of AV node reentry tachycardia, or Maze procedure; and also tricuspid valve surgery. *The tricuspid valve should be repaired, and when the tricuspid valve is not amenable to repair or the repair result is not satisfactory, tricuspid valve replacement approach is adopted using a mechanical or heterograft bioprosthesis.* Right atrial reduction is often considered.

Selected patients with severe RV dysfunction and preserved LV function with low left atrial pressure may benefit from a bidirectional cavopulmonary anastomosis. In patients with significant LV dysfunction (ejection fraction less than 30 %) and symptoms of heart failure, heart transplantation may be considered.

Reoperations are usually performed for tricuspid valve replacement or re-replacement (tissue or mechanical). Re-repair of the tricuspid valve is seldom successful [14].

Tricuspid Atresia/Single Ventricle

Surgical options for the treatment of adults with tricuspid atresia/single ventricle consist of the following.

Systemic-to-Pulmonary Artery Shunt

This operation is rarely performed as an isolated procedure and often connects the ascending aorta and the main or right pulmonary artery (central shunt). It is considered only if the Glenn shunt is contraindicated.

Bidirectional Glenn (Bidirectional Cavopulmonary Anastomosis [BDCPA])

This is a term to describe end-to-side anastomosis of the divided superior vena cava to the undivided right pulmonary artery. This operation directs superior vena cava blood to both right and left pulmonary arteries. This is most commonly performed in infancy or early childhood as a staged procedure toward the Fontan completion. The current procedure provides a stable source of pulmonary blood flow without volume loading the SV. It generally should not be the only source of pulmonary blood flow (except as the stage II procedure for hypoplastic left-sided heart syndrome).

BDCPA Plus Additional Pulmonary Blood Flow

The most reliable source of additional pulmonary blood flow is through the native RVOT with native PS or with a pulmonary artery band. A simultaneous systemic-to-pulmonary artery shunting may be performed if an increase in systemic oxygenation is needed, but this is at the expense of an increase in volume load on the SV and often elevated superior vena cava pressure.

Single-Ventricle Repair

When the rudimentary pulmonary ventricle is less than 30 % of its normal volume, a Fontan operation is performed.

The Fontan operation was introduced in 1968 and is a palliative operation for patients with a functional or anatomic single-ventricle or complex anomaly who are not considered appropriate for a biventricular reparative operation [19]. In patients with univentricular circulation, the Fontan operation results in diversion of systemic venous return directly to the pulmonary artery, usually without the interposition of a subpulmonary ventricle. The operation has gone through several modifications to the procedure; each provides the systemic venous return to enter the pulmonary circulation directly leading to improvement of systemic oxygen saturation and elimination of volume overload of th e systemic ventricle.

Modified Fontan Procedures

The most commonly used procedures in modified Fontan operation include bidirectional Glenn shunt plus conduit from inferior vena cava to right pulmonary artery/main pulmonary artery (extracardiac conduit) and bidirectional Glenn shunt plus intra-atrial conduit from inferior vena cava to right pulmonary artery/main pulmonary artery (intra-atrial conduit). The latter is preferred in patients that the ventricular mass would lie on top of an extracardiac conduit, such as in isolated dextrocardia or isolated levocardia with situs inversus [8, 14].

One-and-a-Half-Ventricle Repair

It is a term used to describe a procedure for patients with cyanotic congenital heart disease performed when the pulmonary ventricle is insufficiently developed to accept the entire systemic venous return. In this operation, a BDCPA is constructed to enable superior vena cava blood to directly enter into the pulmonary arteries, while the inferior caval blood is directed to the lungs via the small pulmonary ventricle.

Two-Ventricle Repair

It is a term used to describe a procedure for patients with cyanotic congenital heart disease with a common ventricle or adequately sized pulmonary ventricles and SVs that communicate via a VSD. The pulmonary and systemic circulations are surgically separated by placement of an interventricular patch (for common ventricle) or a VSD patch (for separate pulmonary and systemic ventricle cavities).

Transplantation

Heart transplantation and heart/lung transplantation are reserved for severe systemic ventricle failure with or without pulmonary artery hypertension (PAH) when there is no conventional surgical option.

Selected adult patients with prior Fontan repair for single-ventricle physiology should be considered for *reoperation*, as described in Chap. 13.

For patients with recurrent atrial fibrillation or flutter without hemodynamically significant anatomic abnormalities, reoperation for Fontan conversion may be useful. *This operation includes revision of an atriopulmonary connection to an intracardiac lateral tunnel, intra-atrial conduit, or extracardiac conduit.* In these patients, a concomitant Maze procedure should also be considered. Reoperation usually consists of a single or combination of the procedures, including valvular repair/replacement in the presence of systemic atrioventricular valve regurgitation, resection of subaortic obstruction, closure of an unintended residual shunt, revision of Fontan pathway obstruction, and Fontan conversion for atrial tachyarrhythmia with or without anatomic abnormalities [20]. A modified Fontan procedure may be applied to ameliorate venous collateral channels or arteriovenous malformations in the right lung in the presence of a classic Glenn shunt. Following this procedure, hepatic venous blood will perfuse the right-sided pulmonary vascular bed [19]. If arteriovenous malformations are not large and have not been long standing, they would regress. Transcatheter occlusion is usually used to treat clinically significant persistent venous collateral channels or systemic aortopulmonary collaterals. Catheter ablation may be beneficial for the treatment of atrial tachycardia. Complete atrioventricular block or sick sinus syndrome commonly necessitates permanent pacing, usually epicardial. In patients suffering from protein losing enteropathy (PLE) in whom medical or catheter therapy is not effective, creation of an atrial septal fenestration or the Fontan conversion may be required. The Fontan communication revision may also be considered in patients with PLE due to the Fontan pathway obstruction.

Heart transplantation is often required for severe ventricular dysfunction [21] or PLE [22], though PLE does not always resolve.

Bicuspid Aortic Valve

There is no general consensus regarding the most appropriate size of the aortic root which necessitates valvular replacement, even though a diameter of greater than 5 cm has been proposed [23]. Furthermore, the beneficial results of aortic root replacement in these patients have remained to be elucidated. The surgical intervention in patients with bicuspid aortic valve may include AV repair or replacement, aortic root reconstruction (valve-sparing techniques or composite graft implantation), or even Ross procedure if indicated.

Subaortic Stenosis

Surgical treatment of discrete subaortic stenosis includes circumferential resection of the fibrous ring and partial resection of the muscular base along the left septal surface. This operation may damage the mitral apparatus or aortic valve, cause a complete heart block necessitating permanent pacemaker implantation, or perforate the interventricular septum (i.e., an acquired VSD). Aortic valve can be repaired simultaneously with subaortic resection in patients with AR. *Against discrete lesions, those with fibromuscular or tunnel-type subaortic stenosis usually need a more extensive septal resection and in some instance a mitral valve replacement.* Subaortic stenosis with long-segment LVOT obstruction may need a Konno-Rastan procedure. It has been demonstrated that the Konno-Rastan procedure is feasible and has acceptable morbidity and mortality in adult patients with diffuse subaortic stenosis, even when associated with other congenital abnormalities such as coarctation of aorta, patent ductus arteriosus, and Shone syndrome [24]. Though the surgical results are satisfactory, restenosis may ensue [8, 14]. In the presence of significant aortic regurgitation, aortic valve replacement may be needed simultaneously with the Konno procedure.

Coronary Arteriovenous Fistula

No treatment is needed for *small arteriovenous shunts*, though IE prophylaxis is advised for patients with more than minimal volume of shunt. In contrast, *large arteriovenous shunts may be associated with significant hemodynamic consequences and should be closed in conditions with a high pulmonary-to-systemic flow (Q_P:Q_S)*. Success rate of the operation would be enhanced if the anatomy of the fistula is clearly defined. In cases with suboptimal anatomic definition, recurrences may ensue, particularly in patients with typically distal fistulous connections which are poorly visualized [14]. Coronary vein bypass grafts may be associated with favorable results, especially in cases with tortuous and aneurysmal fistula which may cause perioperative myocardial infarction due to their potential risk of turbulent flow, clot formation, and extension of the thrombosis [25].

References

1. Zomer AC, Verheugt CL, Vaartjes I, et al. Surgery in adults with congenital heart disease. Circulation. 2011;124(20):2195–201.
2. Carole A, Warnes C, Liberthson R, et al. Task Force 1: the changing profile of congenital heart disease in adult life. J Am Coll Cardiol. 2001;37(5):1170–5. doi:10.1016/S0735-1097(01)01272-4.
3. Khoshbin E, Prayaga S, Kinsella J, et al. Mini-sternotomy for aortic valve replacement reduces the length of stay in the cardiac intensive care unit: meta-analysis of randomised controlled trials. BMJ Open. 2011;1(2):e000266.
4. Masiello P, Coscioni E, Panza A, et al. Surgical results of aortic valve replacement via partial upper sternotomy: comparison with median sternotomy. Cardiovasc Surg. 2002;10(4):333–8.
5. Ding C, Wang C, Dong A, et al. Anterolateral minithoracotomy versus median sternotomy for the treatment of congenital heart defects: a meta-analysis and systematic review. J Cardiothorac Surg. 2012;7:43.
6. Kogon BE, Daniel W, Fay K, et al. Is the liberal use of preoperative 3-dimensional imaging and presternotomy femoral cutdown beneficial in reoperative adult congenital heart surgery? J Thorac Cardiovasc Surg. 2013 Sep 23. pii: S0022-5223(13)00907-0. doi: 10.1016/j.jtcvs.2013.07.074.
7. Nikolaou K, Vicol C, Vogt F, et al. Dual-Source computed tomography of the chest in the surgical planning of repeated cardiac surgery. J Cardiovasc Surg (Torino). 2012;53(2):247–55.
8. Warnes CA, Williams RG, Bashore TM, et al. ACC/AHA 2008 guidelines for the management of adults with congenital heart disease: a report of the American College of Cardiology/American Heart Association Task Force on Practice Guidelines (Writing Committee to Develop Guidelines on the Management of Adults With Congenital Heart Disease). J Am Coll Cardiol. 2008;52(23):e143–263.
9. Tabatabaei MB, Ghavidel AA, Yousefnia MA, et al. Classic Konno-Rastan procedure: indications and results in the current era. Asian Cardiovasc Thorac Ann. 2006;14:377–81.
10. Celermajer DS, Sholler GF, Hughes CF, et al. Persistent ductus arteriosus in adults. A review of surgical experience with 25 patients. Med J Aust. 1991;155:233–6.
11. Wang R, Sun LZ, Hu XP, et al. Treatment of complex coarctation and coarctation with cardiac lesions using extra-anatomic aortic bypass. J Vasc Surg. 2010;51(5):1203–8.
12. Knyshov GV, Sitar LL, Glagola MD, et al. Aortic aneurysms at the site of the repair of coarctation of the aorta: a review of 48 patients. Ann Thorac Surg. 1996;61:935–9.
13. Atik FA, Atik E, da Cunha CR, et al. Long-term results of correction of tetralogy of Fallot in adulthood. Eur J Cardiothorac Surg. 2004;25(2):250–5.
14. Baumgartner H, Bonhoeffer P, De Groot NM, et al. ESC Guidelines for the management of grown-up congenital heart disease (new version 2010). Eur Heart J. 2010;31(23):2915–57.
15. Murphy JG, Gersh BJ, Mair DD, et al. Long-term outcome in patients undergoing surgical repair of tetralogy of Fallot. N Engl J Med. 1993;329:593–9.
16. Nollert G, Fischlein T, Bouterwek S, et al. Long-term survival in patients with repair of tetralogy of Fallot: 36-year follow-up of 490 survivors of the first year after surgical repair. J Am Coll Cardiol. 1997;30:1374–83.
17. Gatzoulis MA, Balaji S, Webber SA, et al. Risk factors for arrhythmia and sudden cardiac death late after repair of tetralogy of Fallot: a multicentre study. Lancet. 2000;356:975–81.
18. Hirata Y, Chen JM, Quaegebeur JM, et al. Should we address the neopulmonic valve? Significance of right-sided obstruction after surgery for transposition of the great arteries and coarctation. Ann Thorac Surg. 2008;86(4):1293–8; discussion 1298. doi:10.1016/j.athoracsur.2008.03.059.
19. Fontan F, Baudet E. Surgical repair of tricuspid atresia. Thorax. 1971;26:240–8.
20. Mavroudis C, Deal BJ, Backer CL, et al. J. Maxwell Chamberlain Memorial Paper for congenital heart surgery. 111 Fontan conversions with arrhythmia surgery: surgical lessons and outcomes. Ann Thorac Surg. 2007;84:1457–65.
21. Gamba A, Merlo M, Fiocchi R, et al. Heart transplantation in patients with previous Fontan operations. J Thorac Cardiovasc Surg. 2004;127:555–62.
22. Marcelletti CF, Hanley FL, Mavroudis C, et al. Revision of previous fontan connections to total

extracardiac cavopulmonary anastomosis: a multicenter experience. J Thorac Cardiovasc Surg. 2000;119: 340–6.
23. Bonow RO, Carabello BA, Chatterjee K, et al. ACC/AHA 2006 guidelines for the management of patients with valvular heart disease: a report of the American College of Cardiology/American Heart Association Task Force on Practice Guidelines (Writing Committee to Revise the 1998 Guidelines for the Management of Patients With Valvular Heart Disease) developed in collaboration with the Society of Cardiovascular Anesthesiologists, endorsed by the Society for Cardiovascular Angiography and Interventions and the Society of Thoracic Surgeons. J Am Coll Cardiol. 2006;48:e1–148.
24. Ghavidel AA, Javadpour H, Tabatabaei MB, et al. Complete surgical repair of Tetralogy of Fallot in adults, is it ever too late? J Card Surg. 2008;23:23–6.
25. Ghavidel AA, Kyavar M, Ojaghi Z, et al. Huge arteriovenous fistula between a giant aneurysmal right coronary artery and coronary sinus. Arch Iran Med. 2012;15(2):1.

Part II

Specific Cardiac Disease

Atrial Septal Defect

19

Anita Sadeghpour, Azin Alizadehasl,
Nehzat Akiash, and Majid Kyavar

Keywords

Atrial Septal Defect (ASD) • Secundum Type ASD • Septum Primum Type ASD • Sinus Venosus Type ASD • Coronary Sinus Type ASD • Echocardiography

Atrial Septal Defect

Atrial Septal Defect: Definition and Classification

One of the most common adult congenital heart defects (CHD) is the atrial septal defect (ASD), which is a true, direct, and permanent communication between two atria. There are four major types of the ASD: ostium secundum, ostium primum, sinus venosus defect (superior and inferior types), and coronary sinus defect or unroofed coronary sinus (CS) [1, 2].

The ostium secundum is a true defect of the atrial septum which involves the fossa ovalis. Atrioventricular septal defects (AVSD) constitute a form of anomalies with defects in the atrioventricular (AV) septum and abnormalities of the AV valves. The sinus venosus ASD usually occurs at the junction of the superior vena cava and the

A. Sadeghpour, MD, FACC, FASE (✉)
Echocardiography Lab, Department of Cardiology, Adult Congenital Heart Disease Clinic, Rajaie Cardiovascular Medical and Research Center, Iran University of Medical Science, Tehran, Iran
e-mail: anita.sadeghpour@gmail.com, asadeghpour@rhc.ac.ir

A. Alizadehasl, MD, FACC
Echocardiography Lab, Department of Cardiology, Rajaie Cardiovascular Medical and Research Center, Iran University of Medical Science, Tehran, Iran
e-mail: alizadeasl@gmail.com, alizadeasl@rhc.ac.ir

N. Akiash, MD
Department of Cardiology, Rajaie Cardiovascular Medical and Research Center, Tehran, Iran

M. Kyavar, MD, FACC
Cardiovascular Imaging Ward, Department of Cardiology, Adult Congenital Heart Disease Clinic, Rajaie Cardiovascular Medical and Research Center, Iran University of Medical Science, Tehran, Iran

Electronic supplementary material The online version of this chapter (doi: 10.1007/978-1-4471-6383-1_19) contains supplementary material, which is available to authorized users.

A. Sadeghpour et al. (eds.), *Comprehensive Approach to Adult Congenital Heart Disease*,
DOI 10.1007/978-1-4471-6383-1_19, © Springer-Verlag London 2014

right atrium (RA) and is almost always associated with partial anomalous pulmonary venous connection (PAPVC). The unroofed CS is a defect between the CS and the left atrium (LA), resulting in a left-to-right shunt [1, 3].

The patent foramen ovale (PFO) is a flap-like communication in which the septum primum, which covers the fossa ovalis, overlays the superior limbic band of the septum secundum. In some cases, the septum primum or septum secundum is aneurysmal and has several small fenestrations [1, 2].

Epidemiology and Associated Lesions

The ASD accounts for about 10–15 % of all CHDs and also is the most common form of CHD in adults. The most common form of the ASD is the ostium secundum type (70 %), and 65–75 % of patients with the secundum ASD are female. The ostium primum type accounts for almost 20 % of all types of the ASD. Complete AV canal accounts for about 3 % of all cardiac malformations, and females are affected slightly more frequently than males. The sinus venosus ASD accounts for approximately 4–11 % of all ASDs, and finally the unroofed CS is a rare type [1, 2, 5].

The ASD can be correlated with additional CHD in approximately 30 % of patients. The primum ASD is almost always seen with a cleft in the anterior mitral valve leaflet. The sinus venosus ASD defect often has PAPVC of the right pulmonary veins. Of course this association exists in a small group of patients with the secundum-type ASD. Also, mitral valve prolapse is often seen in cases with the ASD. Valvular pulmonic stenosis may be seen in patients with the ASD; however, sometimes, mildly increased right ventricular outflow tract gradient is present only due to a greater passing flow.

The CS septal defect may be complemented by PAPVC or total anomalous pulmonary venous connection (TAPVC) or a persistent left superior vena cava draining into the CS [1–3, 6].

Pathophysiology

In the ASD, the defect allows the crossing of the blood through the atrial septum. The extent of the shunt depends on size of the defect, end-diastolic pressures of both ventricles, and function of the atrioventricular valves.

Regarding the lower right ventricular end-diastolic pressure (RVEDP) compared to the left ventricular end-diastolic pressure (LVEDP), the ASD usually creates a left-to-right shunt.

In case of significant tricuspid regurgitation, elevated RVEDP due to the abnormal compliance of the RV, and pulmonary hypertension, a right-to-left shunt can occur. In the ASD with significant left-to-right shunting, pulmonary artery pressure increases mildly, despite normal pulmonary vascular resistance. Nevertheless, Eisenmenger's syndrome with a right-to-left shunt occurs in about 5 % of the secundum-type ASD, mostly in women [1, 4, 5].

Clinical Signs and Symptoms for All Types

Patients with the ASD frequently remain asymptomatic until adulthood. The most frequent signs and developed symptoms are reduced functional class, exertional dyspnea and tachycardia (supraventricular tachyarrhythmias), and less frequently pulmonary infections and right-sided heart failure [2].

A large ASD [pulmonary artery blood flow relative to systemic blood flow (Q_p/Q_s >2.0)] may cause congestive heart failure and failure to thrive in an infant or child. An undetected ASD with a significant shunt (Q_p/Q_s >1.5) possibly causes symptoms over time in adolescence or adulthood, and symptomatic cases frequently become progressively more physically limited as they age. Clinical findings are the fixed splitting of the second heart sound (S2) without respiratory variation (although this finding is not invariable), systolic murmur in the pulmonary area, and diastolic murmur across the tricuspid valve due to an increased flow across the pulmonary valve and tricuspid valve [6–8].

Effort dyspnea is seen in about 30 % of patients by the third decade and in more than 75 % of cases by the fifth decade of life. Supraventricular arrhythmias such as atrial fibrillation or atrial flutter and right-sided heart failure develop by 40 years of age in about 10 % of cases and become more frequent with aging. Paradoxical embolism resulting in a transient ischemic attack or stroke can call attention to the diagnosis. The development of pulmonary hypertension, though probably not as common as originally thought, can happen at an early age. If pulmonary hypertension is severe, a second causative diagnosis must be sought.

The CS ASD usually does not show important symptoms in childhood. Occasionally, even infants develop clinically significant symptoms of congestive heart failure with other contributing factors. The symptoms that occasionally happen in the CS ASD include mild exercise intolerance, frequent respiratory infections, exertional dyspnea, systemic emboli, cerebral abscess, transient ischemic attacks, and cyanosis [1–3, 5].

Electrocardiography

The electrocardiogram (ECG) may be normal with an uncomplicated ASD and a small shunt. Most affected individuals have a normal sinus rhythm, but atrial arrhythmias often occur beyond the third decade. The ECG hallmark of an ASD is an rSr' or rsR' pattern in the right precordial leads. RV volume overload is responsible for enlargement and increased thickness, which causes the terminal force of the QRS to be directed to the right, superior, and anterior sides.

A notch near the apex of the R wave in the inferior leads of the ASD is referred to as "crochetage." It correlates with the severity of the shunt, and the sensitivity and specificity of this sign are prominent when it is associated with an incomplete right bundle branch block or when it is present in all the inferior limb leads [1, 2, 4, 9].

Chest Radiography

Cardiomegaly may be present from right heart dilation (in all types of the ASD) and occasionally from left heart dilation if significant mitral regurgitation is present in the patient with the ostium primum ASD or in older adults with atrial fibrillation rhythm.

The central pulmonary arteries are characteristically enlarged with increased pulmonary vascular markings due to pulmonary arterial overflow. Shunt vascularity is apparent by uniformly distributed vascular markings with the absence of the normal lower lobe vascular predominance and right descending pulmonary artery diameter >17 mm.

In a significant ASD, the chest X-ray film is often (but not always) abnormal.

The sinus venous ASD may be accompanied by the localized enlargement or ampullary dilation of the superior vena cava proximal to its attachment to the RA.

In comparison to the classic chest X-ray findings, the radiographic appearance in patients diagnosed at a later age (mostly after age 50) may be atypical. The atypical findings include normal vasculature, evidence of pulmonary venous hypertension, LA enlargement, and even pulmonary edema.

On the chest X-ray, the ascending aorta is seldom border-forming because the shunt does not traverse the aortic root [1–4, 9–11].

Echocardiography

Echocardiography can document the presence, type, and size of the ASD besides the direction of the shunt.

Subcostal view, parasternal short-axis view, and off-axis four-chamber view are the most useful views for the evaluation of the ASD. The interatrial septum in the fossa ovalis region is thin and is parallel with the ultrasound beam; accordingly, in apical four-chamber view finding, a dropout in the septum would be misleading.

Color Doppler study and contrast echocardiography using agitated saline can confirm the presence of the communication [2–6].

Echocardiography is particularly useful for the evaluation of the morphology of the AV valves. The vast majority of the AV canal defects are diagnosed by echocardiography alone. Echocardiographic assessment is required for the evaluation of the associated anomalies and can determine their significance. Transthoracic echocardiography (TTE) can show the hemodynamic significance of the shunt based on right-sided volume overload, presence/absence of paradoxical septal motion (RV volume overload), and ventricular septal orientation. TTE is the primary diagnostic imaging modality for the evaluation of the ASD in that it can reveal right heart dilation. Enlargement of the RA and RV with diastolic flattening and paradoxical interventricular septal motion are the evidence of a significant left-to-right shunt and RV volume overload. False-negative diagnoses are relatively common in adults with poor-quality transthoracic images, especially patients with the sinus venosus ASD. Even a bubble study may be falsely negative because the shunt is usually completely left to right. Transesophageal echocardiography (TEE) may be necessary to identify the presence and type of the ASD and confirm the normal connection of all pulmonary veins to the LA. Also in patients with pulmonary artery hypertension, the low velocity of the shunt flow may be difficult to diagnose.

All associated lesions should be considered during the echocardiographic study too [2, 6–8].

Cardiac Catheterization

Cardiac catheterization is not required in younger patients with an uncomplicated ASD and adequate noninvasive imaging. Cardiac catheterization remains essential in case of pulmonary hypertension (pulmonary artery pressure 50 % of systemic pressure) documented by Doppler echocardiography. Cardiac catheterization is generally required for the evaluation of coronary artery disease in patients at risk and reactivity in patients with significant pulmonary artery hypertension [2, 4, 5].

Septum Secundum-Type Atrial Septal Defect

The most common form of the ASD is the ostium secundum type (70 %). The secundum-type ASD involves the fossa ovalis. More often than not, the deficiency of the infolding of the atrial wall results in the extension of the defect to the outside of the true limits of the fossa ovalis. It is called the secundum defect due to its presence at the site of the embryologic ostium secundum. The shape of the defect varies, but it is often oval shaped and sometimes irregular. Less often, the secundum defect with multiple perforations of the membrane creates a fenestrated appearance, which suggests multiple defects (Video 19.1). Infrequently, a defect can extend posteriorly and inferiorly, approaching the site of the inferior vena cava entering into the RA [1–3].

The ECG and chest X-ray demonstrate the aforementioned findings (Figs. 19.1 and 19.2).

TTE and TEE have the main role in diagnosis as well as the study of the associated disease and evaluation of the presence and indeed the size of the defect and the presence and size of rims for determining the possibility of device closure [6] (Figs. 19.3, 19.4, 19.5 and 19.6. Video 19.2).

In adults, TTE shows false-positive two-dimensional dropout, mostly in four-chamber view in the fossa ovalis region. Consequently, pulsed wave Doppler study and color flow imaging can be drawn upon to identify the true defect [2, 3] (Figs. 19.7 and 19.8. Video 19.3).

Contrast echocardiography with agitated saline is used to detect atrial shunt and shows positive and negative contrasts [2, 6]. (To be demonstrated in (Figs. 19.9 and 19.10).

During early systole, there can be a minor reversal of the shunt flow, resulting in a positive contrast study (Video 19.4). Three-dimensional TEE affords precise anatomic detail of the ASD regarding the morphology, size, and surrounding rims (Fig. 19.11).

Right heart catheterization in the secundum-type ASD shows that the catheter enters the LA and the left upper pulmonary vein via the ASD (Video 19.5).

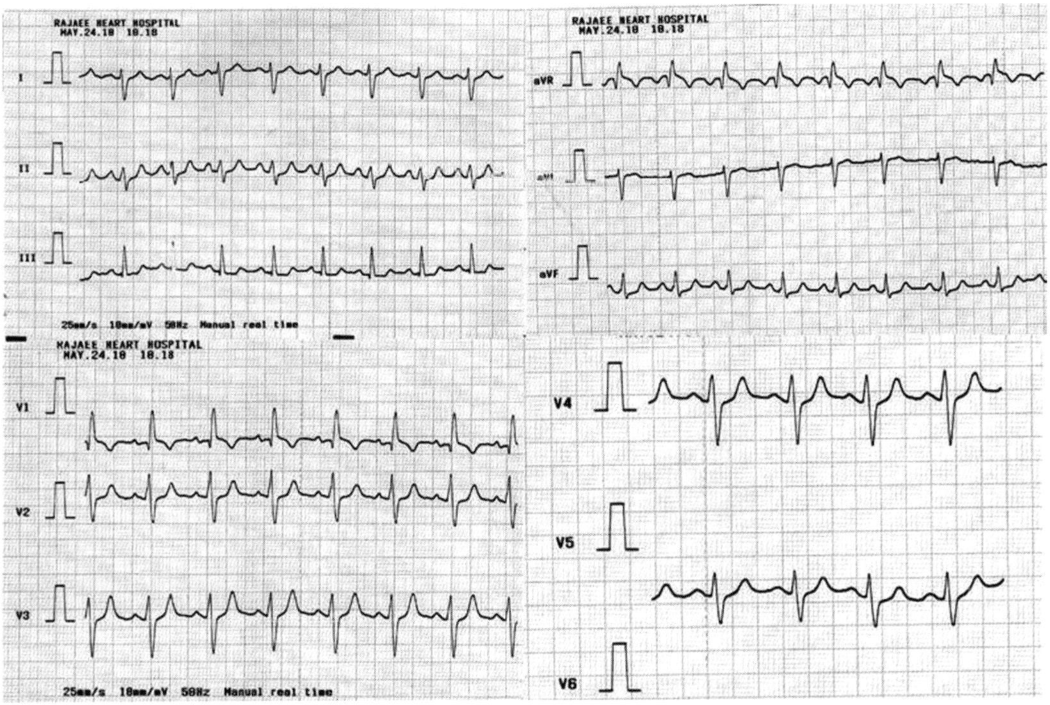

Fig. 19.1 Right-axis deviation: peaked P wave in lead II, rsR' in lead V_1, tall R wave in leads V_1–V_2, and deep S wave in leads I, AVL, and V_4–V_6 are noted in this electrocardiogram

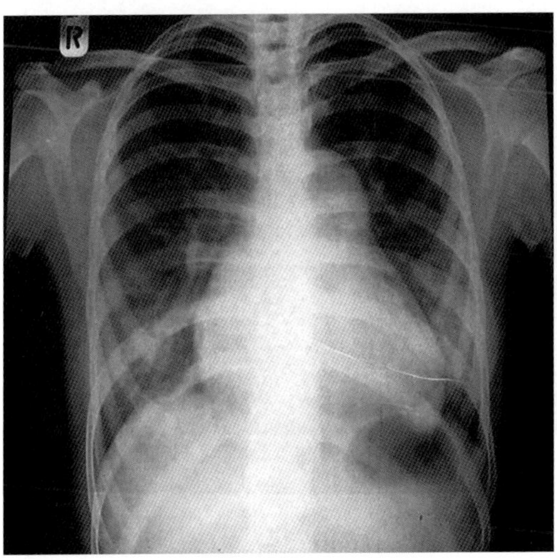

Fig. 19.2 Chest X-ray in posteroanterior projection, demonstrating levocardia, situs solitus, prominent pulmonary artery segment, shunt vascularity, small aortic knob, increased cardiothoracic ratio, and cardiomegaly due to right ventricular and right atrial enlargement

Currently, the majority of secundum ASDs can be closed with a percutaneous catheter technique. When this is not possible or not suitable, however, surgical closure of the ASD is recommended. In the postoperative evaluation, the patch should appear in proper position without any residual shunt or any mass [1, 2, 6–8] (Figs. 19.12 and 19.13, Videos 19.6 and 19.7).

Septum Primum-Type Atrial Septal Defect

The ostium primum type accounts for almost 20 % of all types of the ASD. An ostium primum ASD is found in the most anterior and inferior portion of the atrial septum (Fig. 19.14a, b. Videos 19.8 and 19.9).

It is the simplest form of the AV canal or AV septal defect (AVSD). In the partial AVSD, a

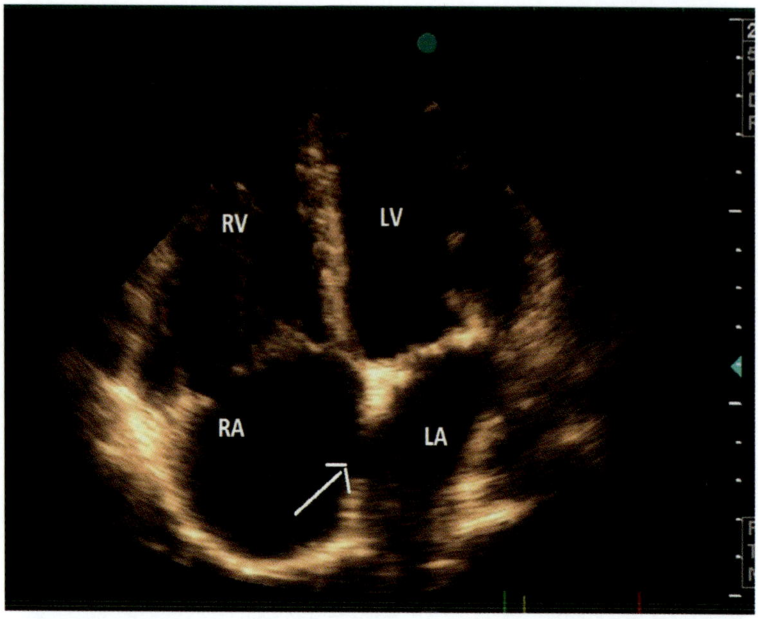

Fig. 19.3 Transthoracic echocardiography in four-chamber view, showing a two-dimensional defect in the atrial septum associated (*arrow*) with right atrial and ventricular enlargement, highly suggestive of the secundum-type atrial septal defect (It should be confirmed in other views). *RV* right ventricle, *LV* left ventricle, *LA* left atrium, *RA* right atrium

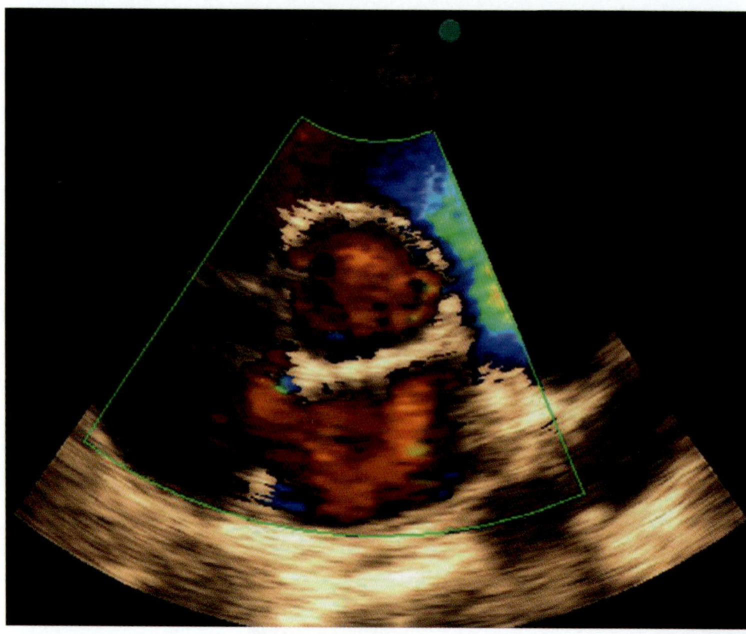

Fig. 19.4 Secundum-type atrial septal defect with a left-to-right shunt by color flow imaging

primum-type ASD is always present with two distinct tricuspid and mitral valve annuli. The left AV valve (mitral valve) is invariably trileaflet with a cleft in the anterior mitral leaflet [1–3] (AML) (Fig. 19.15 Video 19.10).

The common pathology in all types of the AVSD is the absence of the AV septum, associated with the abnormalities of the AV valves. On echocardiographic examination, the AV valves are at the same level (Video 19.11) with an elongated LV outflow tract, which is called the "goose neck deformity" [1, 2, 4–6] (Figs. 19.16 and 19.17).

The complete form also includes a primum ASD, but it is contiguous with an inlet ventricular

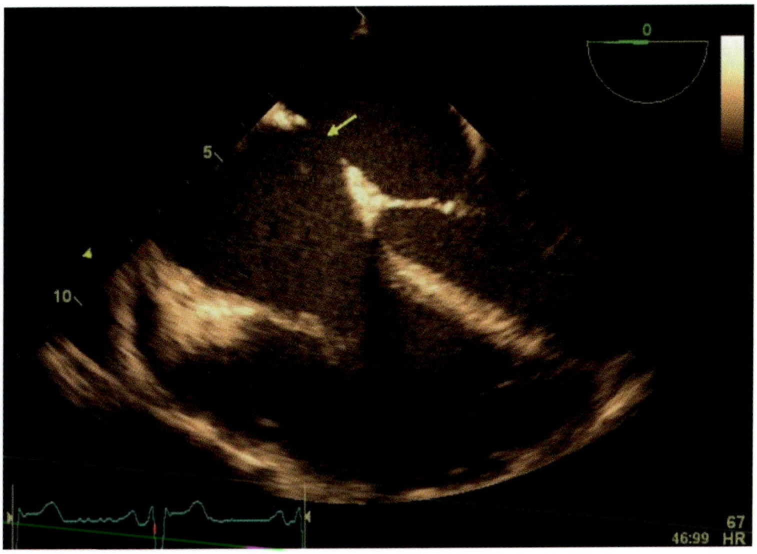

Fig. 19.5 Two-dimensional transesophageal echocardiography, demonstrating a secundum-type atrial septal defect (*arrow*) The surrounding rims are noted as posterosuperior and anteroinferior (mitral) rims

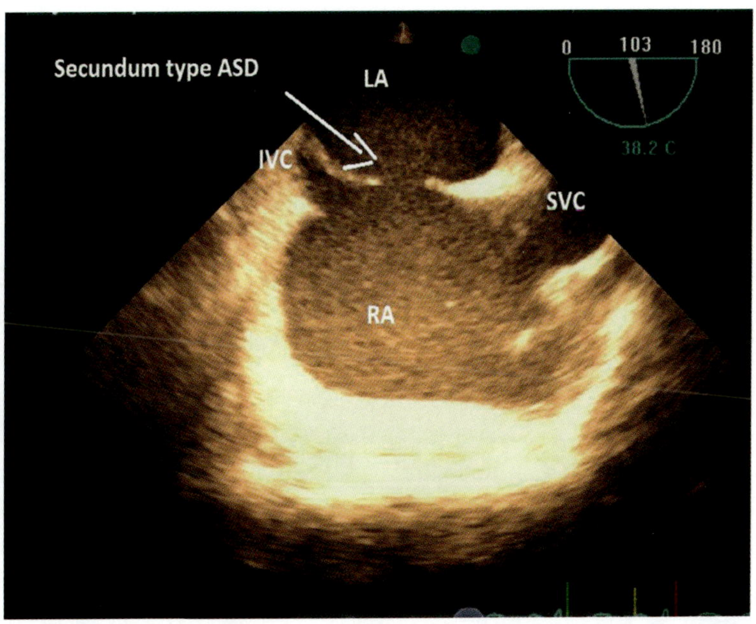

Fig. 19.6 Bicaval view, confirming the location and type of the atrial septal defect (*arrow*) with superior (superior vena cava) and inferior (inferior vena cava or inferoposterior) rims. *LA* left atrium, *IVC* inferior vena cava, *RA* right atrium, *SVC* superior vena cava

septal defect (VSD) and the common AV valve has a single annulus. During fetal growth, the rudimentary and primary atrium is divided by the septum primum, except for the anterior and inferior part, which is the ostium primum. Of course, it is sealed by the fusion of the superior and inferior endocardial cushions around the fifth week of fetal development; if this development fails to happen, an ostium primum ASD is created [1, 3, 5, 8]. The endocardial cushions are also important in the completion, formation, and separation of the two separate AV valves in tandem with the inlet interventricular septum. For this reason, the ostium primum ASD is generally allied to the malformations of these parts. The ostium primum ASD may happen alone, but most frequently it is

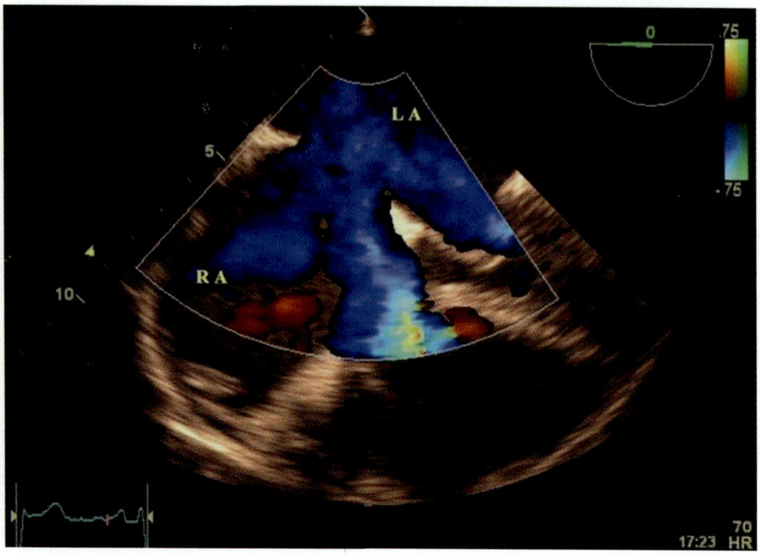

Fig. 19.7 Color flow imaging on the two-dimensional defect, showing a low-velocity *blue color jet* representing a left-to-right flow across the atrial septal defect

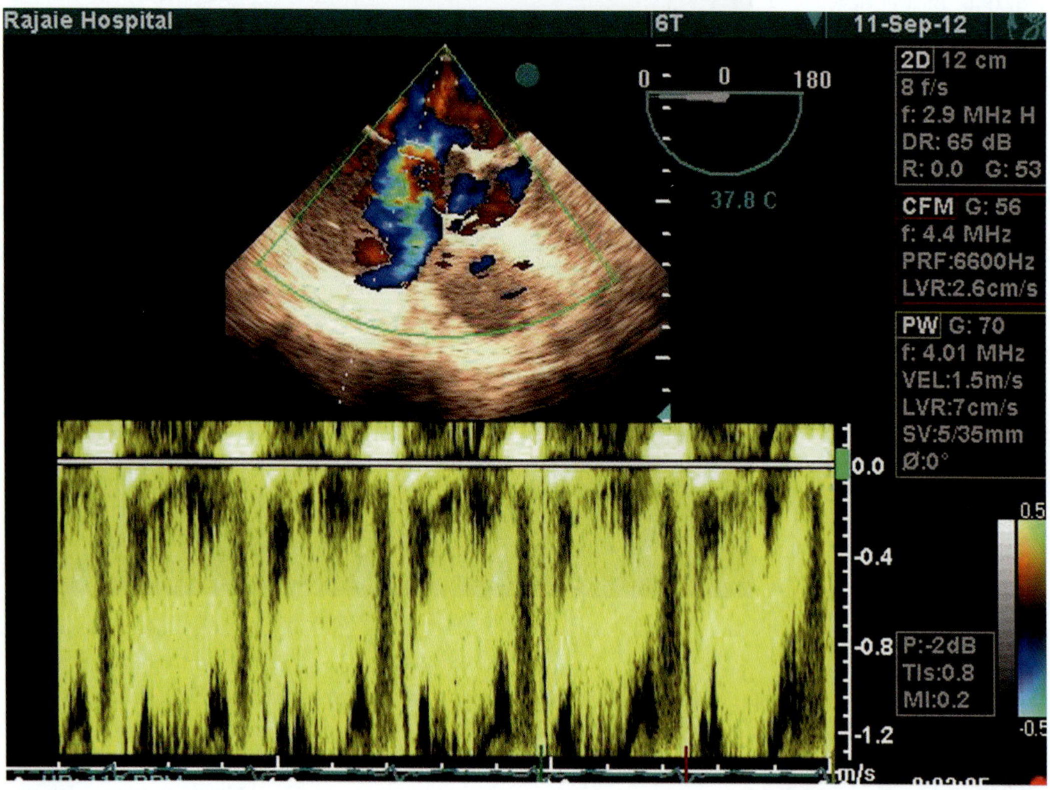

Fig. 19.8 Pulsed wave Doppler study on the *blue color jet*, confirming the left-to-right flow across the atrial septal defect

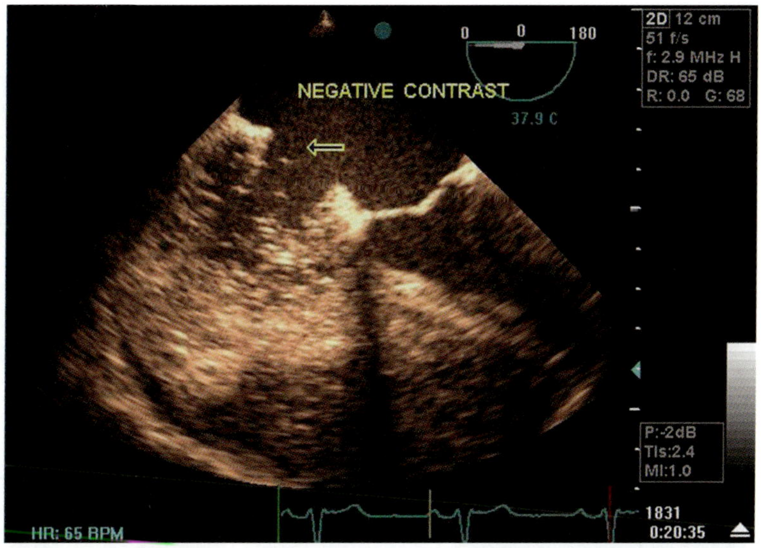

Fig. 19.9 Contrast echocardiography by the rapid injection of the agitated saline, confirming the presence of an atrial septal defect. Non-contrast blood that crosses the atrial septal defect results in negative contrast in the right atrium

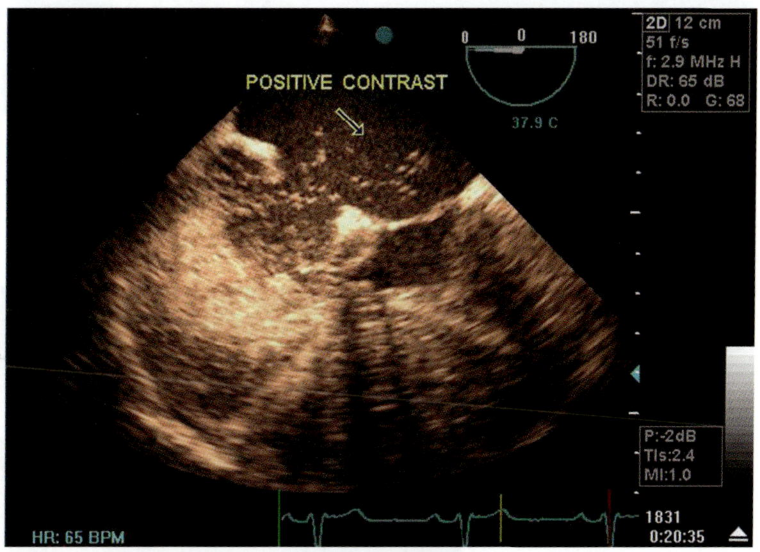

Fig. 19.10 Right heart contrast study, showing the passage of a few bubbles from the right atrium to the left atrium

present with a cleft in the anterior leaflet of the mitral valve. This is referred to as a partial AV canal defect or a partial AVSD. In the chest X-ray of these patients, left heart dilation may be present (concomitant with right heart dilation) if there is significant mitral regurgitation.

TTE and TEE are the major diagnostic tools in the diagnosis of the AVSD spectrum, divided into the partial or the complete AVSD [4, 6].

Sinus Venosus-Type Atrial Septal Defect

The sinus venosus ASD accounts for approximately 4–11 % of ASDs. Sinus venosus ASD differs from secundum-type ASD; sinus venosus ASD is an interatrial defect outside the fossa ovalis, in the unfolding wall which separates the LA and the superior vena cava or the inferior vena cava.

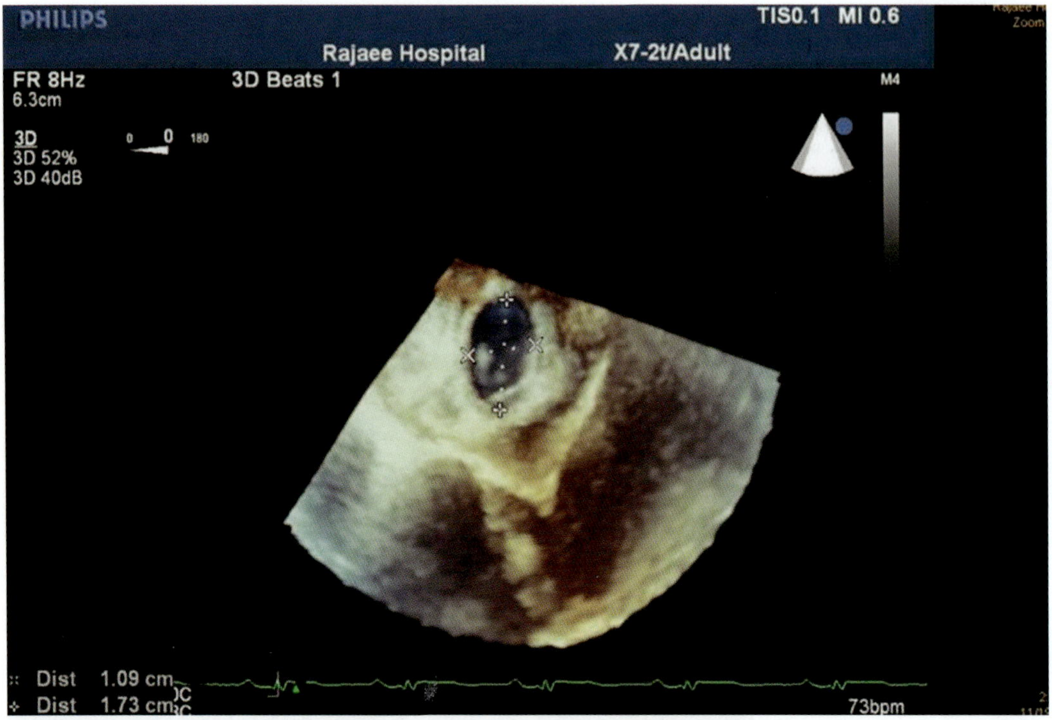

Fig. 19.11 Three-dimensional transesophageal echocardiography, affording precise anatomic detail of the atrial septal defect's morphology, size, and surrounding rims

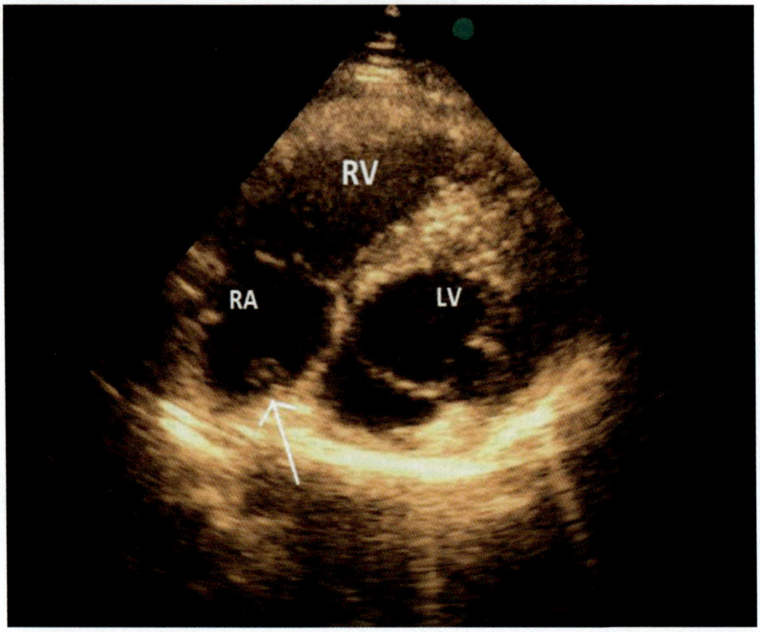

Fig. 19.12 Postoperative echocardiography in an adult patient with atrial septal defect repair by pericardial patch, showing an echogenic mass attached to the right side of the interatrial septum, suggestive of thrombosis (*arrow*). *RV* right ventricle, *RA* right atrium, *LV* left ventricle

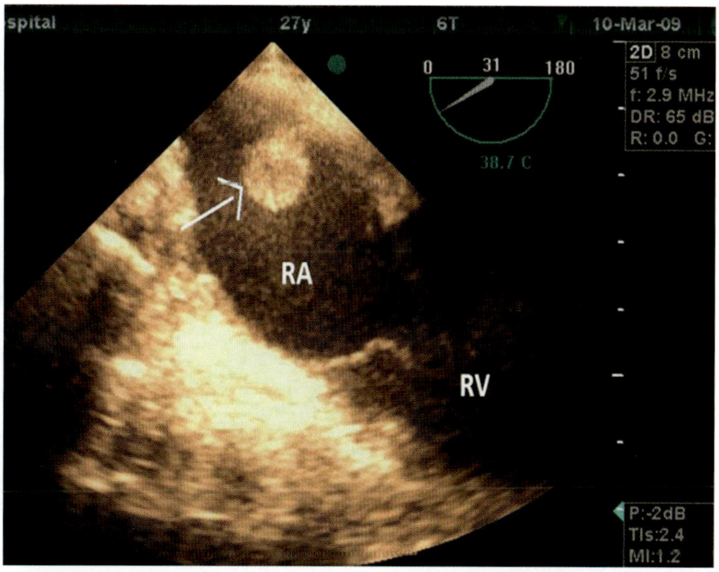

Fig. 19.13 Transesophageal echocardiography in the same patient, showing the round echogenic mass attached to the inferoposterior side of the interatrial septum, suggestive of thrombosis (*arrow*), which was subsequently resolved by anticoagulation therapy

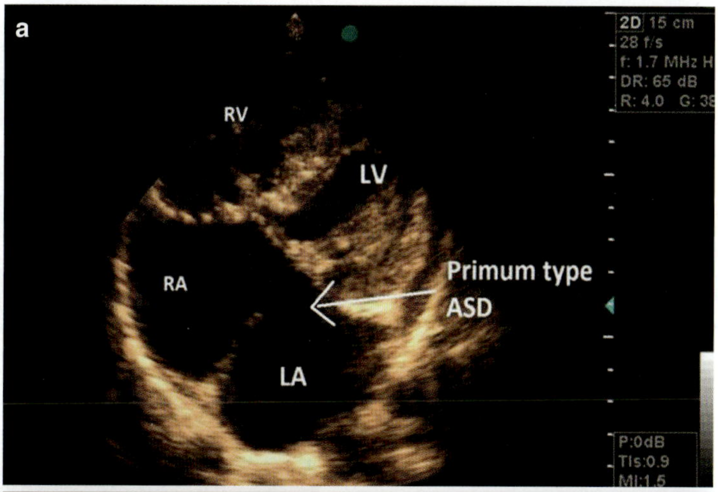

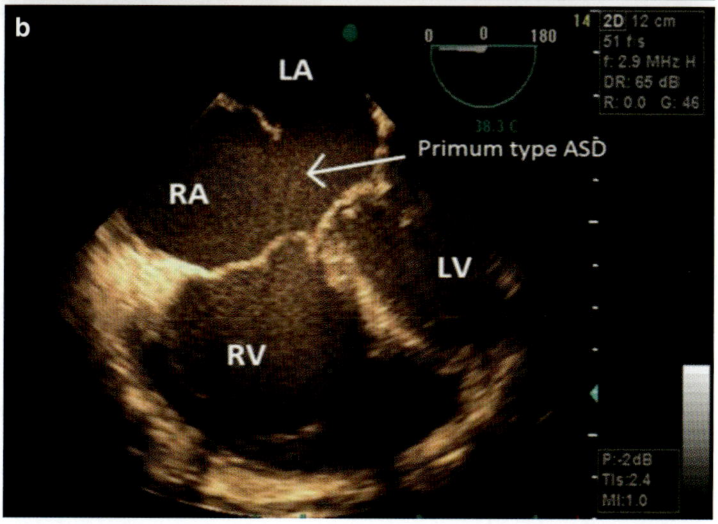

Fig. 19.14 (**a**, **b**) Transthoracic and transesophageal echocardiography in four-chamber view, showing the same level atrioventricular valves associated with a large defect in the most anteroinferior portion of the atrial septum suggestive of primum-type ASD and partial AVSD. *RA* right atrium, *RV* right ventricle, *LV* left ventricle, *LA* left atrium

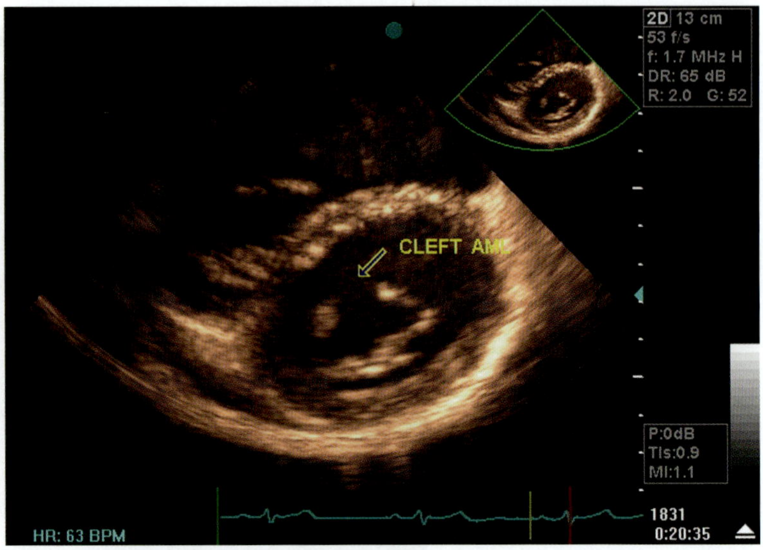

Fig. 19.15 The trileaflet left AV valve (mitral valve) with a cleft in the anterior mitral leaflet (*AML*)

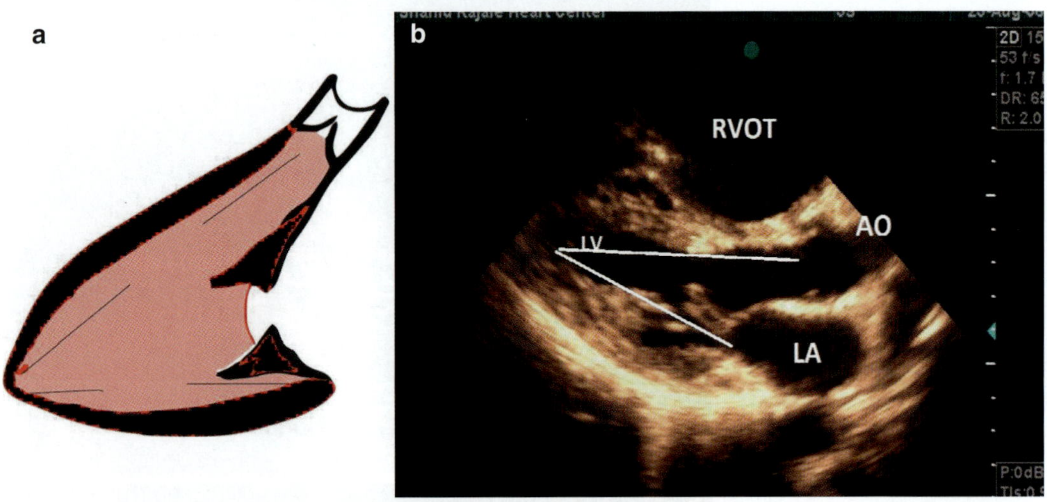

Fig. 19.16 (**a**, **b**) Elongated LVOT with shorter distance from MV annulus to LV apex than AV annulus to the apex. *AO* aorta, *RVOT* right ventricular outflow tract, *LV* left ventricle *LA* left atrium

The superior form of the sinus venosus ASD is more common than the inferior type and accounts for 5–10 % of all ASDs. Posterior aspect is the RA free wall, and its superior border is often absent because of an overriding superior vena cava. As a result of defect, superior vena cava or less commonly the inferior vena cava overrides across interatrial septum; its superior border is often absent. Anomalous connection of some or all of the right pulmonary veins, especially the right upper pulmonary vein (RUPV), to the superior vena cava or the right atrium is very common in sinus venosus ASD [1–3, 12].

In the ECG of the sinus venosus ASD patients, sinus node dysfunction can cause persistent sinus bradycardia (<50 bpm), ectopic atrial rhythm (inverted inferior P wave), junctional rhythm, and a wandering pacemaker rhythm [1, 2] (Fig. 19.18).

A sinus venosus ASD may or may not be accompanied by localized enlargement of the superior vena cava proximal to its attachment to the RA (Fig. 19.19).

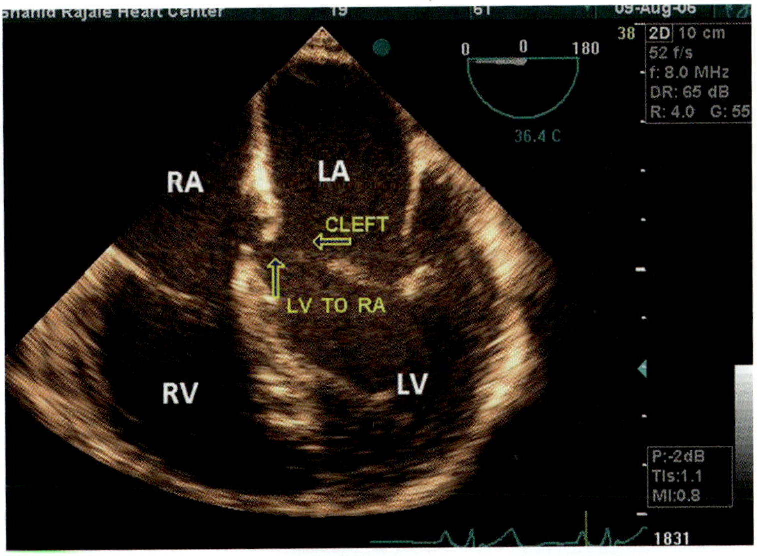

Fig. 19.17 Transesophageal echocardiography in four-chamber view, showing multiple defects in the internal cardiac crux (including the atrial septum, ventricular septum, and septal portions of the AV valves). *Arrows* showing a cleft in the anterior mitral valve and direct LVOT to RA communication. *RA* right atrium, *RV* right ventricle, *LV* left ventricle, *LA* left atrium, *LV* to RA left ventricle to right atrium

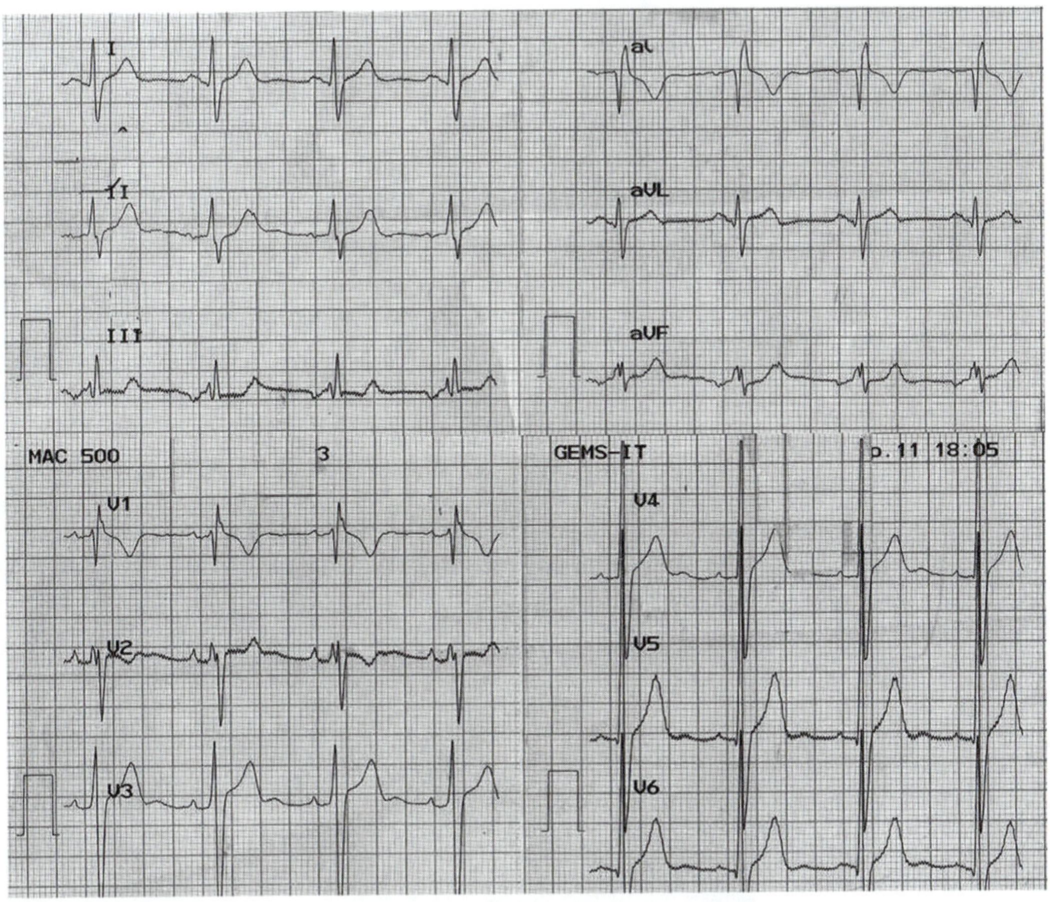

Fig. 19.18 Electrocardiogram, revealing right axis deviation; incomplete right bundle branch block (RBBB); rSR pattern in lead V1; deep S wave in leads I, AVL, and V4-V6; a notch on the R wave in lead AVF ("crochetage pattern"); and ectopic atrial rhythm (negative P wave in leads III and AVF and positive in leads I and AVL), highly suggestive of a sinus venous-type atrial septal defect (ASD) due to absent or deficient sinus node or ASD located near the sinus node

The important, false-negative diagnosis in TTE is sinus venosus ASD although it can be visualized in off-axis view [6–8] (Fig. 19.20, Video 19.12).

TEE plays a major role in the diagnosis of the sinus venosus ASD (Figs. 19.21 and 19.22a, b, Videos 19.13 and 19.14).

PAPVC, especially the abnormal drainage of the right upper pulmonary vein into the superior vena cava, may be present, which is detected well by TEE (Figs. 19.23 and 19.24, Video 19.15), and also by contrast echocardiography; it interestingly shows negative contrast in the site of the right upper pulmonary vein drainage into the superior vena cava (Fig. 19.25 and Video 19.16).

Cardiac CT confirms the diagnosis [2, 6, 8] (Fig. 19.26).

Cardiac catheterization is generally required for the evaluation of coronary artery disease in patients at risk and reactivity in patients with significant pulmonary artery hypertension.

The right catheter course: right femoral vein → inferior vena cava → RA → superior vena cava → right upper pulmonary vein [3–5, 13, 14, 15] (Fig. 19.27, Videos 19.17 and 19.18).

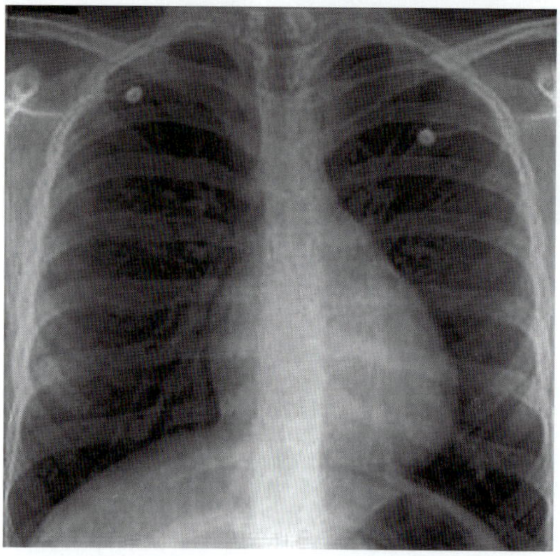

Fig. 19.19 Chest X-ray, demonstrating increased pulmonary blood flow and shunt vascularity, central pulmonary artery enlargement, small aortic knob, and enlargement of the right heart chambers

Coronary Sinus-Type Atrial Septal Defect

The unroofed CS is a communication between the CS and the LA. The most common anomaly associated with this type of the ASD is the left superior vena cava. The unroofed CS is classified into four types: type I, completely unroofed CS with the left superior vena cava; type II, completely unroofed CS without the left superior vena cava; type III, partial unroofed midportion

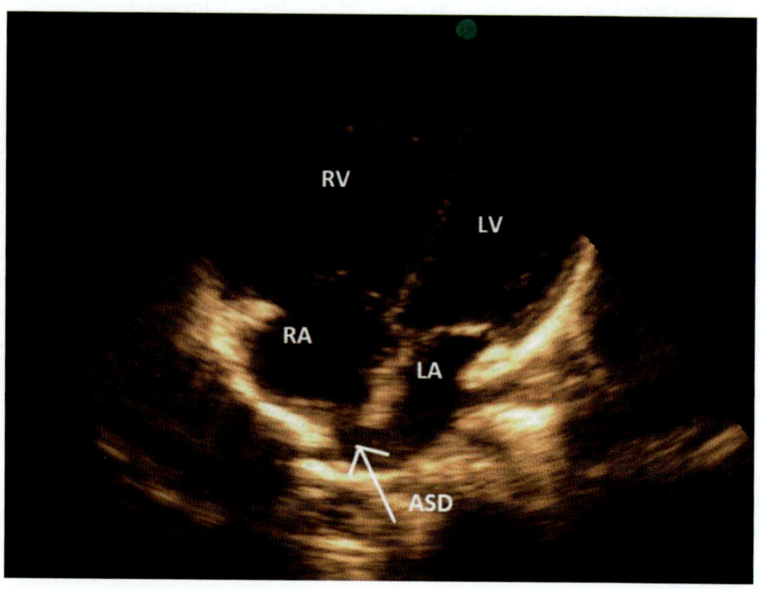

Fig. 19.20 Transthoracic echocardiography (TTE), showing an atrial septal defect (*ASD*) located at the superior region of the interatrial septum adjacent to the to the right pulmonary veins

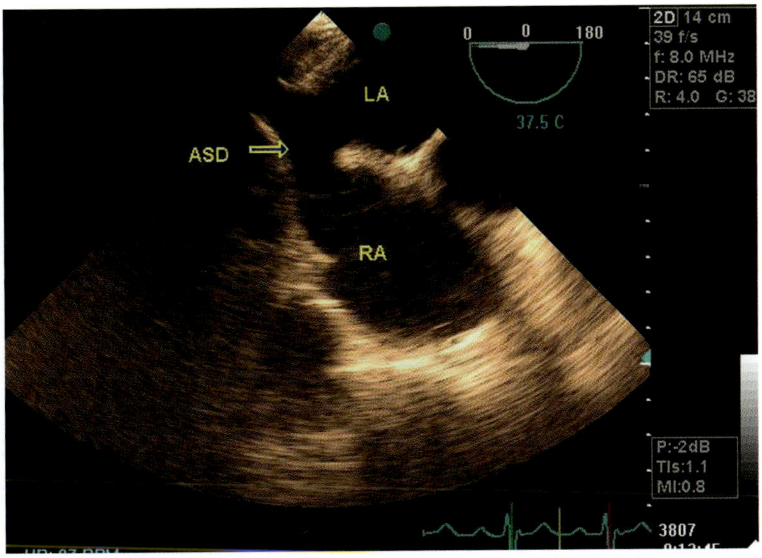

Fig. 19.21 Transesophageal echocardiography (TEE) (0°) in high esophageal view, demonstrating a two-dimensional defect at the superior vena cava to the right atrium and left atrium junction

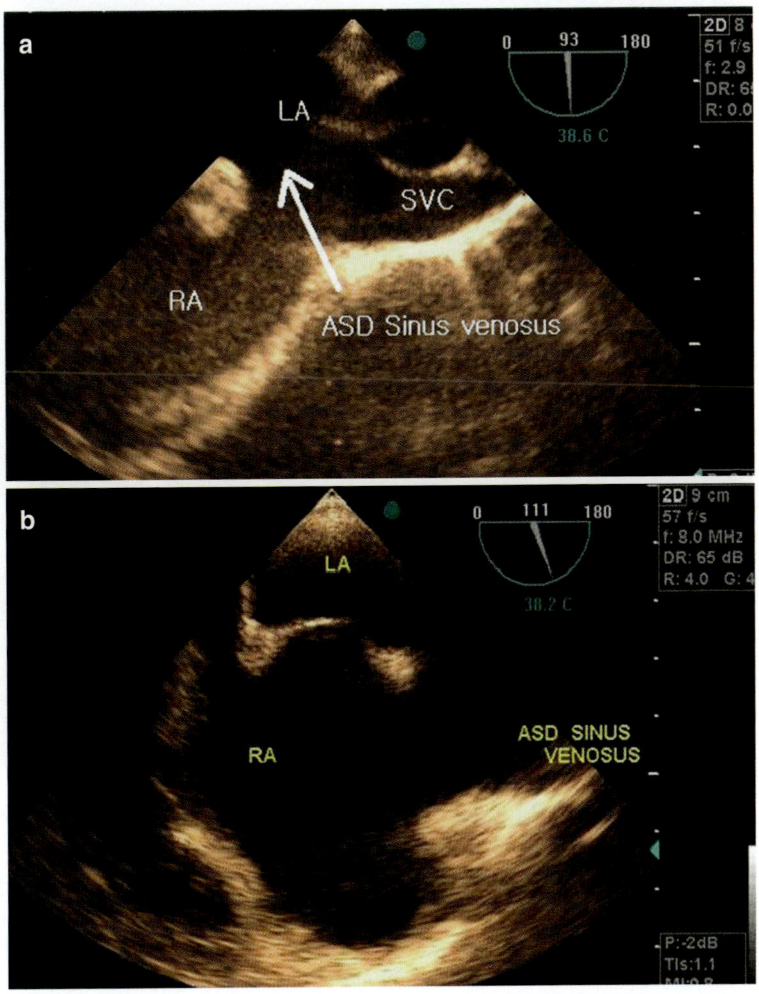

Fig. 19.22 (**a**, **b**) Transesophageal echocardiography (TEE) in bicaval view (90°), confirming the sinus venous-type atrial septal defect diagnosis. *RA* right atrium, *LA* left atrium, *SVC* superior vena cava, *ASD* atrial septal defect

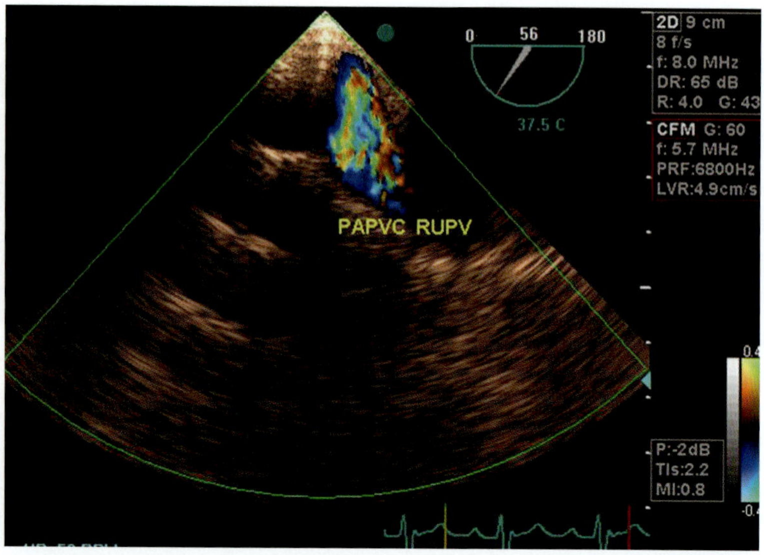

Fig. 19.23 Color Doppler imaging, showing abnormal drainage of the right upper pulmonary vein to the right atrium. *PAPVC* partial anomalous pulmonary venous connection, *RUPV* right upper pulmonary vein

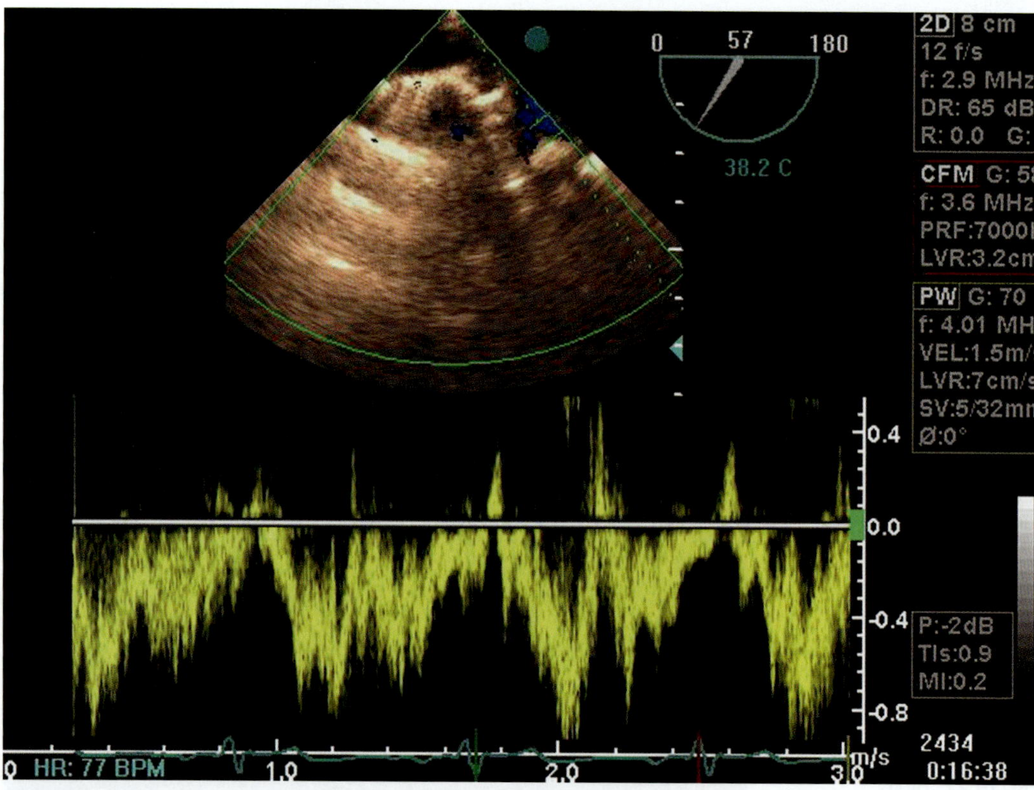

Fig. 19.24 Doppler study, confirming the abnormal drainage of the right upper pulmonary vein to the right atrium

of the CS; and type IV, partial unroofed terminal portion [2–6].

The clinical presentation is largely determined by the size of the defect and the degree of left-to-right shunting. These patients may not exhibit important symptoms, although some can even develop clinically significant symptoms of congestive heart failure. The symptoms that

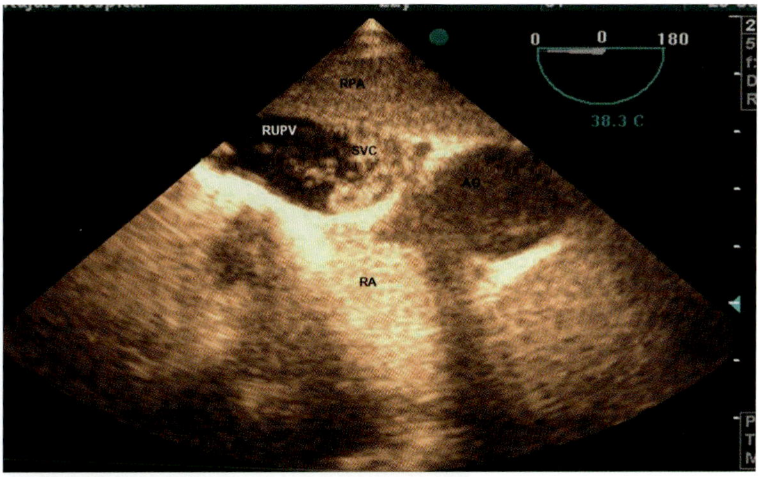

Fig. 19.25 Contrast injection in the high esophageal view (0°), demonstrating the negative contrast in the site of the right upper pulmonary vein draining into the superior vena cava. *RA* right atrium, *SVC* superior vena cava, *RUPV* right upper pulmonary vein, *AO* aorta, *RPA* right pulmonary artery

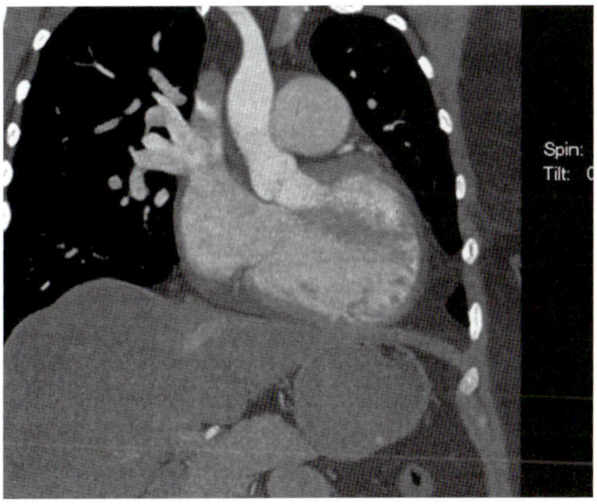

Fig. 19.26 Cardiac CT showing the abnormal drainage of the right upper and middle pulmonary veins to the right atrium

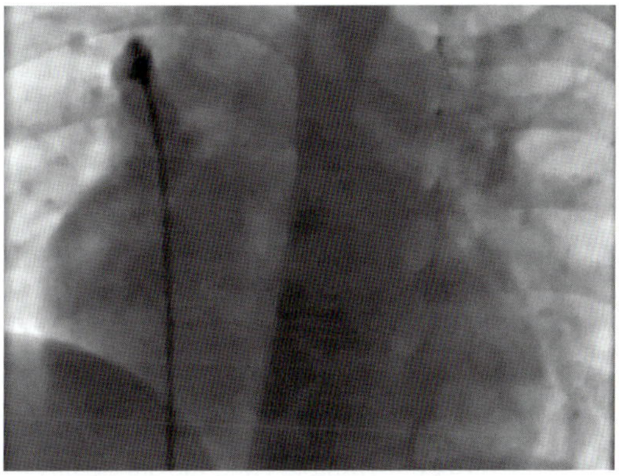

Fig. 19.27 Right catheter course: Right femoral vein → inferior vena cava → right atrium → superior vena cava → right upper pulmonary vein

occasionally happen in the CS ASD include mild exercise intolerance, frequent respiratory infections, exertional dyspnea, systemic emboli, cerebral abscess, transient ischemic attacks, supraventricular arrhythmia, and cyanosis.

The unroofed CS is often seen in association with other CHDs. Apart from the left superior vena cava, other kinds of CHD such as cor triatriatum, pulmonary atresia, Tetralogy of Fallot, and PAPVC have also been reported in patients with CS defects [1, 3, 7, 9].

TTE is typically used as the first imaging modality for a suspected unroofed CS. Nonetheless, inability to visualize the posterior cardiac structures such as the CS and pulmonary veins is a major disadvantage of TTE. In contrast, TEE can assess these posterior structures more accurately, particularly in mid-esophageal long-axis views, and can confirm the anomaly [2, 6, 8] (Fig. 19.28, Videos 19.19 and 19.20).

Importantly, in echocardiography, a large CS orifice with signs of atrial shunting may specify a defect in the roof of the CS. As a result, the entire CS roof must be imaged when this is suspected. Cardiac catheterization can confirm the diagnosis (Video 19.21). When a CS defect is a related

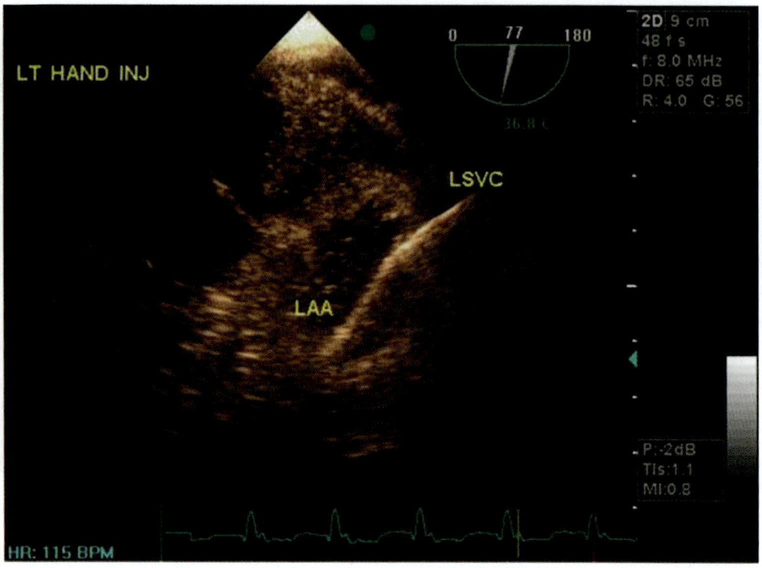

Fig. 19.28 Unroofed coronary sinus with persistent LSVC (agitated saline contrast injection via the left antecubital vein shows rapid LA opacification via the persistent LSVC to LA connection) *LAA* left atrial appendix. *LSVC* left superior vena cava

disease that causes right-to-left shunting, the orifice of the CS may not be enlarged, and the defect may not be documented until after definitive surgery and the occurrence of left-to-right shunting [1–4].

Diagnostic Pitfalls for All Types

The slow onset of symptoms and the subtle physical findings with the ASD frequently lead to late diagnosis, which puts the patient at superior risk of creating and developing pulmonary artery hypertension, arrhythmia, and paradoxical embolism. False-positive detection of the ASD can result from apparent interatrial septal dropout on two-dimensional echocardiography. By using TEE or contrast echocardiography, false-positive interpretations may be reduced. Patients with PAPVC without an ASD, which will have RV volume overload, should be considered as a false-positive diagnosis for a concomitant ASD [1, 3, 7].

False-negative diagnoses are common too, especially in adults with poor window transthoracic images, and particularly the sinus venosus ASD because of its superior location. Accordingly, all patients with an unexplained RV volume overload by TTE should be assessed further by TEE or other imaging modalities not only to completely evaluate the intra-atrial septum and all pulmonary veins but also to rule out defects in the roof of the CS [2–6, 8].

Management and Follow-Up

Patients with small shunts and a normal RV size are usually asymptomatic and need no medical therapy. Follow-up of patients with a small ASD without pulmonary artery hypertension or RV enlargement should include evaluation of symptoms (arrhythmias and probable paradoxical embolic events) and echocardiography every 2–3 years to assess the RV size and function and pulmonary hypertension. Atrial arrhythmias must be treated to maintain the sinus rhythm. If atrial fibrillation occurs, both antiarrhythmic and anticoagulation therapies are recommended [1–4, 16].

ASDs that are large and cause pulmonary artery hypertension should be closed if there is evidence of pulmonary vascular reactivity and left-to-right shunting. Medical therapy for the ASD with pulmonary artery hypertension is planned only for irreversible pulmonary artery hypertension. Medical therapy for congestive heart failure improves the signs and symptoms and can be a bridge until surgery. Medications for heart failure include digitalis, diuretics, and vasodilators and some new generations of pulmonary vasodilators. Surgery consists of ASD repair and also repair of the concomitant diseased valves before the occurrence of pulmonary hypertension. Also, cardioversion, rate control, and anticoagulation are suggested for atrial fibrillation [1, 4, 16–18].

Indications for ASD closure include cases with significant shunts and signs of RV volume overload besides pulmonary vascular resistance <5 Wood units. These patients should undergo ASD closure. Device closure is the treatment of choice for most secundum-type ASDs except for patients with Eisenmenger's physiology. After ASD closure by device, the risk of arrhythmia such as atrial flutter and atrial fibrillation and sick sinus syndrome is very low. Antiplatelet therapy is necessary for at least 6 months.

Surgical closure is essential for cases with the ostium primum and the sinus venosus ASD and also patients with the secundum ASD whose anatomy is not suitable for device closure. Device closure is the first choice for the secundum-type defect. If morphology is appropriate and the process is supported by TEE or intracardiac echocardiography, this type of treatment minimizes hospitalization and recovery period. After device closure, some small residual shunts are likely to persist; however, these are not hemodynamically significant and many will close spontaneously within 1 year. Other complications such as atrial tachyarrhythmias, erosion of the atrial wall or aorta, and thromboembolic events are rare.

Surgical repair of the sinus venosus ASD can be associated with postoperative sinus node dysfunction, venous obstruction, and right-to-left shunting. The precise evaluation of the extraseptal nature of the interatrial communication reduces the risk of sinus node dysfunction during surgery. The sinus venosus ASD repair with PAPVC is associated with low morbidity and mortality even in old age, and severe complications such as sinus node dysfunction are rare [2, 10, 11, 17].

Of note, small ASDs (diameter <5 mm) with no evidence of RV volume overload do not affect the natural history; thus, they may not need closure except when they are correlated with paradoxical embolism.

It is not uncommon to detect the ASD in adults, which raises the question regarding the benefit of ASD closure in these patients, particularly when the patient is 40 years of age or more. In a randomized clinical trial, surgical closure of the ASD was performed in patients >40 years and the results showed reduced morbidity (but not mortality). In contrast, another study reported survival improvement even in patients older than 60 years [2, 4, 16] (Tables 19.1 and 19.2).

Endocarditis Prophylaxis

Endocarditis does not happen in cases with isolated ASDs and is typically related with concomitant valvular disease, such as a cleft MV. So endocarditis prophylaxis is not needed for isolated ASDs before or after any surgery except for the first 6 months after closure procedure [3, 7].

Pregnancy

Pregnancy in cases with ASDs is usually well tolerated, without maternal mortality and no important maternal or fetal morbidity. Though the left-to-right shunt may increase with the rise in cardiac output in pregnancy, of course, this is counterbalanced by the reduction in peripheral resistance.

Mothers with large shunts and also PAH may have arrhythmias and ventricular dysfunction and also progression in PAH. It is important that pregnancy in patients with ASD and Eisenmenger's syndrome is contraindicated due to high maternal and fetal mortality and must be strongly discouraged. Paradoxical embolism may infrequently be faced in small or large ASDs [1, 3, 7].

Activity

Cases with small ASDs and with no PAH have normal exercise capability and do not need any limitation in physical activity. In patients with large left-to-right shunts, exercise is frequently self-limited due to reduced cardiopulmonary

Table 19.1 Recommendations for interventional and surgical therapy (ACC/AHA Guidelines 2008)

Class I
1. Closure of an ASD either percutaneously or surgically is indicated for RA and RV enlargement with or without symptoms *(level of evidence: B)*
2. A sinus venosus, CS, or primum ASD should be repaired surgically rather than by percutaneous closure *(level of evidence: B)*
3. Surgeons with training and expertise in CHD should perform operations for various ASD closures *(level of evidence: C)*
Class IIa
1. Surgical closure of secundum ASD is reasonable when concomitant surgical repair/ replacement of a tricuspid valve is considered or when the anatomy of the defect precludes the use of a percutaneous device *(level of Evidence: C)*
2. Closure of an ASD, either percutaneously or surgically, is reasonable in the presence of: a. Paradoxical embolism *(level of evidence: C)*
3. b. Documented platypnea-orthodeoxia *(level of evidence: B)*
Class IIb
1. Closure of an ASD, either percutaneously or surgically, may be considered in the presence of net left-to-right shunting, pulmonary artery pressure less than two thirds systemic levels, PVR less than two thirds systemic vascular resistance, or when responsive to either pulmonary vasodilator therapy or test occlusion of the defect (patients should be treated in conjunction with providers who have expertise in the management of pulmonary hypertensive syndromes) *(level of evidence: C)*
2. Concomitant Maze procedure may be considered for intermittent or chronic atrial tachyarrhythmias in adults with ASDs *(level of evidence: C)*
Class III
Patients with severe irreversible PAH and no evidence of a left-to-right shunt should not undergo ASD closure *(level of evidence: B)*

Table 19.2 Recommendations for postintervention follow-up (ACC/AHA 2008 Guidelines)

1. In early postoperative symptoms of undue fever, fatigue, vomiting, chest pain, or abdominal pain may represent postpericardiotomy syndrome with tamponade and should prompt immediate evaluation with echocardiography *(level of evidence: C)*
2. Annual clinical follow-up is recommended for patients postoperatively if their ASD was repaired as an adult and the following conditions persist or develop: (a) PAH *(level of evidence: C)* (b) Atrial arrhythmias *(level of evidence: C)* (c) RV or LV dysfunction *(level of evidence: C)* (d) Coexisting valvular or other cardiac lesions *(level of evidence: C)*
3. Evaluation for possible device migration, erosion, or other complications is recommended for patients 3 months to 1 year after device closure and periodically thereafter *(level of evidence: C)*
4. Device erosion, which may present with chest pain or syncope, should warrant urgent evaluation *(level of evidence: C)*

function. Symptomatic supraventricular or ventricular arrhythmias might also compromise the exercise capacity. Also patients with significant PAH must limit their activities to low intensity sports. Severe PAH with right-to-left shunting is typically self-limiting, and active physical efforts should be avoided [3].

References

1. Bonow RO, Mann DL, Zipes DP, Libby P. Braunwald's heart disease: a textbook of cardiovascular medicine. 9th ed. Philadelphia: Elsevier – Health Sciences Division; 2011. p. 1435–50.
2. Gatzoulis MA, Webb GD, Broberg CS, Uemura H. Cases in adult congenital heart disease. Philadelphia: Churchill Livingstone; 2010.
3. Warnes C, Williams RG, Bashore TM, et al. ACC/AHA, guidelines for the management of adults with congenital heart disease. JACC. 2008;52(23):2008.
4. Warnes CA, American Heart Association. Adult congenital heart disease, AHA clinical series. Hoboken: 2009. p. 9–24. Chapter 2.

5. Allen HD, Driscoll DJ, Shaddy RE. Moss and Adams' heart disease in infants, children, and adolescents: including the fetus and young adults. 7th ed. Philadelphia: Lippincott Williams & Wilkins; 2008.
6. Eidem BW, Cetta F, O'leary PW. Echocardiography in pediatric and adult congenital heart disease. Philadelphia: Lippincott Williams & Wilkins; 2012.
7. Baumgartner H, Bonhoeffer P, De Groot NM, et al. ESC guidelines for the management of grown-up congenital heart disease (new version 2010). Eur Heart J. 2010;31(23):2915–57.
8. Houston A, Hillis S, Lilley S, et al. Echocardiography in adult congenital heart disease. Heart. 1998;80 Suppl 1:S12–26.
9. Perloff JK. The clinical recognition of congenital heart disease. 5th ed. Philadelphia: WB Saunders; 1994. p. 300–25.
10. S Yamaki , T Horiuchi, M Miura, et al. Pulmonary vascular disease in secundum atrial septal defect with pulmonary hypertension. Chest. 1986;89:694–698.
11. Reading M. Chest x-ray quiz: an atrial septal defect. Aust Crit Care. 2000;13:96–119.
12. Oliver JM, Gallego P, Gonzalez A, et al. Sinus venosus syndrome: atrial septal defect or anomalous venous connection? A multiplane transoesophageal approach. Heart. 2002;88(6):634–8.
13. Jesinger RA, Strollo DC. Radiology corner. Sinus venosus atrial septal defect. Mil Med. 2010;175(4): 52–83.
14. Sojak V, Sagat M, Balazova E, et al. Outcomes after surgical repair of sinus venosus atrial septal defect in children. Bratisl Lek Listy. 2008;109(5):215–9.
15. Attenhofer Jost CH, Connolly HM, Danielson GK, Bailey KR, Schaff HV, Shen WK, et al. Sinus venosus atrial septal defect: long-term postoperative outcome for 115 patients. Circulation. 2005;112(13): 1953–8.
16. Humenberger M, Rosenhek R, Gabriel H. Benefit of atrial septal defect closure in adults: impact of age. Eur Heart J. 2010.
17. Attie F, Rosas M, Granados N, Zabal C, Buendia A, Calderon J. Surgical treatment for secundum atrial septal defects in patients.40 years old. A randomized clinical trial. J Am Coll Cardiol. 2001;38: 2035–42.
18. Gatzoulis MA, Redington AN, Somerville J, Shore DF. Should atrial septal defects in adults be closed? Ann Thorac Surg. 1996;61:657–9.

Partial Anomalous Pulmonary and Systemic Venous Connection (PAPVC)

20

Anita Sadeghpour and Azin Alizadehasl

Keywords
Partial Anomalies of the Pulmonary Venous Connections (PAPVC) • Atrial Septal Defect (ASD) • Sinus Venosus Type ASD • Right upper pulmonary vein • Echocardiography

Morphology

In the normal anatomy four separate pulmonary veins (PVs) directly connect to the left atrium. However, normal variations in the number of PVs are not uncommon. Partial anomalous pulmonary venous connection (PAPVC) is a condition in which a segment or all of one lung drain into a site other than the left atrium. Sinus venosus type defects are correlated with PAPVC classically from the right upper and right middle lobe pulmonary veins to the superior vena cava. PAPVC can be directed to the superior vena cava at the level or above the right pulmonary artery, left vertical vein, and azygos vein and also to the coronary sinus. PAPVC to the inferior vena cava (scimitar syndrome) can be related to right lung hypoplasia and pulmonary sequestration with an abnormal collateral supply [1–4].

PAPVC can be seen in <10 % of patients with a secundum type atrial septal defect (ASD). When there is PAPVC to the right atrium and the pulmonary veins in the normal position, the septum primum is deviated to the left. This lesion is seen more often in hearts with visceral heterotaxia [1, 2, 5].

Clinical Findings

In the absence of related abnormalities, the number of anomalous veins, their site of junction, size of ASD (if present), and pulmonary vascular resistance determine the physiologic disturbance. Usually, in patients with an isolated connection or with connections between two anomalous veins, the hemodynamic status and the physical findings bear striking similarities to those of patients with ASD [1, 6].

A. Sadeghpour, MD, FACC, FASE (✉)
Echocardiography Lab, Department of Cardiology, Adult Congenital Heart Disease Clinic, Rajaie Cardiovascular Medical and Research Center, Iran University of Medical Science, Tehran, Iran
e-mail: anita.sadeghpour@gmail.com, asadeghpour@rhc.ac.ir

A. Alizadehasl, MD, FACC
Echocardiography Lab, Department of Cardiology, Rajaie Cardiovascular Medical and Research Center, Iran University of Medical Science, Tehran, Iran
e-mail: alizadeasl@gmail.com, alizadeasl@rhc.ac.ir

Electronic supplementary material The online version of this chapter (doi: 10.1007/978-1-4471-6383-1_20) contains supplementary material, which is available to authorized users.

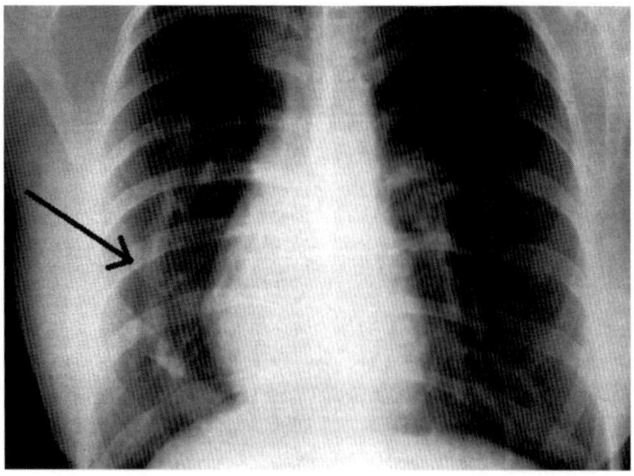

Fig. 20.1 In the scimitar syndrome, one or all of the right PVs connect to the IVC making a curved sword appearance (resembles Turkish sword) on the chest X-ray associated with right lung hypoplasia and dextroposition of the heart. Abnormal pulmonary vein connecting IVC (*arrow*)

Electrocardiography

In isolated PAPVC cases, the electrocardiographic (ECG) findings are similar to those in secundum type ASD [2, 6].

Chest Radiography

Most cases reveal cardiomegaly involving the right ventricle, with increased and prominent pulmonary vascular markings. In the scimitar syndrome, one or all of the right lung PVs connect to the IVC. These anomalous PVs orientation are more vertical and dilated making a curved sword appearance mainly on the Chest X Ray.

In the scimitar syndrome, there is dextroposition associated with right lung hypoplasia [1, 2, 5] (Fig. 20.1).

Echocardiography

Echocardiography plays an important role in detection of the PAPVC and associated hemodynamic effect on the chambers (as the right ventricular enlargement with paradoxical septal motion in the significant left-to-right shunt). When there is left-sided PAPVC with connection to the innominate vein through the vertical vein, the suprasternal long-axis view is very useful. *In the suprasternal long-axis view, leftward angulation can identify the left vertical vein as a red color flow toward the innominate vein. The left vertical vein connects the left pulmonary veins to the innominate vein which drains to the SVC* [1, 2] (Fig. 20.2a, b. Videos 20.1, 20.2 and 20.3). Transesophageal echocardiography (TEE) may also be helpful in the diagnosis of PAPVC. In the scimitar syndrome, the abnormal pulmonary vein drainage is observed in subcostal view during evaluation of the inferior vena cava (Fig. 20.2. Videos 20.4, 20.5 and 20.6). It is also likely to detect the stenosis of the pulmonary vein. In PAPVC to the coronary sinus, what can usually be seen is a dilated coronary sinus [1, 4].

Cardiovascular Magnetic Resonance Imaging

TEE can be employed with a considerable degree of accuracy and precision in older patients with poor echocardiographic window; nevertheless, it is practically less invasive to find data by cardiovascular magnetic resonance imaging (CMR), which yields outstanding images of the course, position, and junction site of the connecting veins. Moreover, CMR is capable of calculating the pulmonary-to-systemic flow [7, 8].

Management

In cases with right ventricular enlargement, it is advisable that surgery be contemplated. Surgery, however, is rendered unnecessary when there is only one anomalously draining vein and no right ventricular enlargement. The surgery type hinges on the site of the abnormal drainage but generally comprises reconnection of the abnormally

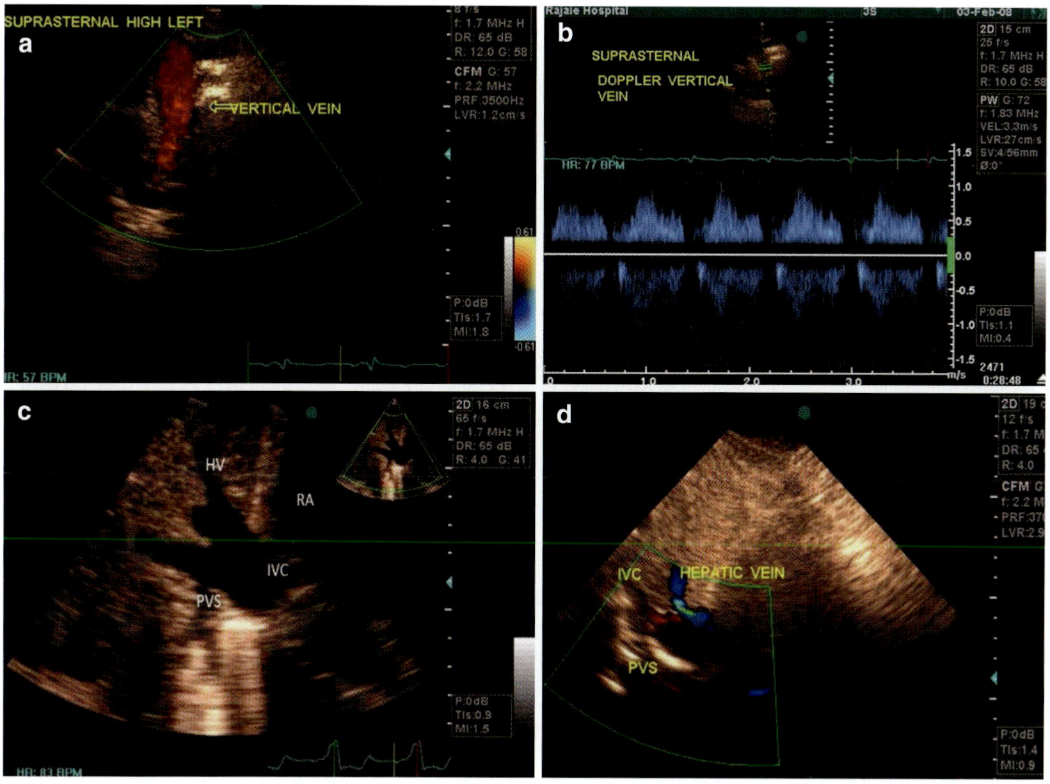

Fig. 20.2 (**a**, **b**) Transthoracic echocardiographic evaluation of PAPVC in the suprasternal view demonstrating a vessel parallel to the aortic arch with red color flow suggestive for vertical vein as it is connecting the left pulmonary veins to the innominate vein and then to the SVC. PW Doppler study showing the low-velocity venous flow of the vertical vein. (**c**, **d**) Subcostal view showing abnormal pulmonary vein drainage to the inferior vena cava suggestive for scimitar syndrome. *IVC* inferior vena cava, *HV* hepatic vein, *RA* right atrium, *PVS* pulmonary veins

draining veins to the left atrium, either directly in the case of a left vertical vein or with a baffle in many other cases. In the scimitar syndrome, it is necessary to block the collateral arteries and redirect the pulmonary veins [1, 4, 9–11].

Outcomes

Overall, patients with repaired PAPVC have a good prognosis, as is the case in those with an isolated ASD. Nonetheless, the exact patency rate of the veins that are reconnected the left atrium has yet to be clearly determined. Patients with the scimitar syndrome have a good outcome if their lesion is relatively isolated, but the existence of other important associated intracardiac diseases significantly compromises the outcome [2, 12, 13].

References

1. Keane JF, Lock JE, Fyler DC, Nadas AS, editors. Nadas' pediatric cardiology. 2nd ed. Philadelphia: Saunders; 2006.
2. Bonow RO, Mann DL, Zipes DP, Libby P, eds. Braunwald's Heart Disease: A Textbook of Cardiovascular Medicine. 9th ed. Philadelphia, PA: Saunders Elsevier; 2011.
3. Perloff JK. Clinical. Recognition of congenital heart disease. 4th ed. Philadelphia, PA: WB Sanuders; 1994.
4. Warnes CA, Williams RG, Bashore TM, et al. ACC/AHA 2008 guidelines for the management of adults

with congenital heart disease. J Am Coll Cardiol. 2008;52(23):e143–263.

5. Lilje C, Weiss F, Weil J. Detection of partial anomalous pulmonary venous connection by magnetic resonance imaging. Pediatr Cardiol. 2005;26(4):490–1.
6. Xue JR, Luo Y, Cheng P, et al. [Diagnosis and treatment of partial anomalous pulmonary venous connection]. Zhonghua Yi Xue Za Zhi. 2008;88(15): 1066–8.
7. Julsrud PR, Ehman RL. The "broken ring" signs in magnetic resonance imaging of partial anomalous pulmonary venous connection to the superior vena cava. Mayo Clin Proc. 1985;60(12):874–9.
8. Kasahara H, Aeba R, Tanami Y, et al. Multislice computed tomography is useful for evaluating partial anomalous pulmonary venous connection. J Cardiothorac Surg. 2010;5(1):40.
9. Paulista MD, Paulista PH, Guerra AL, et al. Surgical treatment of partial anomalous pulmonary venous connection to the superior vena cava. Rev Bras Cir Cardiovasc. 2009;24(2):133–7.
10. Jemielity M, Perek B, Paluszkiewicz L, et al. Results of repair of partial anomalous pulmonary venous connection and sinus venosus atrial septal defect in adults. J Heart Valve Dis. 1998;7(4):410–4.
11. Nakahira A, Yagihara T, Kagisaki K, et al. Partial anomalous pulmonary venous connection to the superior vena cava. Ann Thorac Surg. 2006;82(3):978–82.
12. Shahriari A, Rodefeld MD, Turrentine MW, et al. Caval division technique for sinus venosus atrial septal defect with partial anomalous pulmonary venous connection. Ann Thorac Surg. 2006;81(1):224–9; discussion 229–30.
13. Vanderheyden M, Goethals M, Van Hoe L. Partial anomalous pulmonary venous connection or scimitar syndrome. Heart. 2003;89(7):761.

Total Anomalous Pulmonary Venous Connection (TAPVC)

21

Anita Sadeghpour and Azin Alizadehasl

Keywords

Total Anomalous Pulmonary Venous Connection (TAPVC) • Atrial Septal Defect (ASD) • Transesophageal Echocardiography (TEE) Pulmonary vein

Total anomalous pulmonary venous connection (TAPVC) is a congenital abnormality in which all pulmonary veins drain into the right atrium, although by varied route. Consequently in the TAPVC, the systemic and pulmonary venous blood drain and will be mixed in the right atrium. An atrial defect or foramen ovale (part of the complex) is important in left ventricular output both in the fetal and in newborn circulation [1, 2].

There are four variants of TAPVC:

1. Supracardiac (50 %): The blood drains into one of the innominate veins (brachiocephalic veins) or the superior vena cava.
2. Cardiac (20 %): The blood drains into the coronary sinus or directly into the right atrium.
3. Infradiaphragmatic (20 %): The blood drains into the portal or hepatic veins.
4. Mixed type (10 %).

Pulmonary venous obstruction happens in virtually all patients with subdiaphragmatic drainage and in about 50 % of patients with supracardiac drainage, and patients with obstruction develop symptoms early, usually at 24–36 h, including tachypnea, tachycardia, and cyanosis. Signs of pulmonary hypertension progress with a decreasing pulmonary blood flow and worsening cyanosis. However, patients with an unobstructed pulmonary venous flow present with symptoms more similar to a very large atrial septal defect (ASD) [1, 2, 4].

Electrocardiography

The electrocardiogram (ECG) resembles a nonrestrictive, secundum-type ASD. The PR interval tends to be prolonged. Atrial fibrillation occurs in older patients as it does with a secundum-type

A. Sadeghpour, MD, FACC, FASE (✉)
Echocardiography Lab, Department of Cardiology, Adult Congenital Heart Disease Clinic, Rajaie Cardiovascular Medical and Research Center, Iran University of Medical Science, Tehran, Iran
e-mail: anita.sadeghpour@gmail.com, asadeghpour@rhc.ac.ir

A. Alizadehasl, MD, FACC
Echocardiography Lab, Department of Cardiology, Rajaie Cardiovascular Medical and Research Center, Iran University of Medical Science, Tehran, Iran
e-mail: alizadeasl@gmail.com, alizadeasl@rhc.ac.ir

Electronic supplementary material The online version of this chapter (doi: 10.1007/978-1-4471-6383-1_21) contains supplementary material, which is available to authorized users.

ASD. Also in the presence of pulmonary hypertension, the ECG exhibits peaked RA, P waves, right axis deviation, tall right precordial R waves, inverted T waves, and deep left precordial S waves of right ventricular hypertrophy [1, 5].

Chest X-Ray

The "snowman" heart is a typical appearance in the chest X-ray. It is not likely to be detected in the first few months of life because it takes time for the unique venous channels to become large and, thus, radiodense enough to be visible on the X-ray. Albeit a rare incidence, it is conceivable for the communicating venous channel to appear within the substance of the lung rather than in the mediastinum. In this scenario, the channel looks rather like "the scimitar sign" of a partial anomalous pulmonary venous connection (PAPVC). Although the agenesis of the right lung is rare with TAPVC, it is common in the scimitar syndrome. Sometimes TAPVC with obstruction results in pulmonary edema, which is striking with the distention of the pulmonary veins and lymphatics and a reticular nodular "ground-glass" appearance. What stand out in contrast here are the abnormality of the lung fields and the ordinariness of the cardiac silhouette. Figure 21.1 *shows a typical snowman appearance in the chest X-ray; the left-sided dilated vertical vein, the prominent innominate vein on the top, and the right-sided superior vena cava all together give form to a specific image called "snowman sign" or figure of eight* [1, 2, 6, 7].

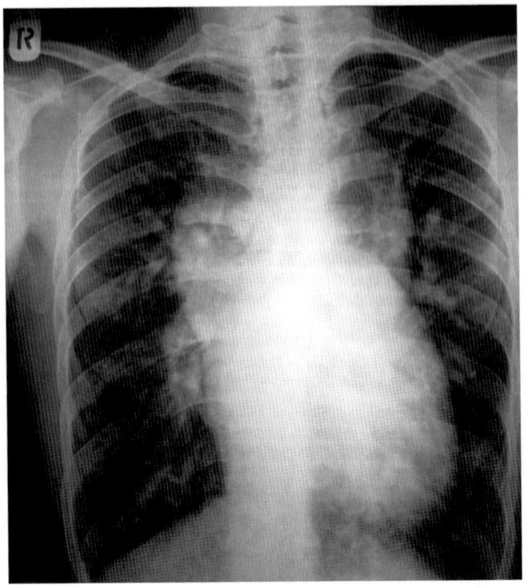

Fig. 21.1 A typical snowman appearance in the chest X-ray. The left-sided dilated vertical vein, the prominent innominate vein on the top, and the right-sided superior vena cava all together give form to a specific image called "snowman sign" or figure of eight

Echocardiography

For patients with TAPVC or PAPVC, echocardiography is the preferred examination. Echocardiographic results usually confirm the diagnosis. In the PAPVC at least one pulmonary vein connects normally to the left atrium. The echocardiography in the TAPVC demonstrates an enlarged right ventricle and a small left atrium. The *common pulmonary venous chamber which receives all pulmonary veins does not enter to the left atrium; instead, this confluence chamber enters the vertical vein and finally drains to the SVC. This is the most common type of TAPVC which is known as supracardiac type* (Fig. 21.2a, b, c; Videos 21.1, 21.2, 21.3 and 21.4). In all types of TAPVC, an obligatory right-to-left shunt almost always is present. All the aforementioned types can be diagnosed by echocardiography [1, 2, 4–6].

When the pattern of the Doppler venous flow of the abdominal veins is obtained, the finding of the venous flow away from the heart is pathognomonic of TAPVC below the diaphragm. Often, shunting occurs almost exclusively from the right atrium to the left atrium, at the atrial level. Sometimes, in anomalous pulmonary venous return, echocardiographic views are limited, but magnetic resonance imaging (MRI) or computed tomography (CT) may be necessary [1–4].

MRI and fast CT scan can also assist with defining pulmonary venous drainage, and cardiac catheterization via selective pulmonary

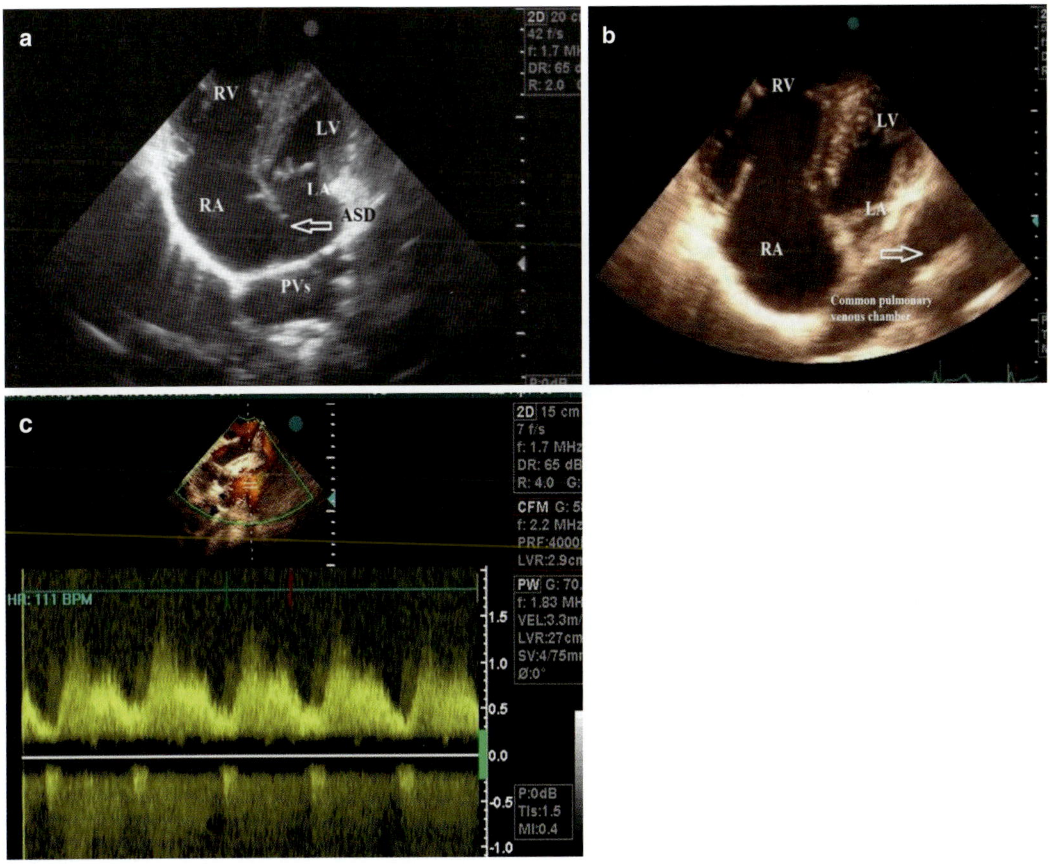

Fig. 21.2 (**a–c**) Echocardiographic evaluation of TAPVC demonstrating enlarged right-side chambers, small left atrium, and common pulmonary venous chamber just behind the left atrium with no connection to the left atrium (as this confluence chamber enters the vertical vein) and associated ASD which is obligatory for TAPVC. Doppler study demonstrating the typical low-velocity pulmonary vein flow pattern. *RV* right ventricle, *LV* left ventricle, *RA* right atrium, *LA* left atrium, *ASD* atrial septal defect, *PVs* pulmonary veins

arteriography can demonstrate the presence of anomalous pulmonary veins.

Cardiac Catheterization

Regarding the high accuracy of 2-D and Doppler echocardiography, the need for diagnostic cardiac catheterization is nearly eliminated. Cardiac catheterization in TAPVC is rarely performed for accurate measurement of systolic pulmonary artery pressure or for what is undiagnosed by echocardiography.

Interestingly the oxygen saturation in the right and left cardiac chambers are nearly identical, and right atrium saturation ranges between 80 and 95 %. Oxygen saturation in pulmonary artery even goes higher than systemic artery. In the *selective* pulmonary angiography, the levophase study shows the anomalous pulmonary veins connection to the innominate vein. The contrast delineates the innominate vein connection to the SVC and right atrium [1, 4, 5] (Fig. 21.3, Video 21.4).

Management

It is vitally important that corrective surgery be undertaken as soon as possible. However, when a child is asymptomatic and without pulmonary hypertension, it is possible to postpone surgery

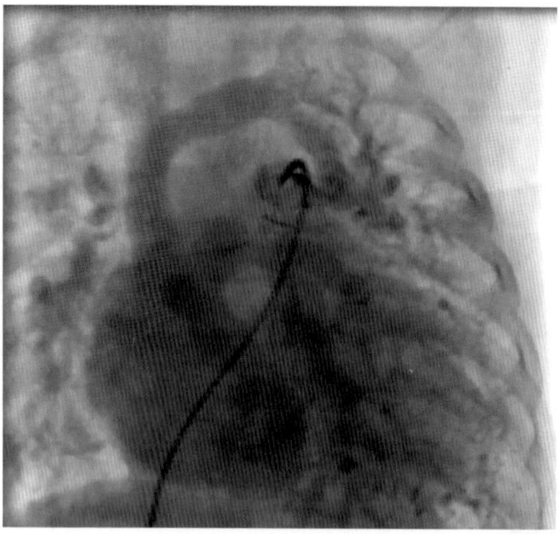

Fig. 21.3 Main pulmonary arteriography shows that contrast collects in the common pulmonary venous chamber and draining into vertical vein and left innominate vein and clearly outlines the right atrium in recirculation opacification

until the child is 3–6 months of age. Finally, it is logical to assume that adult patients have invariably undergone surgical repair in their childhood [1, 2, 7, 8].

References

1. Keane JF, Lock JE, Fyler DC, Nadas AS, editors. Nadas' pediatric cardiology. 2nd ed. Philadelphia: Saunders; 2006.
2. Bonow RO, Mann DL, Zipes DP, Libby P, eds. Braunwald's Heart Disease: A Textbook of Cardiovascular Medicine. 9th ed. Philadelphia, PA: Saunders Elsevier; 2011.
3. Perloff JK. Cilinical. Recognition of congenital heart disease. 4th ed. Philadelphia: WB Sanuders; 1994.
4. Warnes CA, Williams RG, Bashore TM, et al. ACC/AHA, guidelines for the management of adults with. Congenit Heart Dis. 2008;52(23):2008.
5. Ritter S, Tani LY, Shaddy RE, et al. An unusual variant of total anomalous pulmonary venous connection with varices and multiple drainage sites. Pediatr Cardiol. 2000;21(3):289–91.
6. Allan LD, Sharland GK. The echocardiographic diagnosis of totally anomalous pulmonary venous connection in the fetus. Heart. 2001;85(4):433–7.
7. Douglas YL, Jongbloed MR, den Hartog WC, et al. Pulmonary vein and atrial wall pathology in human total anomalous pulmonary venous connection. Int J Cardiol. 2009;134(3):302–12.
8. Vahanian A, Baumgartner H, Bax J, Butchart E, et al. Guidelines on the management of valvular heart disease: the Task Force on the Management of Valvular Heart Disease of the European Society of Cardiology. Eur Heart J. 2007;28(2):230–68.

22 Isolated Ventricular Septal Defect

Azin Alizadehasl, Anita Sadeghpour, and Mitra Chitsazan

Keywords
Ventricular Septal Defect (VSD) • Perimemberanous • Sub-arterial VSD Muscular VSD • Echocardiography

Definition

Ventricular septal defect (VSD), as the most common congenital heart disease (CHD) at birth [1], is found less in older infants and in the adults since most of small VSDs will close spontaneously over the time [2, 3].

Four anatomic types of VSDs have been described (with various nomenclature and synonyms) [2–6]:

- *Type 1:* Outlet supracristal, sub-arterial, subpulmonary, infundibular, supracristal, or conal VSD is located in the outflow tract of the right ventricle (RV), under the semilunar valves in conal or outlet septum, and has a variable prevalence ranging from approximately 6 % of defects in non-Asian patients to up to 33 % in Asian populations [4]. *Spontaneous closure in type 1 VSD is uncommon.* This type of VSD is often related to the progressive aortic regurgitation (AR) secondary to prolapse of the aortic valve cusps (usually right cusp).
- *Type 2:* Perimembranous, paramembranous, or conoventricular VSD constitutes almost 80 % of defects in the membranous septum. This defect might also extend into inlet, trabecular, or outlet septum. Perimembranous VSD is near to the tricuspid septal leaflet, which can frequently adhere to the defect and create a pouch or "aneurysm" in the ventricular septum. This pouch limits left-to-right shunting and may result in partial or complete closure of septal defect. This type of defect is also close to the aortic valve on the LV side of interventricular septum.
- *Type 3:* Inlet, atrioventricular (AV) canal, or AV-type VSD lies in the lower portion of RV, near to the tricuspid valve, and just inferior of

A. Alizadehasl, MD, FACC (✉)
Echocardiography Lab, Department of Cardiology, Rajaie Cardiovascular Medical and Research Center, Iran University of Medical Science, Tehran, Iran
e-mail: alizadeasl@gmail.com, alizadeasl@rhc.ac.ir

A. Sadeghpour, MD, FACC, FASE
Echocardiography Lab, Department of Cardiology, Adult Congenital Heart Disease Clinic, Rajaie Cardiovascular Medical and Research Center, Iran University of Medical Science, Tehran, Iran
e-mail: anita.sadeghpour@gmail.com, asadeghpour@rhc.ac.ir

M. Chitsazan, MD
Research Lab, Rajaie Cardiovascular Medical and Research Center, Tehran, Iran

Electronic supplementary material The online version of this chapter (doi: 10.1007/978-1-4471-6383-1_22) contains supplementary material, which is available to authorized users.

A. Sadeghpour et al. (eds.), *Comprehensive Approach to Adult Congenital Heart Disease*, DOI 10.1007/978-1-4471-6383-1_22, © Springer-Verlag London 2014

AV valve apparatus. This type of VSD is typically seen in patients with Down syndrome.
- *Type 4:* Muscular or trabecular VSD is completely surrounded by muscle. It may have a central position (midmuscular) or an apical position or may be located at the margin of septum and RV free wall. This type of VSD is frequently multiple in number. Spontaneous closure is particularly common in this type, and although these lesions account for up to 15–20 % of VSDs in infancy, the incidence is much less in adults.

Associated Lesions

Although VSD is most often an isolated lesion, multiple defects can also be seen. Moreover, VSD is a common part of complex cardiac lesions such as tetralogy of Fallot (TOF) and transposition of great arteries (TGA). VSD also occurs in association with left-sided obstructive anomalies such as subvalvular aortic stenosis and coarctation of the aorta. Spontaneous closure of VSD most often occurs in muscular/trabecular type but is uncommon in perimembranous and outlet defects [7]. Although small defects can close spontaneously at any age, this most commonly happens during infancy [8, 9].

Pulmonary vascular resistance (PVR), size of the defect, LV and RV systolic/diastolic function, and presence of RV outflow tract obstruction (RVOTO) are the main determinants of the shunt direction and magnitude.

Clinical Presentation and Natural History

Possible scenarios for adults with an isolated VSD might contain:
- An asymptomatic patient with a systolic murmur
- Fever and bacteremia caused by infective endocarditis (IE)
- Progressive pulmonary vascular disease in patients with large VSD with originally large left-to-right shunting eventually resulting in cyanosis and exercise intolerance secondary to shunt reversal (Eisenmenger complex)

Clinical presentation of isolated VSDs is mainly determined by the defect size and PVR:
- Small VSDs (less than or nearly equal to 25 % of the aortic annulus diameter) have small left-to-right shunts, no LV volume overload, and no pulmonary artery hypertension (PAH) and present as systolic murmurs.
- Moderate VSDs (more than 25 % but less than 75 % of the aortic annulus diameter) have small to moderate left-to-right shunts, mild to moderate LV volume overload, and mild or no PAH. These patients may remain asymptomatic or experience symptoms of mild congestive heart failure. Symptoms generally subside with the medical management and with time as VSD diameter decreases in absolute terms or relative to the increasing size of the body.
- Large VSDs (greater than or equal to 75 % of the aortic diameter) are associated with a moderate to large left-to-right shunts, LV volume overload, and PAH. A history of congestive heart failure during infancy might be noted in most of adult patients with large VSDs.
- In patients with a small VSD, endocarditis (IE) may be complicated by pulmonary embolism or cerebral abscess.
- Postsurgical presentation consists of signs and symptoms associated with IE, aortic regurgitation, heart block, LV dysfunction, PAH, tricuspid regurgitation (TR), recurrent VSDs, and ventricular arrhythmias.

Clinical Examination

Clinically, VSD is characterized by a systolic murmur maximal at the left lower sternal border. A precordial thrill may also be palpable. The VSD murmur is "blowing" and "pansystolic" if the RV pressure is low. With higher RV pressures, the murmur becomes "shorter," "softer," and "lower pitched." Small muscular VSDs are usually very high pitched and are heard only in early systole due to the closure of the defect by muscular contraction.

Diagnostic Workup

Clinical Examination

Clinically, VSD is characterized by a systolic murmur that is usually maximal at the left lower sternal border. A precordial thrill may also be palpable. The VSD murmur is blowing and pansystolic in the presence of a low pressure RV. With higher RV pressure, the murmur is shorter, softer, and lower pitched. Small, muscular VSDs are usually very high pitched and are heard only in early systole due to the closure of the defect by muscular contraction.

Electrocardiogram

The ECG may show biventricular hypertrophy or isolated RV hypertrophy in patients with a large VSD and significant PAH (Fig. 22.1).

Chest X-Ray

Patients with a small VSD have a normal chest x-ray. In the presence of significant left-to-right shunt, evidences of left atrial (LA) and LV enlargement and increased pulmonary vascular markings can be seen on CXR (Fig. 22.2). Patients with significant PAH do not demonstrate LV enlargement but will have a prominent pulmonary artery and diminished pulmonary vascular markings at the periphery of the lung.

Echocardiography

Echocardiography is the mainstay diagnostic technique used in both the diagnosis and assessment of disease severity. The large VSDs are easily detected by 2D echocardiography, as the small VSDs may be difficult to visualize. Most of the VSDs in adults have small flow; consequently a

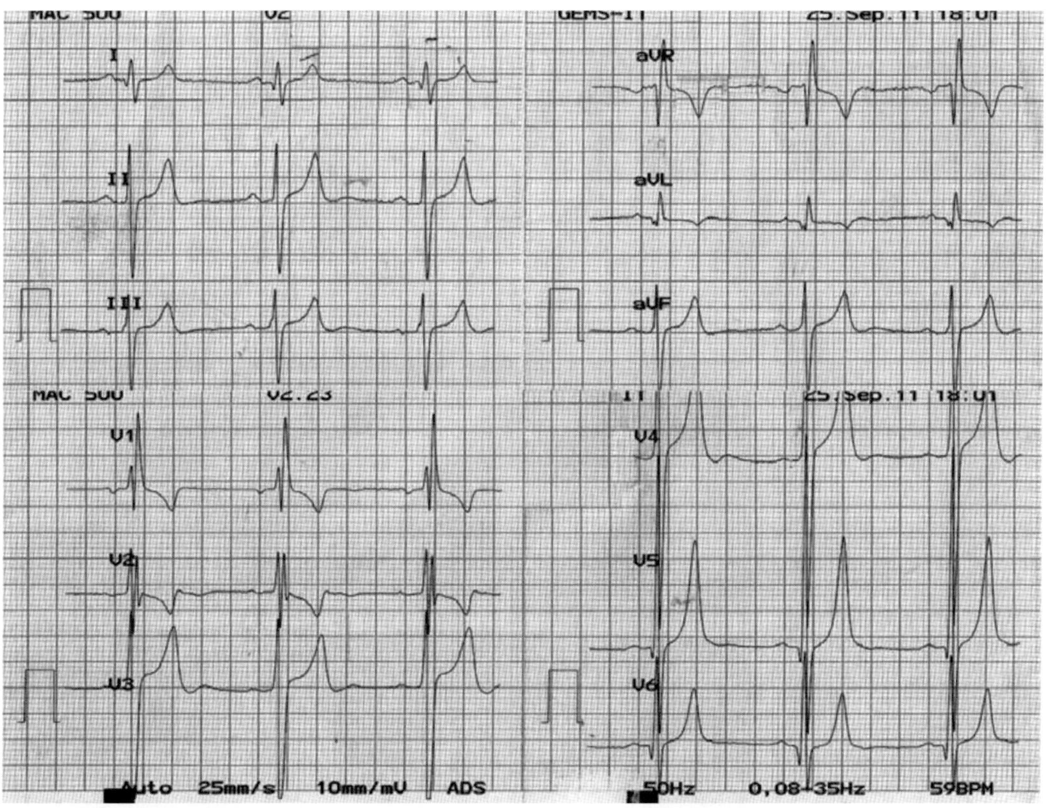

Fig. 22.1 Electrocardiography showing left atrium enlargement associated with biventricular hypertrophy

complete 2D and color flow imaging study besides the physical exam would be helpful.

Key findings on echocardiographic examination include the number of defects, location of defects, chamber size, ventricular function and the severity of LV volume overload, presence or absence of aortic valve prolapse and/or regurgitation especially in the case of outlet (supracristal) and high perimembranous VSDs, presence or absence of RV or LV outflow obstruction, and presence or absence of TR and estimated PAP.

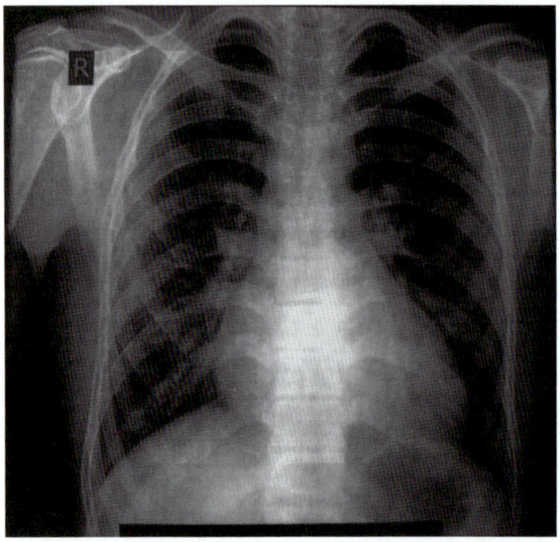

Fig. 22.2 Shunt vascularity with left-to-right shunt; left ventricular and left atrial enlargement are suggestive for ventricular septal defect (VSD)

VSDs that are categorized earlier will be described based on the adjacent structure:

A. *Perimembranous VSD* which is the most common type of VSD is seen *adjacent to the aortic valve and tricuspid valve*. Usually it is imaged in parasternal view (both long axis and short axis), apical 5-chamber view, and subcostal view (Fig. 22.3).
B. *Subarterial or doubly committed VSD* which is more common in Asian population is seen *adjacent to the both aortic valve and pulmonic valve (doubly committed VSD)* in the short-axis view (Fig. 22.4).
C. *Inlet-type VSD* usually is seen as a part of atrioventricular septal defect (AVSD) although it can be seen as isolated defect. It is *adjacent to both the mitral and tricuspid valves and best seen in the apical 4-chamber view* and short-axis view.
D. *Muscular-type VSD* which is surrounded by muscle is located anterior, posterior, apical, or midmuscular. Sometimes the muscular VSD has multiple defects known as "Swiss cheese" septum. Detection of muscular VSDs needs precise sweeping of the whole septum by 2D and color Doppler study (Fig. 22.5, Video 22.1).

Estimation of RV systolic pressure from TR jet, VSD jet, and/or septal configuration should also be performed.

Echocardiographic evaluation of VSD consists of the precise sweeping of the whole septum

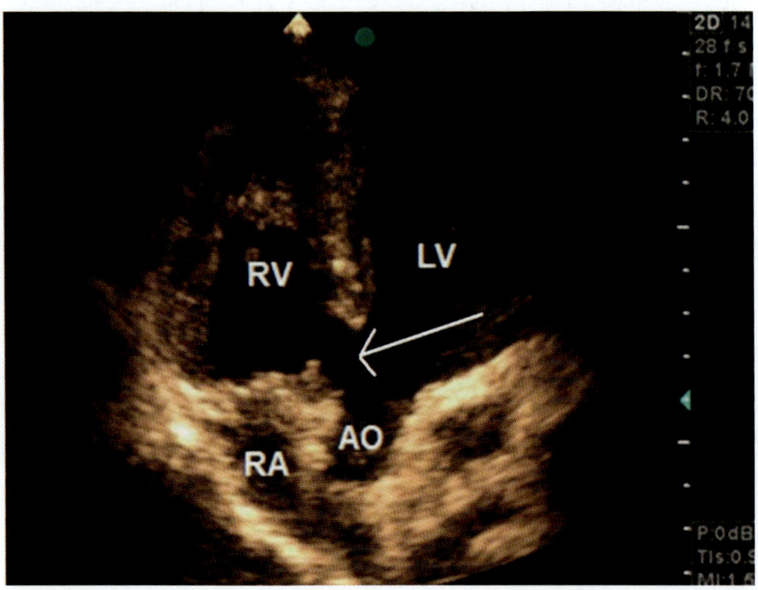

Fig. 22.3 Transthoracic echocardiography in five-chamber view showing large perimembranous VSD (*white arrow*). *RV* right ventricle, *LV* left ventricle, *RA* right atrium, *Ao* aorta

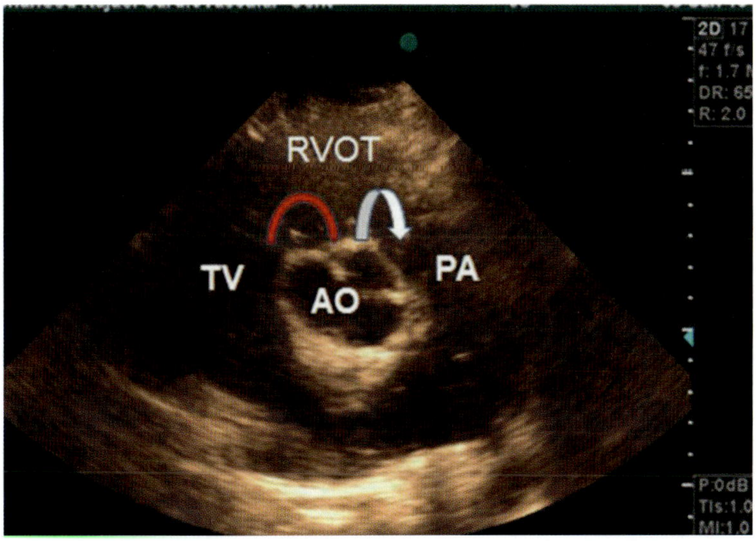

Fig. 22.4 *White arrow* demonstrating the subarterial location of the VSD and *red line* showing the location of the perimembranous VSD. *RVOT* right ventricular outflow tract, *TV* tricuspid valve, *AO* Aorta *PA* pulmonary artery

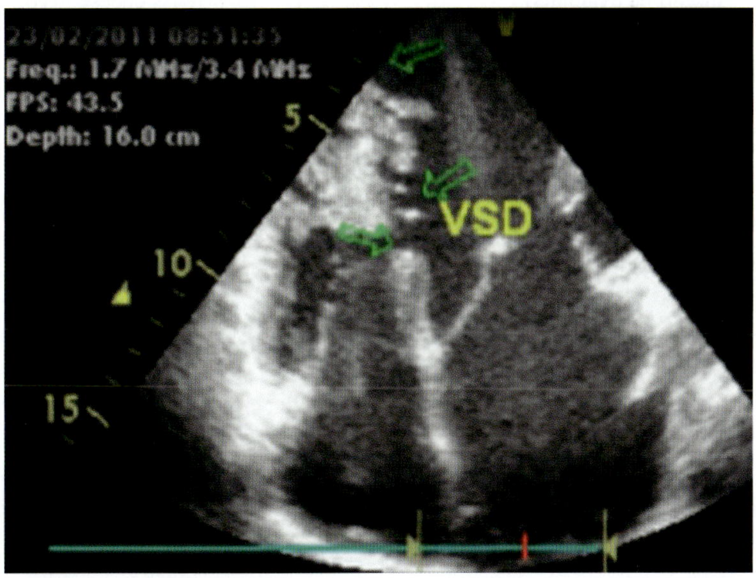

Fig. 22.5 Transthoracic echocardiography in 4-chamber view showing multiple midmuscular VSD (Swiss cheese septum) associated with left heart enlargement

by 2D and color flow imaging from the base to apex in multiple views.

Cardiac Magnetic Resonance

CMR may be useful, particularly for the following:

- Assessment of pulmonary artery, pulmonary venous, and aortic anatomy in the presence of coexisting lesions
- Assessment of LV volume overload and shunt quantification
- Assessment of the anatomy of unusual VSDs such as inlet or apical defects which are not well seen by echocardiography

Cardiac Catheterization

In patients with high PAP based on echocardiography data, cardiac catheterization is required to measure PVR. Moreover, ACC/AHA recommends to use cardiac catheterization for the assessment of the operability of adults with VSD and PAH (Class I, *Level of Evidence: C)* [10].

Cardiac catheterization provides the following data in adults with VSD:

- Quantification of shunting.
- Assessment of pulmonary pressures and resistance in patients with suspected PAH. Using

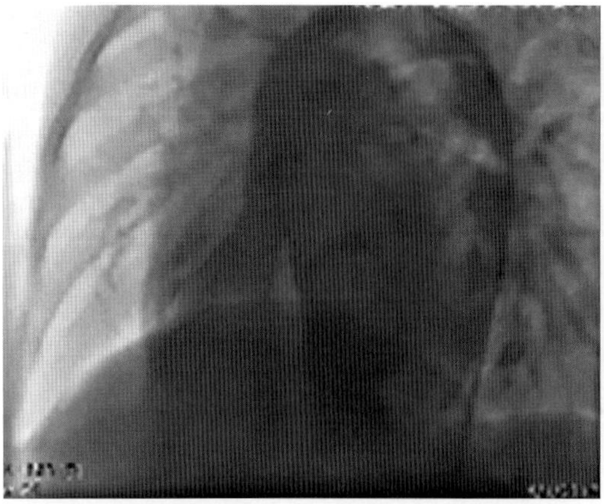

Fig. 22.6 LV injection showing subaortic VSD

pulmonary vasodilators, reversibility of PAH should be evaluated.
- Assessment of concomitant lesions such as aortic regurgitation and double-chambered right ventricle.
- Evaluation of VSD anatomy, particularly for patients in whom device closure is planned (Video 22.2) (Fig. 22.6).

Coincident opacification of the left and right ventricles indicates the presence of a VSD.

Management Strategies [10]

Medical Therapy

Adults with VSDs and severe PVD may benefit from pulmonary vasodilator therapy.

Surgical Ventricular Septal Defect Closure

In patients with a Qp/Qs (pulmonary to systemic blood flow ratio) of 2.0 or more and clinical evidence of LV volume overload, VSD should be closed surgically. Patients with a history of IE should also undergo surgical closure of the VSD. However, VSD closure is not recommended for patients with severe irreversible PAH.

Interventional Catheterization

Device closure may be considered in muscular VSDs, especially if the VSD is remote from the tricuspid valve and the aorta. Catheter device closure of VSD is performed in patients with residual defects following prior surgical closure, restrictive VSDs with a significant left-to-right shunt, traumatic VSDs, or iatrogenic VSDs after surgical replacement of the aortic valve. Restrictive VSDs in the adults may be closed in patients with a history of bacterial endocarditis or a hemodynamically significant left-to-right shunting (Qp/Qs >1.5:1). Percutaneous closure of VSD provides an alternative to surgery in patients with increased surgical risk factors, multiple previous cardiac surgeries, poorly accessible muscular VSDs, or "Swiss cheese"-type VSDs (Video 22.3).

Follow-up

Adults with VSD with residual heart failure, shunts, PAH, AR, or RVOT or LVOT obstruction should visit at least annually at an adult CHD center. In patients with a small residual VSD and no other lesions, 3- to 5-year intervals may be reasonable. Adults undergoing device closure of a VSD should be seen every 1–2 years depending on the location of the VSD. Continued follow-up is not required in adults with no residual VSD, no associated lesions, and normal pulmonary artery pressure.

Bifascicular block or transient trifascicular block after VSD closure increases the risk of development of complete heart block in later years. Thus, these patients should be followed up yearly by history, ECG, ambulatory monitoring, and/or exercise testing [10].

Additional Considerations

Pregnancy

Pregnancy in asymptomatic women with small VSDs, normal LV function, no PAH, and no associated lesions is generally well tolerated and not accompanied by increased maternal mortality or cardiovascular risk for pregnancy. It is believed that although the increase in cardiac output during pregnancy may accentuate the left-to-right shunt, the decrease in peripheral resistance would counterbalance this effect. Pregnancy is contraindicated in patients with severe PVD (Eisenmenger physiology) since arrhythmias, ventricular dysfunction, and progression of PAH might occur in these patients leading to maternal and fetal mortality [10, 11].

Activity/Exercise

No activity restrictions are requisite for patients with small VSDs without associated lesions, pulmonary hypertension, significant arrhythmias, and normal left ventricular function and also after VSD closure. However, in the presence of PAH, activity is usually self-restricted, but patients should be advised to limit themselves to low-intensity recreational activity/sports and to avoid travel to altitudes above 5,000 ft. In long-distance air travel, dehydration should be prevented, and the need for supplemental oxygen must be consulted with an adult CHD specialist.

IE Prophylaxis

The European Society of Cardiology and also AHA/ACC recommend IE prophylaxis only for high-risk VSD patients.

References

1. Hoffman JI, Kaplan S. The incidence of congenital heart disease. J Am Coll Cardiol. 2002;39:1890–900.
2. Du ZD, Roguin N, Wu XJ. Spontaneous closure of muscular ventricular septal defect identified by echocardiography in neonates. Cardiol Young. 1998;8:500–5. 277.
3. Kidd L, Driscoll DJ, Gersony WM, et al. Second natural history study of congenital heart defects. Results of treatment of patients with ventricular septal defects. Circulation. 1993;87:I38–51.
4. Graham Jr TP, Gutgesell HP. Ventricular septal defects In: Emmanouilides GC, Riemenschneider TA, Allen HD, Gutgesell HP, editors. Moss and Adams heart disease in infants, children and adolescents. Baltimore: Williams & Wilkins; 1989. p. 724–46.
5. Prosad S. Ventricular septal defects. In: Gatzoulis MA, Webb GD, Daubeney PE, editors. Diagnosis and management of adult congenital heart disease. London: Churchill Livingstone; 2003. p. 171–8.
6. Jacobs JP, Burke RP, Quintessenza JA, Mavroudis C. Congenital heart surgery nomenclature and database project: ventricular septal defect. Ann Thorac Surg. 2000;69:S25–35.
7. Miyake T, Shinohara T, Fukuda T, Ikeoka M, Takemura T. Spontaneous closure of perimembranous ventricular septal defect after school age. Pediatr Int. 2008;50:632–5.
8. Neumayer U, Stone S, Somerville J. Small ventricular septal defects in adults. Eur Heart J. 1998;19:1573–82.
9. Onat T, Ahunbay G, Batmaz G, Celebi A. The natural course of isolated ventricular septal defect during adolescence. Pediatr Cardiol. 1998;19:230–4.
10. Warnes CA, Williams RG, Bashore TM, et al. ACC/AHA 2008 guidelines for the management of adults with congenital heart disease: a report of the American College of Cardiology/American Heart Association Task Force on Practice Guidelines (Writing Committee to Develop Guidelines on the Management of Adults With Congenital Heart Disease). Developed in Collaboration With the American Society of Echocardiography, Heart Rhythm Society, International Society for Adult Congenital Heart Disease, Society for Cardiovascular Angiography and Interventions, and Society of Thoracic Surgeons. J Am Coll Cardiol. 2008;52(23):e143–263.
11. Baumgartner H, Bonhoeffer P, De Groot NM, et al. ESC Guidelines for the management of grown-up congenital heart disease (new version 2010). Task Force on the Management of Grown-up Congenital Heart Disease of the European Society of Cardiology (ESC); Association for European Paediatric Cardiology (AEPC); ESC Committee for Practice Guidelines (CPG). Eur Heart J. 2010;31(23):2915–57.

Atrioventricular Septal Defect (AVSD)

23

Azin Alizadehasl, Anita Sadeghpour, and Nehzat Akiash

Keywords

Atrioventricular Septal Defect (AVSD) • Complete AVSD • Partial AVSD • Transitional AVSD • Primum ASD

Atrioventricular septal defect (AVSD) consists of a group of anomalies with the common main pathology of the absence of the atrioventricular (AV) septum associated with the abnormalities of the AV valves [1]. AVSD has been divided into the two main categories as the partial and complete forms and two other subtypes as the transitional (which is the subtype of partial AVSD) and intermediate (which is the subtype of complete AVSD). In complete AVSD, a primum ASD is concomitant with an inlet-type ventricular septal defect (VSD), and a common AV valve has only single annulus. In addition, transitional AVSD is used when a partial AVSD also has a small inlet-type VSD that is partially obstructed via chordal attachments to the intraventricular septum. Also, intermediate subtype of AVSD has separate right and left AV valve orifices even though having only one common annulus. These distinct orifices are referred to as right and left AV valve orifices rather than mitral and tricuspid [2, 3].

A. Alizadehasl, MD, FACC (✉)
Echocardiography Lab, Department of Cardiology, Rajaie Cardiovascular Medical and Research Center, Iran University of Medical Science, Tehran, Iran
e-mail: alizadeasl@gmail.com; alizadeasl@rhc.ac.ir

A. Sadeghpour, MD, FACC, FASE
Echocardiography Lab, Department of Cardiology, Adult Congenital Heart Disease Clinic, Rajaie Cardiovascular Medical and Research Center, Iran University of Medical Science, Tehran, Iran
e-mail: anita.sadeghpour@gmail.com; asadeghpour@rhc.ac.ir

N. Akiash, MD
Department of Cardiology, Rajaie Cardiovascular Medical and Research Center, Tehran, Iran

Partial Atrioventricular (AV) Septal Defect: Primum ASD + Cleft Anterior Leaflet of the Mitral Valve

Azin Alizadehasl, Anita Sadeghpour, and Nehzat Akiash

Partial AVSD is characterized by the defect in both interatrial septum and the left atrioventricular valve (mitral valve) with two distinct MV and tricuspid valve (TV). Mitral and tricuspid annuli insert in the same level on the interventricular septum due to the absence of the atrioventricular (AV) septum and consequently

Electronic supplementary material The online version of this chapter (doi: 10.1007/978-1-4471-6383-1_23) contains supplementary material, which is available to authorized users.

A. Sadeghpour et al. (eds.), *Comprehensive Approach to Adult Congenital Heart Disease*, DOI 10.1007/978-1-4471-6383-1_23, © Springer-Verlag London 2014

apical displacement of the left AV annulus. In partial AV canal, left ventricular outflow tract (LVOT) is elongated resulting in goose neck deformity [3, 4].

Lack of fusion of the atrial septum primum with the endocardial cushion causes the primum atrial septal defect (ASD), and there is abnormal development of the septum secundum. Most primum ASDs are large and located anteroinferior to the fossa ovalis. The abnormal attachment of the left AV valve causes malcoaptation of leaflets and mitral valve regurgitation. The papillary muscles are also abnormal and occasionally close to each other and sometimes create single papillary muscles [1, 4].

Clinical Presentation

The presentation of patient with AVSD and no diagnosis in childhood occurs in adulthood due to symptoms of exercise intolerance or dyspnea on exertion and also palpitations from a new atrial arrhythmia. The patients may present the typical findings of an ASD's physical findings including systolic ejection-type murmur at the left sternal border (LSB), a widely split or fixed second heart sound (S2), and a diastolic rumble along the lower LSB from greater flow across the TV. Seldom, mitral stenosis will develop in an adult with unrepaired partial AVSD. These cases usually have a single LV papillary muscle [1, 5, 6].

Electrocardiogram

The following ECG is showing the classic findings of the patient with partial AVSD [1, 2] (Fig. 23.1).

Chest X-ray

In uncomplicated forms of partial AVSD, atrial septal defect causes the dilation of the right heart and mitral valve results in the left atrium and left ventricle enlargement [1, 3, 6] (Fig. 23.2).

Echocardiography

The typical echocardiographic findings in partial AVSD are as follows:

A. Same level insertion of the left and right AV valves (MV and TV); lack of offsetting septal insertion of the AV valves (Fig. 23.3).
B. Primum-type interatrial septal defect (usually large) (Fig. 23.4).
C. Cleft anterior mitral valve leaflet or left AV valve cleft associated with insufficiency, which is best seen in parasternal and subcostal short-axis views (Fig. 23.5).
D. Elongated left ventricular outflow tract (LVOT). Normally, the AV annulus to LV apex distance is equal to the MV annulus to the LV apex. In AVSD, the distance from MV annulus to LV apex is shorter than AV annulus to the apex [2, 3, 6] (Fig. 23.6).

Systemic and pulmonary venous return usually is normal. Importantly, there is inferior displacement of the AV valves and attachment of a portion of the left AV (mitral) valve to the septum. The free edges of the cleft do not insert on the papillary muscles, but may attach to the septum. Infrequently, a parachute or a double-orifice MV also happens. The anterior component of the septal leaflet of tricuspid valve is abnormal and results in widening of anteroseptal commissure. The papillary muscles that are closer to each other can be evaluated in the left parasternal short-axis view. There is myxomatous appearance in AV valves, and apical 4-chamber view is suitable for evaluation of AV valves. Evaluation of LVOT, MV displacement, and subaortic component is possible in the apical long-axis or left parasternal views. Also we should be aware in our echocardiographic assessment that progressive LVOT obstruction may happen in up to 15 % of cases after repair of partial AVSD. Indeed, it occurs more frequently in patients with the partial form of AVSD than in patients with the complete form; this is due to the special LVOT anatomy in these patients. For this reason, after repair surgery, these patients require lifelong periodic echocardiographic study for development or progression of LVOT obstruction as well as aortic valve regurgitation and MV regurgitation (MR) [1–3, 6].

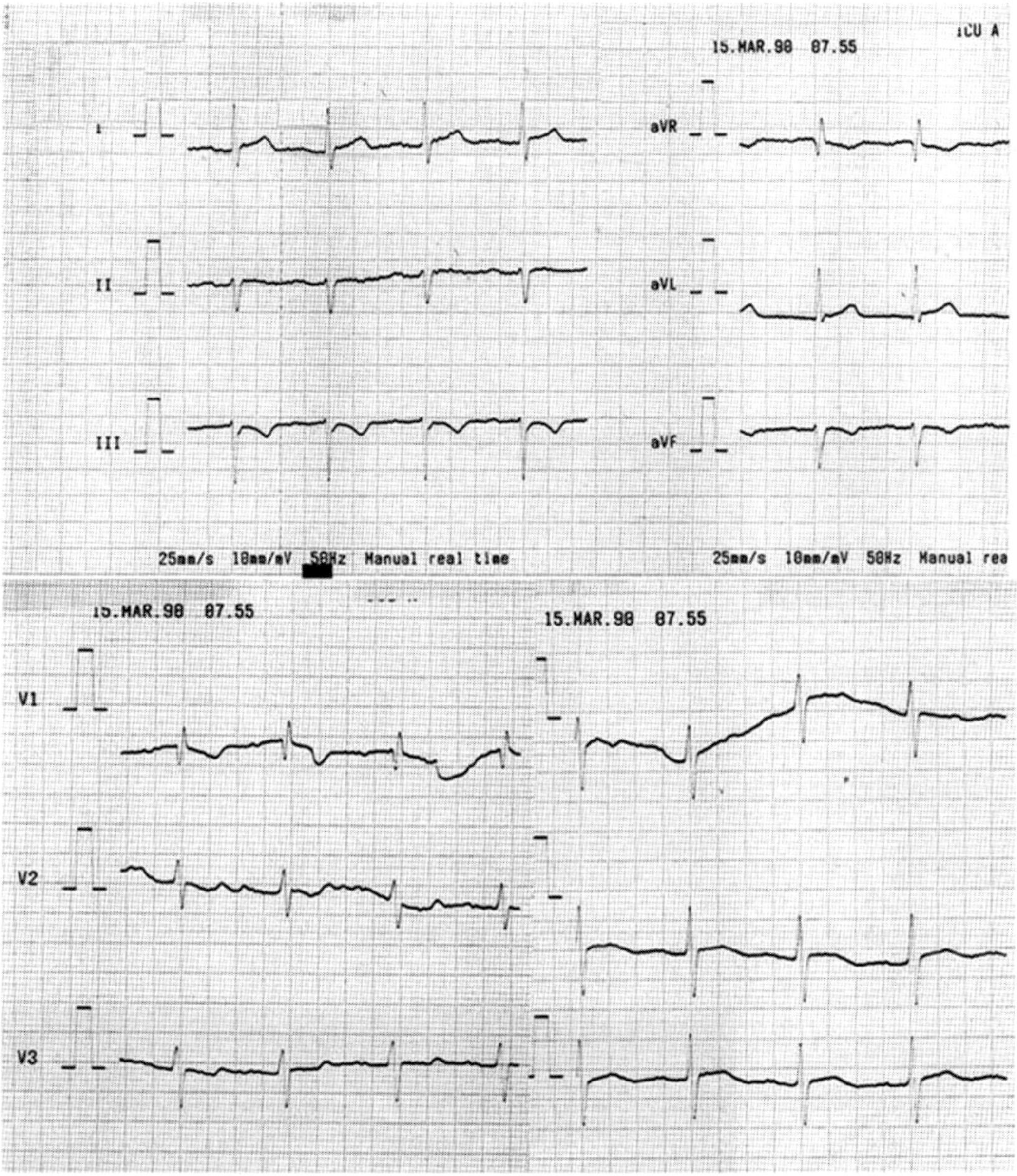

Fig. 23.1 Sinus rhythm, left atrial abnormality, left axis deviation, biventricular hypertrophy, and right ventricular volume overload pattern due to left-to-right shunt

In echocardiographic assessment, the associated lesions should be evaluated as the most common ones are secundum-type ASD and persistent left superior vena cava connecting to the coronary sinus and the less frequent ones are tetralogy of Fallot, double-outlet RV, pulmonary valve atresia, anomalous pulmonary venous connections, LV hypoplasia, and coarctation of the aorta [3, 4, 7].

Cardiac Catheterism

There is a limited role of cardiac catheterization in these patients unless the suspicion exists regarding the pulmonary vascular resistance. Classically, we would prefer pulmonary vascular resistance to be less than six units for successful and safe repair. In patients aged 40 years or older, noninvasive methods and coronary angiography are performed for assessment of coronary artery disease prior to surgery. In addition, it should be mentioned that primum ASDs are not appropriate to closure with transcatheter devices [1–4, 7, 8] (Fig. 23.7).

Management

Once diagnosed, repair of partial AVSD is classically suggested due to volume overload of the right heart chambers that caused by left-to-right shunt at the atrial level. In addition, closure of the MV cleft is indicated to stop progression of MR severity. Reoperation is performed in at least 25 % of patients due to progressive MR or development of LVOT obstruction [1, 3, 8–10].

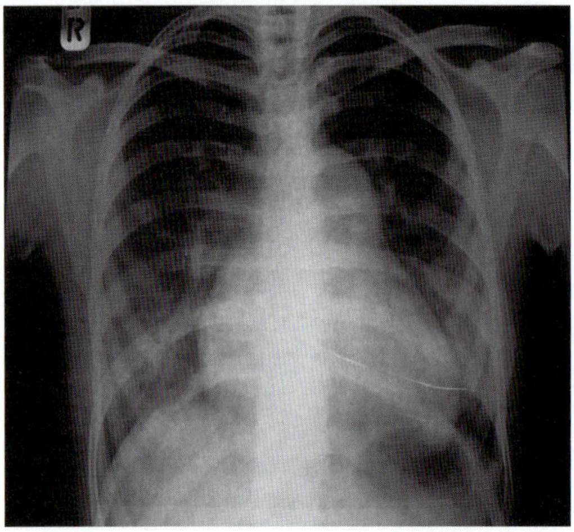

Fig. 23.2 Cardiomegaly and shunt vascularity with left-to-right shunt in AVSD pattern

Complete AV Canal: Common AV Valve + Large Primum ASD + Large Inlet-Type VSD

Azin Alizadehasl and Anita Sadeghpour

Complete AVSD consists of a common AV valve, ostium primum atrial septal defect, and interventricular septum defect (usually large size) (Fig. 23.8, Video 23.1).

Common AV valve is the key point for the anatomic classification in all types of complete AVSD. Complete AVSD is basically built up of five leaflets (superior bridging, left mural, inferior bridging, right mural, and right anterosuperior) [1, 2, 6] (Fig. 23.9, Videos 23.2).

According to the morphology of the superior leaflet of the common AV valve, three types of CAVC have been classified (types A, B, and C, according to Rastelli's classification) (Videos 23.3 and 23.4) (Figs. 23.10 and 23.11) (Table 23.1).

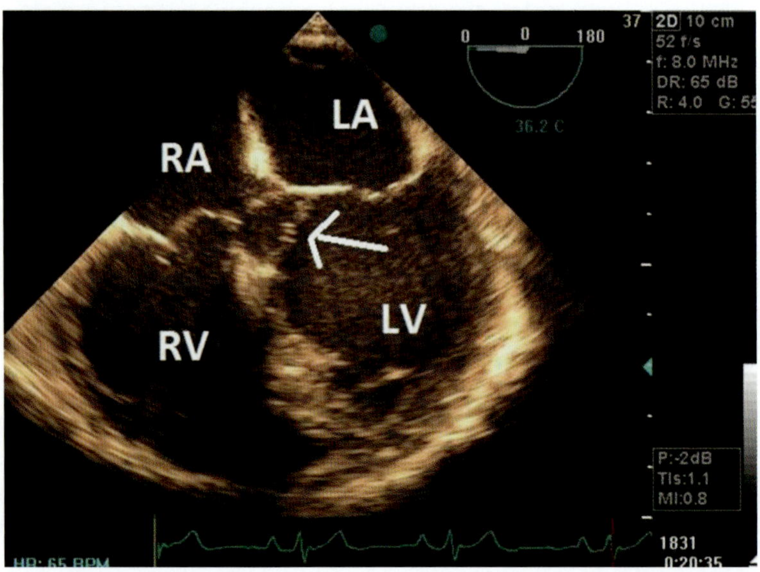

Fig. 23.3 Same level atrioventricular valves associated with septal attachment of left AV valve (*white arrow*). *RA* right atrium, *LA* left atrium, *RV* right ventricle, *LV* left ventricle

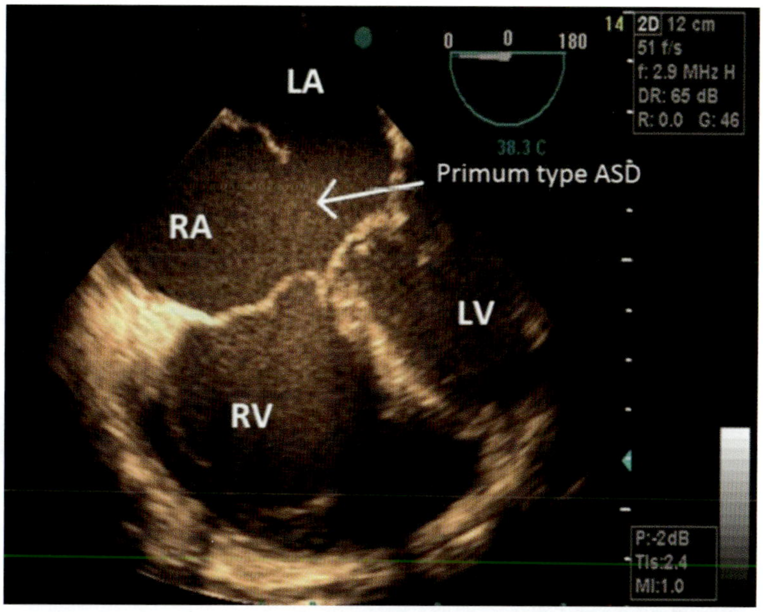

Fig. 23.4 Transesophageal echocardiography in four-chamber view, showing large defect in the most anteroinferior portion of the atrial septum associated with right-sided enlargement suggestive of primum-type ASD and partial AVSD. *RA* right atrium, *LA* left atrium, *RV* right ventricle, *LV* left ventricle

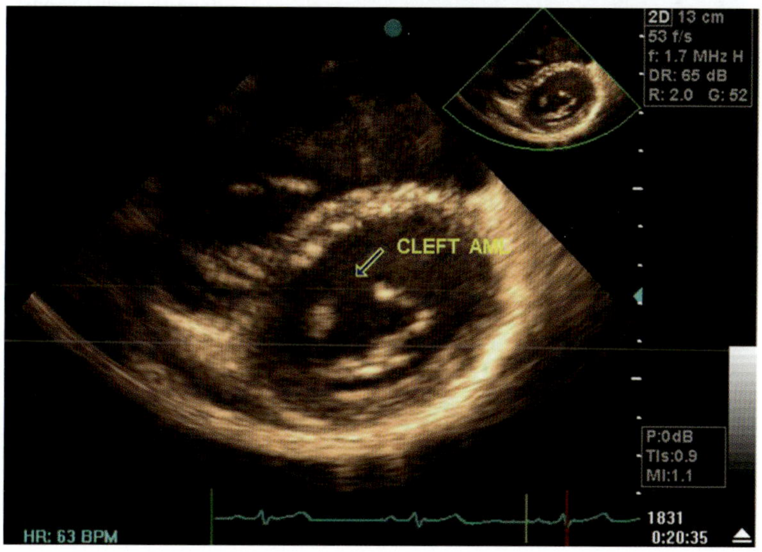

Fig. 23.5 The trileaflet left AV valve (mitral valve) with a cleft in the anterior mitral leaflet (*AML*) that is directed to the mid-part of ventricular septum. In isolated cleft of MV, the cleft is directed to the LVOT

The least common form of complete AVSD is type B. Type A is most frequently accompanied with left-sided obstructions. Type C is often associated with other complex cardiac anomalies. Anomaly of the left component of the common AV valve causes the LV inflow and outflow obstructions. Although in the modern era, this classification's clinical and surgical significance has become less important. The common AV valve may be divided into distinct right and left orifices by a tongue of tissue that connects the two bridging leaflets, representing the intermediate form of AVSD [2–6].

Chest Radiography

Classically demonstrates cardiomegaly and significantly increased pulmonary vascularity consistent with the large left-to-right shunt [1–3].

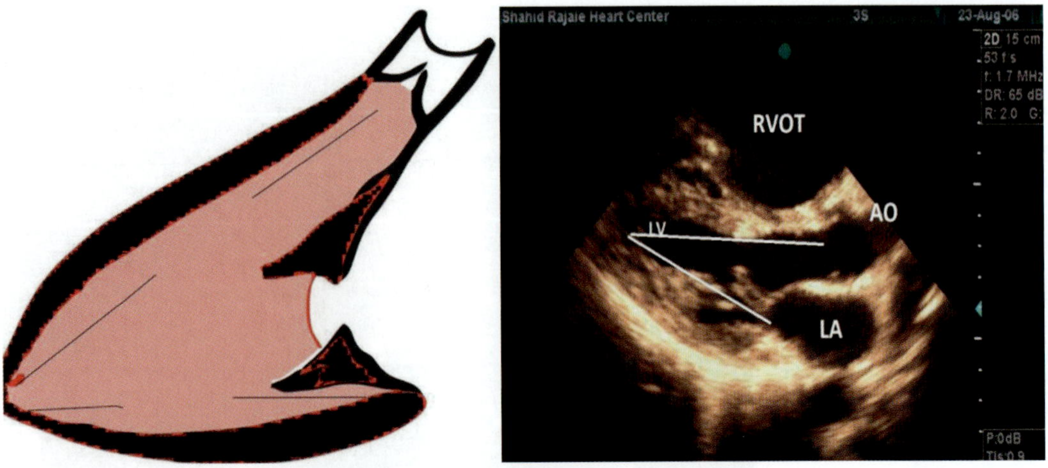

Fig. 23.6 Parasternal long-axis view showing elongated LVOT with shorter distance from MV annulus to LV apex than AV annulus to the apex. *AO* aorta, *LA* left atrium, *RVOT* right ventricular outflow tract, *LV* left ventricle (LV is right)

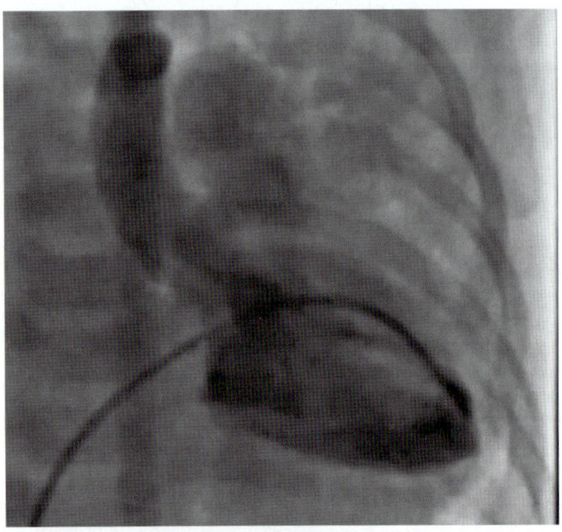

Fig. 23.7 Elongated LVOT, gooseneck deformity in cardiac catheterism

Electrocardiography

Characteristically demonstrates a superior frontal plane axis (extreme left axis deviation) and voltage criteria for ventricular hypertrophy [1–3, 5].

Clinical Presentation

Classically, children with complete AVSD should have surgical repair at 3–6 months of their age. Patients with Down syndrome may have insistent pulmonary artery hypertension (PAH) even despite early repair. Similarly, cases with complete AVSD who were not repaired in the first 9 months of their life are expected to have persistent PAH. The patients with complete AVSD that followed in an adult congenital heart disease clinic classically had repair of lesion in early childhood and need continued careful observation for development of important left AV valve regurgitation or stenosis. Also, some of them may need reoperation in adulthood, for example, the left AV valve is frequently replaced, and however, the surgery should be done by a congenital cardiac surgeon [2, 4].

Echocardiography

In echocardiographic assessments, all of the patients show AV septal defects. Cases with a common AV valve have five leaflets pattern: two (right and left) anterosuperior leaflets, two (right and left) lateral leaflets, and a common posterior leaflet. Hearts with two AV valves reveal pattern of three leaflets [2].

The classification of Rastelli type in AVSD with a common AV valve and a VSD is determined by the mode of insertion of the left and right anterior leaflets. In the common valve, echocardiographic findings show ostium primum

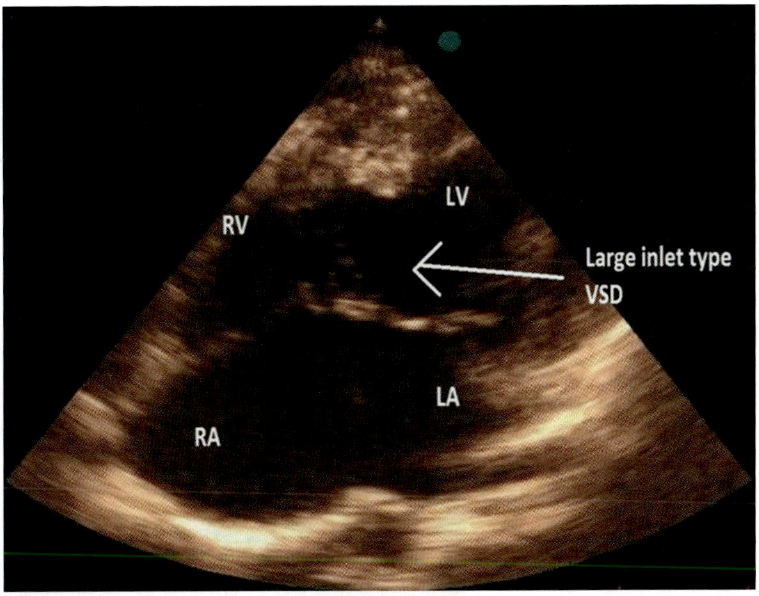

Fig. 23.8 Complete AVSD with a common AV valve, large ostium primum-type atrial septal defect, and large inlet-type interventricular septum defect. *RA* right atrium, *LA* left atrium, *RV* right ventricle, *LV* left ventricle, *VSD* ventricular septal defect

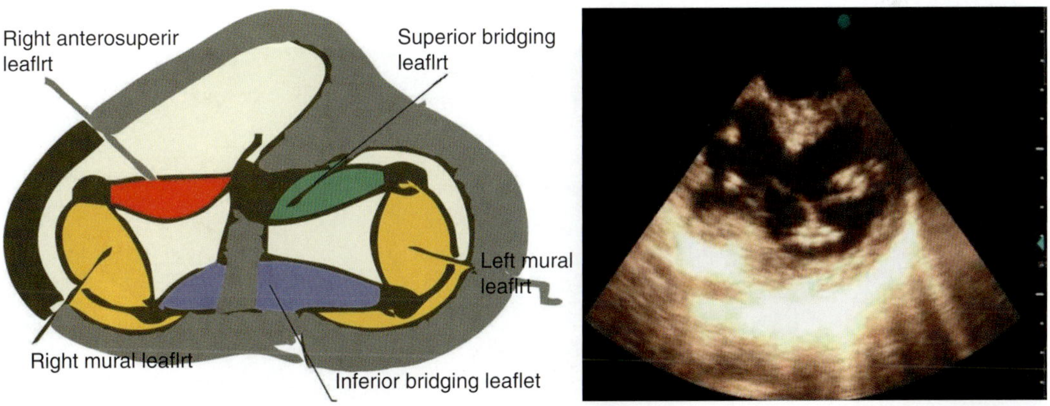

Fig. 23.9 Complete AVSD with common AV valve and its five leaflets

ASD and VSD. In Rastelli type A, the chordae tendineae of the anterior leaflets attach to the crest of the ventricular septum; apical 4-chamber echocardiographic view shows the confluent septal defects, common AV junction with attachment of the anterior leaflets in the crest of the septum, and ventricular septal defect; and the VSD is continuous with the ostium primum. Type B of complete AVSDs, which is rare, is characterized by chordal attachments from the left AV valve to papillary muscles in the RV. In a Rastelli type C defect, the superior bridging leaflet is said to be "free floating" because it is undivided and unattached to the crest of the VSD [1, 3].

In echocardiography studies in complete AVSD, the common AV valve may be positioned equally over both ventricles (balanced) or unequally over the right or left ventricle (unbalanced). MV abnormalities are seen in complete forms of AVSD; in parasternal and short-axis view analysis, cleft is the most common abnormality of MV. Rarely, double-orifice MV and parachute MV are detected in echocardiography study. LVOT obstruction may occur in all forms of AVSD, and it is more common when there are two atrioventricular valve orifices than common orifice. Evaluation of LVOT is performed in apical four-chamber echocardiographic view [2, 5, 6].

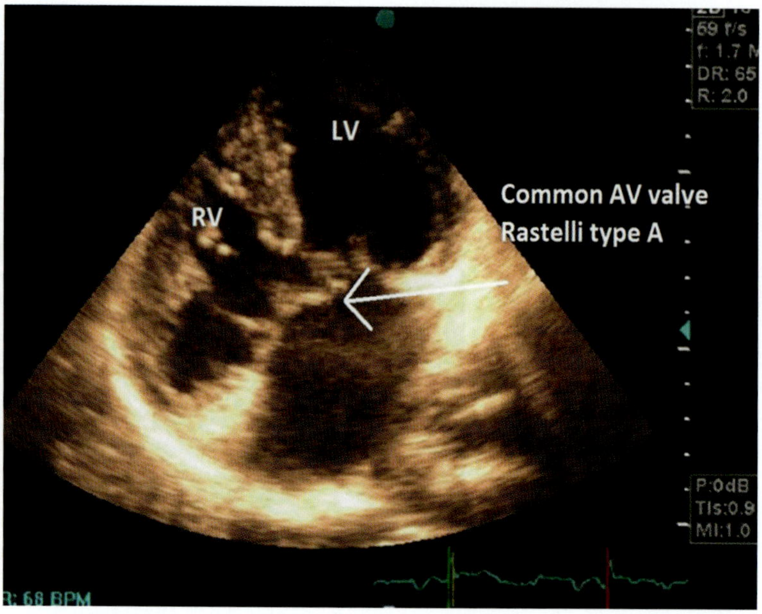

Fig. 23.10 Rastelli type A; the superior bridging leaflet is attached to the crest of ventricular septum. *RV* right ventricle, *LV* left ventricle

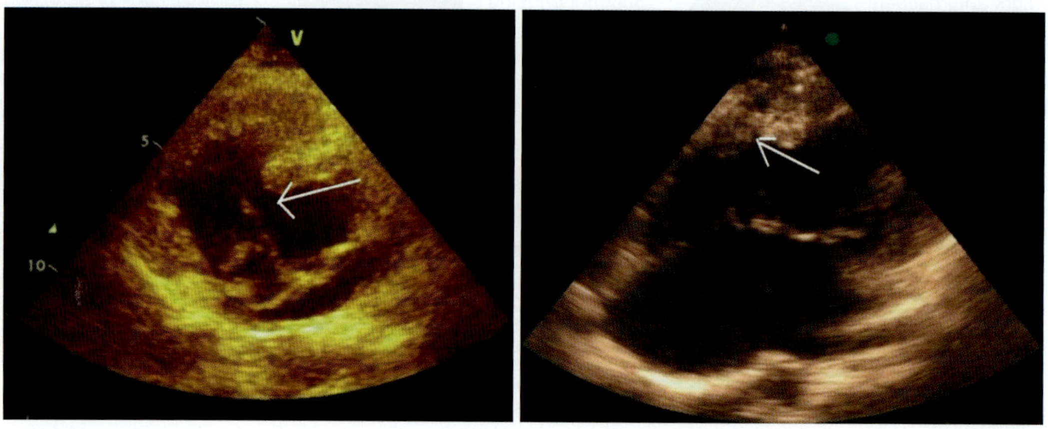

Fig. 23.11 Rastelli type C in short-axis and four-chamber views; the superior bridging leaflet is attached to the papillary muscle on RV free wall (*white arrow*)

Table 23.1 Anatomic classification of CAVC

Type A
The superior bridging leaflet is almost completely adherent to the left ventricle and is firmly attached on the crest of ventricular septum by multiple chordal insertions
Type B
The superior bridging leaflet is attached over the ventricular septum by an anomalous papillary muscle (PM) of the right ventricle (RV)
Type C
The superior bridging leaflet is not attached to the ventricular septum (free-floating leaflet) as it is attached to the PM of RV free wall

Calabrò and Limongelli [17]
PM papillary muscle, *RV* right ventricle, *CAVC* complete AV canal

Spectral and color Doppler help to assess the sites of shunting, severity of AV valve regurgitation, and also connections of the pulmonary veins. In addition, secundum ASDs, a properly common associated finding, can be identified from the subcostal four-chamber view and via clockwise rotation of the transducer in subcostal imaging view. Anomalous pulmonary venous connections are rarely associated with complete AVSDs and may be assessed with two-dimensional Doppler echocardiography or trans-esophageal echocardiography from multiple imaging views and planes [1, 2, 6].

Management

The aims of surgical repair are closure of inter-atrial and interventricular septal defects, construction of two separate and competent AV valves from obtainable leaflet tissues, and also repair of associated lesions. Infrequently, these cases will have hemodynamically important residual shunts after surgery. These shunts are classically not amenable to closure with devices due to the proximity of the AV valves [10–13].

Patients with late repaired or unrepaired lesions or patients with Down syndrome may develop PAH; these cases with PAH can be treated with pulmonary vasoactive agents, such as sildenafil or bosentan, and improvement in symptoms and functional class may happen. These patients also face with progressive left and right AV valves regurgitation and also progressive RV and LV systolic dysfunction. Survival for this subgroup beyond the fifth decade has been reported but is rare. These patients need management for secondary erythrocytosis, urate nephropathy, hemoptysis, thromboembolic events, and sometimes arrhythmia [12–14].

Pregnancy in AVSD

Outcomes for pregnancy in women with AVSD have been good, even if recent studies indicated that atrial arrhythmia can complicate as many as 10 % of pregnancies in women with AVSD. It is overall suggested that women with unrepaired AVSD undergo repair prior to pregnancy; however, in women with partial AVSD, pregnancy is generally well tolerated. Of course, pregnancy is contraindicated in women with unrepaired AVSD who have Eisenmenger physiology [15, 16].

References

1. Bonow RO, Mann DL, Zipes DP, Libby P, eds. Braunwald's Heart Disease: A Textbook of Cardiovascular Medicine. 9th ed. Philadelphia, PA: Saunders Elsevier; 2011.
2. Gatzoulis MA, Webb GD, Broberg CS, Uemura H. Cases in adult congenital heart disease. Philadelphia: Churchill Livingstone; 2010.
3. Warnes C, Williams RG, Bashore TM, et al. ACC/AHA, guidelines for the management of adults with congenital heart disease. J Am Coll Cardiol. 2008;52(23):e143–263.
4. Warnes CA. Adult congenital heart disease, American Heart Association. AHA clinical series. Wiley Blackwell; 2009. Chapter 2. p. 9–24.
5. Allen HD, Driscoll DJ, Shady RE. Moss and Adams' heart disease in infants, children, and adolescents: including the fetus and young adults. 7th ed. Philadelphia: Lippincott Williams & Wilkins; 2008.
6. Eidem BW, Cetta F, O'leary PW. Echocardiography in pediatric and adult congenital heart disease. Philadelphia: Lippincott Williams & Wilkins; 2012.
7. Aubert S, Henaine R, Raisky O, et al. Atypical forms of isolated partial atrioventricular septal defect increase the risk of initial valve replacement and reoperation. Eur J Cardiothorac Surg. 2005;28:223–8.
8. Bergin ML, Warnes CA, Tajik AJ, et al. Partial atrioventricular canal defect: long-term follow-up after initial repair in patients >40 years old. J Am Coll Cardiol. 1995;25:1189–94.
9. McGrath LB, Gonzalez-Lavin L. Actuarial survival, freedom from reoperation, and other events after repair of atrioventricular septal defects. J Thorac Cardiovasc Surg. 1987;94:582.
10. Vet TW, Ottenkamp J. Correction of atrioventricular septal defect. Results influenced by Down syndrome? Am J Dis Child. 1989;143(11):1361–5.
11. Carpentier A. Surgical anatomy and management of the mitral component of atrioventricular canal defects. In: Anderson RH, Shinebourne EA, editors. Paediatric cardiology. Edinburgh: Churchill Livingstone; 1978. p. 477–90.
12. Piccoli GP, Wilkinson JL, Macartney FJ, et al. Morphology and classification of complete atrioventricular defects. Br Heart J. 1979;42:633–9.
13. Atz AM, Hawkins JA, Lu M, et al. Surgical management of complete atrioventricular septal defect: asso-

ciations with surgical technique, age, and trisomy 21. J Thorac Cardiovasc Surg. 2011;141(6):1371–9.
14. Nicholson IA, Nunn GR, Sholler GF, et al. Simplified single patch technique for the repair of atrioventricular septal defect. J Thorac Cardiovasc Surg. 1999;118(4):642–6.
15. Drenthen W, Pieper PG, van der Tuuk K, et al. Cardiac complications relating to pregnancy and recurrence of disease in the offspring of women with atrioventricular septal defects. Eur Heart J. 2005;26:2581–7.
16. Drenthen W, Pieper PG, Roos-Hesselink JW, et al. Outcome of pregnancy in women with congenital heart disease. J Am Coll Cardiol. 2007;49:2303–11.
17. Calabrò R, Limongelli G. Complete atrioventricular canal. Orphanet J Rare Dis. 2006;1:8.

Patent Ductus Arteriosus

24

Azin Alizadehasl, Anita Sadeghpour, and Majid Kyavar

Keywords

Patent Ductus Arteriosus (PDA) • Silent PDA • Continuous Murmur • Differential Cyanosis • Echocardiography

The ductus arteriosus originates from the left sixth primitive aortic arch and links the proximal left pulmonary artery to the descending aorta, just beneath to the left subclavian artery.

In the normal fetus, the ductus is patent. Functional closure of the ductus from vasoconstriction happens shortly after a term birth, while anatomic closure occurred several weeks later from intimal proliferation and fibrosis. In some disease, the circulation depends on the ductus for pulmonary blood flow, such as in severe aortic coarctation, hypoplastic left heart syndrome, and sometimes d-TGA. If spontaneous closure of this ductus happens in such neonates, clinical deterioration and even death may happen [1–3].

Usually patent ductus arteriosus (PDA) is classified based on the degree of left-to-right shunting, which is determined by both the size of the duct and the difference between systemic and pulmonary vascular resistances, as follows:

1. Silent: Tiny PDA detected only by paraclinical means (generally by echocardiography).
2. Small: Continuous murmur is common; Qp/Qs <1.5:1.
3. Moderate: Continuous murmur is common; Qp/Qs of 1.5 to 2.2:1.
4. Large: Continuous murmur is present always; Qp/Qs >2.2:1.
5. Eisenmenger: Continuous murmur is absent; considerable pulmonary hypertension, differential hypoxemia, and cyanosis (pink fingers with blue toes) [1, 4–6].

A. Alizadehasl, MD, FACC (✉)
Echocardiography Lab, Department of Cardiology, Rajaie Cardiovascular Medical and Research Center, Iran University of Medical Science, Tehran, Iran
e-mail: alizadeasl@gmail.com, alizadeasl@rhc.ac.ir

A. Sadeghpour, MD, FACC, FASE (✉)
Echocardiography Lab, Department of Cardiology, Adult Congenital Heart Disease Clinic, Rajaie Cardiovascular Medical and Research Center, Iran University of Medical Science, Tehran, Iran
e-mail: anita.sadeghpour@gmail.com, asadeghpour@rhc.ac.ir

M. Kyavar, MD, FACC
Cardiovascular Imaging Ward, Department of Cardiology, Adult Congenital Heart Disease Clinic, Rajaie Cardiovascular Medical and Research Center, Iran University of Medical Science, Tehran, Iran

Electronic supplementary material The online version of this chapter (doi: 10.1007/978-1-4471-6383-1_24) contains supplementary material, which is available to authorized users.

A. Sadeghpour et al. (eds.), *Comprehensive Approach to Adult Congenital Heart Disease*,
DOI 10.1007/978-1-4471-6383-1_24, © Springer-Verlag London 2014

Natural History

Patency of a ductus arteriosus is prevalent in a preterm newborn who has no normal mechanisms for postnatal ductal closure due to immaturity. A PDA is, therefore, a predictable finding in a premature infant, and delayed spontaneous closure of the ductus may be expected.

Although some full-term newborns have persistent patency of the ductus arteriosus because of their relative hypoxemia, in a full-term newborn, usually patency of a ductus is a true congenital malformation [2, 5, 7, 8].

Children and adults with silent PDAs are identified by nonclinical means, usually echocardiography, and face almost no long-term complications. Of course an exception happens if the patient's murmur is inaudible because of obesity or other anatomic factors. A small ductus accompanied by a small shunt does not cause a significant hemodynamic imbalance but may dispose to endarteritis, especially when a murmur is audible. A moderate-sized duct usually poses a volume load on the left atrium and left ventricle (LV) with resulting dilation and dysfunction of LV and maybe sometimes atrial fibrillation. A large duct sometimes results firstly in LV volume overload but progresses a rise in pulmonary artery pressures and finally irreversible pulmonary vascular changes by 2 years [3–5].

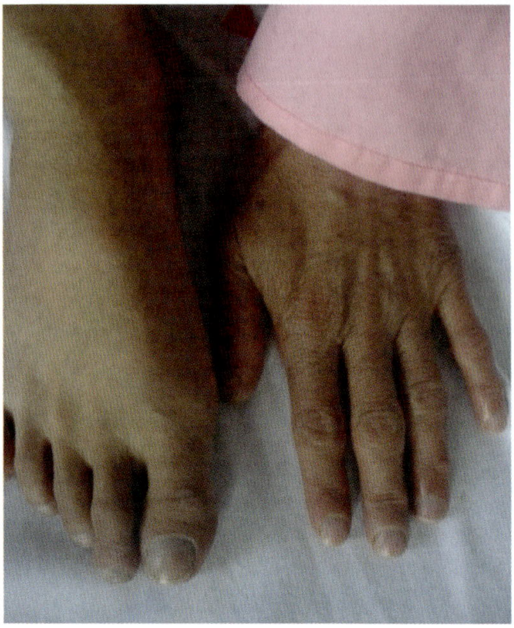

Fig. 24.1 Differential cyanosis in a patient with PDA-related Eisenmenger syndrome. Cyanosis and clubbing of the toe are more profound than the fingers. In this setting, blood bypasses the lungs via the PDA, which results in direct perfusion of the lower limbs with the desaturated blood

Clinical Findings

Most preterm infants with a birth weight less than 1,500 g have a PDA, and about one-third have a large enough shunt to cause important cardiopulmonary worsening. Clinical findings in these patients contain bounding peripheral pulses, interscapular systolic murmur (infrequently a machinery murmur), precordial hyperactivity, and hepatomegaly [1, 2].

But in full-term infants, children, and adults, a small audible duct frequently produces no symptoms but may rarely be manifested as an end arthritis. Physical examination may reveal a grade 1 or 2 continuous murmur peaking in late systole. Patients with a moderate-sized duct may produce with dyspnea or palpitations from atrial arrhythmias. A loud machinery murmur in the first or second left intercostal space is typically accompanied by a wide systemic pulse pressure from aortic diastolic flow into the pulmonary trunk and signs of left ventricular volume overload, such as an emigrant left ventricular apex and even a left-sided S3. With a moderate degree of pulmonary artery hypertension, the diastolic part of the murmur disappears and just leaves a systolic murmur. Adults with a large uncorrected PDA finally present with a short systolic ejection murmur, hypoxemia in the feet more than in the hands (differential cyanosis) (Fig. 24.1), and Eisenmenger syndrome [1, 3, 4, 9].

Electrocardiography

A small duct produces a normal ECG. A moderate duct may display left ventricular volume overload with broad, notched P waves composed with deep Q waves, tall R waves, and peaked T waves

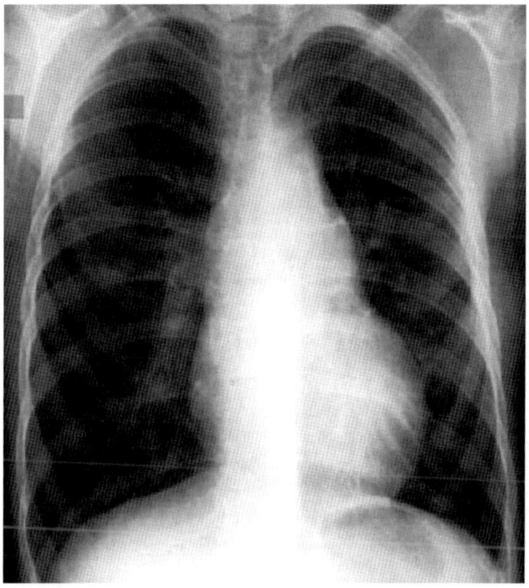

Fig. 24.2 Cardiomegaly, left ventricular enlargement, prominent aortic knob, and left-to-right shunt differential diagnosis: (1) patent ductus arteriosus and (2) ventricular septal defect

in V5 and V6. A large duct with Eisenmenger physiology produce findings of right ventricular hypertrophy [1, 2].

Chest Radiography

A small duct creates a normal chest radiograph. A moderate-sized duct produces moderate cardiomegaly with left heart enlargement, a prominent aortic knuckle, and increased pulmonary perfusion. Calcification of the ductus can be seen through the soft tissue density of the aortic arch or pulmonary trunk in older adults. The large PDA creates an Eisenmenger appearance with a prominent aortic knuckle [1, 2, 5] (Fig. 24.2).

Echocardiography

In adults, direct visualization of PDA may be difficult as they usually have larger body habitus. However, the hemodynamic effect on LA and LV, color flow imaging (CFI), and Doppler study in parasternal short-axis and suprasternal view are important keys for diagnosis.

Detection of diastolic ductal flow in the pulmonary artery (PA) along the lateral wall of main PA has high sensitivity and specificity for diagnosis of a PDA [2, 10].

Echocardiography may be normal or demonstrate right or left ventricular hypertrophy or both; left ventricular dilation or dysfunction depends on the volume of left-to-right shunting and the degree of associated pulmonary artery hypertension.

In echocardiography, PDA may be imaged completely and its size well estimated (Figs. 24.3, 24.4, 24.5, 24.6, 24.7 and 24.8, Videos 24.1, 24.2, 24.3, 24.4 and 24.5). Also Doppler study proves the shunt and documents an accurate assessment of mean pulmonary artery pressure. Measurements of the left atrial and left ventricular size provide indirect evidence of the degree of left-to-right shunting [1, 4, 10, 11].

This determines the presence, size, and degree of shunting and the also the physiologic outcomes of the shunt. The PDA is seen with difficulty in an Eisenmenger context. A bubble study may help in diagnosis of communication [1, 2] (Fig. 24.7, Videos 24.6 and 24.7).

Indications for Treatment

Management of preterm infants with a PDA varies with the degree of shunting and the severity of hyaline membrane disease since the ductus may contribute prominently to mortality in newborns with respiratory distress syndrome. However, closing in asymptomatic infants with a small left-to-right shunt is needless because the PDA virtually experiences spontaneous closure. Those infants with significant left-to-right shunt during the period of respiratory distress syndrome are often unresponsive to medical treatment to control heart failure and need closure of the PDA to live. Often, these newborns are treated by pharmacologic inhibition of prostaglandin synthesis with "indomethacin or ibuprofen." Surgical closure is needed in the estimated 10 % of infants who are nonresponsive to indomethacin [1–3].

But sometimes the ductus reserves pulmonary blood flow, and the spontaneous closure of the

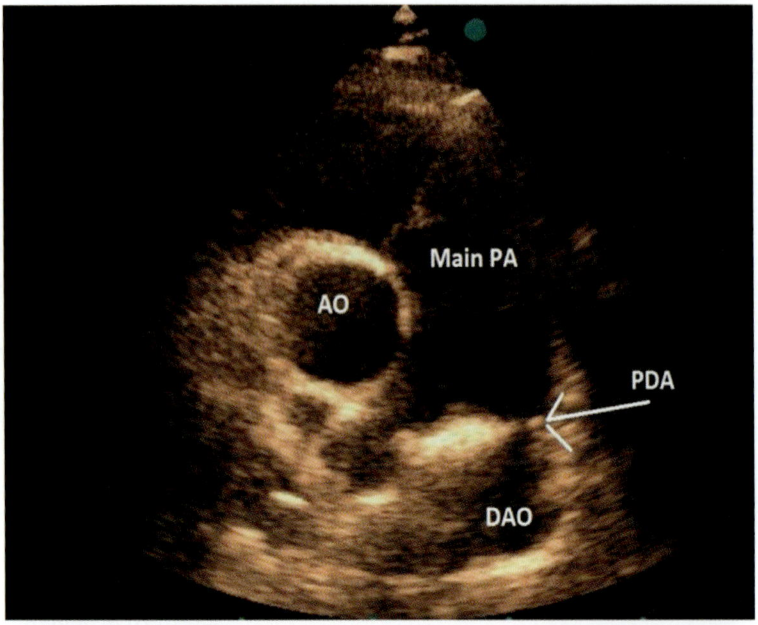

Fig. 24.3 Parasternal SAX view demonstrating 2D dropout between the left pulmonary artery (*LPA*) and descending aorta (*DAO*) suggestive of PDA. *LPA* left pulmonary artery, *PDA* patent ductus aretriosus, *Main PA* main pulmonary artery, *AO* aorta, *DAO* descending aorta

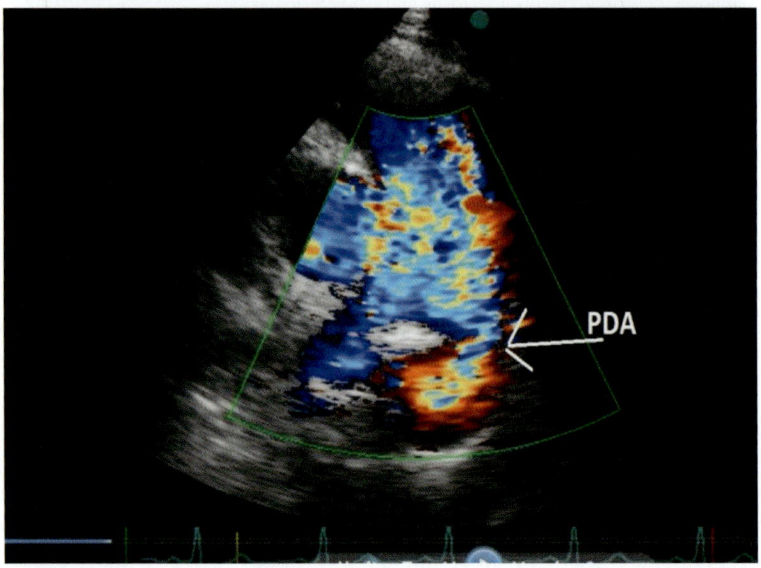

Fig. 24.4 Color Doppler flow imaging in parasternal short-axis view showing high-velocity continuous turbulent flow entering to the pulmonary artery (PA) near the LPA origin

PDA is associated with deep clinical deterioration and even death. By an infusion of prostaglandin E1, unwanted ductal closure may be reversed. By dilation of the constricted PDA, a temporary increase in arterial blood oxygen may occur. But in children and adults closing a hemodynamically significant PDA is necessary (Fig. 24.9). There is discussion about the facts of closing a silent or small PDA to reduce the risk of endarteritis. Even in the presence of severe pulmonary artery hypertension, closure is rarely indicated. Contraindications include irreversible pulmonary artery hypertension and active endarteritis [2, 4, 12].

Management

Transcatheter Treatment

In centers with appropriate properties and also experience, transcatheter device closure should be the method of choice. During the past 20 years, the

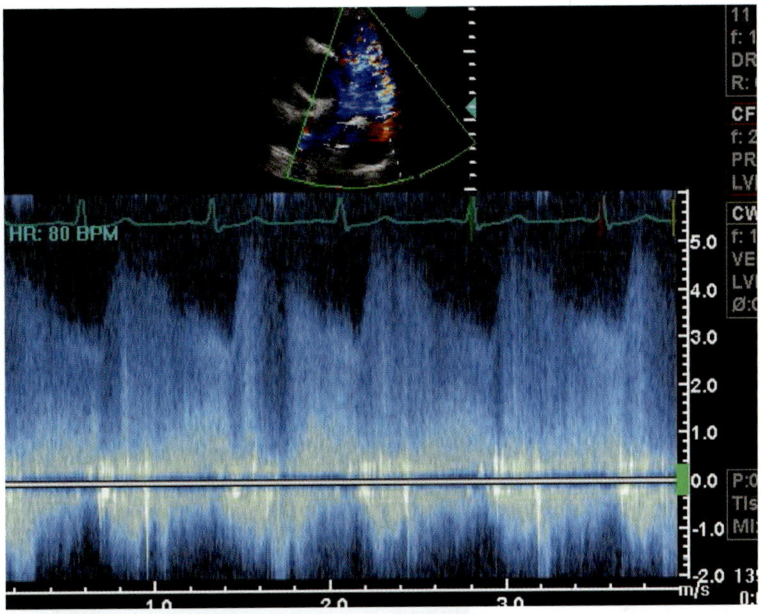

Fig. 24.5 Continuous wave Doppler tracing showing high-velocity continuous (systolic and diastolic) turbulent flow across the PDA with late systolic peal velocity

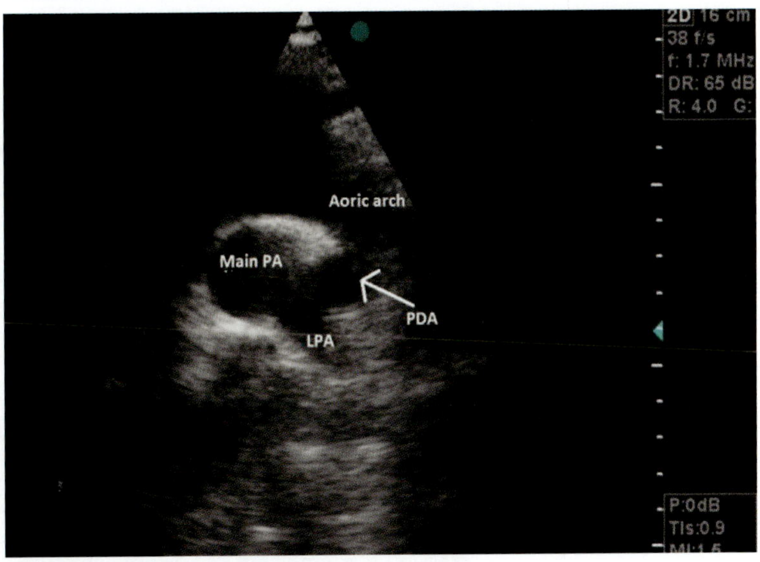

Fig. 24.6 Suprasternal long-axis view showing a large PDA between the LPA origin and proximal DAO

efficiency and safety of transcatheter device closure for ducts smaller than 8 mm have been well known, with complete ductal closure reached in more than 85 % of patients by 1 year after device engagement with a mortality rate of less than 1 % [2, 3, 12–14].

Surgery

Surgical closure (ductal ligation or division) has been performed for more than 50 years with a higher closure rate than by devices but with slightly bigger morbidity and mortality. Surgical closure is a low-risk procedure in children. Surgical mortality in adults is 1–3.5 % and relates to the presence of pulmonary arterial hypertension or hard ductal morphology (calcified or aneurysmal) that is frequently seen in adults. Surgical closure should be kept for those in whom the PDA is too large for device closure or at centers without experience for device closure [2, 4, 13, 14].

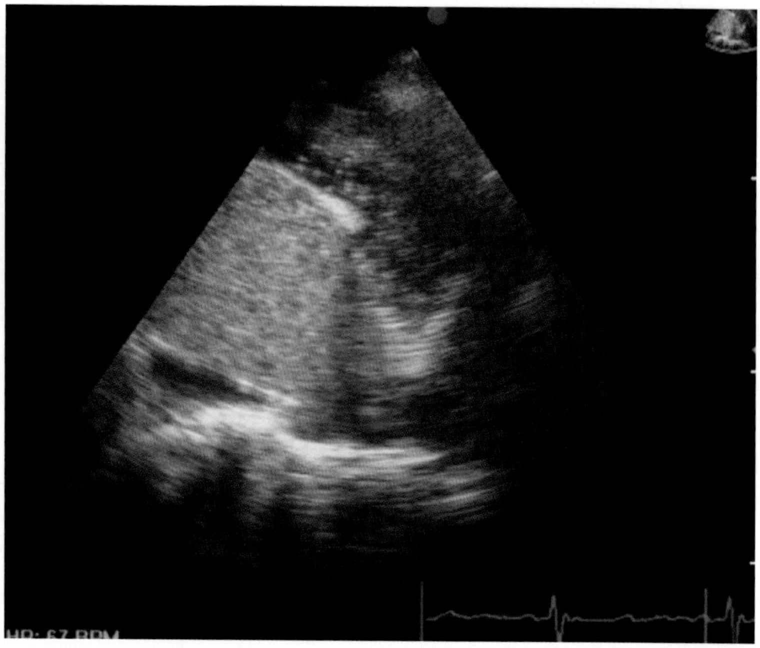

Fig. 24.7 Right-sided contrast injection (agitated saline injection) in the antecubital vein showing the bubble transmission from pulmonary artery to the descending aorta (DAO) in a patient with PDA and high pulmonary vascular resistance

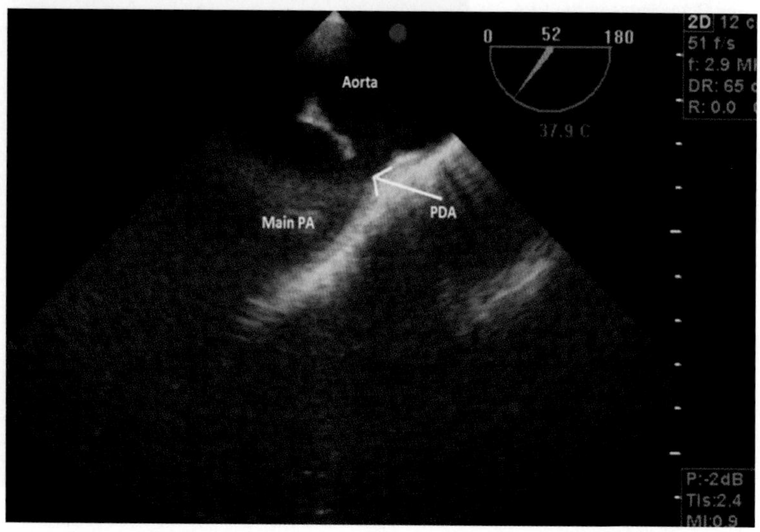

Fig. 24.8 Large PDA in transesophageal echocardiography study. *PDA* patent ductus arteriosus

Follow-up

Patients with device closure or after surgical closing should be examined intermittently for possible recanalization. Endocarditis prophylaxis is recommended for 6 months after PDA device closure or for lifelong if any residual defect persists. Patients with a silent or small PDA perhaps do not need endocarditis prophylaxis or even follow-up [1, 2, 15–17].

Pregnancy is well tolerated in women with silent and small PDAs and in all patients who were asymptomatic before pregnancy. But in women with a hemodynamically significant PDA, pregnancy may initiate or worsen heart failure. We all know pregnancy is contraindicated in Eisenmenger

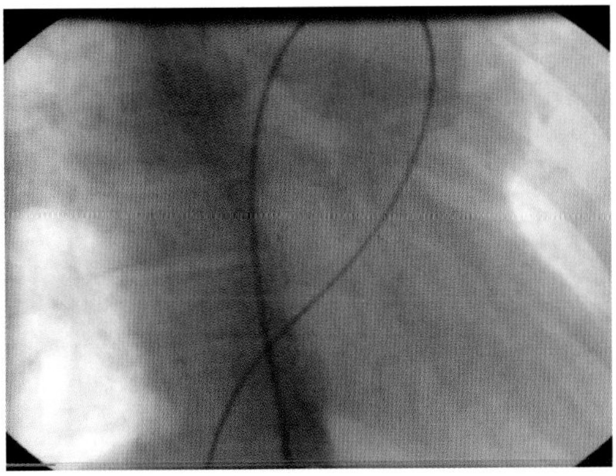

Fig. 24.9 Catheter passes from the inferior vena cava (IVC) through the right atrium (RA) and the right ventricle (RV) into the pulmonary trunk and enters the descending thoracic aorta via patent ductus arteriosus (PDA)

syndrome due to the high maternal (≈50 %) and fetal (≈60 %) mortality (Videos 24.8 and 24.9) [16, 17].

Conclusions

PDA is a congenital disorder found in patients of all ages and sizes, from premature infants to older adults. The clinical findings vary depending on the anatomy of the ductus arteriosus, associated disease, and the underlying cardiovascular status of the patient.

During the past three decades, transcatheter methods have replaced surgical therapy in most patients with PDA. Concomitantly, advances in diagnostic echocardiography and the widespread availability of echocardiography have resulted in improved diagnosis and characterization of PDA in patients of all ages. Complications of PDA can be avoided or amended by proper diagnosis and management.

References

1. Bonow RO, Mann DL, Zipes DP, Libby P. Braunwald's heart disease: a textbook of cardiovascular medicine. 9th ed. Philadelphia: Elsevier/Saunders; 2011. p. 1435–50.
2. Gatzoulis MA, Webb GD, Broberg CS, Uemura H. Cases in adult congenital heart disease. Philadelphia: Churchill Livingstone; 2010.
3. Warnes C, Williams RG, Bashore TM, et al. ACC/AHA, guidelines for the management of adults with congenital heart disease. J Am Coll Cardiol. 2008;52(23):2008.
4. Warnes CA, American Heart Association. Adult congenital heart disease, AHA clinical series. Hoboken: Wiley; 2009. p. 9–24. Chapter 2.
5. Allen HD, Driscoll DJ, Shaddy RE. Moss and Adams' heart disease in infants, children, and adolescents: including the fetus and young adults. 7th ed. Philadelphia: Lippincott Williams & Wilkins; 2008.
6. Record FG, McKeown T. Observations relating to the aetiology of patent ductus arteriosus. Br Heart J. 1953;15:376–86.
7. Hoffman JIE, Kaplan S. The incidence of congenital heart disease. J Am Coll Cardiol. 2002;39:1890–900.
8. Cassels DE. The ductus arteriosus. Springfield: Charles C. Thomas; 1973.
9. Gittenberger-de Groot AC, Moulaert AJ, Hitchcock JF. Histology of the persistent ductus arteriosus in cases of congenital rubella. Circulation. 1980;62:183–6.
10. Eidem BW, Cetta F, O'leary PW. Echocardiography in pediatric and adult congenital heart disease. Philadelphia: Lippincott Williams & Wilkins; 2012.
11. Becker TE, Ensing GJ, Darragh RK, et al. Doppler derivation of complete pulmonary artery pressure curves in patent ductus arteriosus. Am J Cardiol. 1996;78:1066–9.
12. Masura J, Gavora P, Podnar T. Transcatheter occlusion of patent ductus arteriosus using a new angled Amplatzer duct occluder: initial clinical experience. Catheter Cardiovasc Interv. 2003;58:261–7.
13. Sideris EB, Rao PS. Sideris' buttoned device for transcatheter closure of patent ductus arteriosus. J Interv Cardiol. 2001;14:239–46.
14. Rao PS. Summary and comparison of patent ductus arteriosus closure methods. In: Rao PS, Kern MJ, editors. Catheter based devices for the treatment of non-coronary cardiovascular disease in adults and children. Philadelphia: Lippincott Williams & Wilkins; 2003. p. 219–28.
15. Pass RH, Hijazi Z, Hsu DT, et al. Multicenter USA Amplatzer patent ductus arteriosus occlusion device trial: initial and one-year results. J Am Coll Cardiol. 2004;44:513–9.
16. Bessinger Jr FB, Blieden LC, Edwards JE. Hypertensive pulmonary vascular disease associated with patent ductus arteriosus: primary or secondary? Circulation. 1975;52:157–61.
17. Yamaki S, Ishidoya T, Osuga T, et al. Progressive pulmonary vascular disease after surgery in a case of patent ductus arteriosus with pulmonary hypertension. Tohoku J Exp Med. 1983;140:279–88.

25 Truncus Arteriosus

Anita Sadeghpour and Azin Alizadehasl

Keywords
Truncus arteriosus • Truncal valve • Eisenmenger syndrome • Aortopulmonary collaterals • Echocardiography

Morphology and Associated Lesions

Persistent truncus arteriosus is an anomaly in which a single vessel makes the outlet of both ventricles and provides blood supply to the systemic, pulmonary, and coronary arteries. It is classified as a type of congenital heart disease (CHD) with great complexity. It is always attended by a VSD and commonly with a right-sided aortic arch. The common trunk classically straddles a defect in the outlet portion of the interventricular septum (or conal septum), but, in sporadic cases, it might originate almost totally from the right or left ventricle [1, 2].

Truncal valve is frequently tricuspid but is quadricuspid in about 30 % of patients. The truncal valve regurgitation and stenosis are each seen in 10–15 % of truncus arteriosus patients. Patients with a history of truncus arteriosus also have a high prevalence of DiGeorge syndrome. Many patients with this chromosome deletion reveal impairment in social function. Coexisting diseases associated with this syndrome include schizophrenia, mental disability, deafness, immune deficiencies, endocrinopathies, and clubbed foot [1, 3].

Also there can be a single coronary artery in truncus arteriosus patients, and also the proximal portion of the coronary arteries is abnormal in many patients.

Other moderately common but minor relations contain right aortic arch, left-sided superior caval vein, aberrant subclavian artery, and also atrial septal defect [3, 4].

A. Sadeghpour, MD, FACC, FASE (✉)
Echocardiography Lab, Department of Cardiology, Adult Congenital Heart Disease Clinic, Rajaie Cardiovascular Medical and Research Center, Iran University of Medical Science, Tehran, Iran
e-mail: anita.sadeghpour@gmail.com; asadeghpour@rhc.ac.ir

A. Alizadehasl, MD, FACC
Echocardiography Lab, Department of Cardiology, Rajaie Cardiovascular Medical and Research Center, Iran University of Medical Science, Tehran, Iran
e-mail: alizadeasl@gmail.com; alizadeasl@rhc.ac.ir

Electronic supplementary material The online version of this chapter (doi: 10.1007/978-1-4471-6383-1_25) contains supplementary material, which is available to authorized users.

A. Sadeghpour et al. (eds.), *Comprehensive Approach to Adult Congenital Heart Disease*,
DOI 10.1007/978-1-4471-6383-1_25, © Springer-Verlag London 2014

Classification

Truncus arteriosus is classified anatomically based on the mode of origin of pulmonary vessels from the common trunk.

Type I: Partially separate pulmonary trunk of variable elongation exists and gives rise to left and right pulmonary arteries (this is the frequent type of truncus arteriosus).

Type II: Each pulmonary artery rises separately but close to each other from the posterior side of the truncus.

Type III: Each pulmonary artery arises from the lateral aspect of the truncus away to each other.

Less commonly, one pulmonary artery may be absent, with aortopulmonary collaterals supplying the lung that does not obtain a pulmonary artery branch from the truncus [1–3, 5].

Pathophysiology and Natural History

Pulmonary blood flow is provided by the size of the pulmonary arteries and the pulmonary vascular resistance. Indeed because the systemic and pulmonary circulations are basically in parallel, pulmonary blood flow classically is at least three-fold higher than systemic blood flow, with pulmonary over-circulation and increased myocardial labor that results in augmented resting oxygen demand and reduced metabolic reserve. However, pulmonary vascular resistance increases with time, increasing the cyanosis. When pulmonary vascular resistance reaches to systemic level, Eisenmenger physiology and bidirectional shunting happen. Significant truncal valve regurgitation creates a volume load on both right and left ventricles [2–4, 7, 8].

Most deaths happen before 1 year of age from heart failure. Unrepaired patients who live past 1 year most likely present with established severe pulmonary hypertension. The occurrence of significant truncal valve regurgitation increases with age, causing biventricular heart failure and increasing probability of endocarditis [1, 2].

Clinical Findings

Newborns with truncus arteriosus usually present with minimal cyanosis concomitant with findings of a large left-to-right shunt. Signs and symptoms of heart failure and poor physical growth usually appear in the first weeks or months of life. The most common physical findings contain cardiomegaly, loud and single second heart sound, harsh systolic murmur with an ejection click, and low-pitched mid-diastolic rumbling murmur and bounding pulses. A decrescendo diastolic murmur suggests related truncal valve regurgitation [1–3].

With increasing age, the physical findings are different, because the pulmonary blood flow is restricted by high pulmonary vascular resistance. Cyanosis is eminent, and only a short systolic murmur can be heard with an ejection click. Pulmonary vascular resistance frequently does not restrict pulmonary blood flow before the first year of age. Older patients with an unrepaired TA are at very high risk of developing pulmonary hypertension, whereas those with VSDs or ASDs are at moderate and relatively low risk, respectively. The variation in these risks is associated with shunt flow or even with an underlying unknown genetic predisposition [3, 4].

The nature of the anatomic abnormality also defines the age at presentation. Patients with AVSD, truncus arteriosus, transposition of the great vessels, large PDA, and VSD present earliest. Adults presenting with an unrepaired truncus arteriosus have Eisenmenger syndrome and its classic findings, and also patients with significant truncal valve regurgitation have a tendency to present with more significant symptoms of congestive heart failure [1, 5, 6].

Electrocardiography

A normal sinus rhythm and normal intervals and also a normal QRS axis or slight right axis deviation are usually observed. Biventricular hypertrophy is a specific finding [2, 4] (Fig. 25.1).

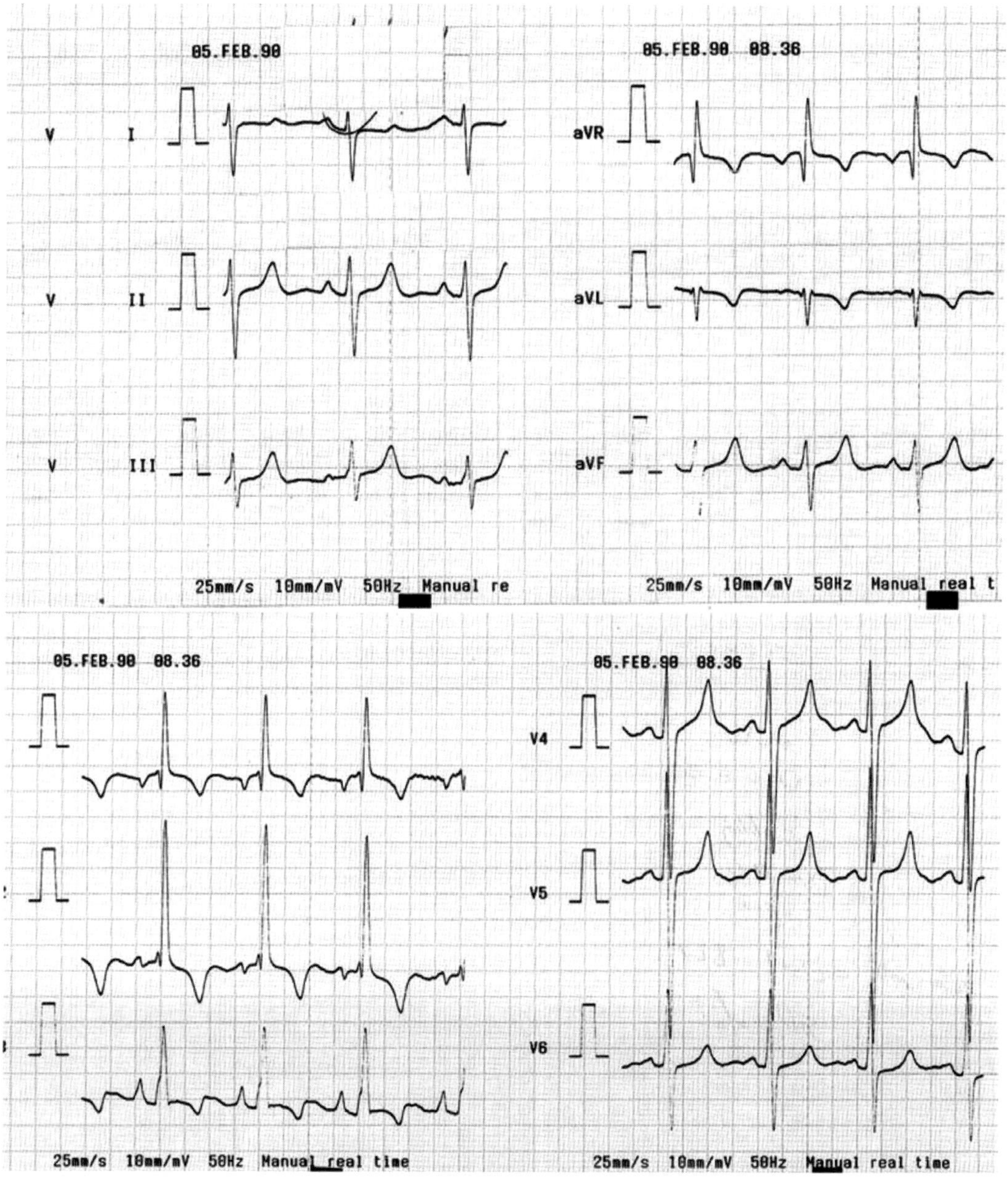

Fig. 25.1 Sinus rhythm, right ventricular hypertrophy, left atrial abnormality, and right atrial abnormality

Chest Radiography

Chest radiography demonstrates cardiomegaly with eminent pulmonary arterial markings and high hilar regions. Fullness in the area of the truncal root may probably be discerned. A right aortic arch happens in half of cases [2, 4] (Fig. 25.2).

Echocardiography

Often 2D echocardiography establishes a complete diagnosis. The study must demonstrate the overriding truncal root, the origin site of the pulmonary arteries, the number of truncal valve cusps, the origin site of the coronary arteries, the regurgitation and stenosis of truncal valve, and the size of the concomitant VSD. Also we can study the all other associated lesions.

The semilunar valve of the truncal artery frequently is abnormal. Usually, the valve leaflet is thickened. It is tricuspid in 61 % and quadricuspid in 31 % of the case. In the echocardiography, truncus arteriosus should be distinguished from the tetralogy of Fallot and pulmonary atresia as both have a large VSD and overriding arterial vessel on them [2, 4, 7] (Figs. 25.3 and 25.4, Videos 25.1, 25.2 and 25.3).

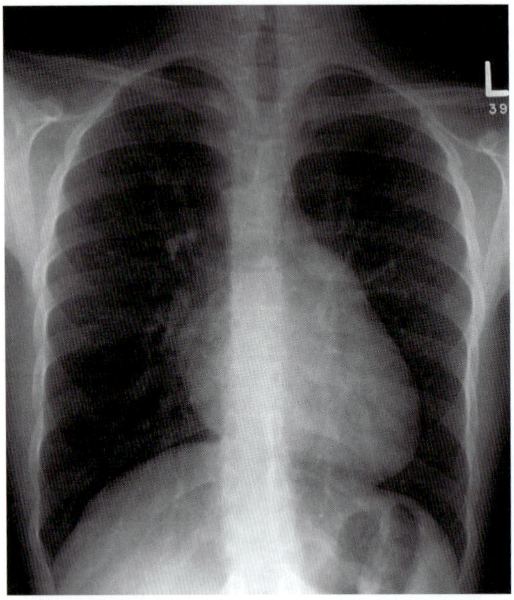

Fig. 25.2 Posteroanterior projection, right aortic arch, bilateral hilar prominence with unusual hilar areas, dilated left pulmonary artery, wide carinal angle cardiomegaly with rounded apex, biventricular and biatrial enlargement, increased pulmonary blood flow, shunt vascularity with left-to-right shunt

MRI

MRI is seldom necessary in patients with truncus arteriosus. MRI provides brilliant imaging modality for characterizing anatomy and may be particularly useful in reconstructing complex pulmonary arterial anatomy in older patients with truncus arteriosus [2, 4, 9].

Catheterization

Cardiac catheterization is generally not necessary prior to repair in neonates and young infants with truncus arteriosus and creates a risk of both morbidity and mortality. In overall, significant arterial desaturation in the absence of pulmonary artery branch stenosis indicates that this patient's lesion cannot be repaired [1, 2, 7] (Fig. 25.5, Video 25.4 and 25.5).

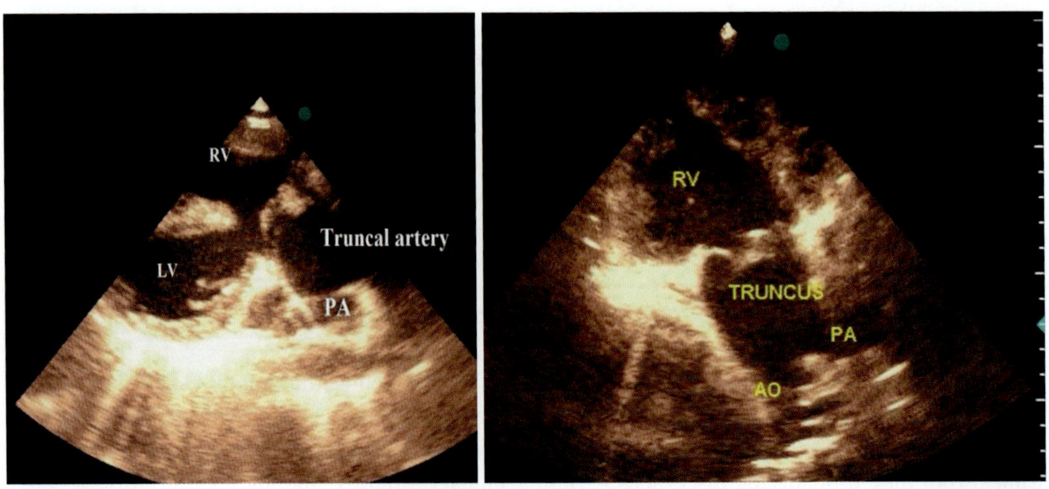

Fig. 25.3 Transthoracic echocardiography in parasternal long-axis and apical off axis view showing a large VSD, overriding truncal artery, and the main pulmonary artery which arises from the posterolateral aspect of the truncus (type I). *RV* right ventricle, *LV* left ventricle, *PA* pulmonary artery, *AO* aorta

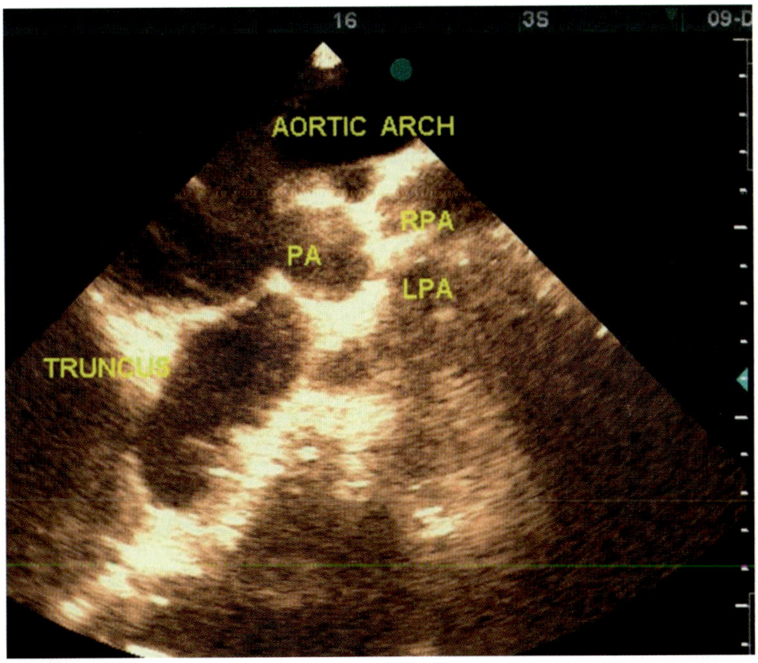

Fig. 25.4 Suprasternal transthoracic echocardiography study showing the truncal artery and the origin of the pulmonary artery and aortic arch that both arise from a single great artery. *PA* pulmonary artery, *RPA* right pulmonary artery, *LPA* left pulmonary artery

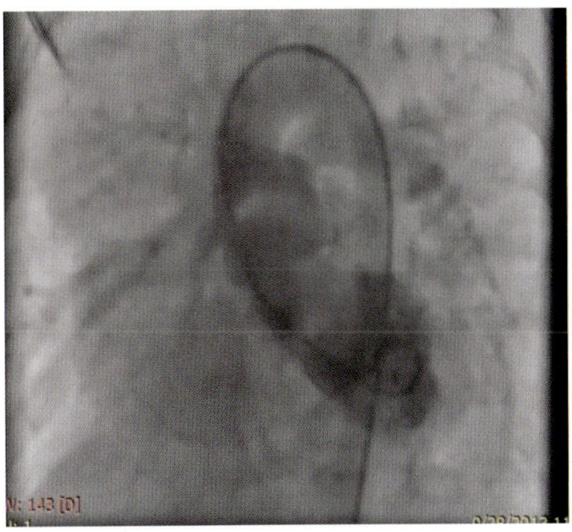

Fig. 25.5 In LV injection at LAO view: there is subaortic VSD concomitant with origination of main PA from the aorta close the left coronary artery origin

Management

Early surgical intervention should be considered in all cases within the first 2 months of life. In the presence of severe pulmonary artery hypertension, surgery is routinely not performed.

Significant risk factors for perioperative mortality are severe truncal valve regurgitation, interrupted aortic arch, coronary artery anomalies, and age at initial operation older than 100 days. Patients with only one pulmonary artery are particularly prone to early development of severe pulmonary vascular resistance [1, 2, 10–12].

Pregnancy

Patients with a repaired truncus arteriosus and no hemodynamically significant residual lesions should tolerate pregnancy well. Patients with important conduit obstruction or significant truncal valve regurgitation need correction of the lesions before pregnancy and careful follow-up throughout pregnancy. Pregnancy is contraindicated in patients with Eisenmenger syndrome that gives 50 % maternal mortality [1, 2, 4].

Follow-up

Patients operated before 1 year of age commonly do well. However, conduit change is frequently indicated within the few years after repair as the patient grows up. Also those cases with significant truncal valve stenosis or regurgitation may finally require truncal valve replacement. Patients operated on >1 year of age need careful follow-up for any signs of pulmonary artery hypertension progression. Endocarditis prophylaxis is obligatory in all truncus arteriosus patients [1, 2, 12, 13].

References

1. Bonow RO, Mann DL, Zipes DP, Libby P, eds. Braunwald's Heart Disease: A Textbook of Cardiovascular Medicine. 9th ed. Philadelphia, PA: Saunders Elsevier; 2011.
2. Gatzoulis MA, Webb GD, Broberg CS, Uemura H. Cases in adult congenital heart disease. Philadelphia: Churchill Livingstone; 2010.
3. Warnes C, Williams RG, Bashore TM, et al. ACC/AHA, guidelines for the management of adults with congenital heart disease. J Am Coll Cardiol. 2008;52(23):e143–263.
4. Warnes CA, American Heart Association. Adult congenital heart disease, AHA clinical series. Hoboken: Wiley; 2009. p. 9–24. Chapter 2.
5. Swanson TM, Selamet Tierney ES, et al. Truncus arteriosus: diagnostic accuracy, outcomes, and impact of prenatal diagnosis. Pediatr Cardiol. 2009;30(3):256–61.
6. Rao PS. Diagnosis and management of cyanotic congenital heart disease: part I. Indian J Pediatr. 2009;76(1):57–70.
7. Bartelings MM, Gittenberger-de Groot AC. Morphogenetic considerations on congenital malformations of the outflow tract. Part 1: Common arterial trunk and tetralogy of Fallot. Int J Cardiol. 1991;32(2):213–30.
8. Calder L, Van Praagh R, Van Praagh S, et al. Truncus arteriosus communis: clinical, angiocardiographic, and pathologic findings in 100 patients. Am Heart J. 1976;92:23–39.
9. Otto CM, editor. The practice of clinical echocardiography. 3rd ed. Philadelphia: W. B. Saunders/Elsevier; 2007.
10. Saxena A. Consensus on timing of intervention for common congenital heart disease. Indian Pediatr. 2008;45(2):117–26.
11. Russell HM, Pasquali SK, Jacobs JP, et al. Outcomes of repair of common arterial trunk with truncal valve surgery: a review of the society of thoracic surgeons congenital heart surgery database. Ann Thorac Surg. 2012;93(1):164–9. discussion 169.
12. Lund AM, Vogel M, Marshall AC, et al. Early reintervention on the pulmonary arteries and right ventricular outflow tract after neonatal or early infant repair of truncus arteriosus using homograft conduits. Am J Cardiol. 2011;108(1):106–13.
13. Barbero-Marcial M, Tanamati C. Alternative nonvalved techniques for repair of truncus arteriosus: long-term results. Semin Thorac Cardiovasc Surg Pediatr Card Surg Annu. 1999;2:121–30.

The Ebstein Anomaly

26

Azin Alizadeasl, Anita Sadeghpour,
and Mohammad Mahdavi

Keywords
Ebstein Anomaly • Atrialization • Atrial septal defect (ASD) • Tricuspid valve • Tricuspid regurgitation

Morphology and Associated Lesions

The *exaggerated apical displacement of the septal and posterior leaflets of the tricuspid valve (TV) in tandem with leaflet dysplasia and adherence of the tricuspid valve leaflets to the underlying right ventricle (RV) myocardium are the diagnostic features of the Ebstein anomaly. Usually, in the normal heart, there is a 10 mm distance between the mitral annulus and tricuspid annulus. In the Ebstein anomaly, the apical displacement of the septal leaflet of the TV is 8 mm/m*^{2} *or more, associated with elongated, tethered anterior TV leaflet* [1–3].

A. Alizadeasl, MD, FACC (✉)
Echocardiography Lab, Department of Cardiology, Rajaie Cardiovascular Medical and Research Center, Iran University of Medical Science, Tehran, Iran
e-mail: alizadeasl@gmail.com, alizadeasl@rhc.ac.ir

A. Sadeghpour, MD, FACC, FASE (✉)
Echocardiography Lab, Department of Cardiology, Adult Congenital Heart Disease Clinic, Rajaie Cardiovascular Medical and Research Center, Iran University of Medical Science, Tehran, Iran
e-mail: anita.sadeghpour@gmail.com, asadeghpour@rhc.ac.ir

M. Mahdavi, MD
Pediatric Ward, Department of Pediatric Cardiology, Rajaie Cardiovascular Medical and Research Center, Iran University of Medical Science, Tehran, Iran

Of course many cases have concomitant displacement of the posterior leaflet too, *but the anterior leaflet is never displaced*, and it may be adherent to the free wall of the right ventricle (RV). *The displacement of the tricuspid valve (TV) leaflets causes "atrialization" of the inflow tract of the RV and subsequently creates a small functional RV*. The spectrum of the abnormality in the Ebstein anomaly may range from only slight displacement of the septal and/or posterior leaflets to an imperforate membranous tissue or muscular layer between the inlet and trabecular regions of the RV. *Related anomalies include patent foramen ovale (PFO) or atrial septal defect (ASD) in about 50 % of patients, accessory conduction pathways in 25 % of patients* (frequently right sided), and infrequently RV outflow tract obstruction in varying degrees, ventricular septal defect (VSD), aortic coarctation, patent ductus arteriosus (PDA), or sometimes mitral valve (MV) disease. Left ventricular (LV) non-compaction syndrome has also been defined in some cases [3–6].

Electronic supplementary material The online version of this chapter (doi: 10.1007/978-1-4471-6383-1_26) contains supplementary material, which is available to authorized users.

A. Sadeghpour et al. (eds.), *Comprehensive Approach to Adult Congenital Heart Disease*,
DOI 10.1007/978-1-4471-6383-1_26, © Springer-Verlag London 2014

Pathophysiology

Variable degrees of tricuspid valve regurgitation (TR) or unusually tricuspid stenosis (TS) are associated with atrialized RA, causing right atrial enlargement. RV volume overload from significant TR can also present. Right-to-left shunting through a PFO or ASD happens if the right atrial (RA) pressure exceeds the left atrial (LA) pressure (usually with severe TR).

The functional impairment of the RV retards the forward flow of blood through the right side of the heart. In addition, during the contraction of the atrium, the atrialized portion of the RV expands out and acts as a passive pool, lessening the volume of the ejected blood. The global effect on the RA is dilation, increasing the size of an interatrial communication. TR is increased via annular dilatation. Related heart disease in the Ebstein anomaly has an additional effect on physiology [4–6].

Clinical Findings

Newborns and infants with severe TV deformity present with right-sided heart failure. Most other pediatric patients with delayed diagnosis (e.g., after the neonatal period) remain asymptomatic until late adolescence or early adult life. Most adult patients present with exercise intolerance, palpitations of supraventricular origin, cyanosis because of right-to-left shunting in the atrial level, and rarely a paradoxical embolus causing a transient ischemic attack or stroke. Right-sided heart failure from severe TR and RV dysfunction is probable. Sudden cardiac death has been described too [4].

Physical Examination

Physical examination classically exposes a non-impressive jugular venous pressure because of the large and compliant RA and atrialized RV, *widely split S1 sound with a loud TV component (sail sound), widely split S2 due to right bundle branch block (RBBB), and right-sided S3*. A pansystolic murmur that increases in inspiration from TR is best heard at the lower left sternal border. Cyanosis from a right-to-left shunt at the atrial level may exist [7, 8].

Natural History

When TR and right ventricular dysfunction are extreme, death in utero is common due to hydrops fetalis. However, when the tricuspid valve deformity is severe, symptoms frequently develop in newborns. In patients with moderate tricuspid valve deformity and dysfunction, symptoms develop during late teenage years or young adult life. Adults with the Ebstein anomaly can rarely remain asymptomatic through their lives if the anomaly is mild [4, 6].

Electrocardiography

The electrocardiography (ECG) (Fig. 26.1) presentation of the Ebstein anomaly varies broadly. *Low voltage is classic. Tall and peaked P waves in leads II and V1 reveal right atrial enlargement. The PR interval is frequently prolonged, but a short PR interval and also a delta wave due to the presence of an accessory pathway can be seen.* The R waves in leads V1 and V2 are small. An RSR' pattern in lead V1 is consistent with RV conduction delay, and RBBB is common in adults. First-degree atrioventricular block (AVB) occurs in 40 % of patients. Atrial flutter and fibrillation are prevalent, and finally, the ECG may be normal [6–9].

Chest Radiography

Right- and leftward convexity together from an enlarged RA, atrialized RV, and dilated infundibulum, respectively, gives the heart *a water-bottle appearance on the chest radiograph. Cardiomegaly in different degrees is the rule with normal or reduced pulmonary vasculature*. The aorta and the pulmonary trunk are unremarkable. Accordingly, the typical Ebstein anomaly configuration is a globe-shaped heart with a narrow waist alike to that seen with massive pericardial effusion [4, 6, 10] (Fig. 26.2).

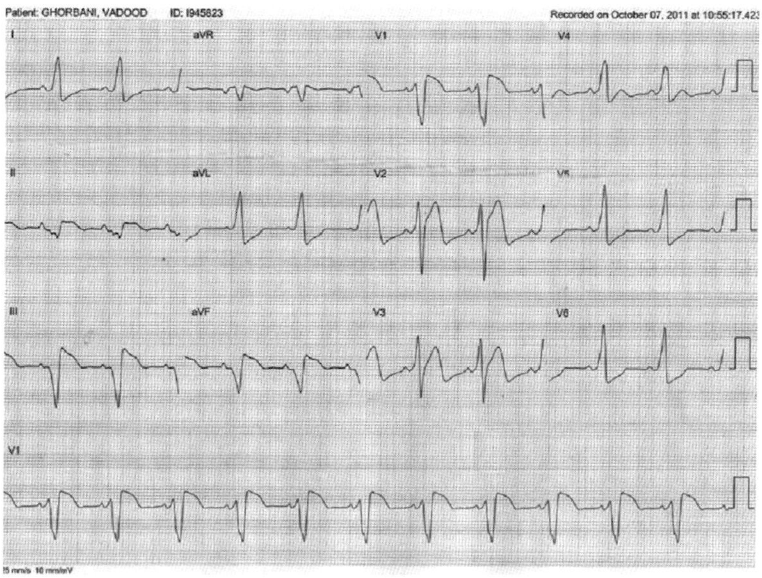

Fig. 26.1 Sinus rhythm and right posteroseptal accessory pathway in the Ebstein anomaly

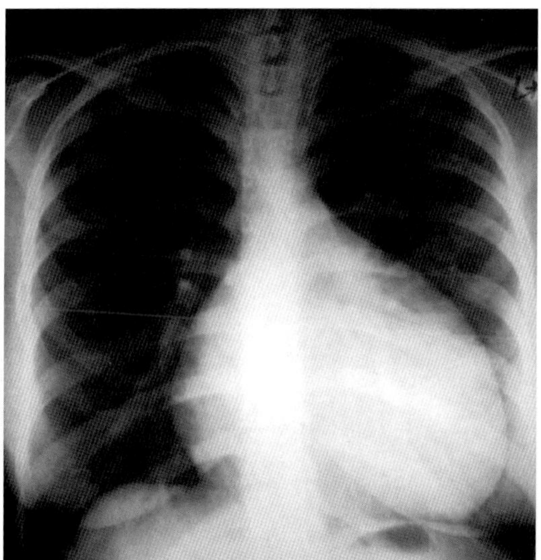

Fig. 26.2 A rightward convexity from an enlarged right atrium and atrialized right ventricle, coupled with a leftward convexity from a dilated infundibulum, gives the heart a "water-bottle" appearance in the Ebstein anomaly

Echocardiography

The diagnosis of the Ebstein anomaly is mostly made by echocardiography. The apical displacement of the septal leaflet of the TV by 8 mm/m^2 or more, with an elongated sail-like appearance of the anterior TV leaflet, proves the diagnosis (Fig. 26.3a, b, Video 26.1).

The size of the atrialized portion of the RV (recognized between the basic place of the TV annulus and the ventricular attachment of the TV leaflets which is a part of anatomic RV and serves as a part of RA) and the systolic performance index of the functional RV can be estimated [10, 11] (Fig. 26.4).

The degree of TR and rarely TS should be evaluated by TTE. Tricuspid regurgitation almost always is present and could be severe. Regarding the low-velocity TR jets, it may be difficult to visualize, so careful investigation in different views will be helpful.

Concomitant displacement of the posterior leaflet should be evaluated by viewing the parasternal RV inflow (Fig. 26.5). A*nterior TV leaflet is never displaced* but usually has adherence to the free wall of the right ventricle (RV). Associated anomalies such as ASD and the presence of shunting can also be recognized [10–14].

Echocardiography should provide comprehensive data regarding the possibility of TV repair. The successful repair is unlikely in the following scoring systems:

1. Extensive adherence of the anterior TV leaflet to the RV myocardium. The assessment is made in apical four-chamber view (more

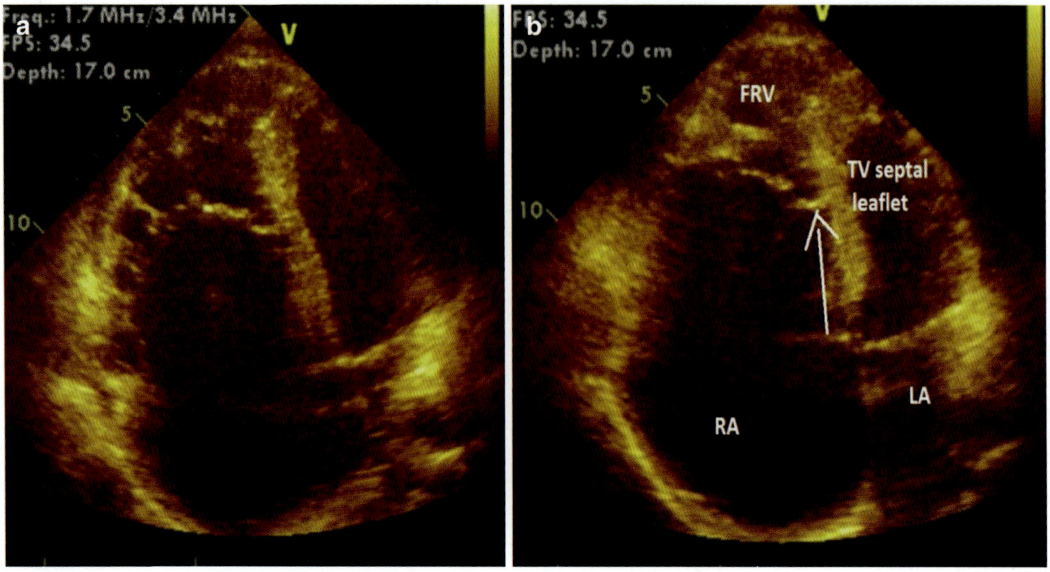

Fig. 26.3 (**a**, **b**) Apical four-chamber view in a typical Ebstein anomaly showing increased apical displacement of septal TV leaflet compared to the mitral leaflet insertion and tethered anterior TV leaflet. *TV* tricuspid valve, *FRV* functional right ventricle, *RA* right atrium, *LA* left atrium (Video 26.2)

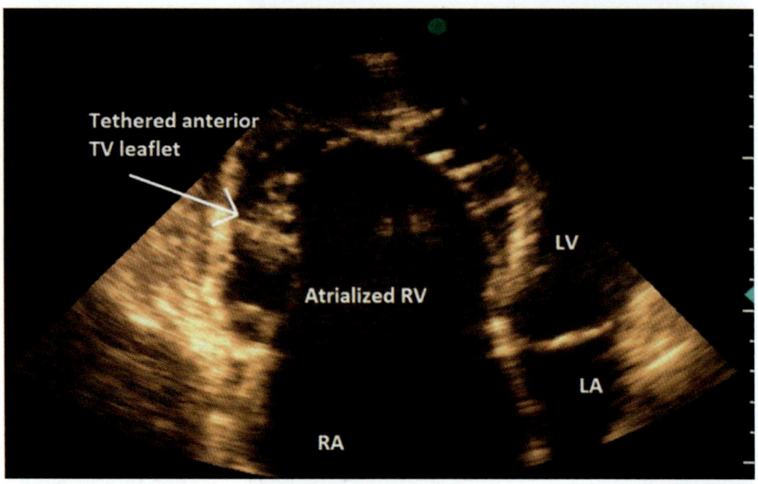

Fig. 26.4 Tethered anterior TV leaflet (ATVL) and atrialized RV tethering have been defined as the restricted motion of the ATVL due to the accessory attachments (at least three attachments) of the ATVL to the RV free wall. *LV* left ventricle, *RA* right atrium, *LA* left atrium

than half of the anterior leaflet should be mobile and moves freely for successful repair).

2. Ratio of the septal TV leaflet apical displacement to the total ventricular septal length more than 0.6 indicates a severe valvular abnormality (Fig. 26.6).
3. Small functional RV (FRV) means FRV less than 35 % of the total RV size (Fig. 26.7).
4. Patients with RA and atrialized RV cavity area compared to the sum of the true RV, LA, and LV area more than 1.5 [14].

Cardiovascular Magnetic Resonance Imaging (CMR)

This study can better assess the functional RV volume and function [6, 7].

Catheterism

Diagnostic cardiac catheterization is seldom needed in patients with the Ebstein anomaly. It is needed when associated coronary artery

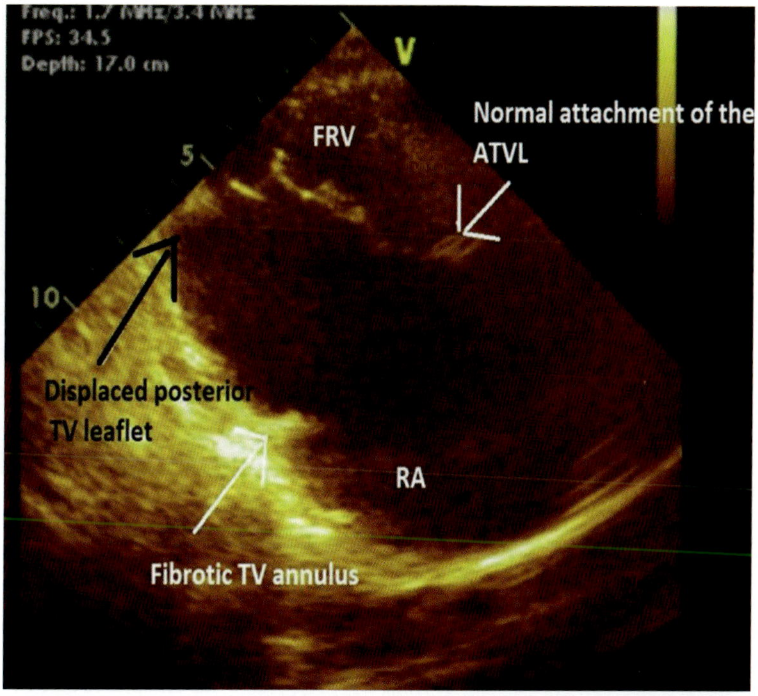

Fig. 26.5 RV inflow study showing significant apical displacement of posterior TV leaflet (*black arrow*) and normal attachment of anterior TV leaflet *ATVL* (*white arrow*). *FRV* functional right ventricle, *RA* right atrium, Another white arrow shows fibrotic TV annulus

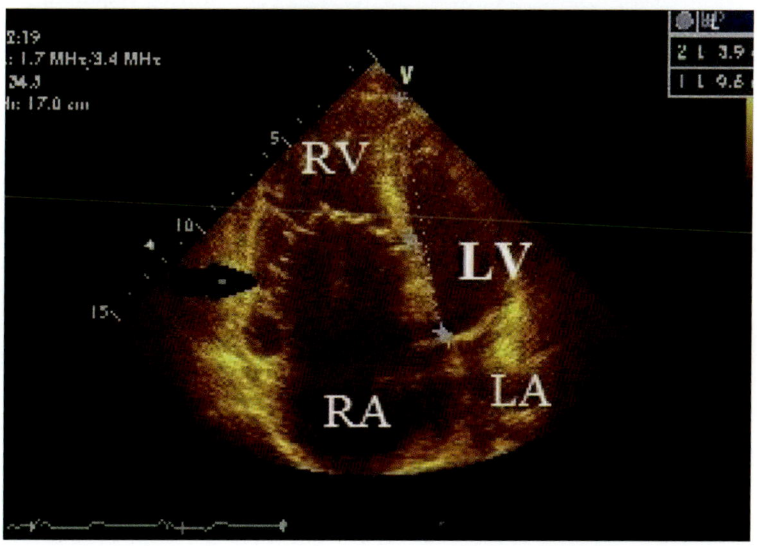

Fig. 26.6 Elongated and tethered anterior TV leaflet (ATVL). *LV* left ventricle, *RV* right ventricle, *RA* right atrium, *LA* left atrium

disease or high pulmonary artery pressure is suspected. Sometimes, selective RV angiography shows the extent of TV displacement, size of the functional RV, and shape of its outflow tract (Fig. 26.8) [4, 6, 15].

Indications for Intervention

Indications for intervention:

1. Considerable cyanosis
2. Right-sided heart failure

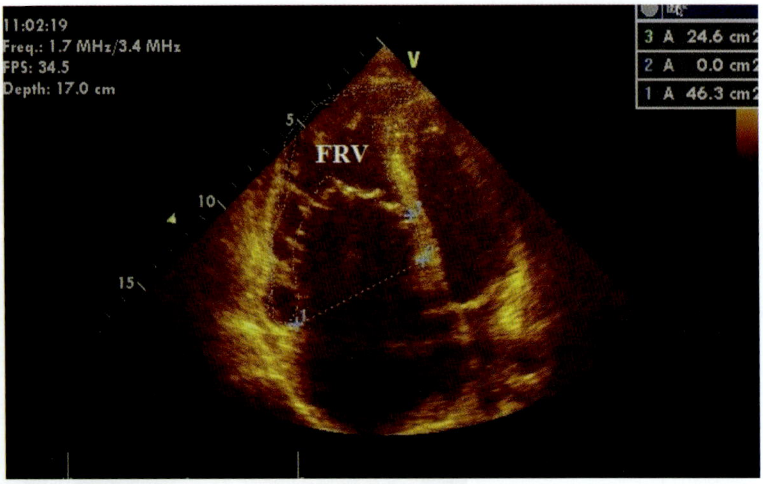

Fig. 26.7 Showing how to measure functional RV compared to the anatomic RV. *FRV* functional right ventricle

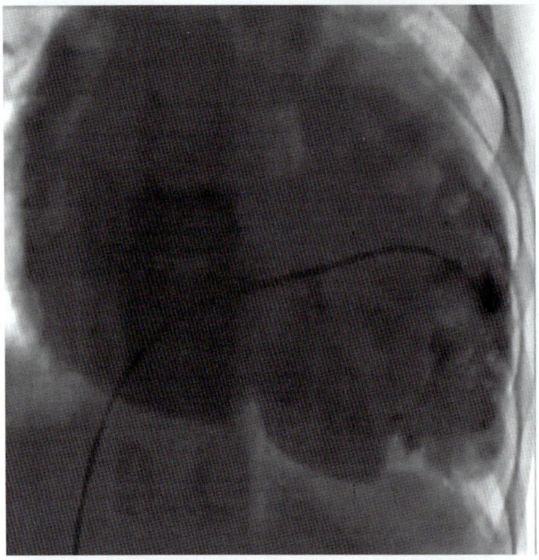

Fig. 26.8 RV injection shows huge cardiomegaly, trilobe sign (arterialized RV), and severe TR (Video 26.3)

3. Poor functional capacity
4. The event of paradoxical emboli

And recurrent supraventricular tachyarrhythmias not managed by medical or ablation therapy and asymptomatic significant cardiomegaly defined by a cardiothoracic ratio >65 % are the relative indications for appropriate treatment [6, 7].

Management Options

TV repair is preferable to the TV replacement. The possibility of TV repair depends primarily on the skill and capability of the surgeon as well as on the adequacy of the anterior leaflet of the TV to make a mono-cusp valve. TV repair is possible if the edges of the anterior leaflet of the TV are not severely tethered to the myocardium and if the functional RV has an acceptable size (>35 % of the total RV size).

If the TV is non-reparable, valve replacement will be required, generally with a bioprosthetic TV [15–18].

For patients with severe TR, an inadequate functional RV, or refractory supraventricular arrhythmias, a bidirectional cavo-pulmonary connection can be used to decrease RV preload if the pulmonary artery pressure is low. In patients with TS or a hypoplastic RV, a Fontan procedure may be the best choice. A concomitant RA or bi-atrial maze procedure at the time of surgery should be considered in patients with long-lasting atrial flutter or fibrillation; and if an accessory pathway is present, this should be eradicated. If there is an ASD, it must be closed.

In specific patients with a resting oxygen saturation >90 % and exercise intolerance due to worsening hypoxemia, the closure of the patent foramen ovale or ASD may be indicated without addressing the TV itself. Prophylaxis for endocarditis is recommended despite its low risk in the anomaly [17–20].

Pregnancy

In the absence of maternal cyanosis, RV failure or arrhythmias during pregnancy are frequently well tolerated [21, 22].

Follow-up

All Ebstein anomaly patients should have regular follow-up visits. Specific attention must be paid to cases with cyanosis, considerable cardiomegaly, poor RV function, and recurrent atrial arrhythmias. All patients with significant TR after TV repair, recurrent atrial arrhythmias, degenerating bioprostheses, or dysfunctional mechanical valves need close follow-up [22, 23].

References

1. Soloff LA, Stauffer HM, Zatuchni J. Ebstein's disease: report of the first case diagnosed during life. Am J Med Sci. 1951;222:554–61.
2. Dearani JA, Danielson GK. Congenital heart surgery nomenclature and database project: Ebstein's anomaly and tricuspid valve disease. Ann Thorac Surg. 2000;69(suppl):S106–17.
3. Lamers WH, Viragh S, Wessels A, et al. Formation of the tricuspid valve in the human heart. Circulation. 1995;91:111–21.
4. Dearani JA, Danielson GK. Ebstein's anomaly of the tricuspid valve. In: Mavroudis C, Backer CL, editors. Pediatric cardiac surgery. 3rd ed. Philadelphia: Mosby; 2003. p. 524–36.
5. Lev M, Liberthson RR, Joseph RH, et al. The pathologic anatomy of Ebstein's disease. Arch Pathol. 1970;90:334–43.
6. Anderson KR, Zuberbuhler JR, Anderson RH, et al. Morphologic spectrum of Ebstein's anomaly of the heart: a review. Mayo Clin Proc. 1979;54:174–80.
7. Celermaje DS, Bull C, Till JA, et al. Ebstein's anomaly: presentation and outcome from fetus to adult. J Am Coll Cordiol. 1994;23:170–6, 994.
8. Khositseth A, Danielson GK, Dearani JA, et al. Supraventricular tachyarrhythmias in Ebstein anomaly: management and outcome. J Thorac Cardiovasc Surg. 2004;128:826.
9. Dearani JA, Danielson GK, et al. Ebstein's anomaly. In: Sellke FW, del Nido PJ, Swanson SJ, editors. Sabiston & Spencer surgery of the chest, vol. 2. 7th ed. Philadelphia: Elsevier Saunders; 2005. p. 2223–35.
10. Snider AR, Serwer GA, Ritter SB. Echocardiography in pediatric heart disease. 2nd ed. St. Louis: Mosby; 1997.
11. Eidem BW, Cetta F, O'leary PW. Echocardiography in pediatric and adult congenital heart disease. Philadelphia: Lippincott Williams & Wilkins; 2012.
12. Shina A, Seward J, Tajik J, et al. Two-dimensional echocardiographic-surgical correlation in Ebstein's anomaly: preoperative determination of patients requiring tricuspid valve plication vs replacement. Circulation. 1983;68(3):534–44.
13. Bonow RO, Mann DL, Zipes DP, Libby P, eds. Braunwald's Heart Disease: A Textbook of Cardiovascular Medicine. 9th ed. Philadelphia, PA: Saunders Elsevier; 2011.
14. Otto CM. The practice of clinical echocardiography. 3rd ed. Philadelphia: W. B. Saunders/Elsevier; 2007.
15. Ullmann MV, Born S, Sebening C, et al. Ventricularization of the atrialized chamber: a concept of Ebstein's anomaly repair. Ann Thorac Surg. 2004;78:918–24.
16. Hancock Friesen CL, Chen R, Howlett JG, Ross DB. Posterior annular plication: tricuspid valve repair in Ebstein's anomaly. Ann Thorac Surg. 2004;77:2167–71.
17. Chen JM, Mosca RS, Altmann K, Printz BF, et al. Early and medium-term results for repair of Ebstein anomaly. J Thorac Cardiovasc Surg. 2004;127:990–8.
18. Boston US, Dearani JA, O'Leary PW, et al. Tricuspid valve repair for Ebstein's anomaly in young children: a 30-year experience. Ann Thorac Surg. 2006;81:690–6.
19. Brown ML, Dearani JA, Danielson GK, et al. Comparison of the outcome of porcine bioprosthetic versus mechanical prosthetic replacement of the tricuspid valve in the Ebstein anomaly. Am J Cardiol. 2009;103:555.
20. Chauvaud S, Berrebi A, d'Attellis N, et al. Ebstein's anomaly: repair based on functional analysis. Eur J Cardiothorac Surg. 2003;23:525–31.
21. Dearani JA, Danielson GK. Surgical management of Ebstein's anomaly in the adult. Semin Thorac Cardiovasc Surg. 2005;17:148.
22. Brown ML, Dearani JA, Danielson GK, et al. Functional status after operation for Ebstein anomaly: the Mayo Clinic experience. J Am Coll Cardiol. 2008;52:460.
23. Attie F, Rosas M, Rijlaarsdam M, et al. The adult patient with Ebstein anomaly. Outcome in 72 unoperated patients. Medicine. 2000;79:27–36.

Tricuspid Atresia

27

Anita Sadeghpour and Azin Alizadeasl

Keywords
Tricuspid atresia • Atrial septal defect (ASD) • Echocardiography • Fontan operation • Hypoplastic right ventricle

Morphology and Associated Lesions

Tricuspid atresia (TA) is best defined as the absence of the right atrioventricular valve in the presence of an atrial septal defect. There is frequently morphologic right ventricular hypoplasia, which connects to the dominant ventricle via a ventricular septal defect.

Patients may be divided into those with concordant ventriculoarterial connections (normally related great arteries in 70–80 % of patients) and cases with discordant connections. Related lesions in the second group consist of subaortic stenosis and aortic arch abnormalities [1].

Pathophysiological and Paraclinical Aspects

The ventriculoarterial connection is of utmost importance in the approach to these patients. All patients have mixing at the atrial level with varying degrees of cyanosis. Patients with concordant ventriculoarterial connections have a tendency to be bluer depending on the size of the ventricular septal defect, whereas those with discordant connections are pinker and more often develop heart failure because of the patent pulmonary circulation originating from the left ventricle. The presentation is sometimes similar to the hypoplastic left heart syndrome due to obstruction at the ventricular septal defect or concomitant aortic arch anomalies [1–3].

Electrocardiography shows left axis deviation, right atrial enlargement, and left ventricular hypertrophy.

Chest radiography usually reveals levocardia with situs solitus and a left-sided aortic arch in 75 % of cases. The cardiac size and also

A. Sadeghpour, MD, FACC, FASE (✉)
Echocardiography Lab, Department of Cardiology, Adult Congenital Heart Disease Clinic, Rajaie Cardiovascular Medical and Research Center, Iran University of Medical Science, Tehran, Iran
e-mail: anita.sadeghpour@gmail.com, asadeghpour@rhc.ac.ir

A. Alizadeasl, MD, FACC
Echocardiography Lab, Department of Cardiology, Rajaie Cardiovascular Medical and Research Center, Iran University of Medical Science, Tehran, Iran
e-mail: alizadeasl@gmail.com, alizadeasl@rhc.ac.ir

Electronic supplementary material The online version of this chapter (doi: 10.1007/978-1-4471-6383-1_27) contains supplementary material, which is available to authorized users.

A. Sadeghpour et al. (eds.), *Comprehensive Approach to Adult Congenital Heart Disease*,
DOI 10.1007/978-1-4471-6383-1_27, © Springer-Verlag London 2014

pulmonary vascular markings vary with the pulmonary blood flow and volume [3, 4].

There is a subclassification for types I and II based on the presence and size of the VSD and associated pulmonary stenosis or atresia [4, 5].

Echocardiography

Echocardiography provides comprehensive information and confirms the diagnosis (Fig. 27.1a, b and Videos 27.1, 27.2 and 27.3).

Typical echocardiographic findings in tricuspid atresia:

A. *The presence of fibromuscular or membranous tissue in the place of the TV with no direct communication between RA and RV*
B. *Obligatory shunt at the level of the atria (right-to-left shunt from ASD or PFO which is obligatory for survival)*
C. *Variable degree of RV hypoplasia*
D. *Direct communication between systemic and pulmonary circulation usually in a form of VSD*

Tricuspid atresia based on the relationship of the great arteries, anatomy of the VSD, and pulmonary valve has been classified as:

Type I: Normally related great arteries (70–80 % of cases and most common type of TA)
Type II: d-transposition of great arteries (d-TGA)
Type III: Associate with more complex lesions (uncommon form of TA, only 3–6 % of patients)

Cardiac Catheterization

Cardiac catheterization is seldom requisite for the initial diagnosis and management (Videos 27.4 and 27.5) (it may be useful to study the degree of subaortic stenosis, if present) of tricuspid atresia and is frequently performed to measure the pulmonary artery pressure and resistance before corrective surgery [4, 5] (Fig. 27.2).

Management

The aim of early palliation (systemic-to-pulmonary shunt, bidirectional Glenn procedure, pulmonary artery banding, and infrequently Norwood stage 1 based on the patient's diagnosis and associated lesions) is to prepare the patient for the Fontan surgery. This should be performed only when there is a good dominant ventricular function, no obstruction in the systemic blood flow, and also minimal atrioventricular valve regurgitation. Candidates for such corrective surgery should also have low pulmonary resistance with a mean pulmonary artery pressure <15 mmHg and acceptable size for the pulmonary arteries [5–7].

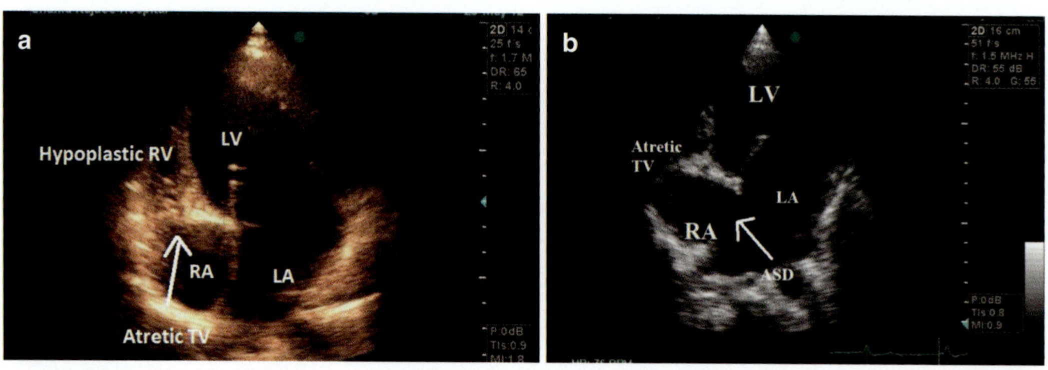

Fig. 27.1 (**a**, **b**) Transthoracic echocardiography in four chamber view showing tricuspid atresia (TA) as a fibromuscular tissue in pace of TV, associated with hypoplastic right ventricle (RV) and large ASD which is an obligatory left to right shunt. *RV* right ventricle. *LV* left ventricle, *RA* right atrium, *LA* left atrium, *ASD* atrial septal defect

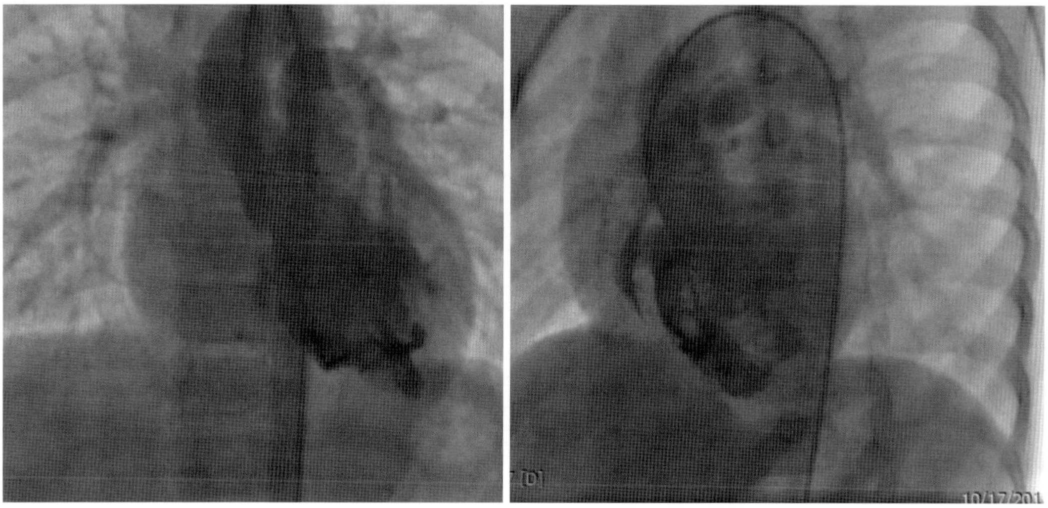

Fig. 27.2 Tricuspid atresia: injection via arterial line in LV shows rudimentary RV with coincident opacification of aorta and pulmonary artery suggestive for tricuspid atresia and VSD

References

1. Jacobs JP, Anderson RH, Weinberg PM, et al. The nomenclature, definition and classification of cardiac structures in the setting of heterotaxy. Cardiol Young. 2007;17 Suppl 2:1–28.
2. Berg C, Lachmann R, Kaiser C, et al. Prenatal diagnosis of tricuspid atresia: intrauterine course and outcome. Ultrasound Obstet Gynecol. 2010;3:183–90.
3. Wald RM, Tham EB, McCrindle BW, et al. Outcome after prenatal diagnosis of tricuspid atresia: a multicenter experience. Am Heart J. 2007;3:772–8.
4. Cohen MS, Anderson RH, Cohen MI, et al. Controversies, genetics, diagnostic assessment, and outcomes relating to the heterotaxy syndrome. Cardiol Young. 2007;17 Suppl 2:29–43.
5. Warnes CA, Williams RG, Bashore TM, et al. ACC/AHA, guidelines for the management of adults with congenital heart disease. J Am Coll Cardiol. 2008;52(23):e143–263.
6. Peer SM, Donofrio MT, Gaur L, Sinha P. Tricuspid atresia with aortopulmonary window: challenges in achieving a balanced circulation. Interact Cardiovasc Thorac Surg. 2013;17:441–3.
7. Sainathan S. Comment. Balancing the pulmonary circulation in tricuspid atresia with an aortopulmonary window. Interact Cardiovasc Thorac Surg. 2013;17:443.

Tetralogy of Fallot

28

Anita Sadeghpour, Azin Alizadehasl,
and Mohammad Mahdavi

Keywords
Tetralogy of Fallot (TOF) • Cyanotic congenital heart disease (CHD) • Right ventricular outflow tract (RVOT) obstruction • Absent pulmonary valve syndrome • Overriding of aortic root

Morphology and Associated Lesions

Tetralogy of Fallot (TOF) as the most common cyanotic congenital heart disease (CHD) is a complex heart defect consisting of four components:

1. Right ventricular outflow tract (RVOT) obstruction, mainly due to anterocephalad deviation of the outlet septum
2. Override of the ventricular septum by the aortic root (rightward malposition of the aortic root)
3. A large nonrestrictive ventricular septal defect
4. Right ventricular (RV) hypertrophy [1]

This combination of lesions happens in 3 of every 10,000 live births and accounts for 7–10 % of all congenital heart diseases. *The fundamental abnormality is the anterior deviation of the outlet septum*; therefore, TOF may happen in the setting of double-outlet right ventricle and may exist with an atrioventricular septal defect. RVOT obstruction is variable. Frequently, a stenotic and bicuspid pulmonary valve with supravalvular hypoplasia is detected. *The main site for the obstruction is typically at the subvalvular level.* In some cases, the RVOT is atretic, and the diagnosis is TOF with pulmonary atresia. While TOF is the most common cyanotic congenital heart defect, TOF with pulmonary valve atresia and major aortopulmonary collateral arteries are considered to be the most extreme type of TOF and account for about 1/5 of all cases of TOF [1, 2].

Also, the size of the ventricular septal defect can vary; in almost all cases, however, the interventricular communication is nonrestrictive and allows bidirectional shunting.

A. Sadeghpour, MD, FACC, FASE (✉)
Echocardiography Lab, Department of Cardiology, Adult Congenital Heart Disease Clinic, Rajaie Cardiovascular Medical and Research Center, Iran University of Medical Science, Tehran, Iran
e-mail: anita.sadeghpour@gmail.com, asadeghpour@rhc.ac.ir

A. Alizadehasl, MD, FACC
Echocardiography Lab, Department of Cardiology, Rajaie Cardiovascular Medical and Research Center, Iran University of Medical Science, Tehran, Iran
e-mail: alizadeasl@gmail.com, alizadeasl@rhc.ac.ir

M. Mahdavi, MD
Pediatric Ward, Department of Pediatric Cardiology, Rajaie Cardiovascular Medical and Research Center, Iran University of Medical Science, Tehran, Iran

Electronic supplementary material The online version of this chapter (doi: 10.1007/978-1-4471-6383-1_28) contains supplementary material, which is available to authorized users.

A. Sadeghpour et al. (eds.), *Comprehensive Approach to Adult Congenital Heart Disease*,
DOI 10.1007/978-1-4471-6383-1_28, © Springer-Verlag London 2014

A right aortic arch happens in nearly 25 % of patients, and anomalies of the course of the coronary arteries occur in about 5 %. The most common one is the origination of the anterior descending artery from the right coronary artery, and it courses anteriorly and crosses the infundibulum of the RV.

Absent pulmonary valve syndrome is a rare form of TOF in which the stenosis and regurgitation of the RVOT are due to a noticeably stenotic pulmonary valve ring with poorly shaped or absent pulmonary valve leaflets. The pulmonary arteries are evidently dilated or aneurysmal and may create airway compression at birth [1, 2].

Pathophysiology

The degree of cyanosis reveals the severity of the RVOT obstruction and the level of systemic vascular resistance (of course in the absence of the other sources of the pulmonary blood flow), and there is right-to-left shunting through the ventricular septal defect. A spell is an acute drop in arterial O_2 saturation, which can be very life-threatening. Its treatment is intended to relieve the obstruction and increase the systemic resistance.

The obstructive muscular sub-pulmonary region created is a dynamic object; accordingly, the degree of stenosis created can be worsened and exacerbated by catecholamines or low intravascular volume, which can predispose the patients to sudden attacks of desaturation and spells [1–3].

Clinical Findings

In unrepaired adult patients, cyanosis of variable degrees is present. The RV heave and systolic thrill are frequently palpable alongside the left sternal border, and an aortic systolic ejection sound is heard at the lower left sternal border and apex. The second heart sound (S2) is typically single. The strength and duration of the systolic ejection murmur (due to subvalvular pulmonary stenosis) vary in reverse with the severity of subvalvular obstruction. With pulmonary atresia, no murmur or only a short and faint murmur may be detected alongside another faint continuous murmur due to aortopulmonary collateral vessels [1, 2].

After palliation surgeries, progressive cyanosis may result from exacerbation in the RVOT obstruction, ongoing stenosis and occlusion of palliative aortopulmonary shunts, or increase in pulmonary artery pressure (sometimes seen after the Waterston or Potts shunts). This situation is likely to give rise to progressive aortic dilation and aortic regurgitation. Moreover, central cyanosis and also clubbing are invariably present [4–6].

After intracardiac repair surgeries, more than 85 % of the patients are well and asymptomatic on follow-up visits. Nevertheless, objective tests show a reduction in maximal exercise capacity. Atrial and ventricular arrhythmias can cause palpitations. Progressive RV dilation due to chronic pulmonary regurgitation or severe residual RVOT stenosis happens in 10–15 % of TOF patients within 20 years after the first repair. Ascending aortic aneurysm and secondary aortic regurgitation may be present. There is also the likelihood of the presence of lower left sternal border RV heave together with low-pitched diastolic murmur from pulmonary regurgitation, systolic ejection murmur from RVOT obstruction, high-pitched diastolic murmur from aortic regurgitation, and pansystolic murmur from a ventricular septal defect residue [1, 6, 7].

Electrocardiography

Right axis deviation with RV and RA overload is common. *In adults with repaired TOF, a complete right bundle branch block post TOF repair is the rule. The QRS width may reveal the degree of RV dilation, and an extreme (>180 milliseconds) or rapid increase in the width can be a risk factor for sustained ventricular tachycardia and sudden cardiac death* (Fig. 28.1) [1, 2].

Chest Radiography

The typical boot-shaped heart (Coeur en sabot) is the hallmark of this disease. Classically, there is a normal-sized and boot-shaped heart with a promi-

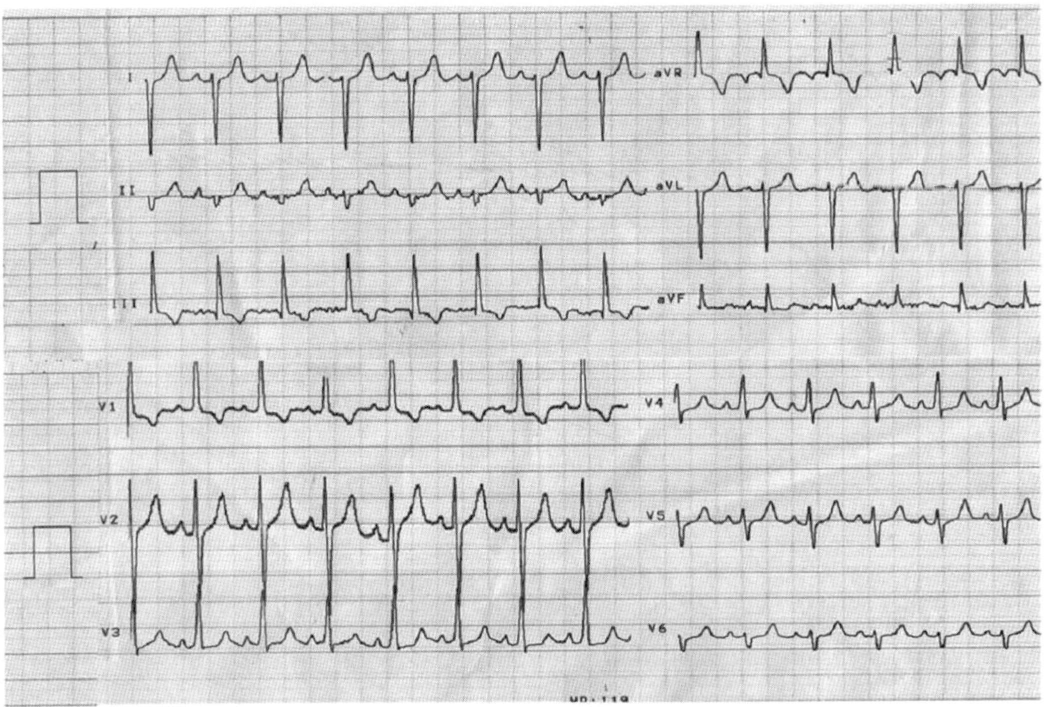

Fig. 28.1 Right axis deviation, right ventricular hypertrophy, right ventricular enlargement with clockwise rotation, and small left-sided chambers; all together, the tetralogy of Fallot should be considered

nent RV and an apparent concavity in the area of the non-developed RVOT and main pulmonary arteries. The pulmonary vascular markings are typically reduced, and the aortic arch might be on the right side in 25 % of the cases (Fig. 28.2) [1, 2].

Echocardiography

Echocardiography confirms the complete diagnosis and typically provides sufficient data for management planning. The echocardiography begins with comprehensive sequential segmental approach. Usually the segmental anatomy is normal. The study should recognize the malaligned and nonrestrictive ventricular septal defect, overriding aorta, and the existence and severity of the RVOT obstruction (infundibular, valvular, and supravalvular as well as pulmonary artery branch stenosis). For further evaluation of associated diseases such as ASD and additional VSD, peripheral pulmonary stenosis is needed (Figs. 28.3 and 28.4, Videos 28.1, 28.2 and 28.3) [4, 8–10].

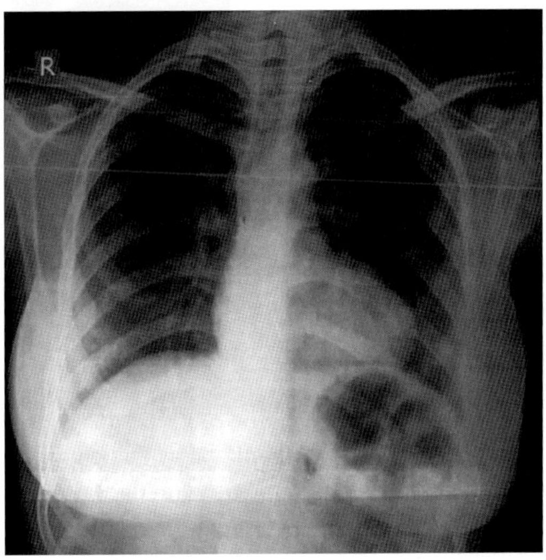

Fig. 28.2 Boot-shaped heart, concave main pulmonary artery segment, and decreased pulmonary vasculature in a tetralogy of Fallot patient

In patients with repaired TOF, residual pulmonary valve stenosis and regurgitation, residual

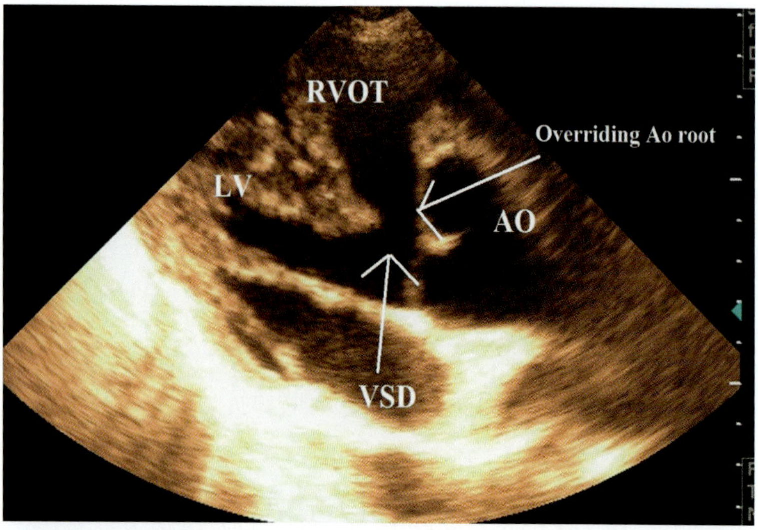

Fig. 28.3 Transthoracic echocardiography in parasternal long-axis view showing overriding aorta on the crest of the ventricular septum and associated VSD. *VSD* ventricular septal defect, *AO* aorta, *LV* left ventricle, *RVOT* right ventricular outflow track

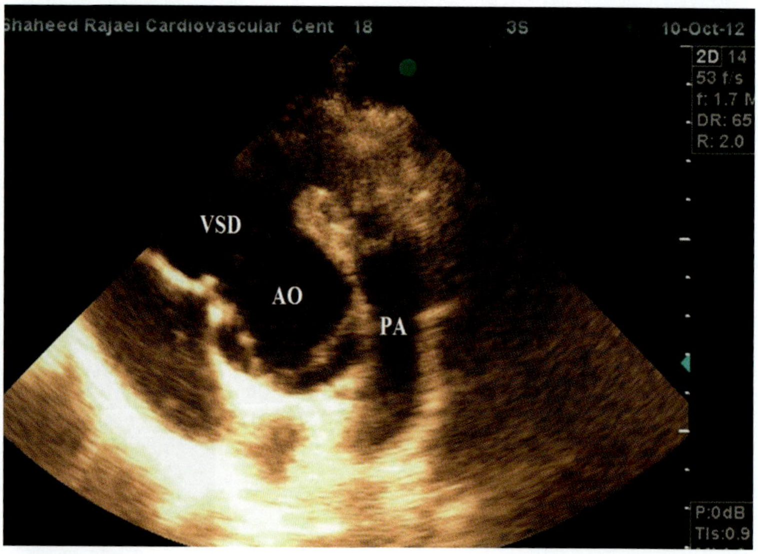

Fig. 28.4 Typical parasternal short-axis view in TOF patient showing anterocephalad deviation of outlet septum with narrow RVOT and large subaortic VSD. *PA* pulmonary artery, *AO* aorta, *VSD* ventricular septal defect

ventricular septal defect, RV and left ventricular (LV) size and function, aortic root size, and degree of aortic regurgitation should be evaluated.

The severity of pulmonary regurgitation in patients with repaired TOF can be measured by pulsed Doppler echocardiographic study of antegrade versus retrograde pulmonary blood flow with a short diastolic flow (pressure half-time <100 ms), suggestive of significant pulmonary regurgitation; this grade of severity can result in a large volume of pulmonary regurgitation and RV dilatation but may also be related with normal or only mildly enlarged RV due to a so-called RV restrictive physiology [1, 8–11].

RV dilatation may also be due to severe residual RVOT obstruction or as a result of surgical scar (in transventricular surgical approach). Significant tricuspid regurgitation can happen in consequence to RV dilatation that begets more RV dilatation.

Aneurysmal dilatation of the RVOT is moderately common in cases with previous pericardial trans-annular patch repair surgery and substantial pulmonary regurgitation. Aneurysmal dilatation of the RVOT can be related with regional RV hypokinesis and may be the arrhythmogenic nidus of sustained ventricular tachycardia. Infrequently LV dysfunction can be detected by echocardiography from a variety of factors [2, 11–13].

Cardiac Catheterization and Angiocardiography

Cardiac catheterization is now rarely needed before corrective surgeries (Video 28.4). Echocardiography, magnetic resonance angiography (MRA), and fast computed tomography (CT) can define the presence and proximal course of the pulmonary blood vessels. Nonetheless, the preoperative study of TOF with pulmonary atresia and major aortopulmonary collateral arteries typically necessitates the delineation of the arterial supply to both lungs via selective catheterization and angiography in order to reveal the course and segmental supply from the collateral arteries and central pulmonary arteries. Major aortopulmonary collateral arteries frequently rise from the descending aorta close to the tracheal bifurcation. These vessels connect the systemic and pulmonary arterial vasculature, thus supplying pulmonary blood flow. Major aortopulmonary collateral arteries are tortuous vessels that arise directly from the aorta or its branches. Major aortopulmonary collateral arteries vary in number and origin; follow circuitous routes to reach central, lobar, and segmental pulmonary arteries; and have variable areas and locations of stenosis [1, 2, 14, 15].

Cardiovascular Magnetic Resonance Imaging

The goals of cardiovascular MRI study after TOF repair consist of the quantitative evaluation of the LV and predominantly RV volumes, stroke volumes, and ejection fraction; the anatomy of the RVOT, pulmonary arteries, aorta, and aortopulmonary collaterals; and quantification of pulmonary, aortic, and tricuspid valve regurgitation [14, 15].

Management

For unrepaired adult patients, surgical repair is still routinely commended inasmuch as the results are satisfying and the operative risk is comparable to that of pediatric cases.

However, palliation is rarely planned as a permanent management approach, and most of these patients must experience surgical repair. Specially, palliated patients with increasing cyanosis and also erythrocytosis (from slow shunt stenosis or elevated pulmonary artery pressure), LV dilation, or aneurysm formation in the shunt should undergo intracardiac repair with shunt closure, unless they have developed irreversible pulmonary artery hypertension [1, 5, 16].

In repaired TOF patients, residual ventricular septal defect with shunt >1.5/1, residual pulmonary stenosis (in the native RVOT region or implanted valved conduit) with RV systolic pressure ≥2/3 the systemic pressure, or severe pulmonary regurgitation correlated with substantial RV dilation or dysfunction (RV diastolic volume index >150 to 170 cc/m^2 or RV ejection fraction <45 %), significant exercise intolerance, and also sustained ventricular arrhythmias need intervention. Surgery is seldom required for significant aortic regurgitation allied to symptoms of progressive LV dilation and for aortic root dilation ≥55 mm. Rapid dilation of an RVOT aneurysm needs surgical attention (Fig. 28.5). Reoperation is required in 10–15 % of patients after reparative surgery during a 20-year follow-up period [2, 17, 18] (Fig. 28.6).

Significant pulmonary regurgitation is almost always encountered when the trans-annular patch

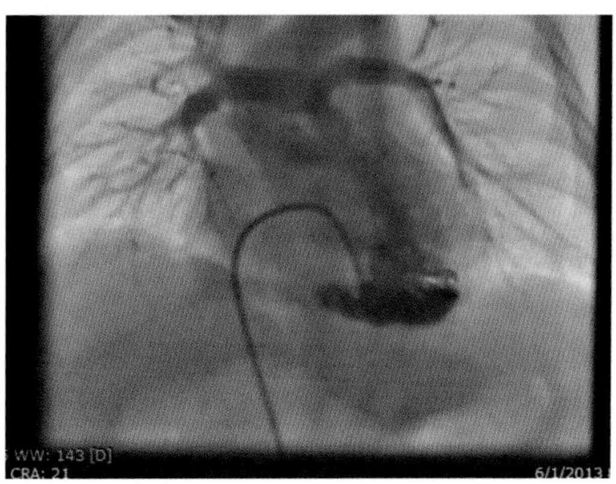

Fig. 28.5 Injection via venous catheter at AP view and in severely hypertrophied RV showed coincident opacification of aorta and pulmonary artery (due to VSD) and overriding aorta. Also there is infundibular, valvular, and supravalvular PS

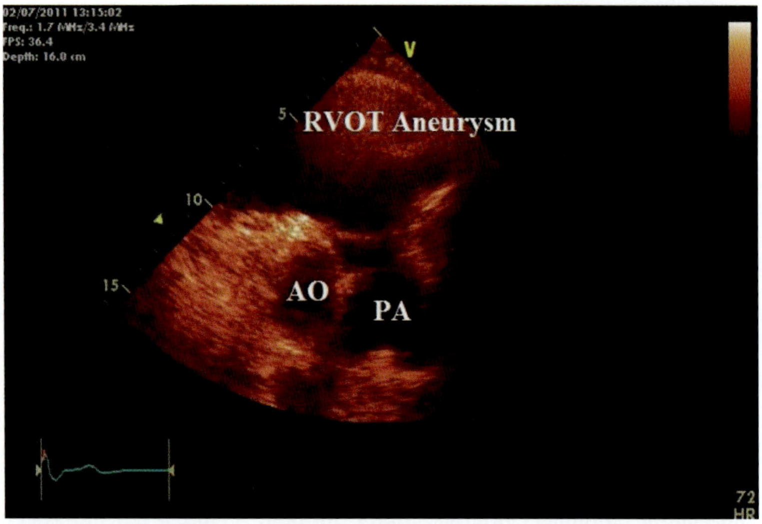

Fig. 28.6 Aneurysmal RVOT in completely repaired tetralogy of Fallot patient due to trans-annular patch repair. *PA* pulmonary artery, *AO* aorta, *RVOT* right ventricular outflow track

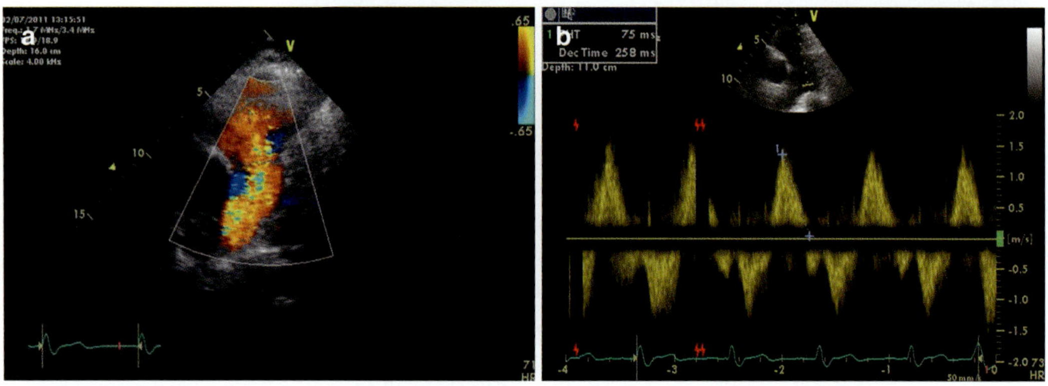

Fig. 28.7 (**a**, **b**) A typical patient with history of repaired TOF and severe pulmonary regurgitation by color flow imaging and Doppler study

repair method has been employed. Pulmonary regurgitation is frequently well tolerated if it is mild to moderate. Severe pulmonary regurgitation, but, may lead to progressive and symptomatic RV dilatation and also dysfunction. The severity of pulmonary regurgitation and its harmful long-term effects are increased by concomitant proximal or distal pulmonary artery obstruction or pulmonary artery hypertension. The severity of pulmonary regurgitation can be measured by pulsed Doppler echocardiographic study of antegrade versus retrograde pulmonary blood flow with a short diastolic flow (pressure half-time <100 ms), suggestive of significant pulmonary regurgitation [1, 5, 18] (Fig. 28.7a, b, Video 28.5).

MRI phase velocity mapping may precisely measure pulmonary regurgitation regurgitant fraction and is used as the gold standard method. Severe pulmonary regurgitation can result in a large volume of pulmonary regurgitation and RV dilatation but may also be related with normal or only mildly enlarged RV due to a so-called RV restrictive physiology [1, 15].

Implantable Cardioverter-Defibrillators

The development of significant cardiac arrhythmias, most commonly atrial flutter or fibrillation or sustained ventricular tachycardia, frequently causes hemodynamic deterioration and must be treated promptly. The reported frequency of sudden cardiac death, seemingly arrhythmic, in late follow-up series differs between 0.5 and 6 % over 30 years, accounting about for 1/3 to 1/2 of late deaths. The selection of suitable candidates for primary prevention and insertion of the implantable cardioverter-defibrillator (ICD) remains controversial. The ICD is probably most beneficial in high-risk patients such as those with a prior palliative shunt, QRS >180 ms, inducible ventricular tachycardia, and LV dysfunction [19, 20].

Outcomes

The overall survival of patients who have had initial repair operation is excellent, when the ventricular septal defect has been closed and the RVOT obstruction has been repaired. In addition, pulmonary valve replacement for severe pulmonary regurgitation or residual RVOT obstruction after the initial repair can be performed securely with a mortality rate of 1 %. Pulmonary valve replacement, when performed for significant pulmonary regurgitation, can improve exercise capacity and create RV remodeling. Be that as it may, the likelihood of sudden cardiac death should not be underestimated. Ventricular tachycardia can rise at the site of the RV surgery line, from the ventricular septal defect sutures or from the RVOT. Patients at high risk for sudden cardiac death include those with RV dilation and QRS duration ≥180 ms. Moderate to severe LV dysfunction is another risk factor for sudden cardiac death. The reported incidence of sudden cardiac death is about 5 %, with nearly 1/3 of late deaths occurring during the first 20 years of follow-up. All patients should have expert cardiology follow-up visits every 1–2 years. And last but by no means least, the risk of the recurrence of TOF in families is 3 % [1, 2, 6].

References

1. Bonow RO, Mann DL, Zipes DP, Libby P. Braunwald's heart disease: a textbook of cardiovascular medicine. 9th ed. Philadelphia: Elsevier/Saunders; 2011. p. 1435–50.
2. Warnes C, Williams RG, Bashore TM, et al. ACC/AHA, guidelines for the management of adults with congenital heart disease. JACC. 2008;52(23):2008.
3. Rauch R, Hofbeck M, Zweier C, et al. Comprehensive genotype-phenotype analysis in 230 patients with tetralogy of Fallot. J Med Genet. 2010;47(5):321–31.
4. Sadeghpour A, Saadatifar H, Kiavar M, et al. Doppler echocardiographic assessment of pulmonary prostheses: a comprehensive assessment including velocity time integral ratio & prosthesis effective orifice area. Congenit Heart Dis. 2008;3:415–21.
5. Al Habib HF, Jacobs JP, Mavroudis C, et al. Contemporary patterns of management of tetralogy of Fallot: data from the Society of Thoracic Surgeons Database. Ann Thorac Surg. 2010;90(3):813–9; discussion 819–20.
6. Park CS, Lee JR, Lim HG, et al. The long-term result of total repair for tetralogy of Fallot. Eur J Cardiothorac Surg. 2010;38(3):311–7.
7. Fox D, Devendra GP, Hart SA, et al. When 'blue babies' grow up: What you need to know about tetralogy of Fallot. Cleve Clin J Med. 2010;77(11):821–8.
8. Tsang FH, Li X, Cheung YF, et al. Pulmonary valve replacement after surgical repair of tetralogy of Fallot. Hong Kong Med J. 2010;16(1):26–30.
9. Kyavar M, Sadeghpour A, Madadi S, et al. Echocardiographic assessment of adults with repaired tetralogy of Fallot: a cardiovascular magnetic resonance comparison study. IHJ. 2012;12:2.
10. Sadeghpour A, Kyavar M, Javani B, et al. Term results of mechanical pulmonary prostheses in adults with congenital heart disease: importance of anticoagulation. Circulation. 2012;125(19), oral presentations WCC 2012.
11. Naderi N, Haghighi ZO, Pezeshki S, Alizadehasl A. Quantitative assessment of right atrial function by strain imaging in adult patients with totally corrected tetralogy of Fallot. Arch Cardiovas Imaging. 2013; 1(1):8–12.
12. Sadeghpour A, Javani B, Peighambari M, et al. Mid-term follow-up of pulmonary valve bioprostheses in adults with congenital heart disease. Anadolu Kardiyol Derg. 2012;12:434–6.
13. Sadeghpour A, Kyavar M, Madadi S, et al. Doppler-derived strain and strain rate imaging assessment of right ventricular systolic function in adults late after tetralogy of Fallot repair: an observational study. Anadolu Kardiyol Derg. 2013;13:536–42.
14. Oosterhof T, van Straten A, Vliegen HW, et al. Preoperative thresholds for pulmonary valve replacement in patients with corrected tetralogy of Fallot using cardiovascular magnetic resonance. Circulation. 2007;116:545.
15. Boechat MI, Ratib O, Williams PL, et al. Cardiac MR imaging and MR angiography for assessment of complex tetralogy of Fallot and pulmonary atresia. Radiographics. 2005;25(6):1535–46.
16. He GW. Current strategy of repair of tetralogy of Fallot in children and adults: emphasis on a new technique to create a monocusp-patch for reconstruction

of the right ventricular outflow tract. J Card Surg. 2008;23(6):592–9.
17. Hörer J, Friebe J, Schreiber C, et al. Correction of tetralogy of Fallot and of pulmonary atresia with ventricular septal defect in adults. Ann Thorac Surg. 2005;80(6):2285–91.
18. Aboulhosn J, Child JS. Management after childhood repair of tetralogy of fallot. Curr Treat Options Cardiovasc Med. 2006;8(6):474–83.
19. Witte KK, Pepper CB, Cowan JC, et al. Implantable cardioverter-defibrillator therapy in adult patients with tetralogy of Fallot. Europace. 2008;10(8): 926–30.
20. Khairy P, Harris L, Landzberg MJ, et al. Implantable cardioverter-defibrillators in tetralogy of Fallot. Circulation. 2008;117(3):363–70.

Double-Outlet Right Ventricle

29

Azin Alizadehasl and Anita Sadeghpour

Keywords

Double-Outlet Right Ventricle (DORV) • Ventricular septal defect (VSD) • Transposition of the great arteries • Conus

Double-outlet right ventricle (DORV) defines malformation in which >50 % of each semilunar valve arises from the morphologic right ventricle (RV). It may coexist with any form of atrial situs or AV connections, and it is independent of conal anatomy. In the normal heart, conus which is a circular tube of muscle lies under the pulmonary valve, and the conus under the aortic valve is resorbed. In the DORV, variable amount of conal septum under the semilunar valves exist [1, 2].

A. Alizadehasl, MD, FACC (✉)
Echocardiography Lab, Department of Cardiology, Rajaie Cardiovascular Medical and Research Center, Iran University of Medical Science, Tehran, Iran
e-mail: alizadeasl@gmail.com, alizadeasl@rhc.ac.ir

A. Sadeghpour, MD, FACC, FASE
Echocardiography Lab, Department of Cardiology, Adult Congenital Heart Disease Clinic, Rajaie Cardiovascular Medical and Research Center, Iran University of Medical Science, Tehran, Iran
e-mail: anita.sadeghpour@gmail.com, asadeghpour@rhc.ac.ir

Morphology and Associated Lesions

According to some previously reported opinions, the anatomic definition of DORV and also other types of congenital heart defects is less important than the study and understanding of the association and relationship between the great vessels and the VSD and also the anatomy of the outlets in relation to great vessels, which are basic and crucial leading points for management and prognosis.

More than 50 % of patients with DORV have associated lesions of the AV valves. Mitral valve stenosis or even atresia related with a hypoplastic left ventricle (LV), Ebstein anomaly of the tricuspid valve (TV), complete AV septal defect, and also overriding or straddling of either semilunar AV valve may happen [3].

Electronic supplementary material The online version of this chapter (doi: 10.1007/978-1-4471-6383-1_29) contains supplementary material, which is available to authorized users.

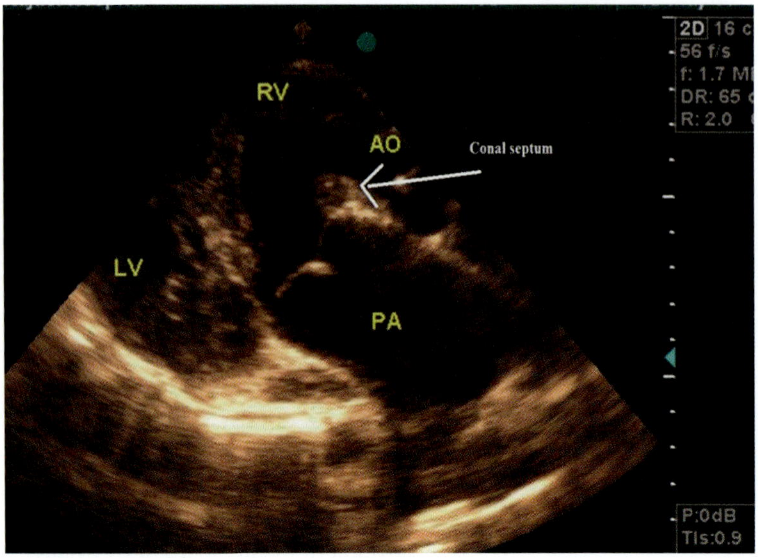

Fig. 29.1 Transthoracic echocardiography in off axis view showing both great arteries arise from the hypertrophied right ventricle, *white arrow* shows conal septum. *RV* right ventricle, *LV* left ventricle, *AO* aorta, *PA* pulmonary artery

Clinical Findings

The common features of the DORV are the following:

1. Overriding of the aorta more than 50 % on the right ventricle (Video 29.1)
2. Mitral-aortic discontinuity (Video 29.2)
3. VSD which is found in most cases (Videos 29.3 and 29.4)
4. Variable amount of conal septum under the semilunar valves

Three main subtypes of DORV exist: DORV with a sub-aortic VSD, DORV with a sub-pulmonary VSD, and DORV with a non-committed VSD [1, 4, 5].

Deviation of the outlet septum and its position modifies the feature and hemodynamics of DORV significantly. Anterior deviation of the outlet septum creates sub-aortic stenosis and aortic anomalies, and posterior deviation causes sub-pulmonary stenosis and limits pulmonary blood flow. It is also important to recognize DORV with a non-committed VSD. This defines hearts in which the VSD is remote from the outlets, making surgical management particularly difficult. Also DORV with a sub-pulmonary VSD (Taussig-Bing anomaly) can be considered as a type like TGA. This is because the natural position of the pulmonary artery (leftward and posterior to the aorta) causes the streaming of oxygenated and deoxygenated blood similar to transposition, although most of the pulmonary valve is linked to the RV [3, 5].

Echocardiography

Echocardiography is the cornerstone of diagnosis. The location of the VSD and the great arteries relationship to the VSD are the leading keys to diagnosis and management.

The relation between semilunar valves and ventricles should be determined carefully (Figs. 29.1 and 29.2).

It should be mentioned that in patients with sub-aortic stenosis, the echocardiographic examination must include the study for abnormalities of the aortic arch. Sub-pulmonary stenosis is often present in a DORV with a sub-pulmonary VSD. And also potential AV valve anomalies should be considered always [1, 4, 5].

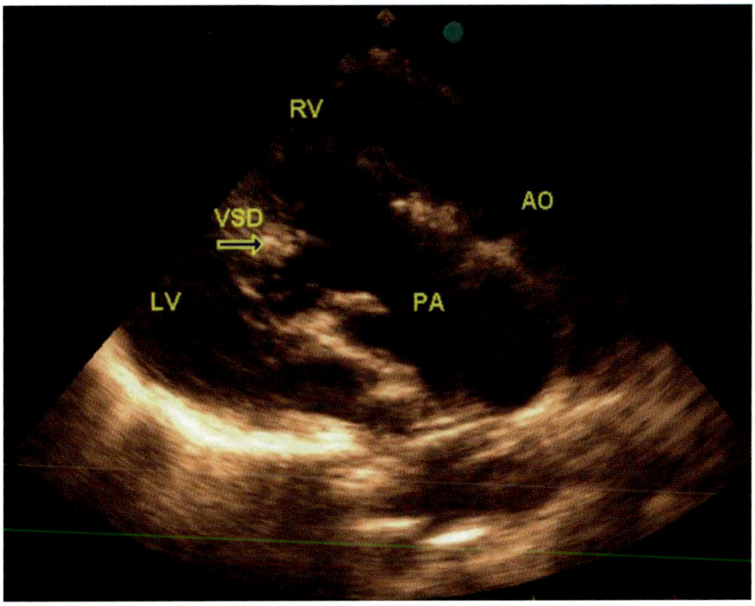

Fig. 29.2 The location of the VSD in relation to the great arteries is shown; sub-pulmonic VSD and DORV are suggestive of Taussig-Bing anomaly. *RV* right ventricle, *LV* left ventricle, *AO* aorta, *PA* pulmonary artery, *VSD* ventricular septal defect

Indications for Intervention

The aims of surgery are as follows: to keep and establish the continuity between the LV and aorta, create sufficient RV with pulmonary continuity, and repair all associated lesions. Palliative surgeries (such as aortopulmonary shunt) are reserved for patients in whom biventricular complete repair is not possible and in cases with noticeably decreased pulmonary blood flow. Of course, nowadays, complete repair is the primary procedure of choice [1, 4].

In DORV patients with a sub-aortic VSD, repair is performed by creation of an intraventricular baffle that directs LV blood to the aorta. If the VSD is sub-pulmonary, without sub-pulmonary stenosis, repair is done by closing of the VSD and also arterial switch. In concomitant sub-aortic stenosis, the aorta is attached to the LV via an intraventricular baffle, and in sub-pulmonary stenosis, the repair is similar to that of tetralogy of Fallot or the insertion of a RV-to-pulmonary artery conduit to complete the repair (Rastelli procedure). Classic surgical methods cannot be performed if the VSD is remote and uncommitted to either semilunar valve. In the best situation the VSD may be baffled toward the aorta; however, when it is not possible, the RV can be used as the systemic and dominant ventricle. This idea needs a Mustard or Senning procedure, closing of the VSD, and an insertion of a conduit between the LV and the pulmonary artery [1, 5–7].

Management

The types of surgical procedures including tetralogy of Fallot-type repair, arterial switch, or Rastelli procedure tend to be less acceptable and pleasing when there is a DORV than when this type of surgery is performed for more classic indications. Creation of sub-aortic stenosis is more likely due to the abnormal geometry of the LV outflow tract. Similarly, Rastelli conduit obstruction is more likely due to difficulties on spatial placement of the conduit and the position of the RV and the sternum.

Because of these complications and difficulties, the choices for catheter interventions are often restricted and limited. But, arch obstruction or distal pulmonary artery obstruction are agreeable to balloon dilation and probable stenting. All of these patients need at least annual visit and study by a CHD cardiologist [1, 4–7].

References

1. Warnes CA, Williams RG, Bashore TM, et al. ACC/AHA, guidelines for the management of adults with congenital heart disease. J Am Coll Cardiol. 2008;52(23):e143–263.
2. Walters HL, Mavroudis C, Tchervenkov CI, et al. Congenital Heart Surgery Nomenclature and Database Project: double outlet right ventricle. Ann Thorac Surg. 2000;69:249–63.
3. Obler D, Juraszek AL, Smoot LB, et al. Double outlet right ventricle: aetiologies and associations. J Med Genet. 2008;45:481–97.
4. Bonow RO, Mann DL, Zipes DP, Libby P, eds. Braunwald's Heart Disease: A Textbook of Cardiovascular Medicine. 9th ed. Philadelphia, PA: Saunders Elsevier; 2011.
5. Lev M, Bharati S, Meng CC, et al. A concept of double-outlet right ventricle. J Thorac Cardiovasc Surg. 1972;64:271–81.
6. Franklin RC, Anderson RH, Daniels O, et al. Report of the Coding Committee of the Association for European Paediatric Cardiology. Cardiol Young. 2002;12:611–8.
7. Lacour-Gayet F. Intracardiac repair of double outlet right ventricle. Semin Thorac Cardiovasc Surg Pediatr Card Surg Annu. 2008;11:39–43.

Double-Inlet Ventricular and Univentricular Heart

30

Anita Sadeghpour and Azin Alizadehasl

Keywords
Double inlet ventricle • Univentricular heart • Single ventricle • Transposition of the great vessels (TGA) • Ventricular septal defect (VSD)

Definition and Clinical Findings

A double-inlet left ventricle (DILV) or single ventricle is a congenital heart defect (CHD) occurring in 5 in 100,000 newborns that both the left atrium (LA) and the right atrium (RA) feed into the LV; indeed, 2 separated atrioventricular ostia open in a morphological LV. The right ventricle (RV) is hypoplastic or sometimes does not exist [1–3].

Cyanosis is present in cases with sub-pulmonary stenosis, but, patients with DILV and aortic arch obstruction are the least cyanotic because they never show sub-pulmonary stenosis; such cases are vulnerable for poor lower body perfusion upon decrease in ductal diameter.

A. Sadeghpour, MD, FACC, FASE (✉)
Echocardiography Lab, Department of Cardiology, Adult Congenital Heart Disease Clinic, Rajaie Cardiovascular Medical and Research Center, Iran University of Medical Science, Tehran, Iran
e-mail: anita.sadeghpour@gmail.com, asadeghpour@rhc.ac.ir

A. Alizadehasl, MD, FACC
Echocardiography Lab, Department of Cardiology, Rajaie Cardiovascular Medical and Research Center, Iran University of Medical Science, Tehran, Iran
e-mail: alizadeasl@gmail.com, alizadeasl@rhc.ac.ir

In physical examination, the first heart sound (S1) is normal. The second heart sound (S2) is often single. A systolic ejection type murmur is present in cases with sub-pulmonary stenosis as well as patients with aortic obstruction [3–5].

Paraclinic

Common findings in electrocardiography consist of septal Q wave in all the right precordial leads (in cases of L-looped single LV) and a steady R/S pattern in all the anterior precordial leads.

Chest X-ray findings vary. In cases with pulmonary stenosis (PS), the cardiac silhouette is normal to only mildly enlarged. Pulmonary vascularity marking is normal and not increased. But in cases with arch obstruction, the cardiac silhouette is generally at least mildly enlarged, and pulmonary vascularity marking usually is increased. A systematic comprehensive approach is essential for optimal diagnosis and management [4, 5] Table 30.1.

Electronic supplementary material The online version of this chapter (doi: 10.1007/978-1-4471-6383-1_30) contains supplementary material, which is available to authorized users.

Table 30.1 Key clinical points of morphology in single ventricle

Atrial arrangement	Situs solitus, inversus, left isomerism, or right isomerism
Atrioventricular connection	Double-inlet ventricle: two patent valves linking to one ventricle (>50 % of both atria and valves joined to this ventricle) Common valve (e.g., unbalanced atrioventricular septal defect) One atretic valve (mitral or tricuspid atresia) One or two straddling valves
Ventricles	Dominant LV, dominant RV, or rarely indeterminate (defined AV valve arrangement, position, trabecular pattern) Left heart hypoplastic syndrome
VA connection	Concordant, discordant, double-outlet
Systemic venous return	Heterotaxy syndromes with variable venous return patterns
Pulmonary circulation	Stenotic, atretic, or normal (unprotected)
Pulmonary venous return	Anomalous pulmonary venous drainage
Conduction system	Sinus node variable in isomerism AV node and His variations
Associated lesions	Cardiac including aortic arch abnormalities and coarctation of aorta Noncardiac: variations in bronchial situs, abdominal abnormalities including asplenia, multiple spleens, biliary atresia

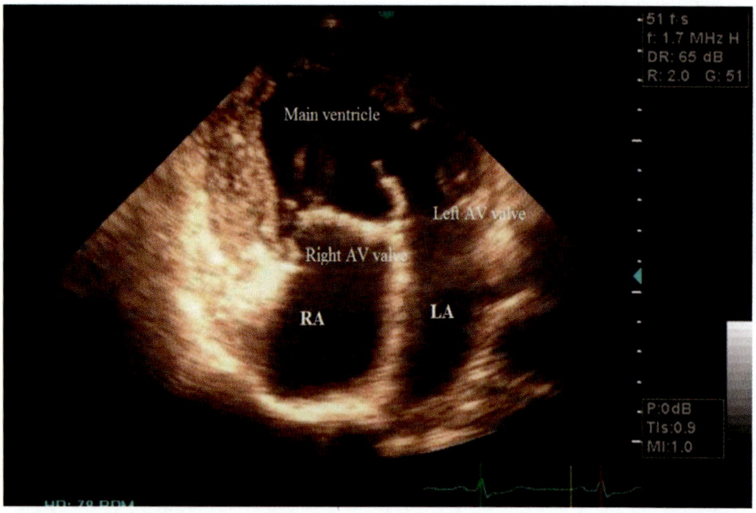

Fig. 30.1 Transthoracic echocardiography in 4-chamber view showing main ventricle with LV morphology (DILV), receiving two separate atrioventricular valves. *RA* right atrium, *LA* left atrium

2D echocardiography is a diagnostic tool for single ventricle. As it was noted before, based on the 50 % rule, a chamber can be termed "ventricle" if it receives 50 % or more of the inlet, even if this inlet is an imperforate fibrotic membrane and is situated over a small right ventricle (RV), as is the case in tricuspid atresia. Note that a chamber need not have an outlet in order to be termed "ventricle" [4, 5].

The atrioventricular connection and also ventriculo-arterial alignment should be evaluated by echocardiography carefully. The two most common types of single ventricle are L-looped single ventricle with LV morphology with transposition of the great arteries (TGA) and subpulmonary stenosis (Figs. 30.1, 30.2, 30.3 and 30.4) and D-looped single LV with TGA and subpulmonary stenosis; also the third most prevalent form is L-looped single LV with TGA and aortic arch hypoplasia. The fourth most common type is D-looped single LV with normally allied great arteries (aorta originated from LV and pulmonary artery from the outlet chamber), which is occasionally referred to as a Holmes heart [6, 7].

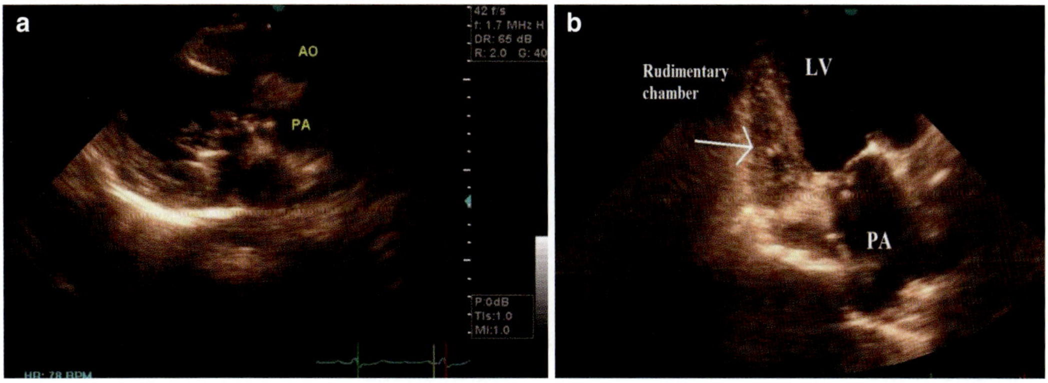

Fig. 30.2 Transthoracic echocardiography in parasternal and apical long axis view showing DILV and transposition of great arteries. *Arrow* indicates rudimentary chamber. *AO* aorta, *PA* pulmonary artery, *LV* left ventricle

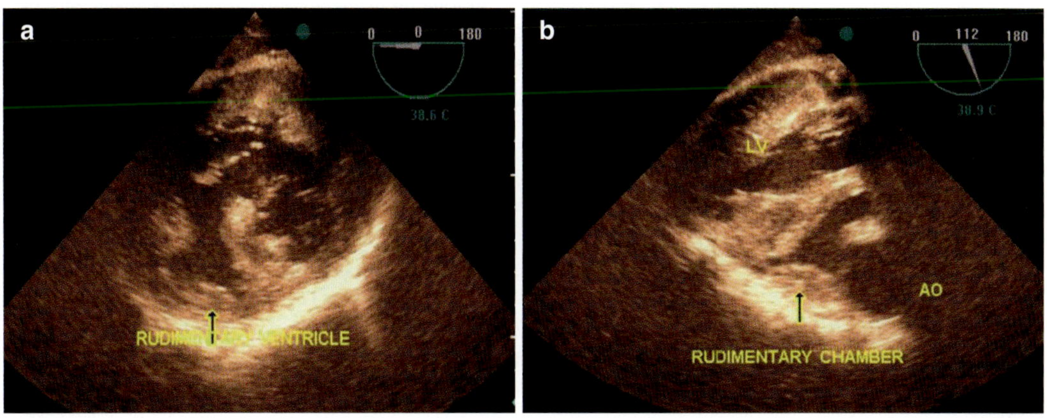

Fig. 30.3 (**a**, **b**): Transesophageal echocardiography in transgastric short axis and long axis view showing main ventricle with LV morphology (DILV) and aorta that arises from the rudimentary anterior chamber. *AO* aorta, *LV* left ventricle

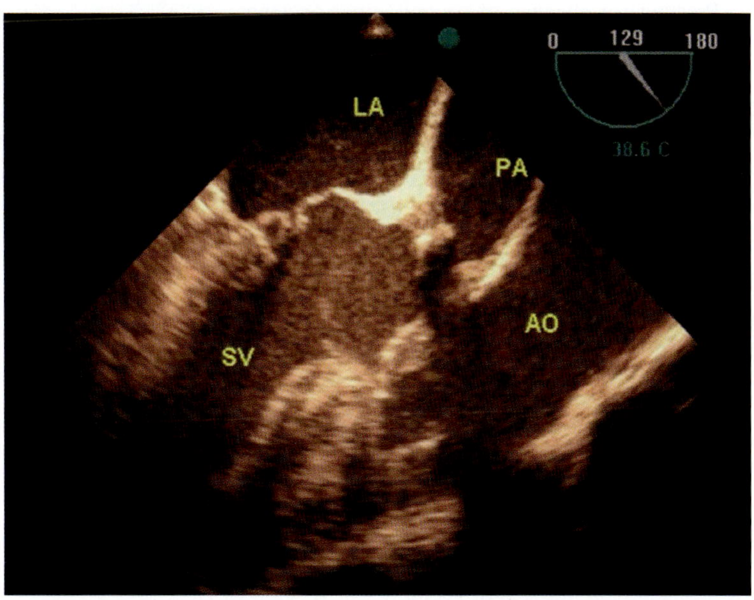

Fig. 30.4 Transesophageal echocardiography in long axis view demonstrating transposition of great arteries and severe pulmonary stenosis. *LA* left ventricle, *AO* aorta, *PA* pulmonary artery, *SV* single ventricle

In single LV with transposition of the great arteries and aortic arch obstruction, the subaortic stenosis that frequently coexists is due to a narrowing at the communication between the LV and the rudimentary right ventricle (outlet chamber). This orifice is frequently referred to as a bulboventricular foramen or outlet foramen [6, 7] (Videos 30.1, 30.2, 30.3, 30.4 and 30.5).

Management

Cardiac catheterization is mostly reserved for study of candidacy for Fontan surgery, evaluating the post-Fontan hemodynamics and also managing supraventricular arrhythmic complications. In single LV with TGA and aortic arch obstruction, the sub-aortic stenosis that often coexists is due to a narrowing at the communication between the LV and the hypoplastic rudimentary RV (outlet chamber). This orifice is often mentioned as a bulboventricular foramen or outlet foramen.

Prior to hemi-Fontan (or bidirectional Glenn) operation, the following data should be obtained by echocardiography:

- Presence or absence of pulmonary artery distortion, either congenital or created inadvertently by prior pulmonary artery surgery
- Presence or absence of second superior vena cava
- Ventricular performance

Creation of a cavo-pulmonary circulation is more safely accomplished in time over 1–2 years because acute volume unloading is related with an acute increase in ventricular wall thickness. This wall thickness increases noticeably and alters the diastolic function of the single ventricle and can restrict cardiac output.

"Cardiac transplantation" is considered for cases who have undergone the Fontan operation and have developed severe complications and for cases whose hemodynamics finding makes them poor and inappropriate candidates for Fontan operation [4, 5, 8, 9].

References

1. Dhanantwari P, Lee E, Krishnan A, et al. Human cardiac development in the first trimester: a high-resolution magnetic resonance imaging and episcopic fluorescence image capture atlas. Circulation. 2009; 120(4):343–51.
2. Sizarov A, Ya J, de Boer BA, et al. Formation of the building plan of the human heart: morphogenesis, growth, and differentiation. Circulation. 2011;123(10):1125–35.
3. Koshiba-Takeuchi K, Mori AD, et al. Reptilian heart development and the molecular basis of cardiac chamber evolution. Nature. 2009;461(7260):95–8.
4. Warnes CA. Congenital heart disease for the adult cardiologist. Transposition of the great arteries. Circulation. 2006;114:2699–709.
5. Warnes CA, Williams RG, Bashore TM, et al. American Heart Association. ACC/AHA 2008 Guidelines for the Management of Adults with Congenital Heart Disease. Circulation. 2008;118:e714–e833.
6. Bruneau BG, Logan M, Davis N, et al. Chamber-specific cardiac expression of Tbx5 and heart defects in Holt-Oram syndrome. Dev Biol. 1999;211(1):100–8.
7. Takeuchi JK, Ohgi M, Koshiba-Takeuchi K, et al. Tbx5 specifies the left/right ventricles and ventricular septum position during cardiogenesis. Development. 2003;130(24):5953–64.
8. Chin AJ, Whitehead KK, Watrous RL. Insights after 40 years of the Fontan Operation. World J Pediatr Congenit Heart Surg. 2010;1:328–43.
9. DeLeval MR, Deanfield JE. Four decades of Fontan Palliation. Nat Rev Cardiol. 2010;7:520–7.

Heterotaxy Syndrome

31

Azin Alizadehasl and Anita Sadeghpour

Keywords
Heterotaxy Syndrome • Isomerism • Asplenia • Polysplenia • Dextocardia

Heterotaxy syndrome subjects with isomerism also usually have concomitant congenital heart defects (CHD). Isomerism is a complex syndrome that happens when the main axis of the body fails to rotate properly during developing in the womb in early embryonic period. Many patients have a variable range of severe CHD, while a lesser percentage have none or mild cardiac problems, and also each individual with heterotaxy is only one of its kind. A number of these patients have pulmonary complications, while for others the main concern is their gastrointestinal or immune systems. Indeed heterotaxy syndrome is characterized by a wide range of cardiac and extra-cardiac congenital defects [1, 2].

A. Alizadehasl, MD, FACC (✉)
Echocardiography Lab, Department of Cardiology, Rajaie Cardiovascular Medical and Research Center, Iran University of Medical Science, Tehran, Iran
e-mail: alizadeasl@gmail.com, alizadeasl@rhc.ac.ir

A. Sadeghpour, MD, FACC, FASE
Echocardiography Lab, Department of Cardiology, Adult Congenital Heart Disease Clinic, Rajaie Cardiovascular Medical and Research Center, Iran University of Medical Science, Tehran, Iran
e-mail: anita.sadeghpour@gmail.com, asadeghpour@rhc.ac.ir

The molecular and cellular reasons of the right-left asymmetry have been expansively studied previously, and the developmental rules of this syndrome have been noticeably explained [1, 3].

The heterotaxy syndrome was known as Ivemark's syndrome, the name of the doctor who first documented the outline of abnormalities, and now, it is known by some different labels. Often it can be submitted as situs inversus ambiguous or is occasionally called left or right atrial isomerism. It frequently appears that the individual has two right-side or two left-side atria. Isomerism means the symmetric morphology of the structures that normally are not symmetric, such as similarity between the right and left atrial appendages and the right and left lung and bronchi [2–4].

It is often categorized based on the number of spleens or the lack of them, asplenia and polysplenia syndromes:

Asplenia Syndrome

This is the type of heterotaxy syndrome that is well known as right atrial isomerism, in that the patient has two right sides, with no spleen. And due to the absence of a spleen, these cases have

A. Sadeghpour et al. (eds.), *Comprehensive Approach to Adult Congenital Heart Disease*,
DOI 10.1007/978-1-4471-6383-1_31, © Springer-Verlag London 2014

an increased risk of infection, so this type of disease is related with higher mortality and morbidity rates and also with more severe associated cardiac malfunctions. These patients may have intra-atrial or intraventricular septal defects, anomalous pulmonary venous connection, and heart valve problems (especially the pulmonary valve) and also two trilobed lungs; the liver and other structures of the body can be on the wrong side of the body too [2, 3].

Polysplenia Syndrome

This type is typically matching with the term left atrial (LA) isomerism, in which the patient has two left sides. Characteristically, multiple spleens or "spleen nodules" may be recognized. It should be mentioned that though these patients might have several spleens, sometimes their spleens may not work well. Howell Jolly Body blood test can determine whether the patient has a functioning spleen or not, so sometimes it is needed that they be managed as functionally asplenic. Patients with this type usually have two-lobed lungs. They are more likely to have none or milder concomitant CHD [2, 3]. Also these cases are more likely to having primary ciliary dyskinesia syndrome [4–6].

These patients may have different types of septal defects: heart valve problems and also heart electrical system disorders. Complete heart block is common and needs pacemakers [2–4].

Interestingly, many cases do not fit exactly into one of these two types. For example, some people with severe CHD may have polysplenia, while others with milder CHD have asplenia. Altogether the common heart malformations that are related with heterotaxy syndrome consist of the following: dextrocardia, single ASD, single VSD, TGA, AVSD, TAPVC, PAPVC, coarctation of the aorta, pulmonary atresia, pulmonary stenosis, and double outlet RV. Of course so many cases with heterotaxy syndrome have a combination of heart anomalies. For this cause, staged surgeries, with the final Fontan surgery, are common in these patients.

As mentioned above, many organs are affected in this syndrome; some of the important ones are noticed as follows:

- The intestine may have malrotation and also volvulus that needs surgery.
- Some cases can have a very severe liver disease that is called biliary atresia. This also may need surgical intervention. Also abdominal defects are common in these patients.
- There may also be abnormalities in musculoskeletal, central nervous, and urinary tract systems.
- IgM and IgE deficiency and many other extracardiac problems may present in these cases [2–4].

The survival rate for heterotaxy syndrome is very different patient by patient. Nowadays, fortunately, with new medication and other less invasive procedural technologies, survival rates have meaningfully increased. Many cases with functional asplenia are on prophylactic antibiotic therapy, such as penicillin or amoxicillin. Of course the most important time for infections is before the age of 5 [2–4, 7].

Cases with heterotaxy syndrome face many other challenges. They need many types of doctors including pediatric cardiologists, pulmonologists, neurologists, immunologists, and gastroenterologists [4, 7].

Medical and surgical management of heterotaxy syndrome have advanced recently. But prognosis of the disease still remains unsatisfactory because the syndrome is frequently associated with a combination of CHD and extra-cardiac disorders. Management and treatment of heterotaxy patients, especially those who have experienced the staged surgeries, is now one of the most important matters in adult CHD clinics [3, 4, 7].

References

1. Zhu L, Belmont JW, Ware SM. Genetics of human heterotaxias. Eur J Hum Genet. 2006;14:17–25.
2. Taketazu M, Lougheed J, Yoo SJ, Lim JS, Hornberger LK. Spectrum of cardiovascular disease, accuracy of diagnosis, and outcome in fetal heterotaxy syndrome. Am J Cardiol. 2006;97:720–4.

3. Lim JS, McCrindle BW, Smallhorn JF, Golding F, Caldarone CA, Taketazu M, Jaeggi ET. Clinical features, management, and outcome of children with fetal and postnatal diagnoses of isomerism syndromes. Circulation. 2005;112:2454–61.
4. Matthew Swisher, Richard Jonas, Xin Tian, et al. Increased postoperative and respiratory complications in patients with congenital heart disease associated with heterotaxy. J Thorac Cardiovasc Surg. 2011;141:637–644.e3.
5. Barbato A, et al. Primary ciliary dyskinesia: a consensus statement on diagnostic and treatment approaches in children. Eur Respir J. 2009;34:1264–76.
6. Kennedy MP, Omran H, Leigh MW, Dell S, Morgan L, Molina PL, Robinson BV, Minnix SL, Olbrich H, Severin T, Ahrens P, Lange L, Morillas HN, Noone PG, Zariwala MA, Knowles MR. Congenital heart disease and other heterotaxic defects in a large cohort of patients with primary ciliary dyskinesia. Circulation. 2007;115:2814–21.
7. Icardo JM, de Vega Sanchez MJ. Spectrum of heart malformations in mice with situs solitus, situs inversus, and associated visceral heterotaxy. Circulation. 1991;84:2547–58.

32 Congenitally Corrected Transposition of the Great Arteries

Azin Alizadehasl, Anita Sadeghpour, and Mohammad Mahdavi

Congenitally corrected transposition of the great arteries (CCTGA) is defined as a disorder with discordant atrioventricular (AV) connections in combination with discordant ventriculoarterial (VA) connections [1, 2].

Morphology and Associated Lesions

CC-TGA is rare (less than 1 % of all CHD). In this anomaly systemic venous blood flow passes from the right atrium (RA) across the mitral valve (MV) to the left ventricle (LV) and then to the posteriorly located pulmonary artery (PA). Pulmonary venous blood flow passes from the left atrium (LA) via the tricuspid valve (TV) to the left-sided right ventricle (RV) and then to the left-sided, anterior aorta. Indeed, this circulation is physiologically corrected, but in this anomaly the morphologic RV should undergo the systemic vascular resistance. Associated lesions happen in up to 95 % of cc-TGA patients and include VSD (in 75 %), pulmonary valvular and subvalvular stenosis (in 75 %), and left-sided TV anomalies (in >75 %). Also 5 % of patients with cc-TGA are born with congenital complete heart block (CHB) [1–3].

A. Alizadehasl, MD, FACC (✉)
Echocardiography Lab, Department of Cardiology, Rajaie Cardiovascular Medical and Research Center, Iran University of Medical Science, Tehran, Iran
e-mail: alizadeasl@gmail.com, alizadeasl@rhc.ac.ir

A. Sadeghpour, MD, FACC, FASE
Echocardiography Lab, Department of Cardiology, Adult Congenital Heart Disease Clinic, Rajaie Cardiovascular Medical and Research Center, Iran University of Medical Science, Tehran, Iran
e-mail: anita.sadeghpour@gmail.com, asadeghpour@rhc.ac.ir

M. Mahdavi, MD
Pediatric Ward, Department of Pediatric Cardiology, Rajaie Cardiovascular Medical and Research Center, Iran University of Medical Science, Tehran, Iran

Natural History

Patients with isolated cc-TGA can live until the seventh or eighth decade. Progressive TV regurgitation and RV dysfunction happen from the fourth decade; atrial tachyarrhythmias are more frequent from the fifth decade. Acquired CHB develops at a rate of 2 % per year. A significant amount of patients are naturally and logically balanced by their VSD in combination with subpulmonary LV outflow tract obstruction. So, they often remain well, with no need of intervention for long time [2].

Clinical Findings

Unrepaired patients with no related lesions may be asymptomatic till late adulthood. Dyspnea, exercise intolerance from varying degrees of

Electronic supplementary material The online version of this chapter (doi: 10.1007/978-1-4471-6383-1_32) contains supplementary material, which is available to authorized users.

A. Sadeghpour et al. (eds.), *Comprehensive Approach to Adult Congenital Heart Disease*, DOI 10.1007/978-1-4471-6383-1_32, © Springer-Verlag London 2014

heart failure, and palpitations from atrial arrhythmias frequently initiate from the fifth decade. In well-balanced patients paradoxical emboli or cyanosis may be present. In physical examination A2 is frequently palpable at the second left intercostal space due to the anterior position of aorta, and P2 is silent due to posterior location of pulmonary artery. The murmur of a VSD or of TV regurgitation or pulmonary stenosis may be present. If there is CHB, cannon a waves may be present too [2–4].

After corrective repair many patients are in functional Class I despite the TV regurgitation and systemic RV dysfunction that usually progress after surgical repair. CHB may complicate surgery [2].

Electrocardiography

Q waves are frequently present in the right precordial leads and absent in the left ones due to abnormal direction of septal depolarization from right to left. First-degree AV block, CHB, and atrial arrhythmias may be present [2, 5, 6] (Fig. 32.1).

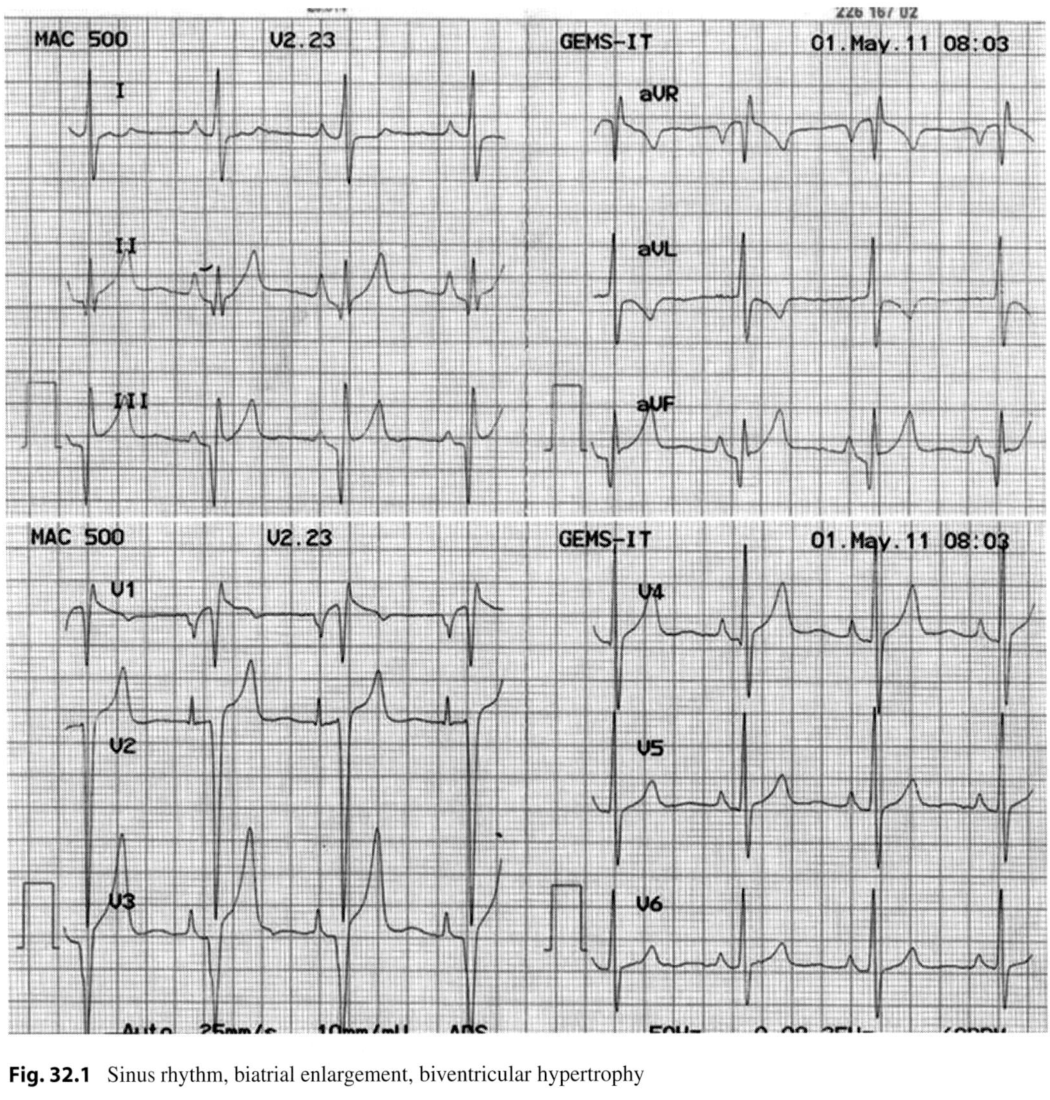

Fig. 32.1 Sinus rhythm, biatrial enlargement, biventricular hypertrophy

Chest Radiography

Chest X-ray typically shows absence of the normal PA segment in the left cardiac border. The right pulmonary hilum is frequently prominent and also elevated compared with the left one, creating a right-sided waterfall appearance [2, 4] (Fig. 32.2).

Echocardiography

Echocardiography allows the detailed diagnosis of the basic anomaly as well as of any related lesions. The right-sided morphologic LV is defined by its smooth endocardium and has bileaflet MV with no direct attachment to septum. The morphologic RV is characterized by its apical trabeculation and also moderator band and has a trileaflet apically displaced AV valve (TV) with direct septal attachment (Fig. 32.3). Ebstein-like anomaly of TV is defined as excessive (>8 mm/m^2 BSA) apical displacement of the TV, with or without dysplasia [1, 2, 5] (Fig. 32.4, Videos 32.1, 32.2, 32.3, 32.4 and 32.5).

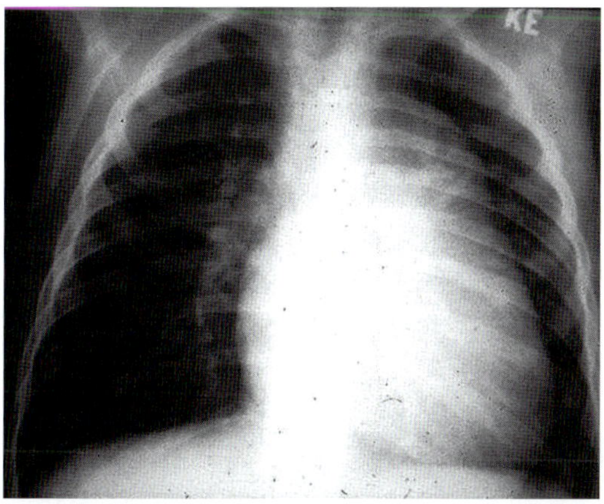

Fig. 32.2 Posteroanterior projection, levocardia, situs solitus, left aortic arch, levo position of the ascending aorta, "waterfall" appearance, straightening of the left heart border, normal pulmonary blood flow, cardiomegaly

CMR

The main role of CMR in cc-TGA patients is to study the systemic RV volume and function as the method of choice (Fig. 32.5). CMR can evaluate conduit function if present and AV valves regurgitation too [4, 6].

Cardiac Catheterization

This is rarely necessary for diagnosis but is indicated for defining of coronary artery anatomy and ventricular end-diastolic and also pulmonary artery pressures before surgery (Fig. 32.6).

Indications for Intervention

In moderate or severe systemic TV regurgitation (TR), valve replacement must be considered before systemic RV's function worsens (at an

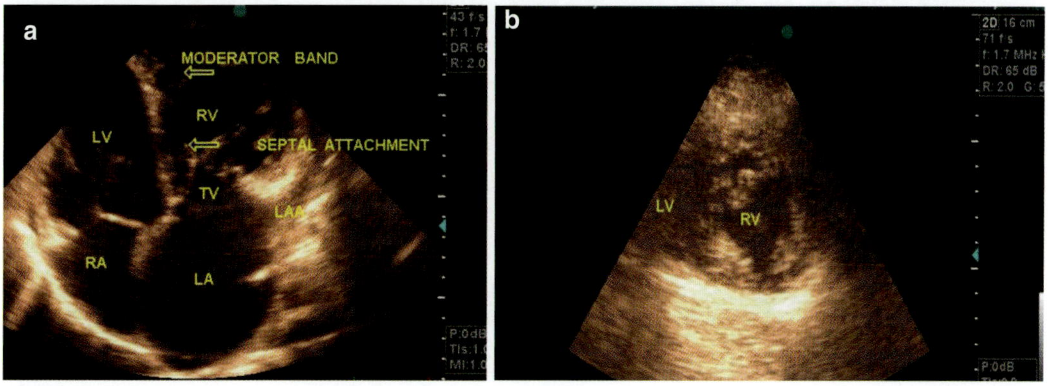

Fig. 32.3 (**a**, **b**) Transthoracic echocardiography in 4-chamber and short axis view showing L-loop ventricle with atrioventricular discordance. Moderator band (*upper arrow*), septal attachment of TV's septal leaflet (*lower arrow*). *LA* left atrium, *LAA* left atrial appendage, *LV* left ventricle, *RA* right atrium, *RV* right ventricle, *TV* tricuspid valve

ejection fraction of 45 % or more). When TR is concomitant with poor RV function, the double-switch surgery must be considered. Patients with end-stage heart failure should be considered for cardiac transplantation. The presence of a native or residual VSD with significant shunting volume (Qp/Qs >1.5: 1) or significant native or conduit pulmonary outflow tract stenosis (mean echocardiographic or catheter gradient >50 mmHg) needs surgical correction; pacemaker implantation (with DDD modality) is needed when CHB is present. Active fixation electrodes are necessary due to the lack of sufficient apical trabeculation in the morphologic LV. Transvenous pacing should be avoided with intra-cardiac shunts due to paradoxical emboli, so epicardial leads are preferred in this situation [1, 2].

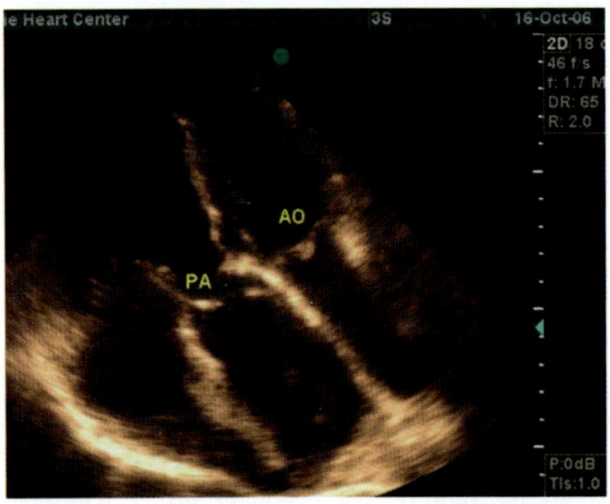

Fig. 32.4 Parallel great arteries in off axis view. *PA* pulmonary artery, *AO* aorta

Management

Medical Therapy

ACE inhibitor or beta-blockers for patients with systemic RV dysfunction may be useful, but the role of them has not been demonstrated. Indeed, patients with deteriorating systemic RV function must be managed aggressively by medical therapy but may require to be considered for cardiac transplantation [5, 7].

Conduit replacement or repair for pulmonary outflow tract stenosis, tricuspid valve replacement, double-switch procedure, and finally cardiac transplantation are options for surgical management [7, 8].

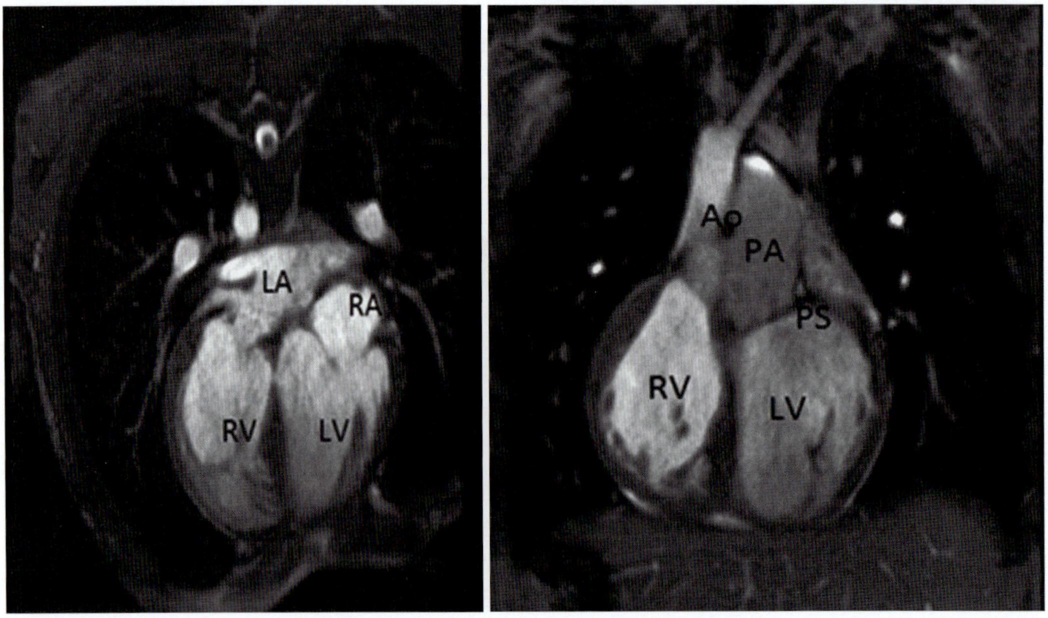

Fig. 32.5 CMR beautifully demonstrates atrioventricular discordance, ventriculoarterial discordance associated with severe subvalve PS, large VSD. Right ventricular size and function accurately is measured by CMR

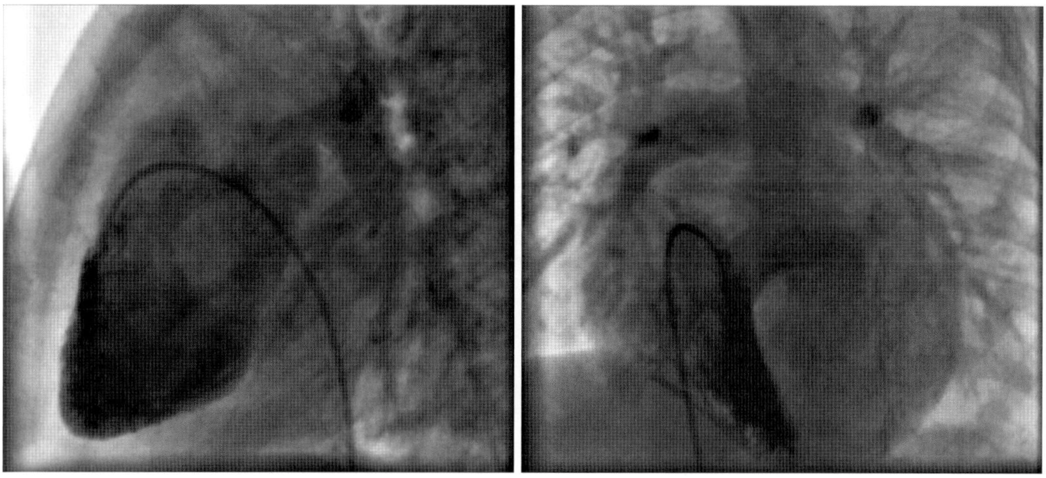

Fig. 32.6 CCTGA, VSD, and PS: Vertical laying of the intraventricular septum, presence of VSD and PS, and also laying of the aorta in anterior position in lateral injection. In addition aorta arises from the morphologic trabeculated RV (Videos 32.6, and 32.7)

Outcomes

The main predictor of poor outcome is the presence of left AV (TV) regurgitation. After complete surgical repair, the median survival of cases that reach adulthood is 40 years. The usual causes of death are sudden arrhythmic death and also, commonly, progressive systemic RV dysfunction with significant TR. Reoperation is common (15–25 %) [7].

Follow-up

All patients must have at least annual follow-up visit with an expert CHD cardiologist considering echocardiography, CMR, and Holter monitoring [7, 8].

References

1. Warnes C, Williams RG, Bashore TM, et al. ACC/AHA 2008 guidelines for the management of adults with congenital heart disease. Circulation 52(23): 2436–438.
2. Warnes CA. Transposition of the great arteries. Circulation. 2006;114:2699–709.
3. Sloth AD, Jensen JK, Steffensen FH, et al. Congenital transposition of the great arteries newly diagnosed in a 76-year-old woman. Ugeskr Laeger. 2009; 171(5):319–21.
4. Kwon SH, Oh JH, Hwang SJ, et al. Congenitally corrected transposition of the great arteries in a 59-year-old man: ECG-gated 64-slice MDCT findings. Int J Cardiol. 2009;13:e6.
5. Van der Bom T, Winter MM, Groenink M, et al. Right ventricular end-diastolic volume combined with peak systolic blood pressure during exercise identifies patients at risk for complications in adults with a systemic right ventricle. J Am Coll Cardiol. 2013;62(10):926–36.
6. Kozelj M, Prokselj K, Berden P, et al. The syndrome of cardiac failure in adults with congenitally corrected transposition. Cardiol Young. 2008;18(6):599–607.
7. Ly M, Belli E, Leobon B, et al. Results of the double switch operation for congenitally corrected transposition of the great arteries. Eur J Cardiothorac Surg. 2009;35(5):879–83; discussion 883–4.
8. Mohite PN, Popov AF, Garcia D, et al. Ventricular assist device outflow graft in congenitally corrected transposition of great arteries – a surgical challenge. J Cardiothorac Surg. 2012;7(1):93.

Complete Transposition of the Great Arteries (d-TGA) and the Senning and Mustard Procedures

33

Anita Sadeghpour, Azin Alizadehasl, and Mohammad Esmaeil Rezaei

Keywords
Complete transposition of the great arteries (d-TGA) • The Senning procedure • Mustard procedures • Transesophageal echocardiography • Arterial switch

Dictionary of Transposition

Atrioventricular discordance: Inappropriate and wrong connections of the morphological right atrium to the morphological left ventricle and the morphological left atrium to the right ventricle.

Ventriculo-arterial discordance: The pulmonary artery arises from the morphological left ventricle, and the aorta arises from the morphological right ventricle.

A. Sadeghpour, MD, FACC, FASE (✉)
Echocardiography Lab, Department of Cardiology, Adult Congenital Heart Disease Clinic, Rajaie Cardiovascular Medical and Research Center, Iran University of Medical Science, Tehran, Iran
e-mail: anita.sadeghpour@gmail.com, asadeghpour@rhc.ac.ir

A. Alizadehasl, MD, FACC
Echocardiography Lab, Department of Cardiology, Rajaie Cardiovascular Medical and Research Center, Iran University of Medical Science, Tehran, Iran
e-mail: alizadeasl@gmail.com, alizadeasl@rhc.ac.ir

M.E. Rezaei, MD
Department of Cardiology, Rajaie Cardiovascular Medical and Research Center, Tehran, Iran

Transposition of the great arteries: Refers to ventriculo-arterial discordance. The aorta arises from the morphological right ventricle, and the pulmonary artery arises from the morphological left ventricle.

D-loop: Refers to the normal rightward (dextro = D) loop of the embryonic heart tube and indicates that the inflow portion of the right ventricle is to the right of the morphological left ventricle.

L-loop: Refers to a leftward (levo = L) loop or bend of the embryonic cardiac tube resulting in the inflow portion of the morphological right ventricle being to the left of the morphological left ventricle.

Morphological ventricles: Morphological right and left ventricles refer to the anatomic features of the chambers and not their positions (e.g., the morphological right ventricle is on the left in congenitally corrected transposition).

Electronic supplementary material The online version of this chapter (doi: 10.1007/978-1-4471-6383-1_33) contains supplementary material, which is available to authorized users.

A. Sadeghpour et al. (eds.), *Comprehensive Approach to Adult Congenital Heart Disease*, DOI 10.1007/978-1-4471-6383-1_33, © Springer-Verlag London 2014

Congenitally corrected transposition (ccTGA): Atrioventricular discordance and ventriculo-arterial discordance. The right atrium enters the left ventricle, which gives rise to the pulmonary artery, and the left atrium enters the right ventricle, which gives rise to the aorta. Therefore, the circulation continues in the appropriate direction but flows through the incorrect, "wrong" ventricles [1, 2].

Definition and Morphology

This common cyanotic congenital heart defect (5–10 % of all CHD cases) is a cono-truncal abnormality characterized by ventriculo-arterial discordance in the presence of atrioventricular concordance. In most patients, the apex of the heart points to the left (levocardia). The aorta is usually located anterior and rightward to the pulmonary artery, but any relationship between great arteries is possible [1, 3].

Almost all patients have an interatrial communication, blood flow across which manages the amount of desaturation. 2/3 have a patent ductus arteriosus, and about 1/3 have an associated ventricular septal defect.

Approximately 2/3 of cases have no major associated anomalies (simple transposition), and 1/3 have associated abnormalities (complex transposition). The most common related abnormalities are ventricular septal defect and pulmonary or sub-pulmonary stenosis. Nowadays, it is increasingly being detected in utero. Without appropriate management, about 30 % of these newborns die within the first week of life, and 90 % of these infants die within the first year [1–4].

Pathophysiology

In this anomaly, the systemic and pulmonary circulation operate in parallel not in series; thus this defect is incompatible with life without some mixing of two circulations (e.g., via ASD, VSD, or PDA). About one third of patients have associated intracardiac anomalies (complex transposition) [1, 2].

Clinical Presentation and Natural History

The history of the patients depends on the severity of cyanosis, presence of associated anomalies, and pulmonary vascular status. Dyspnea and cyanosis are usually present at birth. Without appropriate surgical treatment, about 90 % of the patients die in infancy, so almost all cases with this anomaly who reach middle age and adulthood have had prior reparative cardiac surgeries, though some with a large VSD and also pulmonary vascular disease occasionally survive with Eisenmenger physiology [5–8].

Imaging

The echocardiography can detect this situation and associated anomalies (Figs. 33.1, 33.2 and 33.3, Videos 33.1, 33.2, 33.3 and 33.4). Prenatal diagnosis can affect morbidity and mortality [8–10].

CMR and radionuclide ventriculography can reliably evaluate the ventricular size and function [1–3, 6] (Fig. 33.4 and Video 33.5).

Treatment

Prostaglandin E1 infusion or atrial septostomy can increase arterial saturation. Surgery in infancy is often necessary for survival.

A. *Atrial switch (Senning and Mustard techniques)*

   These operations were the first techniques that were developed for this anomaly. In the Senning procedure, atrial redirection is made by atrial tissue, but in Mustard procedure, it is made by a Dacron or pericardium. The atrial switch produces "physiologic correction"; thus the morphological RV undergoes systemic circulation. Potential sequelae of this procedure are baffle obstruction, baffle leak, systemic RV dysfunction, systemic AV valve regurgitation, and arrhythmias. In patients suffering from significant systemic RV

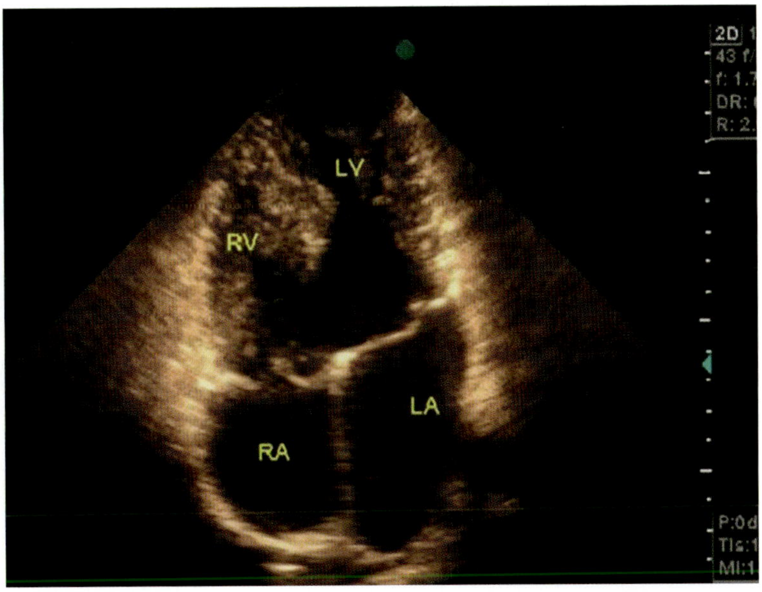

Fig. 33.1 Apical 4-chamber view showing D-loop ventricle associated with a large VSD. *RV* right ventricle, *LV* left ventricle, *LA* left atrium, *RA* right atrium

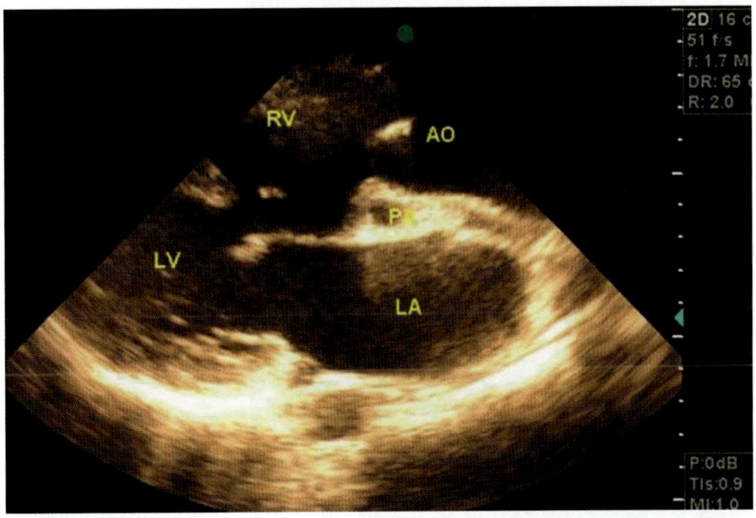

Fig. 33.2 Showing D-loop ventricle associated with transposed great arteries and anteriorly located aorta (AO). *RV* right ventricle, *LV* left ventricle, *LA* left atrium, *RA* right atrium, *PA* pulmonary artery

dysfunction after atrial switch operation, conversion to arterial switch may be considered. Atrial switch is now rarely performed and has been largely replaced by arterial switch operation.

B. *Arterial switch:* In this newer technique, the arterial trunks are transected above the sinus and reconnected to the contralateral roots. The coronary arteries are also anastomosed to the neoaorta. This is a challenging technique but produces "anatomic correction," and incidence of complication is lower than atrial switch. Potential sequelae of the procedure are coronary occlusion, supravalvular aortic or pulmonary stenosis, aneurysm of ascending aorta, and neoaortic valve regurgitation.

C. *Rastelli procedure:* This operation may be performed in infants with d-TGA plus VSD and pulmonary obstruction and consists of a RV to PA conduit plus LV to aorta tunneling. Potential sequelae are RV conduit and LV tunnel obstruction [1, 6, 13].

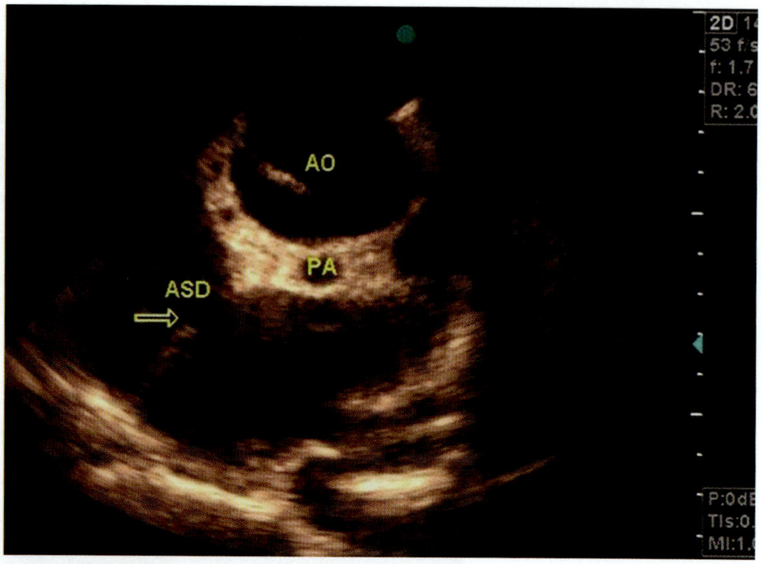

Fig. 33.3 D-loop transposed great arteries as anterior aorta and posterior pulmonary artery associated with ASD. *ASD* atrial septal defect, *AO* aorta, *PA* pulmonary artery

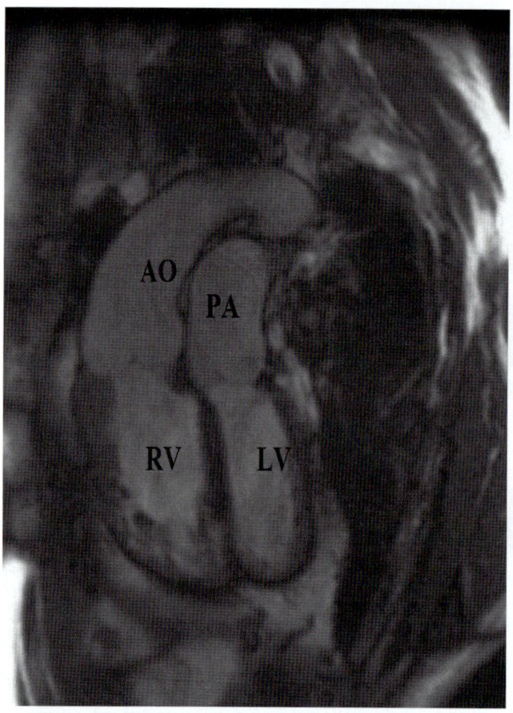

Fig. 33.4 CMR reliably demonstrates the ventricular and arterial looping besides the ventricular size and function. *RV* right ventricle, *LV* left ventricle, *AO* aorta, *PA* pulmonary artery

Follow-up

All patients, irrespective of the type of prior surgery, must have a clinical evaluation yearly or at least every 2 years. Imaging study by echocardiography (or MRI) allows an anatomic and hemodynamic precise assessment and also exercise testing for detection of some arrhythmias, occult coronary artery disease, and also functional capacity. Intermittent Holter monitoring permits detection of sinus node disease and also atrial arrhythmias. Most patients require endocarditis prophylaxis unless they have had an atrial switch surgery and have no residual valve disease or outflow tract stenosis and disturbance [6–8].

Mustard and Senning Procedures

The Mustard and Senning repair procedures for transposition of great arteries (TGA) are similar which were named after the surgeons who first did the operation. In both operations, the surgeons make a two-way baffle at the top portion of the heart. This baffle does as a bridge between two sides of the heart. In the Senning surgery, the baffle is created via patient's own tissue; however in the Mustard surgery, a synthetic and artificial material is used. These are called atrial switch surgeries, because they allow the blood to reach the ventricles [1, 10, 11].

Dr. Ake Senning of Sweden performed Senning procedure in 1957 for the first time, and also Dr. William Mustard performed the first

Mustard procedure in Canada, in 1963. In overall, Senning was more common in Europe, and the Mustard was more used in the United States and Canada. Of course nowadays, the operation that is performed for TGA is called an arterial switch in which the surgeon detaches and reattaches the heart's great arteries to generate more normal flow [4, 6, 13].

There are three types of complications and problems that patients with a history of Mustard and Senning repair face with them:

1. Arrhythmia
2. Baffle complications
3. Heart failure

Arrhythmias

In addition to congenital heart's electrical system abnormalities in TGA patients, the scar lines from previous surgery can also cause important electrical problems. Sometimes the sinus node is damaged and causes sick sinus syndrome. Up to 1/4 of Mustard-Senning cases have a pacemaker by adulthood. On the other hand, some TGA patients experience tachycardia, due to firing of some electrical system parts after surgery.

Ablation or appropriate medication can be used to manage heart rhythm problems. If the problem is life-threatening, a defibrillator can be implanted.

Radio-frequency ablation for atrial arrhythmias is technically more challenging because of the complex anatomy, atrial scar, and presence of artificial tissue. The reported success rates are about 70 % [3, 4, 13, 14].

Baffle Complications

Over time the made baffles in the Mustard-Senning repairs can develop some problems. Sometimes they become too stenotic. Nowadays it can be treated nonsurgically by an insertion of stent. Of course if a stent cannot fix the problem, surgery is needed. Also, importantly, baffles can leak over time. Usually, these leaks do not need treatment, unless they are large; it is possible to use a covered stent to stop blood leaks in the baffle. Echocardiography has a main role in diagnosis and management of these mechanical baffle complications as is explained as follows [4, 13–15].

Heart Failure

After a Mustard or Senning repair, the right ventricle acts as a systemic ventricle. So, over time, the heart failure symptoms and signs can develop; according to previous studies, about 10 % of TGA post Mustard-Senning patients experience heart failure in follow-up [1, 13, 14].

Echocardiography

In the d-TGA patients who are repaired by atrial baffle procedure, comprehensive echocardiographic imaging is needed in a regional ACHD center to evaluate the anatomy and hemodynamics.

The SVC anastomosis is patent if contrast injected into a peripheral arm vein promptly enters the SVA. In obstruction at the SVC, azygous or other collaterals to IVC will cause contrast to first enter the IVC and then to SVA.

- IVC obstruction may cause hepatic congestion or even cirrhosis.
- Baffle leaks occur in up to 25 % of patients.
- Pulmonary venous obstruction may also occur but is less common.
- In many mature patients, the SVC pathway is not visible on any surface scans, and TEE is required to assess this pathway.

Apical 4C view is usually the most informative initial scan by 2D, CFI, Doppler, and also contrast study (Figs. 33.5 and 33.6, Videos 33.6 and 33.7).

Contrast injection help detect baffle leaks which commonly occurs after atrial switch.

The most common early structural complications include baffle obstruction, which most commonly affects the superior limb rather than the IVC that may result in "superior vena cava syndrome" [1, 6, 9, 10] (Video 33.8 and 33.9).

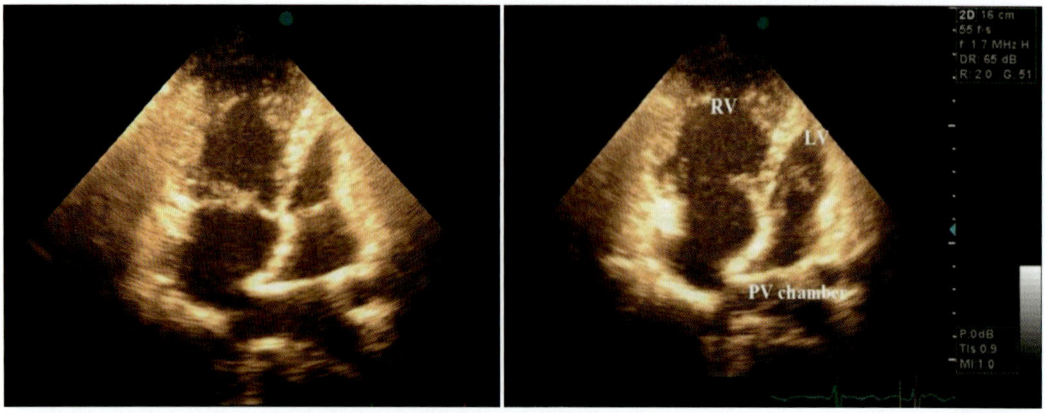

Fig. 33.5 Transthoracic echocardiography in 4-chamber view showing pulmonary venous chamber drains to the morphological RV with no obstruction in 2D study. *RV* right ventricle, *LV* left ventricle

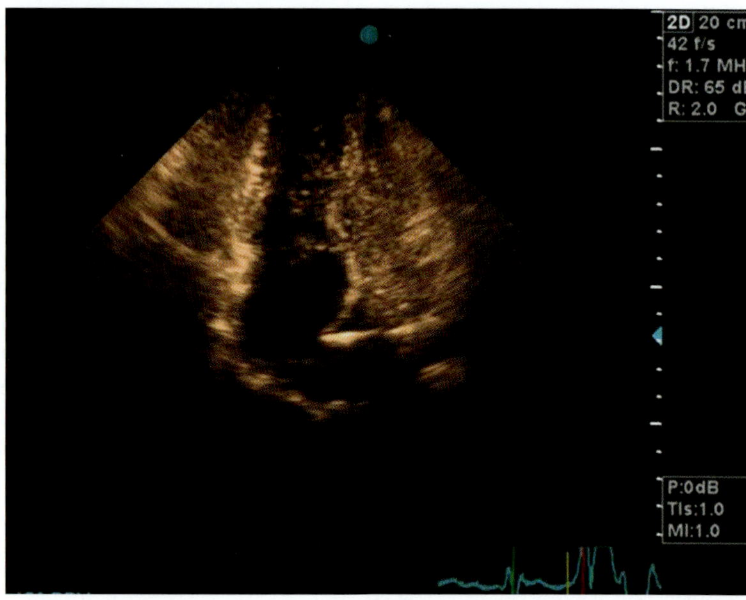

Fig. 33.6 Patent systemic venous chamber with no leakage as demonstrated in right-hand contrast injection

- CFI is useful to confirm laminar flow through the reconstruction and to detect stenoses or residual shunts.
- Successful procedures have larger RV resembling LV with small LV resembling RV.
- Vena cava and pulmonary venous obstruction (defined as turbulent non-phasic flow in the baffles with peak velocity >1 m/s and mean PG > 2–3 mmHg) is best assessed from apical 4C.

The assessment of RV function is challenging, and the most commonly used modality is still 2D echocardiography (TTE), though qualitative rather than quantitative due to the complex geometry and anatomy of the RV. Other echo-Doppler parameters can also be measured, such as the myocardial performance index and the dP/dT (by the use of the tricuspid valve regurgitant velocity). Nowadays, a tissue Doppler measurement of myocardial acceleration during isovolumic contraction (isovolumic myocardial acceleration) has been reported and can be a sensitive, reliable, and noninvasive method of studying the RV contractility that is less load dependent compared to other echocardiographic parameters. Other imaging modalities consist of radionuclide methods and angiography or magnetic resonance imaging [3, 6, 9].

Contrast echocardiography was also used in postoperative assessments. The technique was useful in identifying patch leaks and also residual defects after Senning and Mustard operations or after closure of atrial and ventricular septal defects and for assessing the patency of superior vena cava course and anastomosis sites. Most patients were found to have no superior vena cava obstruction by contrast echocardiography after the Senning or Mustard procedure [9, 10, 15, 16].

Pregnancy

Most women with TGA post Mustard-Senning can safely undergo pregnancy and also delivery. The exceptions are when there is heart failure, pulmonary hypertension, and uncontrolled rhythm problems. All pregnant women with TGA should be followed up by a special maternal fetal health team and also ACHD team that are working together. Of course a few number of women with TGA experience new problems with heart failure or arrhythmia during pregnancy [2, 3, 11, 12].

References

1. Warnes CA. Adult congenital heart disease. Chichester: Wiley-Blackwell; 2009. p. 128–37; chapter 9.
2. Perloff JK. The clinical recognition of congenital heart disease. 5th ed. WB Saunders; 1994. p. 300–25.
3. Warnes C, Williams RG, Bashore TM, et al. ACC/AHA 2008 guidelines for the management of adults with congenital heart disease. JACC. 2008;52(23): e143–e263.
4. Oechslin E, Jenni R. 40 Years after the first atrial switch procedure in patients with transposition of the great arteries: long-term results in Toronto and Zu-rich. Thorac Cardiovasc Surg. 2000;48: 233–7.
5. Williams WG, Mc Crindle BW, Ashburn DA, et al. Out-comes of 829 neonates with complete transposition of the great arteries 12–17 years after repair. Eur J Cardiothorac Surg. 2003;24:1–9.
6. Bonow RO, Mann DL, Zipes DP, Libby P, eds. Braunwald's Heart Disease: A Textbook of Cardiovascular Medicine. 9th ed. Philadelphia, PA: Saunders Elsevier; 2011.
7. FusterV, Walsh RA, Harrington RA. Hurst's the heart. 13th ed. McGraw Hill Medical; 2011. p. 1906–7; chapter 84.
8. Nihoyannopoulos P, Kisslo J. Echocardiography. Dordrecht/New York: Springer; 2009. p. 529–32; chapter 27.
9. Eidem BW, Cetta F, O'Leary PW. Echocardiography in pediatric and adult congenital heart disease. Philadelphia: Lippincott Williams & Wilkins; 2010. p. 249–68; chapter 16.
10. Lai WW, Mertens LL, Cohen M, et al. Echocardiography in pediatric and congenital heart disease. Wiley-Blackwell; 2010. p. 398–14; chapter 24.
11. Gatzoulis MA, Webb GD, Daubeney PEF. Diagnosis and management of adult congenital heart disease. 2nd ed. Philadelphia: Elsevier/Saunders; 2011. p. 37; chapter 5.
12. Gatzoulis MA, Swan L, Therrien J, et al. Adult congenital heart disease, a practical guide. Malden, Mass: Blackwell; 2005. p. 103–7; chapter 13.
13. Moons P, Gewillig M, Sluysmans T, et al. Long term outcome up to 30 years after the Mustard or Senning operation: a nationwide multicentre study in Belgium. Heart. 2004;90:307–13.
14. Kirjavainen M, Happonen JM, Louhimo I. Late results of Senning operation. J Thorac Cardiovasc Surg. 1999;117:488–95.
15. Agnetti A, Carano N, Cavalli C, et al. Long-term outcome after Senning operation for transposition of the great arteries. Clin Cardiol. 2004;27:611–4.
16. Wells WJ, Blackstone E. Intermediate out-come after Mustard and Senning procedures: a study by the Congenital Heart Surgeons Society. Semin Thorac Cardiovasc Surg Pediatr Card Surg Annu. 2000;3: 186–97.

34 Fontan Operation

Anita Sadeghpour, Mohammad Esmaeil Rezaei, and Azin Alizadeasl

Keywords
Fontan operation • Single ventricle • Bidirectional Glenn • Lateral tunnel • Transesophageal echocardiography

Definition

The Fontan operation is a palliative surgical procedure for patients suffering from univentricular circulation, although initially it was designed for patients with tricuspid atresia. The Fontan operation has several variations that connecting the whole systemic venous return to the pulmonary artery is common point between them:

A. Classic Fontan (atriopulmonary connection): It is a direct connection between the right atrium and the pulmonary artery.

B. Extracardiac Fontan: In this subtype, the inferior vena cava (IVC) is connected to the pulmonary artery using an extracardiac conduit, and the superior vena cava (SVC) is connected to the pulmonary artery as in the bidirectional Glenn.

C. Lateral tunnel: The difference between this subtype and the extracardiac Fontan is that the IVC is connected with a baffle within the right atrium to the right atrial appendage or the lower portion of the SVC, which is connected to the pulmonary artery.

D. Fenestrated Fontan: In this subtype, a fenestration is created in the atrial patch or baffle allowing right-to-left shunting and decompression of the Fontan circuit and maintaining adequate cardiac output.

E. Right atrial-right ventricular Fontan: In this operation, a conduit is created between the right atrium and the right ventricle [1, 2].

A. Sadeghpour, MD, FACC, FASE (✉)
Echocardiography Lab, Department of Cardiology, Adult Congenital Heart Disease Clinic, Rajaie Cardiovascular Medical and Research Center, Iran University of Medical Science, Tehran, Iran
e-mail: anita.sadeghpour@gmail.com, asadeghpour@rhc.ac.ir

M.E. Rezaei, MD
Department of Cardiology, Rajaie Cardiovascular Medical and Research Center, Tehran, Iran

A. Alizadeasl, MD, FACC
Echocardiography Lab, Department of Cardiology, Rajaie Cardiovascular Medical and Research Center, Iran University of Medical Science, Tehran, Iran
e-mail: alizadeasl@gmail.com, alizadeasl@rhc.ac.ir

Electronic supplementary material The online version of this chapter (doi: 10.1007/978-1-4471-6383-1_34) contains supplementary material, which is available to authorized users.

A. Sadeghpour et al. (eds.), *Comprehensive Approach to Adult Congenital Heart Disease*, DOI 10.1007/978-1-4471-6383-1_34, © Springer-Verlag London 2014

Complications of the Fontan Procedure

Some of the more common complications in Fontan patients include arrhythmias, thrombosis and stroke, protein-losing enteropathy, right pulmonary artery compression or obstruction due to an enlarged right atrium, Fontan obstruction, ventricular dysfunction and valvular regurgitation, hepatic dysfunction, and cyanosis [3].

Postoperative Work-up

The postoperative work-up for Fontan patients consists of electrocardiography, exercise testing, imaging modalities [echocardiography, computed tomography (CT), magnetic resonance imaging (MRI), and occasionally cardiac catheterization], and blood tests (serum albumin, liver function tests, and, if the protein-losing enteropathy is suspected, alpha1-antitrypsin clearance) [4, 5].

Electrocardiography

Sinus rhythm, atrial flutter, atrial fibrillation, junctional rhythm, and also complete heart block can be present. The QRS complex width and vector reflect the basic underlying cardiac malformation. In patients with tricuspid atresia, left-axis deviation is the role. In patients with univentricular hearts, the conduction pattern varies extensively and depends on the morphology and relative position of the small and rudimentary chamber.

Imaging

Imaging of the Fontan anastomoses is often difficult. Evaluation is facilitated by knowing the specific procedure subtype. Echocardiography generally is the first-line diagnostic modality for the evaluation of Fontan patients and is employed for the assessment of Fontan connections, fenestrations, baffle leaks, thrombi, pulmonary veins, valvular and ventricular functions, and aortic to pulmonary collateral flows. Normally the pulmonary arterial flow is biphasic with one peak in systole and another larger peak in diastole. The velocities are augmented with inspiration. The hepatic veins are always dilated to some extent, particularly in the presence of a systemic venous obstruction [6, 7].

Also TTE can help in assessing of systemic ventricle function; of course, all studies show reduced parameters of systolic and diastolic function including strain and strain rate and also tissue velocities in all patients with single ventricle physiology irrespective of procedure performed or patient's condition; AV valve regurgitation is studied by TTE too [8, 9].

The imaging of the classic Fontan by transthoracic echocardiography is generally difficult. Transesophageal echocardiography is frequently done to assess the patency of anastomosis sites and to detect thrombus within the right atrium (Videos 34.1, 34.2, 34.3, and 34.4). An extracardiac Fontan is even more difficult to assess with echocardiography.

Superior and inferior venae cavae biphasic and pulmonary artery triphasic flow patterns indicate unobstructed flow in the Fontan circuit [9], while a mean gradient between the Fontan circuit and the pulmonary artery of 2 mmHg or more can represent important obstruction. Study of the pulmonary vein flow pattern is important in detecting pulmonary vein obstruction (right pulmonary veins > left pulmonary veins) occasionally caused by an enlarged right atrium.

The all mentioned characteristics of Fontan circuit and also fenestration can be visualized by 2D and color flow imaging study by TTE and TEE [10] (Video 34.5) (Figs. 34.1 and 34.2a, b).

Other imaging modalities such as CT and MRI may be used in these patients insofar as they assist with the evaluation of the pulmonary veins, differential pulmonary flow, and the collaterals (Fig. 34.3).

Cardiac catheterization in Fontan patients can evaluate ventricular and valvular function, hemodynamics such as pulmonary vascular resistance, and Fontan obstruction (Figs. 34.4 and 34.5).

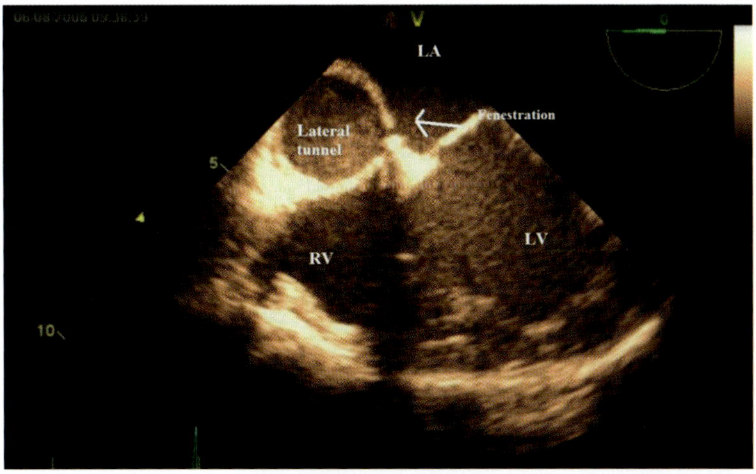

Fig. 34.1 Transesophageal echocardiography showing circular structure which is a cross section of the lateral tunnel with significant stagnant flow through it. *LA* left atrium, *LV* left ventricle, *RV* right ventricle

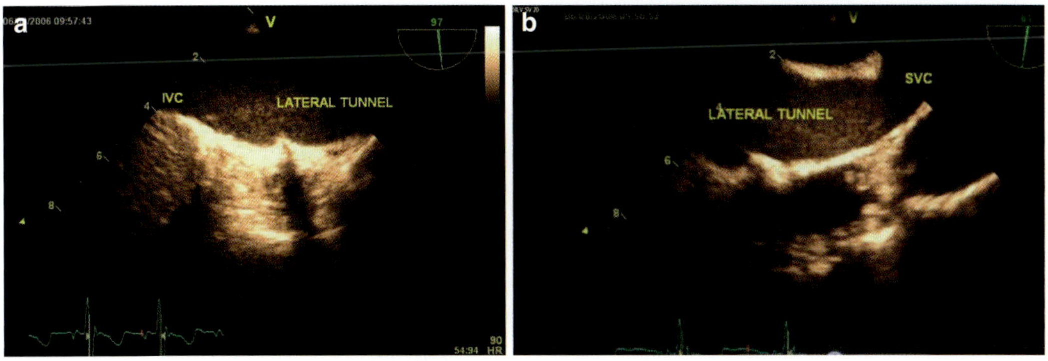

Fig. 34.2 (**a**, **b**) Transesophageal echocardiography is frequently done to assess the patency of the SVC and IVC anastomosis and to detect any thrombus within the right atrium. *SVC* superior vena cava, *IVC* inferior vena cava

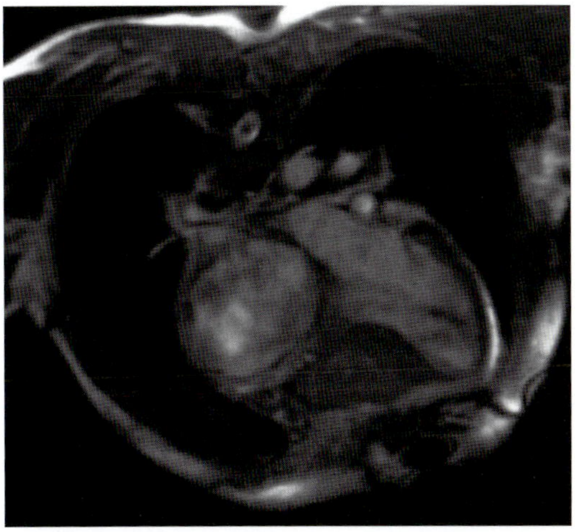

Fig. 34.3 CMR in a patient with lateral tunnel denotes significant stasis with no thrombosis (Video 34.6)

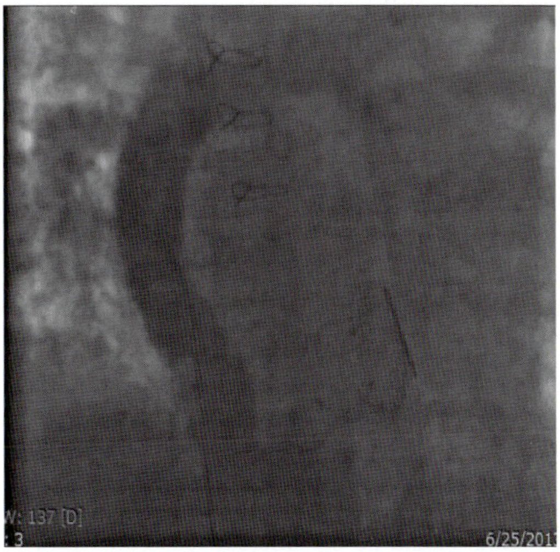

Fig. 34.4 Injection in Fontan pathway shows jaggy and toothed borders of extracardiac conduit; also there is negative washout in Glenn shunt course suggestive of patent Fontan circuit

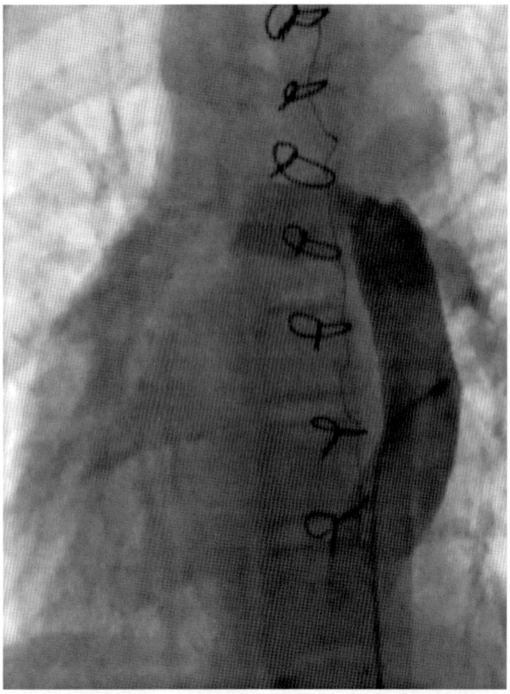

Fig. 34.5 Levocardia, no shunt through the fenestration that this issue can be a vindication for no cyanosis. Also there are three markers in fenestration site in Fontan, and there is a clip anastomosis site between the previous shunt and *LPA* left pulmonary artery

Medical Treatment

There is no consensus about the use of anticoagulation in all Fontan patients. Nevertheless, anticoagulation is definitely indicated when there is right atrial thrombosis, atrial arrhythmias, or thromboembolism. Sustained arrhythmias should be considered a medical emergency. Treatment for protein-losing enteropathy comprises salt restriction, protein diet, diuretics, and ACE inhibitors. Other modalities include steroid use, albumin infusion, and creation of fenestration [3, 5].

Surgical Treatment

For patients with a failing Fontan, surgical intervention should be considered. It is comprised of conversion of the classic Fontan to a total cavopulmonary connection (using a lateral tunnel or an extracardiac connection). These reoperations, however, have significant mortality and morbidity. Catheter intervention may be used for the closure of the fenestration in patients suffering from flow obstruction. As the final resort in some patients, cardiac transplantation may be required [5].

Follow-up

Close and expert follow-up is suggested, with specific attention to ventricular function and systemic AV valve regurgitation presence and severity. The development of atrial tachyarrhythmia must prompt a search for probable obstruction at the Fontan anastomosis, right pulmonary vein stenosis, or also thrombus within the right atrium [3].

References

1. Li W, Henein M, Gatzoulis MA. Echocardiography in adult congenital heart disease. London: Springer; 2007. p. 157; Glossary.
2. Chan K-L, Veinot JP. Anatomic basis of echocardiographic diagnosis. London: Springer; 2011. p. 391; Chapter 14.
3. Bonow RO, Mann DL, Zipes DP, Libby P, eds. Braunwald's Heart Disease: A Textbook of Cardiovascular Medicine. 9th ed. Philadelphia, PA: Saunders Elsevier; 2011.
4. Bax JJ, Kramer CM, Marwich TH, et al. Cardiovascular imaging; a handbook for clinical practice. Malden: Blackwell Publishing; 2005. p. 283–5; chapter 22.
5. Springer News ESC guidelines desk reference: compendium of abridged ESC guidelines 2011. Springer healthcare. p. 147–148; chapter 1.
6. Lai WW, Mittens LL, Cohen MS, et al. Echocardiography in pediatric and congenital heart disease. Wiley-Blackwell; 2010. p. 470–71; chapter 27.
7. Nihoyannopoulos P, Kisslo J. Echocardiography. Dordrecht/New York: Springer; 2009. p. 552; chapter 28.
8. Gatzoulis MA, Webb GD, Daubeney PEF. Diagnosis and management of adult congenital heart disease. 2nd ed. Philadelphia: Elsevier/Saunders; 2011. p. 40–1; chapter 5.
9. Armestrong WF, Ryan T. Feigenbaum's echocardiography. 7th ed. Lippincott Williams & Wilkins; 2010. p. 629–30; chapter 20.
10. Eidem BW, Cetta F, O'Leary PW. Echocardiography in pediatric and adult congenital heart disease. Philadelphia: Lippincott Williams &Wilkins; 2010. p. 457–66; chapter 38.

Congenital Aortic Valve Stenosis

35

Azin Alizadehasl and Anita Sadeghpour

Keywords

Aortic valve stenosis • Echocardiography • Bicuspid aortic valve Unicuspid aortic valve • Aortic insufficiency (AI)

Definition and Morphology

Congenital aortic valve stenosis (AS) is a relatively common anomaly. Congenital AS occurs much more commonly in men, with a male to female ratio of 4:1. Related cardiac anomalies have been seen in up to 1/5 of patients. Patent ductus arteriosus (PDA) and coarctation of the aorta happen most often with AS [1].

Aortic valve (AV) may be unicuspid, bicuspid, or tricuspid or even a dome-shaped diaphragm. Unicuspid valves produce severe stenosis and are the most common anomaly found in valvular AS in children younger than 1 year. Congenitally bicuspid valves might be stenotic due to commissural fusion at birth, but more often they don't create severe stenosis in childhood and adolescence. A subgroup of cases with a bicuspid AV develops important aortic regurgitation (AR) demanding valve surgery. But most patients have normal function of valve till late in life, and superimposed calcific changes result in valve stenosis. When the AV obstruction is hemodynamically important, concentric hypertrophy of the left ventricular (LV) wall and also dilatation of the ascending aorta occur gradually.

Aortic dilation is present in more than 1/2 of young patients with normally functioning bicuspid AV. Aortic dilation must be monitored carefully with echocardiography. The section of maximal dilatation frequently involves the mid-part of ascending aorta but can also contain the aortic sinuses [1–3].

Clinical Findings and Physical Examination

In overall the children are asymptomatic; exercise fatigue and chest pain are unusual complaints and happen only when the stenosis is severe. The

A. Alizadehasl, MD, FACC (✉)
Echocardiography Lab, Department of Cardiology, Rajaie Cardiovascular Medical and Research Center, Iran University of Medical Science, Tehran, Iran
e-mail: alizadeasl@gmail.com, alizadeasl@rhc.ac.ir

A. Sadeghpour, MD, FACC, FASE
Echocardiography Lab, Department of Cardiology, Adult Congenital Heart Disease Clinic, Rajaie Cardiovascular Medical and Research Center, Iran University of Medical Science, Tehran, Iran
e-mail: anita.sadeghpour@gmail.com, asadeghpour@rhc.ac.ir

Electronic supplementary material The online version of this chapter (doi: 10.1007/978-1-4471-6383-1_35) contains supplementary material, which is available to authorized users.

fundamental manifestations in adults are exertional dyspnea, angina, syncope, and finally heart failure. Most of the patients now are diagnosed before the onset of symptoms according to the finding of a systolic murmur on physical examination, with confirmation by echocardiography. In cases with bicuspid AV stenosis, symptoms typically occur at age 50–70 years though even in older age group, about 40 % of AS patients have a congenital bicuspid valve [1, 2].

The most common clinical presentation is a gradual decrease in exercise tolerance, fatigue, or dyspnea on exertion because of LV diastolic dysfunction, with too much rise in end-diastolic pressure leading to pulmonary congestion, and also due to restricted ability to increase cardiac output with exercise. More severe exertional dyspnea, orthopnea, paroxysmal nocturnal dyspnea, and finally pulmonary edema are late symptoms in cases with untreated AS [1–3].

Angina happens in approximately 2/3 of cases with severe AS, about 1/2 of them have associated significant coronary artery disease; angina usually results from the combination of the increased oxygen needs of hypertrophied myocardium and decrease of oxygen delivery secondary to the excessive compression of coronary vessels.

Syncope is most commonly produced by the reduced cerebral perfusion that happens during exertion when arterial pressure declines resulting in systemic vasodilation in the presence of a fixed cardiac output and also due to baroreceptor malfunction in severe AS. Syncope at rest may be caused by transient atrial fibrillation (AF) or due to transient atrioventricular block created by extension of the calcification of the AV into the conduction system [1–4].

Other late findings in patients with isolated AS include AF, pulmonary hypertension, and systemic venous hypertension. Of course, AS may be responsible for sudden cardiac death; this typically happens in cases who had formerly been symptomatic.

On physical examination, a sustained LV apical impulse with a fourth heart sound (S4) is a marker of severe stenosis. The slowly rising and low-volume carotid arterial pulse of severe AS can be noted in younger patients, but changes in arterial compliance frequently mask these findings in older patients. In younger patients with congenital AS, the flexible valve can result in an accentuated A2, and S2 may be normally split, even with severe valve obstruction. In addition, an aortic ejection sound can be audible due to halting upward motion of the AV and disappears when the leaflets become severely calcified. So, it is frequent in children and young adults with congenital AS but is unusual in adults with acquired calcific and rigid AS [1, 2].

The harsh systolic murmur of AS, loudest at the base of the heart and radiating to both carotids, is frequently but not always prominent and noticeable. Low-output states and also obesity can mask the findings. The murmur may radiate toward the apex, but the harsh component is vanished [1].

Electrocardiography

LV hypertrophy with or without strain is the hallmark point [1].

Chest Radiography

Cardiac ratio is overall normal or slightly increased in patients with congenital AS [1, 2].

Echocardiography

2D echocardiography delivers detailed information about the morphology of the AV, the LV function, and the presence or absence of related left-sided lesions. Doppler echocardiography is used to determine the severity of AS and the presence of associated AI.

Also comprehensive echocardiographic assessment should be done for patients with bicuspid AV; echocardiographic characteristic features include systolic doming with eccentric closing line of two visible cusps in the parasternal long-axis view and a single commissural line with two functional cusps in the parasternal short-axis view. Specific care should be taken in studying the valve in both systole and diastole. Because in some patients with asymmetric leaflets and a noticeable and evident raphe, the valve can seem tricuspid in diastole; but the oval football shape of the systolic appearance of orifice indicates bicuspid AV [1, 4, 5] (Fig. 35.1).

The leaflets often are thickened and fibrotic and calcified with increasing age. With extensive calcification, it may be difficult to distinguish stenotic tricuspid from bicuspid AV [4, 5] (Fig. 35.2).

Also, Doppler provides peak instantaneous gradients which are higher than the peak-to-peak gradients derived from cardiac catheterization. Mean gradients as determined by Doppler and catheterization associate closely (Fig. 35.3).

Also, importantly, aortic dilation is present in more than 1/2 of young patients with normally functioning bicuspid AV in echocardiographic study. Aortic dilatation must be monitored and followed up carefully by echocardiography. The section of maximal dilatation frequently is seen in the mid-part of ascending aorta but can also contain the aortic sinuses. If the images of transthoracic echocardiography are limited, alternative imaging studies should include TEE, CT, or CMR. According to ACC/AHA guidelines, aortic root replacement is suggested for cases with a bicuspid AV whose aortic root size is 5 cm or larger [1, 5].

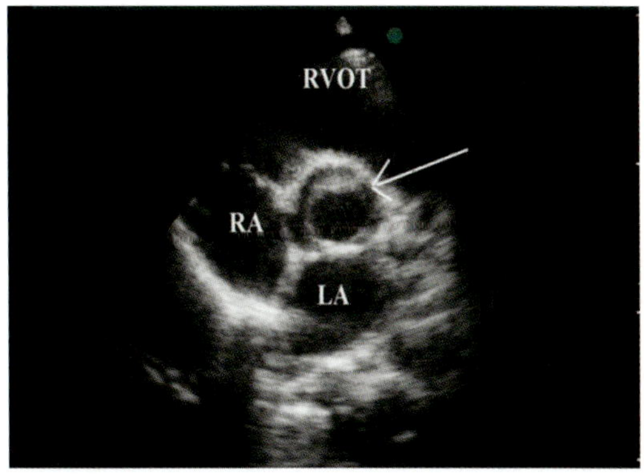

Fig. 35.1 Oval-shaped opening of the bicuspid aortic valve (BAV) in parasternal short-axis view; note the evaluation was done in systole (*arrow*). *LA* left atrium, *RA* right atrium, *RVOT* right ventricular outflow tract (Video 35.1)

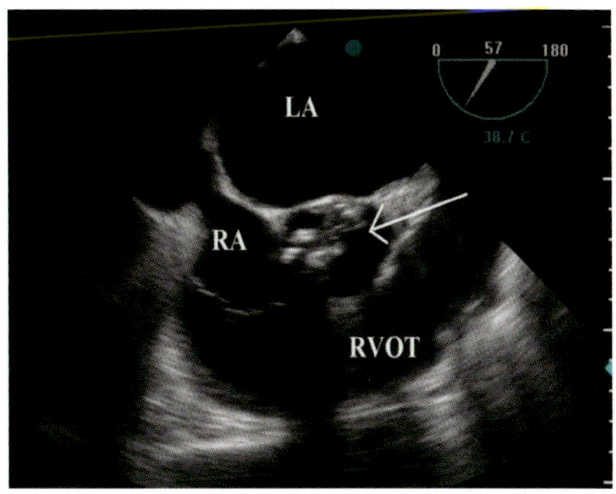

Fig. 35.2 Transesophageal echocardiography showing thickened and calcified BAV in short-axis view (*arrow*). *LA* left atrium, *RA* right atrium, *RVOT* right ventricular outflow tract (Video 35.2)

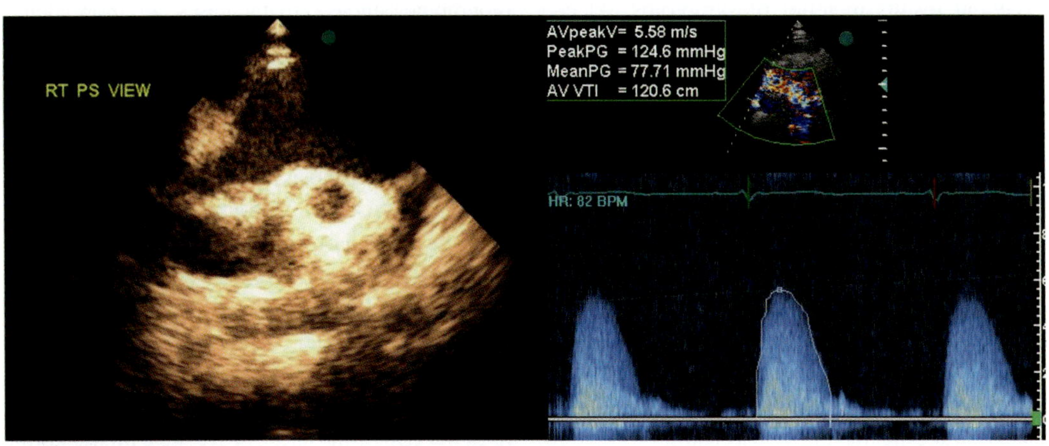

Fig. 35.3 (**a**, **b**) The max gradients should be evaluated by searching in all available windows. *RT PS* right parasternal always should be used

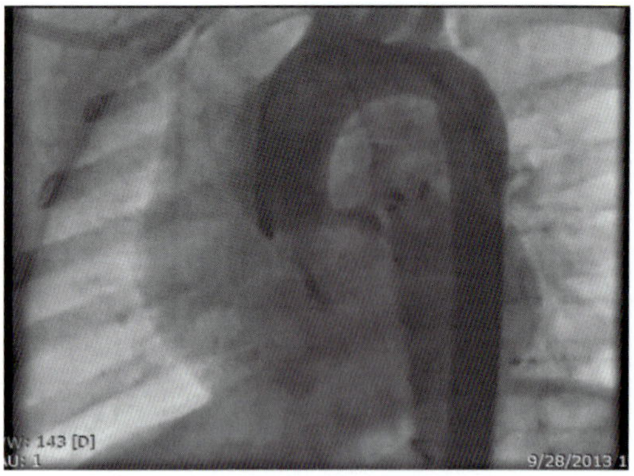

Fig. 35.4 The catheter course is arterial; injection was performed in aortic root and showed doming of AV cusps due to bicuspid aortic valve (Video 35.3)

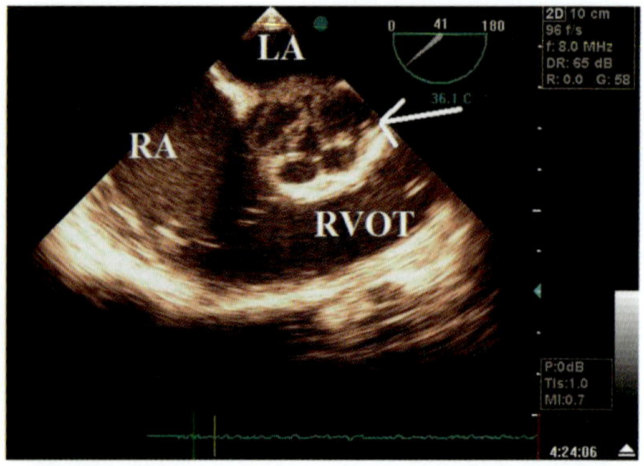

Fig. 35.5 Quadricuspid aortic valve in short-axis transesophageal echocardiography associated with significant aortic regurgitation

Catheterization

Nowadays, cardiac catheterization is rarely used to confirm the site and grade of severity of obstruction to LV outflow. Of course, catheterization is carried out when interventional therapeutic balloon aortic valvuloplasty is planned [5–7] (Fig. 35.4).

Management and Follow-up

Nowadays, therapeutic balloon aortic valvuloplasty has virtually replaced primary surgical valvotomy in children. Of course, aortic valvotomy is a so safe and effective palliative surgery with excellent results in relief of symptoms. AI can infrequently be progressive and need valve replacement. Furthermore, after valve commissurotomy, the valve leaflets remain deformed, and progressive degenerative changes containing calcification will cause important stenosis in future years. So prosthetic AV replacement is needed in about 35 % of cases within 15–20 years of the first operation. For those adolescents requiring AV replacement, the surgical options consist of replacement with a mechanical AV, an aortic homograft, or a pulmonary autograft in the aortic position (Ross procedure). Collecting evidence shows that the pulmonary autograft may be better than the aortic homograft. In the Ross technique, the patient's pulmonary valve is removed and used to replace the diseased AV, and the right ventricular outflow tract is recreated with a pulmonary valve homograft [6–8].

Quadricuspid Aortic Valve

Definition and Diagnosis

Quadricuspid aortic valves (QAV) are infrequent but well-recognized reason of important aortic valve insufficiency (AI). The first instance was reported in 1862. Generally QAV cases traditionally have been exposed incidentally in surgery or postmortem study; however, with advances in echocardiographic studies, many cases are now being diagnosed antemortem. The preoperative identification of QAVs is important as they can be related with abnormal coronary arteries' ostium. Using the transesophageal echocardiography (TEE) is so helpful in the diagnosis, because a higher-frequency transducer is used, and also it is at closer proximity to the heart. In diastole, in the short-axis view of the aortic valve (AV), the commissural lines of adjacent cusps result in an X conformation rather than the Y shape of the normal tricuspid AV [9–11] (Fig. 35.5; Videos 35.4 and 35.5).

Though the echocardiographic studies may propose the size of the cusps of AV, they do not correlate with surgical findings, always. TEE has also revealed displacement of coronary ostium. Newly, cine magnetic resonance imaging (MRI) has also been used for the diagnosis of QAV and the associated lesions. Hurwitz and Roberts defined the seven common anatomic variants of QAV depending on the size of the leaflets. Of course, more than 85 % of the reports are of type A, B, and C [12].

Presentation and Outcome

AI usually develops due to fibrotic thickening with incomplete coaptation of leaflets. Indeed, with the unequal distribution of stress on cusps and also abnormal leaflet coaptation, AI may occur. AI is not frequently seen in young cases with QAVs. Aortic stenosis (AS) may be present but is uncommon and rare. In one of the previously reported studies, of 108 patients with QVA, 73 had pure AI and 28 cases were normal, and in 7 cases there was evidence of mixed AI and AS; in no case there was pure AS (Video 35.6). Of course, it appears that valvular dysfunction has a tendency to deteriorate in adult life and often needs surgery around the sixth decade. The definite risk of infective endocarditis (IE) is not clear, but there have been documented cases of IE affecting a QAV [13, 14].

Associated Abnormalities

Anomalies of coronary artery ostium and course represent in less than 1 % of all congenital heart disease and can associate with QAV. So for surgeon, it is important to be aware and conscious of any displacement of the coronary artery origin to prevent ostial obstruction during fixing of the prosthetic AV ring. Also, QVAs have been reported in association with other abnormalities, including nonobstructive hypertrophic cardiomyopathy, ventricular septal defect, pulmonary valve stenosis, fibro-muscular subaortic stenosis, supravalvular stenosis, and left coronary artery atresia. Fenestrations of the aortic cusps in QAV are seen with advancing age. In addition, QVA has also been reported in association with Ehlers-Danlos syndrome [14].

Management

When a QAV is found on echocardiography, follow-up study is needed as progress to severe AI is to be expected. Valves with four equal cusps are not less likely to develop significant AI. There are a few confirmed cases of IE affecting a QAV, so IE prophylaxis is recommended [12–14].

References

1. Maganti K, Rigolin VH, Enriquez-Sarano M, Bonow RO. Heart valve disease: diagnosis and management. Mayo Clin Proc. 2010;85:453.
2. Ten Harkel AD, Berkhout M, Hop WC, et al. Congenital valvular aortic stenosis: limited progression during childhood. Arch Dis Child. 2009;94(7):531–5.
3. Braverman AC, Guven H, Beardslee MA, et al. The bicuspid aortic valve. Curr Probl Cardiol. 2005;30:470.
4. Lewin MB, Otto CM. The bicuspid aortic valve: adverse outcomes from infancy to old age. Circulation. 2005;111:832.
5. Braverman AC. The bicuspid aortic valve. In: Otto CM, Bonow RO, editors. Valvular heart disease: a companion to Braunwald's heart disease. Philadelphia: Saunders/Elsevier; 2009. p. 169–86.
6. Egito ES, Moore P, O'Sullivan J, et al. Transvascular balloon dilation for neonatal critical aortic stenosis: early and midterm results. J Am Coll Cardiol. 1997; 29(2):442–7.
7. Mc Elhinney DB, Lacro RV, Gauvreau K, et al. Dilation of the ascending aorta after balloon valvuloplasty for aortic stenosis during infancy and childhood. Am J Cardiol. 2012;110(5):702–8.
8. Weber HS, Mart CR, Myers JL. Transcarotid balloon valvuloplasty for critical aortic valve stenosis at the bedside via continuous transesophageal echocardiographic guidance. Catheter Cardiovasc Interv. 2000; 50(3):326–9.
9. Hwang DM, Feindel CM, Butany JW. Quadricuspid semilunar valves: report of two cases. Can J Cardiol. 2003;19:938–42.
10. Tutarel O. The quadricuspid aortic valve: a comprehensive review. J Heart Valve Dis. 2004;13(4):534–7.
11. Feldman BJ, Khandheria BK, Warnes CA, et al. Incidence, description and functional assessment of isolated quadri-cuspid aortic valves. Am J Cardiol. 1990;65:937–8.
12. Barbosa MM, Motta MS. Quadricuspid aortic valve and aortic regurgitation diagnosed by Doppler echocardiography: report of two cases and review of the literature. J Am Soc Echocardiogr. 1991;4:69–74.
13. Timperley J, Milner R, Marshall AJ, et al. Quadricuspid aortic valves. Clin Cardiol. 2002;25:548–52.
14. Hurwitz LE, Roberts WC. Quadricuspid semilunar valve. Am J Cardiol. 1973;31:623–6.

Subaortic Stenosis

36

Anita Sadeghpour, Azin Alizadehasl,
and Majid Kyavar

Keywords

Sub-aortic stenosis • Echocardiography • Discrete fibromuscular • Left ventricular outflow tract (LVOT) • Left ventricular hypertrophy (LVH)

Morphology

Discrete Fibromuscular

This lesion includes a ridge or fibrous ring encircling the left ventricular (LV) outflow tract in varying distances from the aortic valve (AV). This fibrous process usually extends onto the AV leaflets and almost always makes contact with the ventricular aspect of the anterior mitral valve (MV) leaflet at its base.

Focal Muscular

Infrequently there is no fibrous component, but a focal muscular obstruction on the ridge of the interventricular septum is present [1, 2].

Associated Lesions

In some patients, valvular and subvalvular aortic stenoses (AS) co-occur with hypoplasia of the AV annulus and thickened AV leaflets, making a tunnellike narrowing of the left ventricular outflow tract (LVOT) and also sometimes a small ascending aorta. Also the combination of discrete fibromuscular subaortic stenosis and VSD should be supposed in VSDs with some concomitant anterior malalignment of the aorta and a more acute aorto-septal angle. These hearts often develop sub-pulmonary stenosis too. Sometimes, accessory endocardial cushion tissue is present in LVOT in concomitant with cleft in anterior MV leaflet; these forms of obstruction are seen more frequently in those cases with abnormal

A. Sadeghpour, MD, FACC, FASE (✉)
Echocardiography Lab, Department of Cardiology, Adult Congenital Heart Disease Clinic, Rajaie Cardiovascular Medical and Research Center, Iran University of Medical Science, Tehran, Iran
e-mail: anita.sadeghpour@gmail.com, asadeghpour@rhc.ac.ir

A. Alizadehasl, MD, FACC
Echocardiography Lab, Department of Cardiology, Rajaie Cardiovascular Medical and Research Center, Iran University of Medical Science, Tehran, Iran
e-mail: alizadeasl@gmail.com, alizadeasl@rhc.ac.ir

M. Kyavar, MD, FACC
Cardiovascular Imaging Ward, Department of Cardiology, Adult Congenital Heart Disease Clinic, Rajaie Cardiovascular Medical and Research Center, Iran University of Medical Science, Tehran, Iran

Electronic supplementary material The online version of this chapter (doi: 10.1007/978-1-4471-6383-1_36) contains supplementary material, which is available to authorized users.

A. Sadeghpour et al. (eds.), *Comprehensive Approach to Adult Congenital Heart Disease*,
DOI 10.1007/978-1-4471-6383-1_36, © Springer-Verlag London 2014

ventriculo-arterial connection and VSD such as double-outlet right ventricle (RV) and transposition of great arteries [2].

Clinical Features

Subaortic stenosis is usually identified as secondary lesions in those cases with important associated lesions. Also other patients are referred with a systolic murmur for study. In patients with a gradient through their LVOT, there is an ejection systolic murmur heard alongside the lower left sternal border (LSB) with the lack of an ejection click [2].

Electrocardiography

Only it showes LV hypertrophy (LVH) if the obstruction is significant [1, 2].

Chest Radiology

CXR is usually unhelpful in these patients [1].

Echocardiography

Echocardiography is the present standard diagnostic instrument in this lesion, it not only can accurate delineation of the causes of obstruction, but it provides comprehensive data regarding related lesions. Generally, the parasternal long-axis view is key to providing a precise diagnosis (Fig. 36.1, Videos 36.1, 36.2 and 36.3).

The probable presence of mitral aortic discontinuity, the distance of a fibromuscular ridge to the AV, the occurrence of accessory obstructive tissue, and the sizes of the aortic annulus and root all are well imaged in this view. In addition, color flow mapping provides the documentation of associated AV regurgitation. The extension of a fibromuscular ridge to the anterior MV leaflet is best seen in the apical five-chamber view. This also permits the best site for pulsed or continuous-wave Doppler assessment of the maximum gradient across the AV and LVOT. Aortic regurgitation is seen in 40–60 % of patients mostly due to leaflet trauma from the high-velocity subaortic jet. Sometimes TEE plays a central role in defining the pathology (Fig. 36.2, Video 36.4) [1–4].

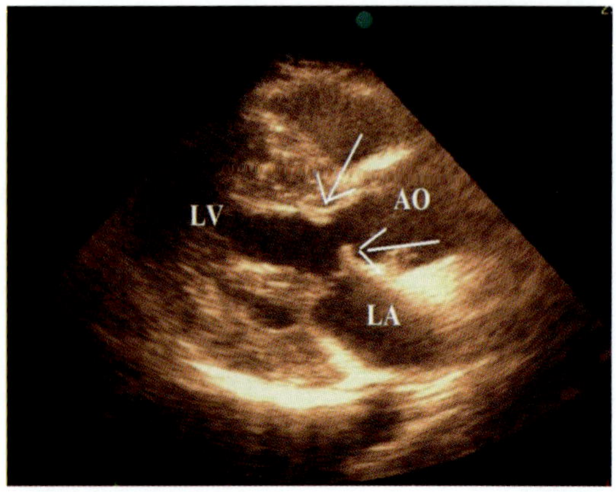

Fig. 36.1 Parasternal long-axis view showing a discrete fibrous ring encircling the left ventricular (*LV*) outflow tract with extension to the anterior MV leaflet (*white arrows*). *LA* left atrium, *AO* aorta

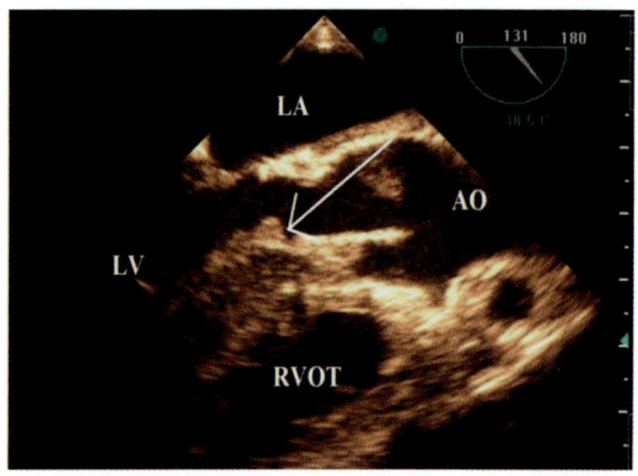

Fig. 36.2 Parasternal long-axis view in transesophageal echocardiography showing fibromuscular ridge encircling the left ventricular (*LV*) outflow tract (*white arrow*) with extension to the anterior MV leaflet. *LA* left atrium, *AO* aorta, *RVOT* right ventricular outflow tract

Cardiac Catheterization

This technique is not important in study of this lesion. Although balloon dilation has been tried, it is in general believed that this is a totally surgical lesion [4, 5] (Fig. 36.3).

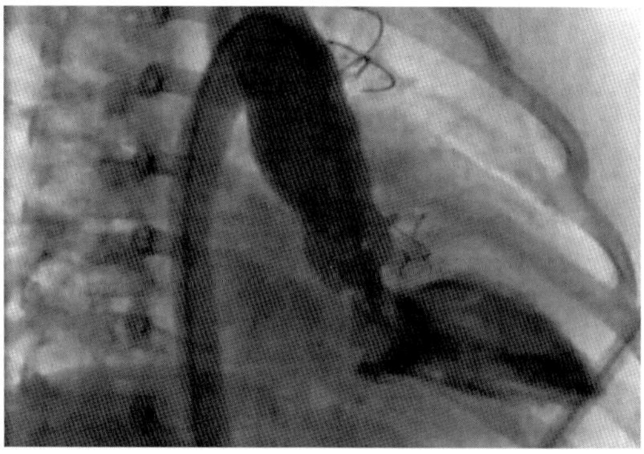

Fig. 36.3 LV injection showing fibromuscular narrowing in LVOT (Video 36.5)

MRI

Generally, MRI is unnecessary, except if there are some problems in obtaining the needed information by echocardiography [4].

Interventional Options

Subvalvular stenosis is mainly a surgical disease, and intervention is necessary. Sixty percent of patients with SAS are assessed in infancy and have undergone surgery by the age of 18. Intervention is best done by a surgeon familiar with the spectrum of subvalvular stenosis and its long-term outcome and complications. It is important that symptoms are not consistently indicative of the severity of stenosis [5–7]. A gradient of >50 mmHg has a poor outcome without treatment, and thus, even in the absence of symptoms, surgery and resection should be suggested when the peak gradient is significantly elevated. In general consensus from multiple surgical studies tends to favor earlier rather than later intervention (>30 mmHg mean gradient). Most procedures are successful in the short term, perfectly with no residual obstruction. Of course, more resection increases the risk of atrioventricular (AV) conduction block, injury to the MV leaflets or its support apparatus, or formation of a ventricular septal defect (VSD). For tunnellike stenosis, LVOT enlargement with placement of a patch is classic [6–8].

Outcomes and Follow-up

Immediate complications post-surgery consist of complete AV block, making a VSD, or mitral regurgitation from intraoperative injury to the MV apparatus. Long term complications consist of recurrence of fibromuscular subvalvular obstruction (up to 20 %). Significant aortic regurgitation is not uncommon (up to 25 % of cases). As a late outcome, in some cases with acquired AV stenosis, balloon dilation is the treatment of choice. Particular attention should be paid to cases with residual or recurrent subaortic stenosis or those with an associated bicuspid AV or important aortic regurgitation because they are most likely to need surgery finally. Endocarditis prophylaxis must be used for prosthetic valves or in the presence of any residual lesions [7–10].

References

1. Freedom RM. The long and the short of it: some thoughts about the fixed forms of left ventricular outflow tract obstruction. J Am Coll Cardiol. 1997;30:1843.
2. Karamlou T, Gurofsky R, Bojcevski A, et al. Prevalence and associated risk factors for intervention in 313 children with subaortic stenosis. Ann Thorac Surg. 2007;84:900.
3. Binet JP, Losay J, Demontoux S, et al. Subvalvular aortic stenosis: long-term surgical results. Thorac Cardiovasc Surg. 1983;31:96.
4. Vogt J, Dische R, Rupprath G, et al. Fixed subaortic stenosis: an acquired secondary obstruction? A twenty-seven year experience with 168 patients. Thorac Cardiovasc Surg. 1989;37:199.
5. Gersony WM. Natural history of discrete subvalvular aortic stenosis: management implications. J Am Coll Cardiol. 2001;38:843.
6. Dodge-Khatami A, Schmid M, Rousson V, et al. Risk factors for reoperation after relief of congenital subaortic stenosis. Eur J Cardiothorac Surg. 2008;33:885.
7. Geva A, McMahon CJ, Gauvreau K, et al. Risk factors for reoperation after repair of discrete subaortic stenosis in children. J Am Coll Cardiol. 2007;50:1498.
8. Giuffre RM, Ryerson LM, Vanderkooi OG, et al. Surgical outcome following treatment of isolated subaortic obstruction. Adv Ther. 2004;21:322.
9. Darcin OT, Yagdi T, Atay Y, et al. Discrete subaortic stenosis: surgical outcomes and follow-up results. Tex Heart Inst J. 2003;30:286.
10. Jahangiri M, Nicholson IA, del Nido PJ, et al. Surgical management of complex and tunnel-like subaortic stenosis. Eur J Cardiothorac Surg. 2000;17:637.

Supravalvular Aortic Stenosis

37

Anita Sadeghpour and Azin Alizadehasl

Keywords
Supravalvular aortic stenosis • Williams syndrome • Hourglass type • Echocardiography • Hypercalcemia

Morphology and Clinical Presentations

Supravalvular aortic stenosis (sup AS) is the least common type of congenital left ventricular outflow tract (LVOT) obstruction. In the most common type of sup AS, there is a fixed aortic narrowing originating from just above the sinus of Valsalva which extends along a variable length of the aorta (hourglass type); the membranous type is the result of a fibrous or fibromuscular semicircular diaphragm with a small central opening in the lumen of the aorta, and diffuse hypoplasia of the ascending aorta illustrates the third type [1].

The clinical aspect of sup AS differs from that observed in the other forms of congenital aortic stenosis. The main difference is the association of sup AS with idiopathic infantile hypercalcemia in the first years of life and it can be related with disturbed vitamin D metabolism; also, sup AS is common in patients with Williams syndrome that will be mentioned as follows. Otherwise, sup AS is usually diagnosed during evaluation for murmur. Adult patients may present with symptoms of LVOT obstruction, systemic hypertension, or myocardial ischemia (owing to insufficient coronary artery blood flow which in turn results from anatomical coronary artery obstruction or limited non-epicardial coronary flow due to myocardial hypertrophy) [1–3].

Findings on physical examination might include any of the unequal pulse volume between the carotid arteries, unequal blood pressures between the upper limbs (blood pressure in right arm > in left arm), left ventricular apical heave, palpable thrill in the suprasternal notch, normal S1, accentuated A2 with the narrowly or

A. Sadeghpour, MD, FACC, FASE (✉)
Echocardiography Lab, Department of Cardiology, Adult Congenital Heart Disease Clinic, Rajaie Cardiovascular Medical and Research Center, Iran University of Medical Science, Tehran, Iran
e-mail: anita.sadeghpour@gmail.com, asadeghpour@rhc.ac.ir

A. Alizadehasl, MD, FACC
Echocardiography Lab, Department of Cardiology, Rajaie Cardiovascular Medical and Research Center, Iran University of Medical Science, Tehran, Iran
e-mail: alizadeasl@gmail.com, alizadeasl@rhc.ac.ir

Electronic supplementary material The online version of this chapter (doi: 10.1007/978-1-4471-6383-1_37) contains supplementary material, which is available to authorized users.

paradoxically split of S2, fourth heart sound, and ejection systolic murmur best heard at the upper right sternal border radiating to the carotids but without an ejection click.

The discordance between the amplitude of the carotid and upper extremity arterial pulsations is caused by "Coanda effect" whereby when a high-velocity jet crosses through a curved obstruction, the direction of the blood flow curves and produces a preferential flow toward the direction of the obstruction [1, 3].

Williams Syndrome

Williams syndrome's picture is created by the coexistence of the cardiac problems in the setting of a multisystem disorder. Beyond infancy in these cases, there is a challenge with vitamin D and calcium-loading abnormalities and also feeding difficulties, failure to thrive, and gastrointestinal problems. The entire spectrum of clinical manifestations throughout their life includes auditory hyperacusis, inguinal hernia, a hoarse voice, a typical personality that is outgoing and engaging, intellectual impairment, narrowing of peripheral systemic and pulmonary arteries especially sup AS, strabismus, elfin facies, and abnormalities in dental development consisting of microdontia, enamel hypoplasia, and malocclusion.

The most common conditions can complicate the course of Williams syndrome including systemic hypertension, gastrointestinal problems, urinary tract abnormalities, progressive joint limitation, and hypertonia. Adult patients are usually handicapped. Williams syndrome was formerly considered to be nonfamilial; however, new information indicates that a genetic defect for supravalvular aortic stenosis is located in the same chromosomal subunit as elastin (on chromosome 7q11.23), and we know that elastin is an important component of the arterial wall [4, 5].

Electrocardiogram

The ECG manifestations of patients with sup AS depend on the severity of LVOT obstruction and the magnitude of coronary artery involvement. Accordingly, patients may show LV hypertrophy and secondary ST-T changes or ischemic abnormalities [5, 6].

Chest X-Ray

The chest x-ray is usually normal; however, there may be evidences of LV hypertrophy or asymmetry of the aortic knob [1, 6].

Echocardiography

This is a valued technique for localizing the location of stenosis in the supravalvular area (Fig. 37.1). Often the sinuses of Valsalva are dilated, but the ascending aorta and arch seem small or of normal size. Always, the size of the aortic annulus is more than that of the sinotubular junction. Color flow Doppler study is helpful for identifying the level of stenosis. In the supra-aortic stenosis, turbulent flow originates above the AV (Video 37.1).

Doppler study defines the site of obstruction but frequently overestimates the maximum gradient compared with that found in cardiac catheterization (due to pressure recovery phenomena) (Fig. 37.2) [5–7].

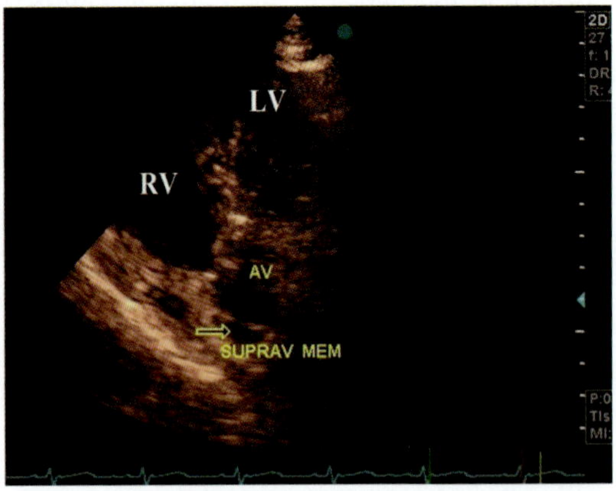

Fig. 37.1 Transthoracic apical 5-chamber view showing a discrete membrane above the aortic valve (*AV*), (Videos 37.2 and 37.3). *RV* right ventricle, *LV* left ventricle

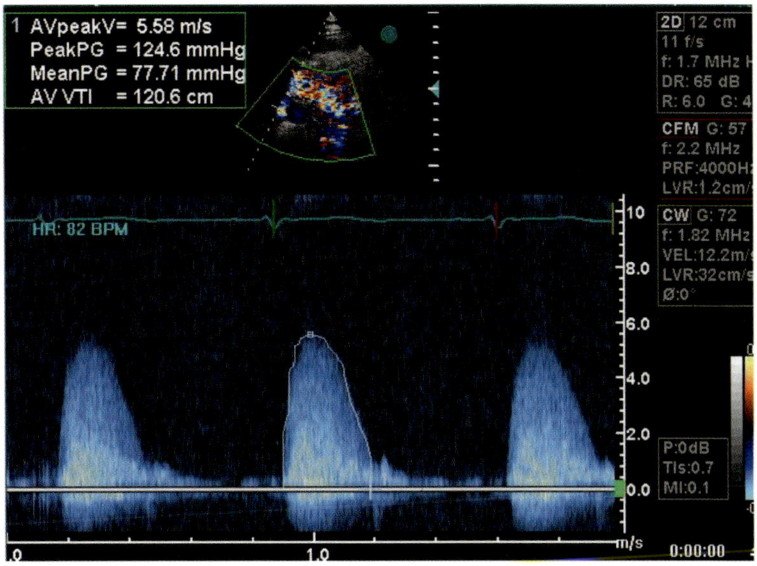

Fig. 37.2 Doppler study defines the site and severity of the obstruction but frequently overestimates the maximum gradient. The max velocity was obtained in suprasternal view

Other Noninvasive Imaging Modalities

MRI/CT also can be used for the assessment of anatomy of aorta and hemodynamic measurements across the obstruction. Assessment of coronary involvement can be performed by noninvasive stress testing or more accurately by myocardial perfusion imaging [5, 7].

Cardiac Catheterization

Cardiac catheterization can be used for delineation of the obstruction anatomy and accurate gradient measurements, as well as to define the status of the coronary arteries. Frequently it also involves a study of the pulmonary artery branches, also the brachiocephalic, renal, and mesenteric arteries; all of them can be stenotic. However, transcatheter balloon angioplasty is not a treatment option for these patients [5, 7].

Treatment

The obstruction (discrete or diffuse) in sup AS can be repaired surgically. No catheter-based techniques have been defined for this lesion. Percutaneous interventions may be applied for the treatment of coronary artery obstruction and also, sometimes, aortic valvuloplasty and subaortic resection in patients with sup AS [7–9].

References

1. Aboulhosn J, Child JS. Left ventricular outflow obstruction: subaortic stenosis, bicuspid aortic valve, supravalvar aortic stenosis, and coarctation of the aorta. Circulation. 2006;114:2412–22.
2. Micale L, Turturo MG, Fusco C, et al. Identification and characterization of seven novel mutations of elastin gene in a cohort of patients affected by supravalvular aortic stenosis. Eur J Hum Genet. 2010;18:317–23.
3. Warnes CA, Williams RG, Bashore TM, et al. ACC/AHA 2008 guidelines for the management of adults with congenital heart disease: a report of the American College of Cardiology/American Heart Association Task Force on Practice Guidelines (Writing Committee to Develop Guidelines on the Management of Adults With Congenital Heart Disease). J Am Coll Cardiol. 2008;52(23):e143–263.
4. Pober BR. Williams–Beuren syndrome. N Engl J Med. 2010;362:239–52.
5. Bonow RO, Carabello BA, Chatterjee K, et al. ACC/AHA 2006 guidelines for the management of patients with valvular heart disease: a report of the American College of Cardiology/American Heart Association Task Force on Practice Guidelines (Writing Committee to Revise the 1998 Guidelines for the Management of Patients With Valvular Heart Disease) developed in collaboration with the Society

of Cardiovascular Anesthesiologists, endorsed by the Society for Cardiovascular Angiography and Interventions and the Society of Thoracic Surgeons. J Am Coll Cardiol. 2006;48:e1–148.
6. Otto CM, editor. Textbook of clinical echocardiography. 4th ed. Philadelphia: Saunders/Elsevier; 2009.
7. Rosenhek R, Baumgartner H. Aortic stenosis. In: Otto CM, Bonow RO, editors. Valvular heart disease: a companion to Braunwald's heart disease. Philadelphia: Saunders/Elsevier; 2009. p. 127–54.
8. Vahanian A, Baumgartner H, Bax J, et al. Guidelines on the management of valvular heart disease: the Task Force on the Management of Valvular Heart Disease of the European Society of Cardiology. Eur Heart J. 2007;28:230.
9. Mc Elhinney DB, Petrossian E, Tworetzky W, et al. Issues and outcomes in the management of supravalvar aortic stenosis. Ann Thorac Surg. 2000;69(2):562–7.

Coarctation of the Aorta

38

Anita Sadeghpour, Azin Alizadehasl, and Mohammad Mahdavi

Keywords

Coarctation of aorta • Bicuspid aortic valve • Echocardiography • Shone syndrome • Aortic stenosis

Background

Coarctation of the aorta (CoA) firstly was described by Morgagni in 1760 during the autopsy of a monkey as a segment of constriction in the distal aorta [1]. Jordan (1827) and Reynaud (1828) provided more detailed pathoanatomic descriptions [2].

The CoA is a common congenital heart disease (CHD) which with a prevalence of isolated forms of ~3 per 10,000 live births accounts for 5–8 % of all CHD [3–5]. The word "coarctation" is taken from the Latin coartare, which means "to press together." The aortic stenosis in CoA may be either localized in a single segment (known as discrete lesions) or fusiform and elongated over a hypoplastic portion of its length with an irregular lumen (known as tubular lesions). However, the latter is less common and its origin is mostly assumed to be inflammatory or autoimmune; thus it may be a variant of *Takayasu arteritis*. The localized constriction may result from a shelf-resembling structure which has an eccentric opening or from a membranous and curtain-resembling structure with an eccentric or central or opening. From the pathological point of view, CoA is defined as a constricted or narrowed segment of aorta resulted by a localized medial layer thickening and medial layer and its superimposed neointimal tissue enfolding [6]. The exact causes of CoA are not known. The most common theories include [1] postnatal constriction in the aberrant ductus tissue and [2] intrauterine alterations of blood flow through the aortic arch.

From pathogenesis perspectives, all types of CoA can be called *juxtaductal*. Whatever the etiology, the present narrowing would restrict normal forward flow across the aorta.

A. Sadeghpour, MD, FACC, FASE (✉)
Echocardiography Lab, Department of Cardiology,
Adult Congenital Heart Disease Clinic,
Rajaie Cardiovascular Medical and Research Center,
Iran University of Medical Science, Tehran, Iran
e-mail: anita.sadeghpour@gmail.com,
asadeghpour@rhc.ac.ir

A. Alizadehasl, MD, FACC
Echocardiography Lab, Department of Cardiology,
Rajaie Cardiovascular Medical and Research Center,
Iran University of Medical Science, Tehran, Iran
e-mail: alizadeasl@gmail.com, alizadeasl@rhc.ac.ir

M. Mahdavi, MD
Pediatric Ward, Department of Pediatric Cardiology,
Rajaie Cardiovascular Medical and Research Center,
Iran University of Medical Science, Tehran, Iran

Electronic supplementary material The online version of this chapter (doi: 10.1007/978-1-4471-6383-1_38) contains supplementary material, which is available to authorized users.

A. Sadeghpour et al. (eds.), *Comprehensive Approach to Adult Congenital Heart Disease*,
DOI 10.1007/978-1-4471-6383-1_38, © Springer-Verlag London 2014

In the typical CoA, obstruction is located in the thoracic aorta, just distal to origin of left subclavian artery and at about the level of the ductus arteriosus insertion site. However, other parts of the aorta such as the transverse aortic arch and the ascending, descending, and abdominal aorta could also be involved. Currently, CoA is assumed to be a part of a generalized arterial pathology and not merely as a circumscribed constriction of the aorta which persists even after treatment as a lifelong disease.

Concomitant cardiac or noncardiac abnormalities could be seen in as high as 50 % of CoA patients [7–9]. Associated cardiac lesions can be found in bicuspid aortic valve (in up to 85 % of patients); supravalvular, valvular, and subvalvular aortic stenosis; mitral valve lesions such as parachute mitral valve stenosis (this complex is defined as Shone syndrome); patent ductus arteriosus; ventricular septal defects; complex CHDs including transposition of the great arteries; Taussig–Bing anomaly; double-inlet left ventricle; tricuspid atresia; hypoplastic left heart syndrome; and circle of Willis cerebral artery aneurysm (berry aneurysm). The latter predisposes affected patients to the cerebrovascular events. CoA may also be seen in a variety of syndromes including Turner syndrome, Williams–Beuren syndrome, Noonan and congenital rubella syndromes, neurofibromatosis, and Takayasu arteritis and also after trauma. Presence of CoA is extremely rare in patients who have severe right ventricular outflow tract obstructions including tetralogy of Fallot and pulmonary atresia with intact ventricular septum. CoA imposes a significant afterload upon left ventricle, which subsequently causes an increased wall stress with compensatory LV hypertrophy and LV dysfunction, and also numerous arterial collaterals would develop proximal to the obstruction. The presence of such abundant collaterals may reduce the pressure gradient thorough the coarctation site and decrease the obstruction severity. A poststenotic dilatation segment which is located immediately distal to the coarctation is usually seen. Several intrinsic abnormalities have been reported in the medial layer of ascending and descending aorta including early fragmentation of elastic fibers, fibrosis, and cystic medial necrosis [10], which may predispose these patients to increased stiffness of aorta and carotid arteries, blunted baroreceptor reflex, and also increased brachial pulse wave velocity and may be related to eventual aneurysm formation and aortic dissection [11].

Pathophysiology

The hemodynamic consequences of CoA depend on the obstruction severity, concomitant cardiac defects, and compensatory cardiovascular mechanisms. Only a little fraction of combined ventricular output (10 %) passes across the isthmus in the fetus, and thus, the minimum hemodynamic difficulties are seen. After birth, ductus arteriosus closes, and hence, several hemodynamic disturbances would develop, which range from systemic hypertension to congestive cardiac failure and cardiogenic shock. Obstruction in the aorta restricts LV output, leading to a significant pressure overload and increased LV end-diastolic pressure.

In the neonates, the development of the pressure load immediately after the ductus closure results in myocardial dilation and congestive cardiac failure symptoms. Myocardial dysfunction, decreased stroke volume, and cardiogenic shock may result from a severe obstruction. Several compensatory mechanisms are activated to improve cardiac output, which include the Frank–Starling mechanism, the renin–angiotensin system, and the sympathetic system [8]. However, these mechanisms may not be effective enough in the neonatal immature myocardium [12] which has lower ß-adrenergic receptor innervation and LV compliance compared with the adult myocardium. LV hypertrophy, as a compensatory mechanism, may also occur with chronic or gradual obstruction. Furthermore, patients with CoA exhibit several vascular abnormalities in the proximal and distal vessels to the obstruction [13]. The vessels proximal to the obstruction have impaired distensibility and enhanced reactivity to norepinephrine in the neonates and children with CoA [14–16]. In these patients plasma renin activity markedly increases and baroreceptor reflexes reset at a higher blood pressure [17, 18]. These abnormalities can persist even after surgical repair and are related to the development of systemic hypertension and premature coronary and cerebrovascular death.

Clinical Presentation

The clinical manifestation of CoA varies and depends on the severity of obstruction and associated lesions. Signs and symptoms of CoA present in early life in patients with serious stenosis, while in particularly mild cases, they may not develop until adulthood. In the neonates and infants, weak femoral pulses and upper-to-lower extremity difference in BP differentiate neonates with CoA [19, 20]. One of the most important differential diagnoses of shock in the neonatal period is left heart obstructing lesions, including CoA. Older children and adolescents exhibit more classic signs of CoA. Key symptoms may include headache, nosebleed, dizziness, tinnitus, shortness of breath, abdominal angina, claudication, leg cramps, exertional leg fatigue, and cold feet legs. Aortic coarctation may be diagnosed in the adult, usually during the work-up of arterial hypertension with discrepant upper and lower extremity pulses. Patients may come to medical attention because of headaches, leg fatigue, and claudication. The CoA may also be complicated by left-sided heart failure, intracranial hemorrhage due to rupture of berry aneurysm, infective endocarditis, aortic rupture or dissection, premature coronary or cerebral artery disease, and associated heart defects [21, 22].

Diagnostic Work-up

The classic clinical features include upper extremity systolic hypertension, relative to the lower extremities, albeit in the absence of an anomalous origin of the right subclavian artery, a blood pressure gradient between upper and lower extremities, brachial–femoral pulse delay, and palpable collaterals. However, in patients with an aortic obstruction of adjacent to left subclavian artery, left arm may not be hypertensive. Also, ACC/AHA 2008 Guidelines for Adults With CHD [23] recommend searching for the "brachial–femoral delay" and upper-to-lower extremity blood pressure gradient in every patient with systemic arterial hypertension (class I, *Level of Evidence: C*). Special attention should also be given to detect a parasternal or apical systolic ejection click reflective of an associated BAV with or without a systolic crescendo–decrescendo murmur of left ventricular outflow tract obstruction or an early diastolic decrescendo murmur suggestive of aortic regurgitation. Other findings may include suprasternal thrills, bruits in the left interscapular position (either due to the CoA or collaterals), continuous murmurs over the parasternal areas (mammary arteries) and around the left scapula (due to collateral vessels), hyperdynamic carotid pulsations, and, occasionally, palpable periscapular collaterals. Repair of aortic coarctation in the late childhood or adulthood often cannot prevent the persistence or late recurrence of systemic hypertension. Hypertension may reappear several years after coarctation repair.

Clinical Evaluation

Electrocardiogram

The electrocardiogram may demonstrate LV hypertrophy with a "strain" pattern of ST segment/T wave depression indicating subendocardial or myocardial ischemia (Fig. 38.1).

Chest X-Ray

Chest X-ray findings may include rib notching of the 3rd and 4th (to the 8th) ribs from collateral vessels, dilated ascending aorta, double contouring of descending aorta ("figure 3" sign) due to localized indentation at the obstruction site, and widening of the left subclavian artery (Fig. 38.2).

Echocardiography and Doppler

Transthoracic echocardiography should be applied in the initial imaging assessment and hemodynamic evaluation of patients with suspected CoA

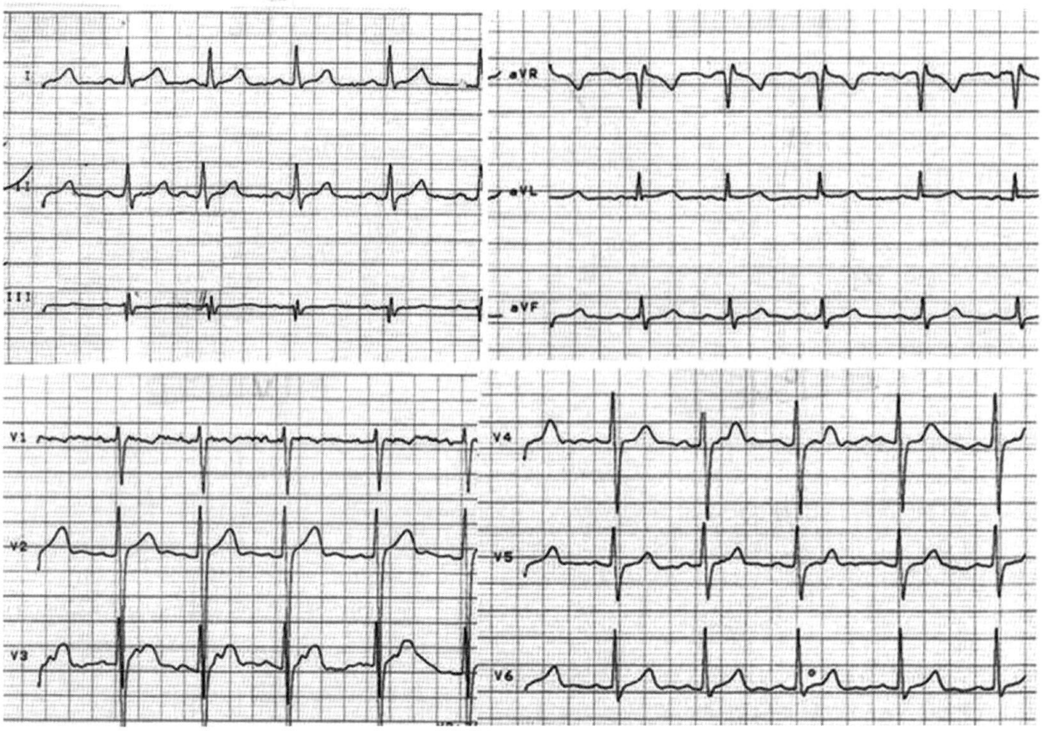

Fig. 38.1 Sinus rhythm and left ventricular hypertrophy, due to long-standing hypertension due to aortic coarctation

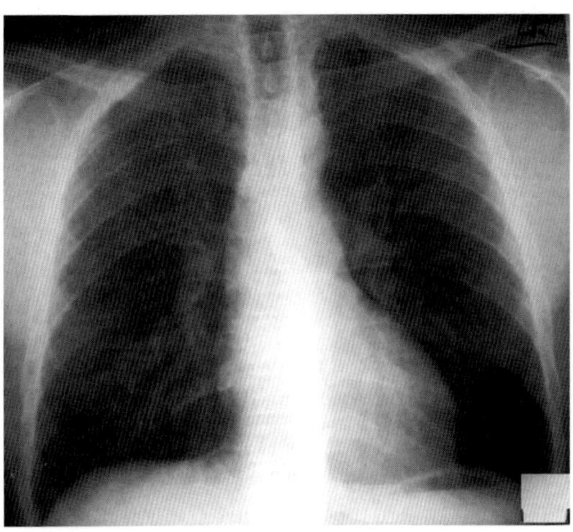

Fig. 38.2 "Figure 3" sign, rounded apex, and rib notching, denoting aortic coarctation

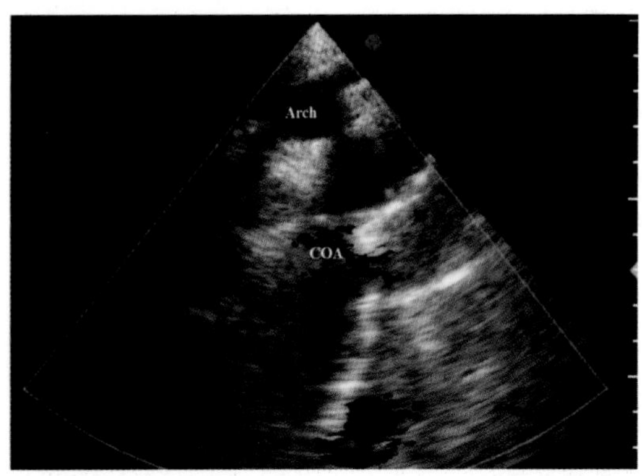

Fig. 38.3 The site of the stenosis may be seen properly in the suprasternal view (Video 38.1)

with making a particular attention to the suprasternal notch acoustic windows (class I, *Level of Evidence: B)* (Fig. 38.3).

The CoA may be diagnosed on suprasternal notch view of aortic arch and proximal descending aorta by a turbulent flow in the proximal descending aorta. However, the presence of extensive collaterals in the native coarctation and the lack of aortic compliance in the postoperative coarctation may limit the utility of Doppler gradient quantification in the assessment of the severity of obstruction. It seems that a diastolic "runoff" flow is the most reliable marker of significant coarctation or

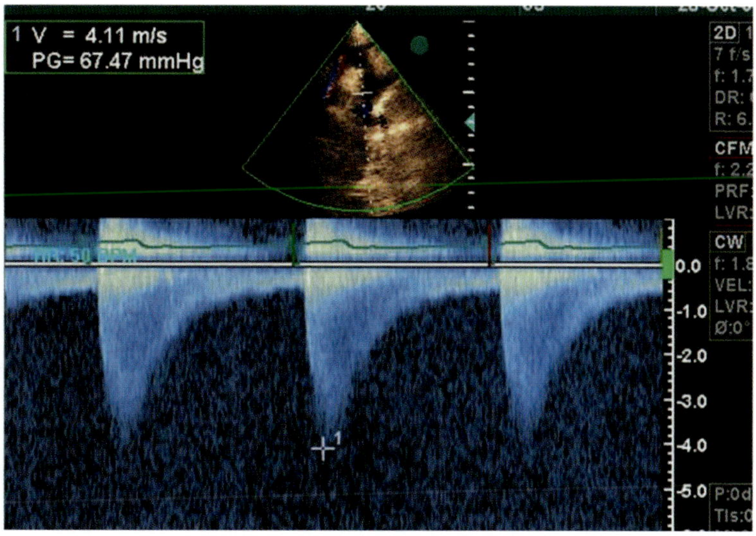

Fig. 38.4 In significant coarctation, there is a turbulent flow in the proximal descending aorta, and continuous-wave Doppler study will reveal increased velocity through the descending aorta, with a diastolic "tail" (high velocities maintained during diastole)

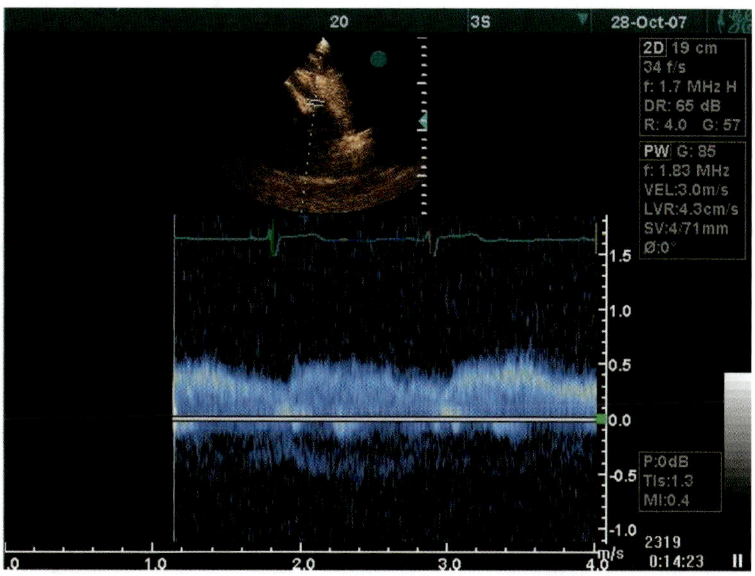

Fig. 38.5 Doppler flow study of the abdominal aorta demonstrating decreased pulsatility and absence of early diastolic flow reversal in the significant CoA

recoarctation (Fig. 38.4). A decreased pulsatility and absence of early diastolic flow reversal may also be demonstrated in the Doppler flow examination of the abdominal aorta (Fig. 38.5).

Echocardiography also aids in the assessment of LV size, mass, and function; the anatomy of the aortic valve and aortic annulus dimensions; associated cardiac abnormalities such as VSD, AS, and mitral valve deformity; and supra-aortic vessel diameters (Fig. 38.6).

So, the cornerstone of diagnosis remains echocardiography. As mentioned before, two-dimensional echocardiography can establish and confirm the diagnosis and delineate the site of obstruction and also associated lesions. Color flow Doppler measures the peak pressure gradient across the obstruction. LV dimensions and function are assessed by 2D echocardiography and M-mode.

Stress Testing

Stress testing may be useful in the assessment of exercise capacity, symptoms, rhythm, and

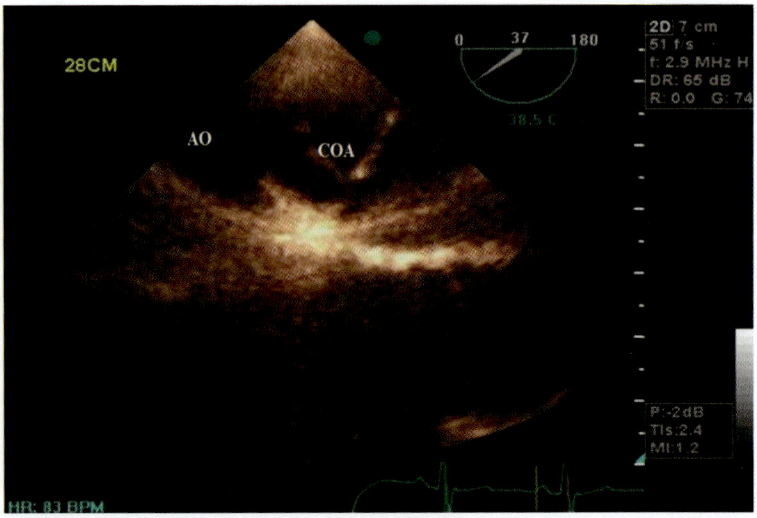

Fig. 38.6 Transesophageal echocardiography showing the CoA site proximal to the descending thoracic aorta (Videos 38.2 and 38.3)

electrocardiography in coarctation patients. However, the most important application of stress testing is to evaluate at rest and exertional systemic arterial blood pressure response, as a surrogate assessment of the CoA gradient.

Magnetic Resonance Imaging/ Computed Tomography with Three-Dimensional Reconstruction

Magnetic resonance imaging and CT angiography with three-dimensional reconstruction are the preferred noninvasive techniques to determine the precise location and anatomy of the coarctation, entire aorta, and collaterals [24]. Magnetic resonance angiography is able to quantify collateral flow. Magnetic resonance angiography may also be useful in the detection of aneurysms of the intracranial arteries. MRI-derived measurements have been shown to be in good correlation with cardiac catheterization gradients and can identify patients who are candidate for transcatheter or surgical treatment [25]. ACC/AHA 2008 Guidelines for Adults With CHD recommend that all patients with native or repaired coarctation should have at least one cardiovascular MRI or CT scan for the evaluation of the thoracic aorta and intracranial vessels (class I, *Level of Evidence: B*).

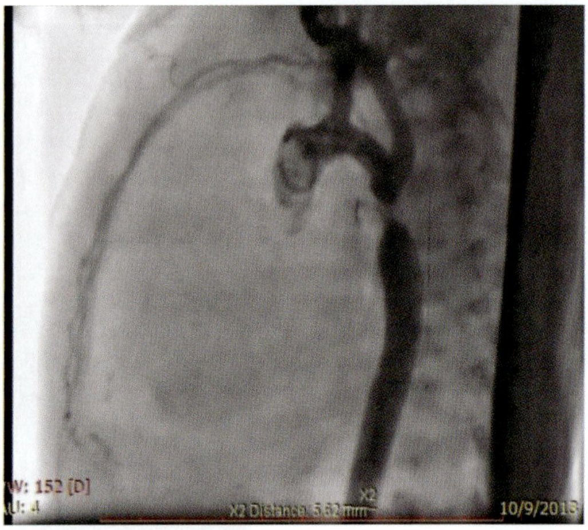

Fig. 38.7 Contrast injection in aortic arch shows discrete CoA with tiny PDA; the relevant movies are showing the balloon angioplasty steps of CoA

Catheterization Hemodynamics/ Angiography

Since MRI/or CT remains the preferred noninvasive means of imaging of the CoA area, a diagnostic cardiac catheterization is mostly required only when associated coronary artery disease is suspected and surgery is planned. However, angiocardiography is still the gold standard method for evaluation of CoA at many centers before and after interventional or surgical treatment (Fig. 38.7). Cardiac catheterization is also indicated for catheter-based interventions (angioplasty or stent implantation). A peak-to-peak gradient of 0.20 mmHg indicates a hemodynamically significant CoA in the absence of well-developed collaterals, while in the presence of extensive collaterals catheter-based gradients may not appropriately measure the severity of obstruction.

Treatment

Medical Therapy

Hypertension should be controlled by beta-blockers, ACE inhibitors, or angiotensin–receptor blockers as first-line medications, with respect to aortic root size, the presence of AR, or both.

Surgical/Catheter Interventional Treatment

In native CoA with appropriate anatomy, stenting is of first treatment choice in adults in many centers. For adults with recurrent or residual CoA, angioplasty with or without stent insertion may be effective [26].

Surgical techniques include the following: (1) resection and end-to-end anastomosis, (2) resection and extended end-to-end anastomosis, (3) prosthetic patch aortoplasty, (4) subclavian flap aortoplasty, (5) interposition of a (tube) graft, and (6) bypass tube (jump) grafts. Ascending-to-descending aorta conduits may be preferred in re-CoA repair in adults with difficult anatomy.

As CoA is a generalized disease of the aorta, concomitant problems which may require intervention include:

- Concomitant significant aortic valve stenosis or regurgitation
- Ascending aorta aneurysm with a diameter of 50 mm (27.5 mm/m^2 body surface area) or rapid increase in its size
- Aneurysm at the previous CoA area
- Symptomatic or large berry aneurysms (aneurysms in the circle of Willis)

Follow-up Recommendations

- At rest or exertional arterial hypertension is common in CoA patients. Arterial hypertension may persist even after successful CoA repair and is an important risk factor for premature CAD, ventricular dysfunction, and rupture of aortic or cerebral aneurysms [27]. The geometry of the aortic arch (such as gothic, crenel or normal) may affect the development of hypertension.
- Patients should be followed-up for the appearance or reappearance of at rest or exertional systemic arterial hypertension. In such cases, after the exclusion of recoarctation, arterial hypertension should be treated aggressively (class I, *Level of Evidence: B*) [23].
- Recurring or residual CoA may induce or deteriorate arterial hypertension and its complications.
- The development of aneurysms in the ascending aorta or the intervention location increases risk of arterial rupture and death [28]. Patients undergoing patch repairs (such as with Dacron) are at particular risk of developing an aneurysm at the repair site, and they should be regularly evaluated using imaging techniques [29].
- Patients should be assessed regarding the presence of associated BAV, mitral valve disease, premature CAD, and berry aneurysms of the circle of Willis. Even though most clinicians do not use routine screening in the asymptomatic patients.

All CoA patients should have regular follow-up at least every second year [29]. ACC/AHA 2008 Guidelines for the Management of Adults With Congenital Heart Disease recommend lifelong cardiology follow-up for all patients with native or repaired aortic coarctation (class I, *Level of Evidence: C*) [23].

However, ACC/AHA 2008 Guidelines for the Management of Adults With Congenital Heart Disease believe that patients who have undergone surgical repair/percutaneous intervention of CoA require at least yearly follow-up (class I, *Level of Evidence: C*) [23]. Depending on the anatomic findings before and after repair, CMR/CT imaging of aorta should be performed in all patients at 5-year intervals or less to evaluate the post-repair or post-intervention anatomy and complications such as restenosis, dilatation, or aneurysm formation (class I, *Level of Evidence: C)*, even in those with satisfactory repair (class I, *Level of Evidence: B)* [23].

Additional Considerations

Exercise/Activity

In patients without residual obstruction who are normotensive at rest and with exercise, no activity restriction is required, except for extensive static sports such as weight lifting at a competition level. In the presence of arterial hypertension, residual obstruction, or other complications, heavy isometric exercises should be restricted in proportion to the severity of the problems [29].

Pregnancy

In women with native and unrepaired CoA, with arterial hypertension despite successful repair, with a residual CoA, or with aortic aneurysms, pregnancy and delivery enhance the potential risk of rupture of the aorta and cerebral aneurysms [29]. However, following a successful repair of CoA, pregnancy can be tolerated without major complication [30].

Infective Endocarditis Prophylaxis

This is recommended for high-risk patients [29] with history of IE or those with a conduit insertion, stent implantation, or surgical repair in less than past 6 months. Patients with uncomplicated native CoA, successfully repaired CoA, and recurrent CoA do not require endocarditis prophylaxis.

References

1. Sinha SN, Kardatzke ML, Cole RB, et al. Coarctation of the aorta in infancy. Circulation. 1969;40:385–98.
2. Perloff JK. The clinical recognition of congenital heart disease. 4th ed. Philadelphia: WB Saunders; 1994.
3. Mitchell SC, Korones SB, Berendes HW. Congenital heart disease in 56,109 births. Incidence and natural history. Circulation. 1971;43:323–32.
4. Rosenthal E. Coarctation of the aorta from fetus to adult: curable condition or life long disease process? Heart. 2005;91:1495–502.
5. Kuehl KS, Loffredo CA, Ferencz C. Failure to diagnose congenital heart disease in infancy. Pediatrics. 1999;103:743–7.
6. Rao PS. Should balloon angioplasty be used instead of surgery for native aortic coarctation? Br Heart J. 1995;74(6):578–9.
7. Kiraly L, Kornyei L, Mogyorossy G, et al. Hypoplastic aortic arch in newborns rapidly adapts to post-coarctectomy circulatory conditions. Heart. 2005; 91:233–4.
8. Beekman RH. Coarctation of the aorta. In: Allen HG, Gutgessell HP, Clark EB, Driscoll DJ, editors. Moss and Adams' heart disease in infants, children, and adolescents including the fetus and young adults. 6th ed. Philadelphia: Lippincott Williams and Wilkins; 2001. p. 988–1010.
9. Paladini D, Volpe P, Russo MG, et al. Aortic coarctation: prognostic indicators of survival in the fetus. Heart. 2004;90:1348–9.
10. Niwa K, Perloff JK, Bhuta SM, et al. Structural abnormalities of great arterial walls in congenital heart disease: light and electron microscopic analyses. Circulation. 2001;103:393–400.
11. Kaemmerer H, Hager A, Hess J. Coarctation of the aorta in adults. SA Heart. 2007;4:4–12.
12. Friedman WF. The intrinsic physiologic properties of the developing heart. In: Friedman WF, Lesch M, Sonnenblick EH, editors. Neonatal heart disease. New York: Grune & Stratton; 1973. p. 21–49.
13. Gupta TC, Wiggers CJ. Basic hemodynamic changes produced by aortic coarctation of different degrees. Circulation. 1951;3:17–31.
14. Vogt M, Kuhn A, Baumgartner D, et al. Impaired elastic properties of the ascending aorta n newborns before and early after successful coarctation repair: proof of a systemic vascular disease of the prestenotic arteries? Circulation. 2005;111:3269–73.
15. Gidding SS, Rocchini AP, Moorehead C, et al. Increased forearm vascular reactivity in patients with hypertension after repair of coarctation. Circulation. 1985;71:495–9.
16. Gardiner HM, Celermajer DS, Sorensen KE, et al. Arterial reactivity is significantly impaired in normotensive young adults after successful repair of aortic coarctation in childhood. Circulation. 1994;89: 1745–50.
17. Parker Jr FB, Streeten DH, Farrell B, et al. Preoperative and postoperative renin levels in coarctation of the aorta. Circulation. 1982;66:513–4.
18. Johnson D, Perrault H, Vobecky SJ, et al. Resetting of the cardiopulmonary baroreflex 10 years after surgical repair of coarctation of the aorta. Heart. 2001;85:318–25.
19. Ward KE, Pryor RW, Matson JR, et al. Delayed detection of coarctation in infancy: implications for timing of newborn follow-up. Pediatrics. 1990;86:972–6.
20. Crossland DS, Furness JC, Abu-Harb M, et al. Variability of four limb blood pressure in normal neonates. Arch Dis Child Fetal Neonatal Ed. 2004;89: F325–7.

21. Campbell M. Natural history of coarctation of the aorta. Br Heart J. 1970;32:633–40.
22. Cohen M, Fuster V, Steele PM, et al. Coarctation of the aorta. Long-term follow-up and prediction of outcome after surgical correction. Circulation. 1989;80:840–5.
23. Warnes CA, Williams RG, Bashore TM, et al. ACC/AHA 2008 guidelines for the management of adults with congenital heart disease: a report of the American College of Cardiology/American Heart Association Task Force on Practice Guidelines (Writing Committee to Develop Guidelines on the Management of Adults With Congenital Heart Disease). J Am Coll Cardiol. 2008;52(23):e143–263.
24. Nistri S, Sorbo MD, Marin M, et al. Aortic root dilatation in young men with normally functioning bicuspid aortic valves. Heart. 1999;82:19–22.
25. Nielsen JC, Powell AJ, Gauvreau K, et al. Magnetic resonance imaging predictors of coarctation severity. Circulation. 2005;111:622–8.
26. Shah L, Hijazi Z, Sandhu S, et al. Use of endovascular stents for the treatment of coarctation of the aorta in children and adults: immediate and midterm results. J Invasive Cardiol. 2005;17:614–8.
27. Hager A, Kanz S, Kaemmerer H, et al. Coarctation Long-term Assessment (COALA): significance of arterial hypertension in a cohort of 404 patients up to 27 years after surgical repair of isolated coarctation of the aorta, even in the absence of restenosis and prosthetic material. J Thorac Cardiovasc Surg. 2007;134: 738–45.
28. Connolly HM, Huston III J, Brown Jr RD, et al. Intracranial aneurysms in patients with coarctation of the aorta: a prospective magnetic resonance angiographic study of 100 patients. Mayo Clin Proc. 2003;78:1491–9.
29. Baumgartner H, Bonhoeffer P, De Groot NM, et al. ESC guidelines for the management of grown-up congenital heart disease (new version 2010). Eur Heart J. 2010;31(23):2915–57.
30. Beauchesne LM, Connolly HM, Ammash NM, et al. Coarctation of the aorta: outcome of pregnancy. J Am Coll Cardiol. 2001;38:1728–33.

39 Sinus of Valsalva Aneurysm and Fistula

Anita Sadeghpour and Azin Alizadehasl

Keywords

Sinus of Valsalva Aneurysm and Fistula • Transesophageal echocardiography Ventricular septal defect (VSD) • Bicuspid aortic valve (BAV) • Coarctation

Morphology

This anomaly forms due to a lack or a separation between the aortic wall media and the aortic valve's annulus fibrosus. The delivery cardiac chamber of a right aortic sinus fistula is typically the right ventricle. However, infrequently, when there is noncoronary cusp involvement, the right atrium becomes the drainage location. The left aortic sinus is rarely involved. Related abnormalities consist of ventricular septal defect, bicuspid aortic valve, and coarctation of the aorta [1, 2].

A. Sadeghpour, MD, FACC, FASE (✉)
Echocardiography Lab, Department of Cardiology, Adult Congenital Heart Disease Clinic, Rajaie Cardiovascular Medical and Research Center, Iran University of Medical Science, Tehran, Iran
e-mail: anita.sadeghpour@gmail.com, asadeghpour@rhc.ac.ir

A. Alizadehasl, MD, FACC
Echocardiography Lab, Department of Cardiology, Rajaie Cardiovascular Medical and Research Center, Iran University of Medical Science, Tehran, Iran
e-mail: alizadeasl@gmail.com, alizadeasl@rhc.ac.ir

Clinical Findings

The congenital aneurysm of an aortic sinus of Valsalva, mostly the right coronary sinus, is a rare abnormality that is three times more frequent in men. Unruptured aneurysms typically do not produce a hemodynamic abnormal effect. Nevertheless, on rare occasions, coronary arterial compression causes myocardial ischemia.

The rupture is frequently sudden onset and gives rise to chest pain, continuous arteriovenous shunting, and acute volume overload of both right and left hearts and quickly results in significant heart failure. Another complication of note is infective endocarditis.

The occurrence of this abnormality should be suspected in a patient with a combination of sudden onset chest pain, resting dyspnea, bounding pulses, and loud and continuous murmur heightened in diastole. The physical findings may prove unable to differentiate this malformation from a coronary arteriovenous fistula [1–3].

Electronic supplementary material The online version of this chapter (doi: 10.1007/978-1-4471-6383-1_39) contains supplementary material, which is available to authorized users.

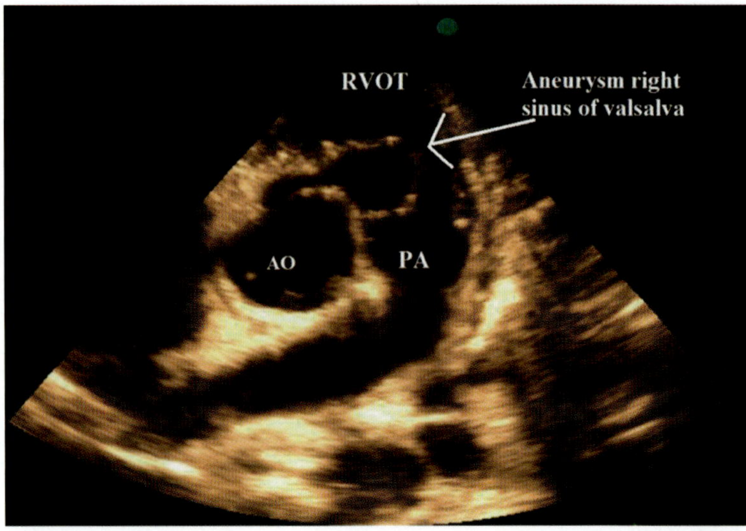

Fig. 39.1 Transthoracic echocardiography in short-axis view showing aneurysmal dilation of right sinus of Valsalva with protrusion to the RVOT. *RVOT* right ventricular outflow track. *AO* aorta, *PA* pulmonary artery

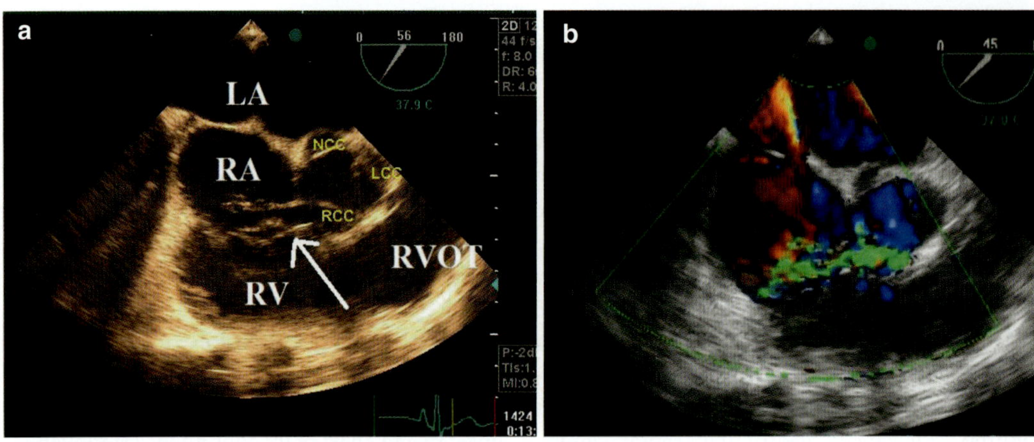

Fig. 39.2 (**a**, **b**) Transesophageal echocardiography in short-axis view revealed a "windsock" dilatation of the right sinus of Valsalva which is ruptured to the RA and color flow imaging showing continuous systolic-diastolic flow. *RVOT* right ventricular outflow track. *RV* right ventricle, *RA* right atrium, *LA* left atrium, *NCC* non coronary cusp, *RCC* right coronary cusp, *LCC* left coronary cusp

Electrocardiography

The electrocardiogram (ECG) is typically normal. On rare occasions, however, the ECG may reveal biventricular hypertrophy [3, 4]

Chest Radiography

Chest X-ray may show cardiomegaly and sometimes heart failure signs [1, 4].

Echocardiography

Two-dimensional and Doppler echocardiographic study can detect the aneurysm and disturbed flow in the coronary sinus as well as the site of perforation (Fig. 39.1, Video 39.1). Transesophageal echocardiography (TEE) may provide more precise information (Fig. 39.2a, b, Videos 39.2 and 39.3). About 90–95 % of the congenital aneurysm originates in the right or noncoronary sinus of Valsalva and project into

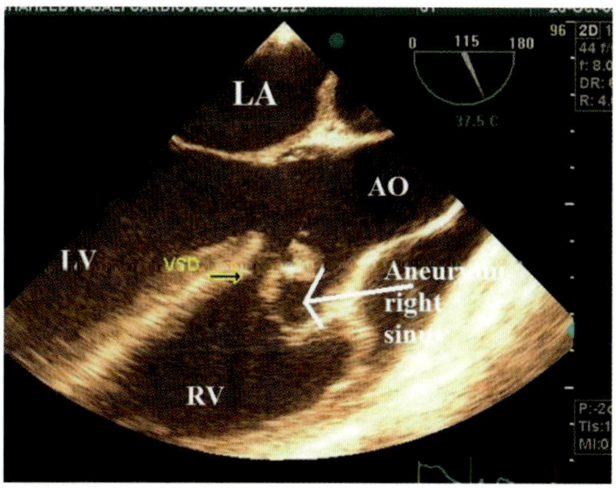

Fig. 39.3 Transesophageal echocardiography in long-axis view revealed a "windsock" dilatation of the right sinus of Valsalva which is ruptured to the RVOT (*white arrow*) and associated VSD (*yellow arrow*). *LA* left atrium, *LV* left ventricle, *AO* aorta, *RV* right ventricle

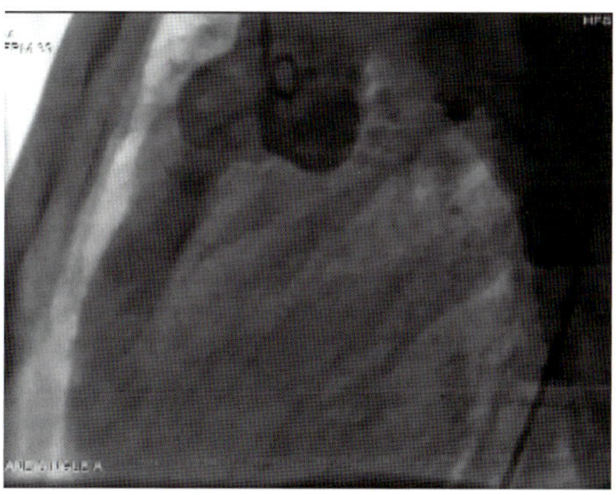

Fig. 39.4 Aortic root injection revealed rupture sinus of Valsalva to the right ventricle, Video 39.6

the RV or RA (Fig. 39.3, Videos 39.4 and 39.5). Aneurysm that arises from the noncoronary sinus ruptures into the RA, and those that arise from the right coronary sinus generally communicate to the RV and occasionally to the RA [5–7].

Cardiac Catheterization

This technique reveals a left-to-right shunt, mostly at the ventricular level (less frequent at the atrial level) (Fig. 39.4, Video 39.6) [8, 9].

Management

Preoperative management includes treatment for heart failure in conjunction with arrhythmias or endocarditis. Surgery consists of closing the aneurysm and repairing the aortic wall either with direct sutures or with prosthesis. Device closure of the ruptured aneurysm has also been reported [8, 9].

References

1. Komoda S, Komoda T, Ivanitskaia-Kuehn E, et al. Giant aneurysm of the right coronary artery and fistula to the coronary sinus. Gen Thorac Cardiovasc Surg. 2010;58:78–81.
2. Hoendermis E, Waterbolk T, Willems T, et al. Large common left and right coronary to coronary sinus fistula. Interact Cardiovasc Thorac Surg. 2006;5:778–9.
3. Gandy KL, Rebeiz AG, Wang A, et al. Left main coronary artery-to-pulmonary artery fistula with severe aneurismal dilatation. Ann Thorac Surg. 2004;77:1081–3.
4. Nakahira A, Sasaki Y, Hirai H, et al. Rupture of aneurysmal circumflex coronary artery into the left atrium after ligation of its arteriovenous fistula. Circ J. 2007;71:1996–8.
5. Davidavicius G, Subkovas E, Abraitis V, et al. Coronary anomalies: single center experience. Semin Cardiol. 2004;10:208–13.
6. Child JS. Echocardiographic evaluation of the adult with postoperative congenital heart disease. In: Otto CM, editor. The practice of clinical echocardiography. 3rd ed. Philadelphia: W. B. Saunders/Elsevier; 2007. p. 1083–109.
7. Snider AR, Serwer GA, Ritter SB. Echocardiography in pediatric heart disease. 2nd ed. St. Louis: Mosby; 1997.
8. Bricker AO, Bindu A, Mohammed TL. Valsalva sinus aneurysms: findings at CT and MR imaging. Radiographics. 2010;30:99–110.
9. El Watidy A, Ismail H, Calafiore AM. Surgical management of right coronary artery coronary sinus fistula causing severe mitral and tricuspid regurgitation. Interact Cardiovasc Thorac Surg. 2010;10:110–2.

Congenital Mitral Stenosis

40

Azin Alizadeasl and Anita Sadeghpour

Keywords
Congenital Mitral Stenosis • Parachute deformity • Supra valvular ring • Mitral valve regurgitation • Balloon valvuloplasty

Morphology and Associated Lesions

Congenital mitral stenosis (MS) refers to the parachute deformity of the valve. In this condition, condensed chordae tendineae join and attach into a single large papillary muscle, usually with thickened leaflets of the mitral valve (MV), fusion of the chordae tendineae, accessory MV tissue, and supravalvular ring of the connective tissue rising at the base of the atrial aspect of the MV leaflets. Associated cardiac lesions are common and consist of coarctation of the aorta, patent ductus arteriosus, left ventricular outflow tract obstruction, and persistent left superior vena cava [1].

A. Alizadeasl, MD, FACC (✉)
Echocardiography Lab, Department of Cardiology, Rajaie Cardiovascular Medical and Research Center, Iran University of Medical Science, Tehran, Iran
e-mail: alizadeasl@gmail.com, alizadeasl@rhc.ac.ir

A. Sadeghpour, MD, FACC, FASE
Echocardiography Lab, Department of Cardiology, Adult Congenital Heart Disease Clinic, Rajaie Cardiovascular Medical and Research Center, Iran University of Medical Science, Tehran, Iran
e-mail: anita.sadeghpour@gmail.com, asadeghpour@rhc.ac.ir

Clinical Findings

Findings and diagnosis are incidental in many cases at the time of the study for other left-sided obstructions such as coarctation of the aorta and/or aortic valve stenosis. The typical auscultatory findings seen with rheumatic MS are frequently absent in the congenital type of this lesion. Classic findings consist of normal S1 and mid-diastolic murmur with or without some presystolic highlighting [1 3].

Electrocardiography

In mild forms, electrocardiography is generally normal. However, there may be left atrial overload and enlargement, with or without right ventricular hypertrophy due to related pulmonary hypertension [1, 4].

Electronic supplementary material The online version of this chapter (doi: 10.1007/978-1-4471-6383-1_40) contains supplementary material, which is available to authorized users.

A. Sadeghpour et al. (eds.), *Comprehensive Approach to Adult Congenital Heart Disease*,
DOI 10.1007/978-1-4471-6383-1_40, © Springer-Verlag London 2014

Chest Radiography

Chest X-ray is normal in mild types, with signs of pulmonary edema in patients with more severe MS [1].

Echocardiography

Two-dimensional and more recently three-dimensional echocardiography, concomitant with color and Doppler assessment, generally provides a comprehensive study of the anatomy and function in patients with congenital MS. The form, shape, and location of the papillary muscles are best seen in the parasternal short-axis view. In congenital MS, if both papillary muscles are present, usually they are closer together than is seen in the normal heart. The four-chamber view and also parasternal long-axis view permit the diagnosis of supravalvular mitral rings. Color flow Doppler helps determine the level of stenosis and obstruction and also confirm the presence of MV regurgitation. Also, Doppler study provides a precise study of the mean gradient and pressure half time through the MV. 2D transthoracic echocardiography in parasternal short-axis view can determine the number of papillary muscles and mitral valve anatomy [1, 3–6] (Figs. 40.1a, b and 40.2).

Management

Clinical and echocardiographic follow-up is all that is required in asymptomatic cases. When the patient begins to have increased pulmonary pressure or develop symptoms, surgical approach is generally indicated. MV balloon valvuloplasty is not as successful as it is in rheumatismal MS. Surgery removes the supra-mitral ring if it is present. Also, the splitting of the papillary muscles and fused chordae is indicated in cases with more common types of congenital MS. In general, surgery provides short-term relief, with many cases demanding MV replacement later [1, 5, 6].

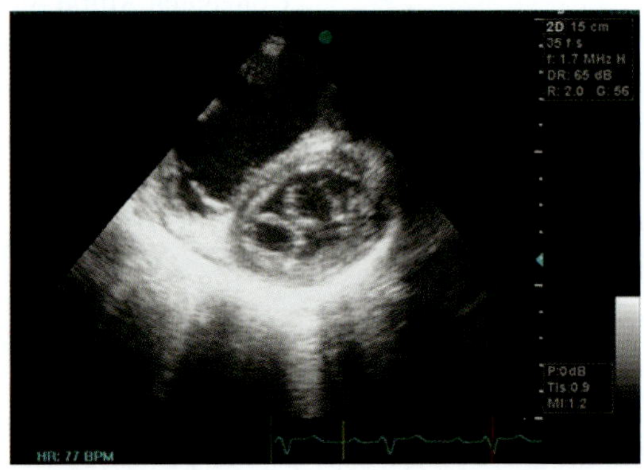

Fig. 40.2 Transthoracic echocardiography in short-axis view showing divided mitral orifice into two components *DOMV* double orifice mitral valve (Video 40.1)

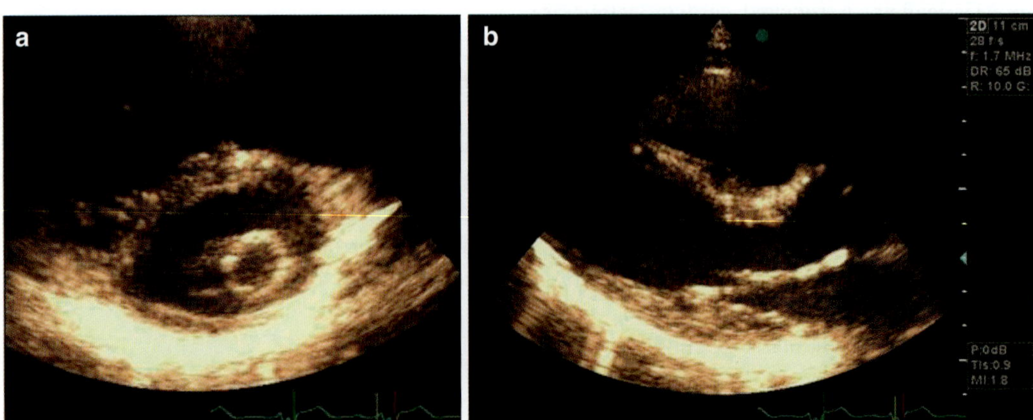

Fig. 40.1 (**a**, **b**) Parachute mitral valve with dominant anterior papillary muscle by 2D echocardiography in short- and long-axis views

References

1. Del Nido PJ, Baird C. Congenital mitral valve stenosis: anatomic variants and surgical reconstruction. Semin Thorac Cardiovasc Surg Pediatr Card Surg Annu. 2012;15(1):69–74.
2. Mc Elhinney DB, Sherwood MC, Keane JF. Current management of severe congenital mitral stenosis: outcomes of transcatheter and surgical therapy in 108 infants and children. Circulation. 2005;112(5):707–14.
3. Delmo Walter EM, Komoda T, Siniawski H, et al. Long-term surgical outcome of mitral valve repair in infants and children with Shone's anomaly. Eur J Cardiothorac Surg. 2013;43(3):473–81; discussion 481–2.
4. Brown JW, Fiore AC, Ruzmetov M, et al. Evolution of mitral valve replacement in children: a 40-year experience. Ann Thorac Surg. 2012;93(2):626–33.
5. Chauvaud S. Congenital mitral valve surgery: techniques and results. Curr Opin Cardiol. 2006;21(2):95–9.
6. Karaci AR, Aydemir NA, Harmandar B, et al. Surgical treatment of infective valve endocarditis in children with congenital heart disease. J Card Surg. 2012;27(1):93–8.

41 Congenital Mitral Regurgitation

Anita Sadeghpour and Azin Alizadeasl

Morphology

Simple Congenital Mitral Valve Regurgitation

This is commonly due to an isolated cleft in the anterior mitral valve (MV) leaflet or the effect of MV leaflets dysplasia with evidence of shortened and fused chordae. In patients with an isolated MV cleft, the defect in the anterior MV leaflet points toward the left ventricular (LV) outflow tract, not like in cases with atrioventricular septal defect (AVSD). As a rule, larger clefts in the anterior MV leaflet will create greater degrees of mitral regurgitation (MR).

In dysplastic MV cases, the chordae apparatus is shortened with variable degrees of dysplasia in both leaflets. Other anatomic deformities such as MV arcade cause MR. Of course, these are usually part of a generalized deformity of the left side of the heart [1, 2].

Complex Congenital Mitral Valve Regurgitation

This is seen more frequently concomitant with the abnormalities of the ventriculoarterial connection such as double-outlet right ventricle (DORV), VSD, and also corrected transposition (cc-TGA). In AVSD, it is common to have a cleft in the anterior MV leaflet with some deformities in the chordal support apparatus. In cc-TGA, the morphologic MV may have an accompanying cleft or be dysplastic or sometimes have multiple papillary muscles. All of these pathologies increase the risk for the MV to be regurgitant [2, 3].

Clinical Findings

Mostly, the signs and symptoms are related to the severity of the MR with different pathologies and also the associated lesions. Exercise intolerance and impaired functional capacity combined with an apical pansystolic murmur with or without a mid-diastolic murmur are the fundamental clinical findings [1–3].

A. Sadeghpour, MD, FACC, FASE (✉)
Echocardiography Lab, Department of Cardiology, Adult Congenital Heart Disease Clinic, Rajaie Cardiovascular Medical and Research Center, Iran University of Medical Science, Tehran, Iran
e-mail: anita.sadeghpour@gmail.com, asadeghpour@rhc.ac.ir

A. Alizadeasl, MD, FACC
Echocardiography Lab, Department of Cardiology, Rajaie Cardiovascular Medical and Research Center, Iran University of Medical Science, Tehran, Iran
e-mail: alizadeasl@gmail.com, alizadeasl@rhc.ac.ir

Electronic supplementary material The online version of this chapter (doi: 10.1007/978-1-4471-6383-1_41) contains supplementary material, which is available to authorized users.

A. Sadeghpour et al. (eds.), *Comprehensive Approach to Adult Congenital Heart Disease*,
DOI 10.1007/978-1-4471-6383-1_41, © Springer-Verlag London 2014

Electrocardiography

Electrocardiography is either normal or proves left atrial (LA) and LV overload [1, 2].

Chest Radiography

This shows cardiomegaly mostly involving the LV and LA [1, 3].

Echocardiography

Doppler and two-dimensional echocardiography provides a precise study of the mechanism and severity of MR. The cleft of the anterior MV leaflet is best seen in the precordial parasternal short-axis view (Fig. 41.1, Videos 41.1 and 41.2). Patients with a dysplastic MV have absence mobility of the valve leaflets and shortened chordae. Color Doppler study helps locate the site of MR and evaluate the severity of MR. Nowadays, three-dimensional echocardiography allows a comprehensive and detailed study of the MV apparatus and mechanisms of regurgitation. Catheterism and magnetic resonance imaging are rarely helpful in management planning [2, 4].

Management

Management plan is determined on the basis of the severity of MR and its influence on the LV function. Surgery should not be postponed until the patient has become symptomatic. For MV cleft, surgery includes suture of an isolated cleft, with or without coincident commissuroplasty. In cases with a dysplastic MV, repair surgery, including leaflet extension with an annuloplasty and commissuroplasty, usually creates effective control of the MR symptoms in the short or medium period. Nevertheless, many of these patients require MV replacement later [5, 6].

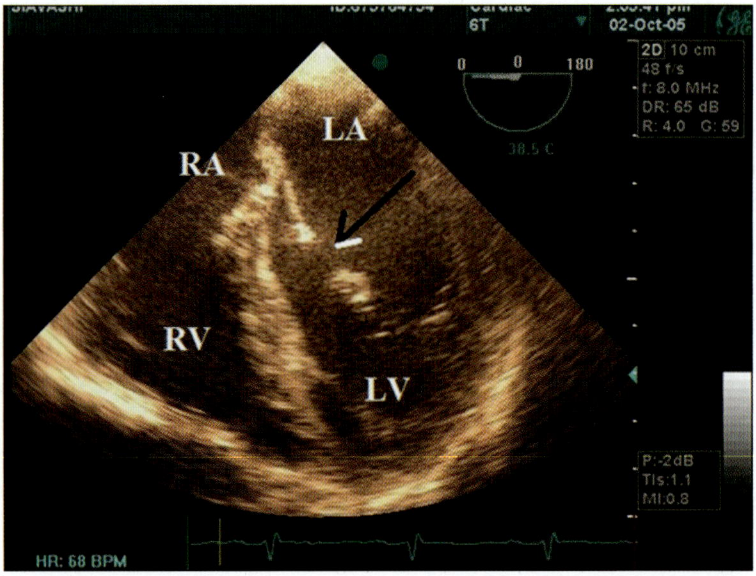

Fig. 41.1 Isolated mitral valve cleft as 2D defect in anterior mitral leaflet in transesophageal echocardiography

References

1. Ahmed MI, Mc Giffin DC, O'Rourke RA, et al. Mitral regurgitation. Curr Probl Cardiol. 2009;34(3):93–136.
2. Rahimtoola SH. The mitral valve is a complex structure. Foreword. Curr Probl Cardiol. 2009;34(3):89.
3. Park SM, Park SW, Casaclang-Verzosa G, et al. Diastolic dysfunction and left atrial enlargement as contributing factors to functional mitral regurgitation in dilated cardiomyopathy: data from the Acorn trial. Am Heart J. 2009;157(4):762.e3–10.
4. Macnab A, Jenkins NP, Ewington I, et al. A method for the morphological analysis of the regurgitant mitral valve using three dimensional echocardiography. Heart. 2004;90:771.
5. Oppido G, Davies B, McMullan DM, et al. Surgical treatment of congenital mitral valve disease: midterm results of a repair-oriented policy. J Thorac Cardiovasc Surg. 2008;135:1313–20.
6. Chauvaud S. Congenital mitral valve surgery: techniques and results. Curr Opin Cardiol. 2006;21:95.

Pulmonary Valve Stenosis

42

Anita Sadeghpour and Azin Alizadehasl

Keywords

Pulmonary valve stenosis (PS) • Intact ventricular septum • Ventricular septal defect (VSD) • Pulmonary atresia • Balloon valvuliplasty

Valvular pulmonary stenosis (PS) frequently presents with an asymptomatic systolic murmur but seldom with exercise intolerance. Mild PS is rarely progressive; however, moderate PS can progress to significant stenosis and secondary hypertrophy in the infundibulum; of coursc, this lesion exists as a continuum, ranging from isolated mild valvular PS to complete atresia of the pulmonary outflow tract [1, 2].

Morphology

The shape of the pulmonary valve (PV) in valvular PS patients varies from a tri-leaflet valve with variable degrees of commissural fusion to even an imperforate membrane. The right ventricle (RV) size is usually normal with different degrees of hypertrophy and sometimes mild hypoplasia [2, 3].

Clinical Findings

Adults with isolated mild to moderate PS usually are asymptomatic. But patients with severe PS may present with dyspnea, exercise intolerance, lightheadedness, and also chest pain (RV angina). Physical examination may show a prominent jugular A wave, an RV heave, and also a thrill on left sternal border (LSB). Auscultation reveals a normal S1, a single or split S2 with a weakened P2, and also a systolic ejection murmur that is best heard on the second intercostal space at LSB. Interestingly if the PV is thin and flexible, a systolic ejection click can be heard and decreases with inspiration. Importantly, as the severity of the PS increases, the interval between S1 and the systolic ejection click develops to be shorter, S2 becomes widely split, P2 weakens or disappears, and also

A. Sadeghpour, MD, FACC, FASE (✉)
Echocardiography Lab, Department of Cardiology, Adult Congenital Heart Disease Clinic, Rajaie Cardiovascular Medical and Research Center, Iran University of Medical Science, Tehran, Iran
e-mail: anita.sadeghpour@gmail.com, asadeghpour@rhc.ac.ir

A. Alizadehasl, MD, FACC
Echocardiography Lab, Department of Cardiology, Rajaie Cardiovascular Medical and Research Center, Iran University of Medical Science, Tehran, Iran
e-mail: alizadeasl@gmail.com, alizadeasl@rhc.ac.ir

Electronic supplementary material The online version of this chapter (doi: 10.1007/978-1-4471-6383-1_42) contains supplementary material, which is available to authorized users.

A. Sadeghpour et al. (eds.), *Comprehensive Approach to Adult Congenital Heart Disease*, DOI 10.1007/978-1-4471-6383-1_42, © Springer-Verlag London 2014

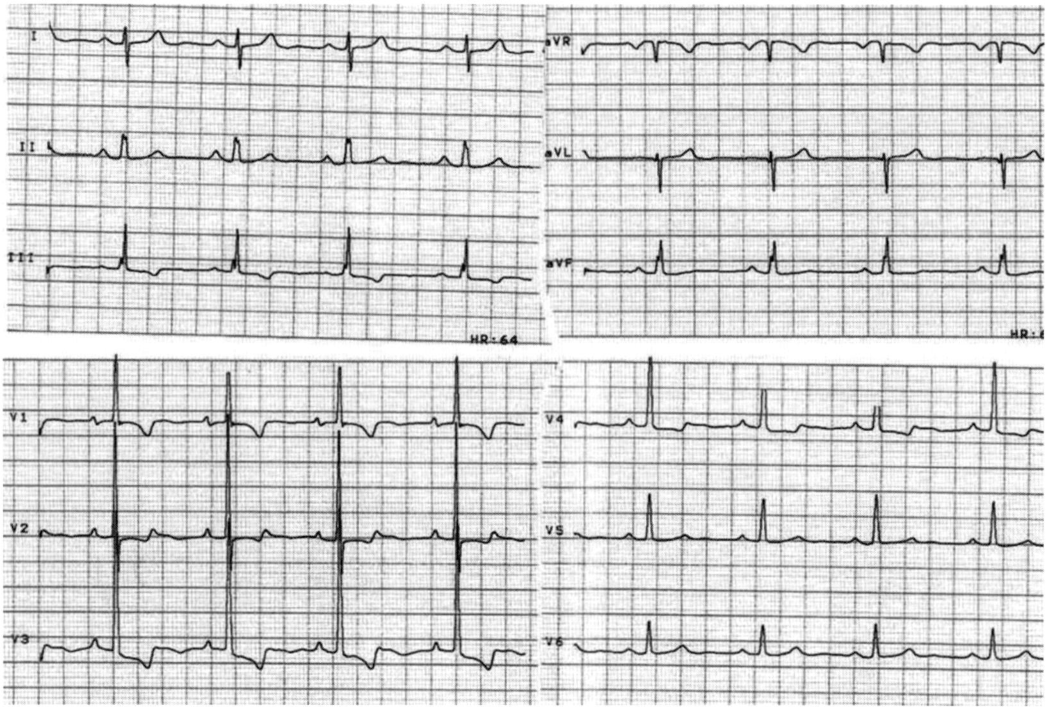

Fig. 42.1 Sinus rhythm, right axis deviation, right ventricular hypertrophy (pressure overload), and right atrial abnormality, suggestive of (1) pulmonary stenosis and (2) pulmonary hypertension

the systolic ejection murmur prolongs and peaks later, frequently till beyond A2. Cyanosis may be present when a PFO or ASD allows to right to left shunting. Atrial arrhythmias resulting from RV pressure overload and tricuspid regurgitation can occur [4, 5].

Electrocardiography

In adults the ECG findings depend on the severity of the PS. In milder PS, the ECG should be normal. As the stenosis progresses, ECG evidence of RV hypertrophy appears. Severe stenosis is seen in the form of tall R wave in lead V4R or V1 with a deep S wave in the V6 lead. The presence of RV strain pattern reflects the severe PS. If an rSR′ pattern is detected in lead V1, usually, lesser RV pressures are present than in patients with a pure R wave even with equal amplitude. Right atrial (RA) overload is related with moderate to severe PS [4, 6] (Fig. 42.1).

Chest Radiography

In adults with mild or moderate PS, chest X-ray often shows a normal size heart and also normal pulmonary vascularity. Poststenotic dilatation of the main and left pulmonary arteries is frequently seen. RA and RV enlargement is detected in patients with severe obstruction and secondary RV failure. The pulmonary vascularity is generally normal without a right to left atrial shunt but may be decreased in patients with severe PS and RV failure (Fig. 42.2) [5, 7].

Echocardiography

Combined 2D echocardiographic and continuous-wave Doppler studies characterize the anatomy of PV and PS severity, and essentially echocardiography has eliminated the requisite for diagnostic cardiac catheterization (Fig. 42.3a, b, Videos 42.1 and 42.2).

Though maximum instantaneous gradients have usually been used in choosing patients for balloon valvuloplasty (Fig. 42.4), recent data would suggest the mean Doppler gradients that correlate better with catheter-derived peak-to-peak gradients and with a value of 50 mmHg being the cut point to start the intervention (Videos 42.3 and 42.4). Invasive assessments are now used for balloon valvuloplasty [1, 8].

RV size, pulmonary artery pressure, tricuspid valve morphology and function, and also the status of the interatrial septum can be addressed by echocardiography (Fig. 42.5) [8, 9].

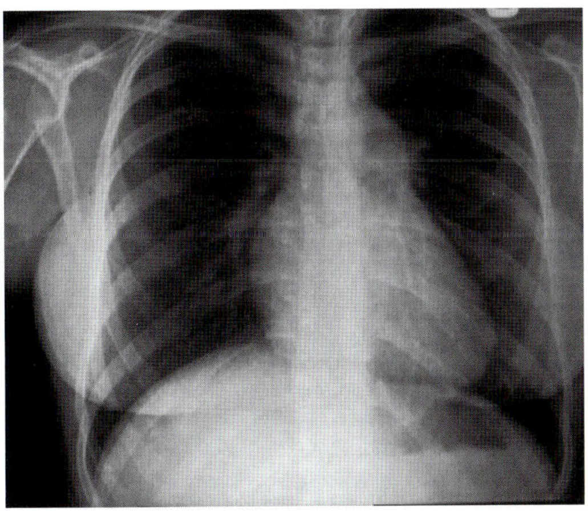

Fig. 42.2 Enlarged main pulmonary artery and left pulmonary artery with normal pulmonary blood flow, denoting severe pulmonary stenosis

Management and Follow-up

Balloon valvuloplasty is suggested when the gradient through the PV is greater than 50 mmHg at rest or when the patient is symptomatic (Video 42.6). Some patients undergo surgery, and despite the excellent survival results from the old studies (survival rate after surgical valvotomy of 95.7 %), recent long-term data indicates that these patients face more challenges. After a mean follow-up period of 33 years, 53 % of patients needed further intervention mostly due to severe pulmonary regurgitation, and 38 % of them had either ventricular or atrial arrhythmias [9–12].

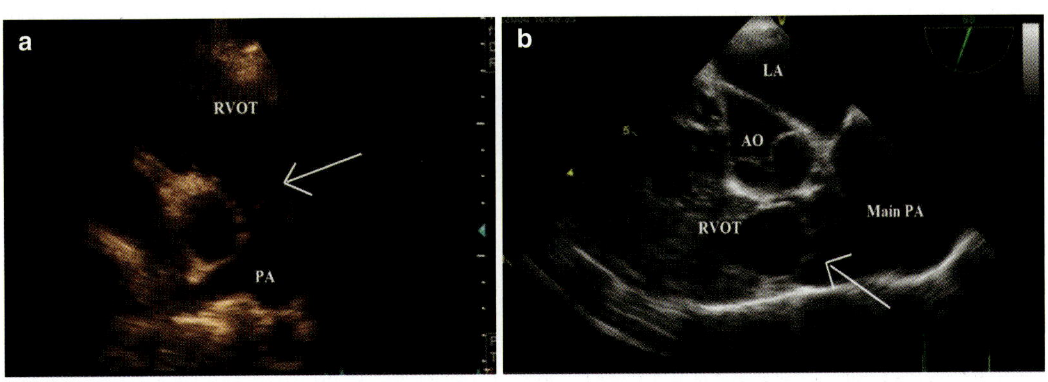

Fig. 42.3 (**a**, **b**) 2D echocardiography imaging of dome-shaped and stenotic pulmonary valve in both transthoracic and transesophageal echocardiography. *RVOT* right ventricular outflow tract, *PA* pulmonary artery, *LA* left atrium, *AO* aorta

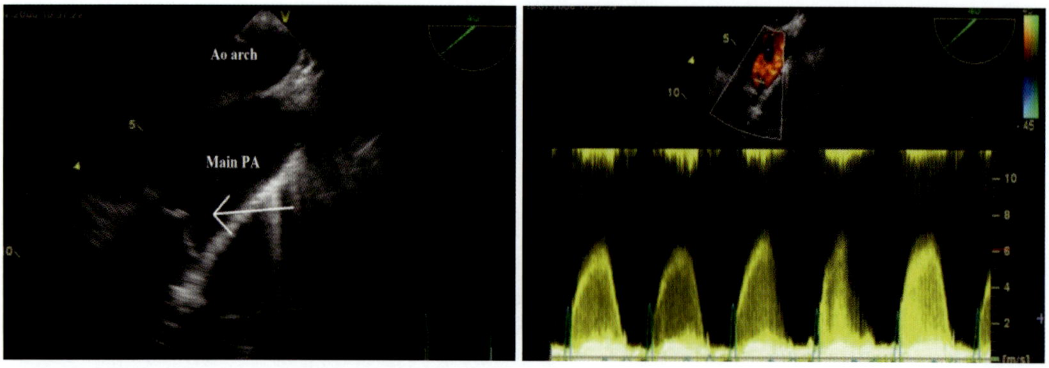

Fig. 42.4 CW Doppler study showing the maximum velocity which is obtained during TEE arch view. *Main PA* main pulmonary artery, *AO arch* aortic arch

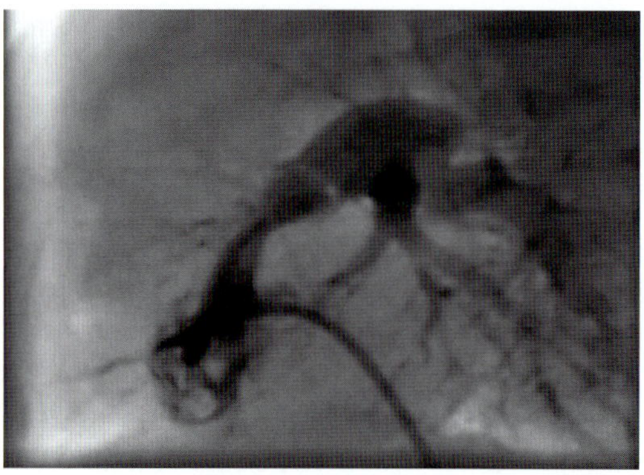

Fig. 42.5 PS: Injection was done by venous catheter at lateral view and in the hypertrophied RV showing doming in PV leaflets and poststenotic dilation, Video 42.5

References

1. Warnes CA, Williams RG, Bashore TM, et al. ACC/AHA 2008 guidelines for the management of adults with congenital heart disease. J Am Coll Cardiol. 2008;52:e1–e121.
2. Broadbent JC, Wood EH, Burchell HB. Left-to-right intra-cardiac shunts in the presence of pulmonary stenosis. Proc Staff Mleet Mayo Clin. 1953; 28:101.
3. Callahan JA, Brandenburg RO, Swan HJC. Pulmonary stenosis and ventricular septal defect with arteriovenous shunts: a clinical and hemodynamic study of eleven patients. Circulation. 1955;12:994.
4. BLount Jr SG, Imccord MC, et al. Isolated valvular pulmonic stenosis: clinical and physiologic response to open valvuloplasty. Circulation. 1954;10:161.
5. Rao PS. Pulmonary valve disease. In: Alpert JS, Dalen JE, Rahimtoola S, editors. Valvular heart disease. 3rd ed. Philadelphia: Lippincott/Raven; 2000. p. 339–76.
6. Gikonyo BM, Lucas RV, Edwards JE. Anatomic features of congenital pulmonary valvar stenosis. Pediatr Cardiol. 1987;8(2):109–16.
7. Campbell M. Simple pulmonary stenosis; pulmonary valvular stenosis with a closed ventricular septum. Br Heart J. 1954;16(3):273–300.
8. Silvilairat S, Cabalka AK, Cetta F, et al. Echocardiographic assessment of isolated pulmonary valve stenosis: which outpatient Doppler gradient has the most clinical validity? J Am Soc Echocardiogr. 2005;18:1137.
9. Bonow RO, Carabello BA, Chatterjee K, et al. ACC/AHA 2006 guideline for the management of patients with valvular heart disease. J Am Coll Cardiol. 2006; 48(3):e1–148.
10. Vahanian A, Baumgartner H, Bax J, et al. Guidelines on the management of valvular heart disease: the task force on the Management of Valvular Heart Disease of the European Society of Cardiology. Eur Heart J. 2007;28(2):230–68.
11. Karagoz T, Asoh K, Hickey E, et al. Balloon dilation of pulmonary valve stenosis in infants less than 3 kg: a 20-year experience. Catheter Cardiovasc Interv. 2009;74:753.
12. Earing MG, Connolly HM, Dearani JA, et al. Long-term follow-up of patients after surgical treatment for isolated pulmonary valve stenosis. Mayo Clin Proc. 2005;80:871.

Dysplastic Pulmonary Valve Stenosis

43

Azin Alizadehasl and Majid Kyavar

Keywords
Dysplastic pulmonary valve stenosis • Noonan syndrome • Hypertrophic cardiomyopathy • Echocardiography • Balloon valvuloplasty

Morphology

Hypoplasia of the pulmonary valve (PV) ring and dysplastic PV may exist in rare patients. PV dysplasia is described by thickened and nodular valvular leaflets with no or minimal commissural fusion, hypoplasia of the valve ring, and absence of poststenotic dilation of the pulmonary artery (PA). This entity is associated with the Noonan syndrome, which in turn may be allied to hypertrophic cardiomyopathy [1, 2].

A. Alizadehasl, MD, FACC (✉)
Echocardiography Lab, Department of Cardiology, Rajaie Cardiovascular Medical and Research Center, Iran University of Medical Science, Tehran, Iran
e-mail: alizadeasl@gmail.com, alizadeasl@rhc.ac.ir

M. Kyavar, MD, FACC
Cardiovascular Imaging Ward, Department of Cardiology, Adult Congenital Heart Disease Clinic, Rajaie Cardiovascular Medical and Research Center, Iran University of Medical Science, Tehran, Iran
e-mail: kiavar@rhc.ac.ir

Clinical Findings

At presentation time, the patient's age is associated with the severity of the stenosis. If the obstruction is severe, the patient may develop symptoms in the neonatal period or in infancy. However, the patient with mild stenosis may present in childhood only with asymptomatic murmurs. The auscultatory finding that differentiates dysplastic valves from simple PV stenosis is the lack of an ejection click. Infants with the Noonan syndrome have short stature, webbed necks, and broad-shaped chests in a style similar to the Turner syndrome. Another unique association in the newborn is pulmonary lymphangiectasia [2, 3].

Adults can be asymptomatic regardless of the degree of their stenosis. However, cases with severe stenosis can present with signs and symptoms of systemic venous congestion, which are similar to the signs of congestive heart failure (CHF). Other possible signs are findings of severe right ventricular (RV) dysfunction or sometimes cyanosis related to a right to left shunt through a patent foramen ovale (PFO) or an atrial septal defect (ASD).

A. Sadeghpour et al. (eds.), *Comprehensive Approach to Adult Congenital Heart Disease*,
DOI 10.1007/978-1-4471-6383-1_43, © Springer-Verlag London 2014

Lightheadedness, syncope, and also chest pain are infrequent; even many cases with moderate or severe pulmonary stenosis (PS) remain asymptomatic [2, 3].

Paraclinical Findings

Chest Radiography

The findings are similar to typical PV stenosis, except for the lack of poststenotic pulmonary artery dilation, even in the presence of severe stenosis. In those with pulmonary lymphangiectasia, the chest radiograph has a ground-glass appearance, which can be difficult to discriminate from pulmonary veins stenosis [3, 4].

Electrocardiography

- Electrocardiography (ECG) findings are frequently normal in mild PS.
- Right-axis deviation and RV hypertrophy happen in moderate and severe PV stenosis.
- Interestingly, the degree of RV hypertrophy is well associated with the severity of PV stenosis.
- There is a good correlation between the height of the R wave in lead V1 and RV peak systolic pressure: the height of the R wave in V1 in mm multiplied by 5 is predictive of RV peak systolic pressure. So, the ECG is a useful noninvasive tool for the assessment of the severity of pulmonary stenosis.
- A superior QRS axis (left-axis deviation) is seen with dysplastic PV and the Noonan syndrome [1, 4–6].

Echocardiography

Echocardiography proves a thickened plump PV, absence of poststenotic dilation, and varying degrees of supravalvular pulmonary stenosis. Doppler echocardiography can define the severity of the obstruction quite well.

The related finding of hypertrophic cardiomyopathy can be confirmed or excluded. If the first echocardiography does not confirm hypertrophic cardiomyopathy, additional studies must be undertaken throughout childhood and adolescence, especially in cases with left-axis deviation [2, 6].

Computed Tomography and Magnetic Resonance Imaging

Computed tomography and magnetic resonance imaging may reveal PV stenosis, but state-of-the-art echocardiography and Doppler studies are more beneficial than CT or MRI in the diagnosis and measurement of PV obstruction [4, 6].

Management

Balloon Valvuloplasty

Although the results of balloon valvuloplasty are less satisfying in dysplastic pulmonary stenosis than in valvular pulmonary stenosis due to commissural fusion, it is worth trying before considering the surgical approach. Furthermore, there are patients that suffer a drop in their gradient, which can postpone surgery [7, 8].

Surgery

If balloon valvuloplasty fails, surgical intervention should be contemplated. This typically comprises a partial valvectomy in combination with patch repair of the supravalvular stenosis.

Adequate relief of the obstruction confers an excellent outlook. The most significant long-term risk factor is the occurrence of hypertrophic cardiomyopathy [7, 8].

References

1. Rao PS. Pulmonary valve disease. In: Alpert JS, Dalen JE, Rahimtoola S, editors. Valvular heart disease. 3rd ed. Philadelphia: Lippincott Raven; 2000. p. 339–76.
2. Gikonyo BM, Lucas RV, Edwards JE. Anatomic features of congenital pulmonary valvar stenosis. Pediatr Cardiol. 1987;8(2):109–16.

3. Koretzky ED, Moller JH, Korns ME, et al. Congenital pulmonary stenosis resulting from dysplasia of valve. Circulation. 1969;40(1):43–53.
4. Jeffery RF, Moller JH, Amplatz K. The dysplastic pulmonary valve: a new roentgenographic entity; with a discussion of the anatomy and radiology of other types of valvular pulmonary stenosis. Am J Roentgenol Radium Ther Nucl Med. 1972;114(2):322–39.
5. Ettinger SJ, Feldman EC. Textbook of veterinary internal medicine. 4th ed. Philadelphia: W.B. Saunders; 1995.
6. Silvilairat S, Cabalka AK, Cetta F, et al. Echocardiographic assessment of isolated pulmonary valve stenosis: which outpatient Doppler gradient has the most clinical validity? J Am Soc Echocardiogr. 2005;18:1137.
7. Karagoz T, Asoh K, Hickey E, et al. Balloon dilation of pulmonary valve stenosis in infants less than 3 kg: a 20-year experience. Catheter Cardiovasc Interv. 2009;74:753.
8. Earing MG, Connolly HM, Dearani JA, et al. Long-term follow-up of patients after surgical treatment for isolated pulmonary valve stenosis. Mayo Clin Proc. 2005;80:871.1.

Peripheral Pulmonary Artery Stenosis

44

Azin Alizadehasl and Anita Sadeghpour

Keywords
Peripheral Pulmonary Artery Stenosis • Main pulmonary artery (PA) Pulmonary atresia • Intact ventricular septum • Right ventricular hypertrophy (RVH)

Morphology

In addition to isolated stenosis in the main pulmonary artery (PA) and its central branches, the stenosis is routinely diffuse and bilateral and extend into the mediastinal or hilar and even the intraparenchymal pulmonary arteries. The term peripheral PA stenosis deals with PA stenosis and an intact ventricular septum, so tetralogy of Fallot and pulmonary atresia with a VSD are excluded [1, 2].

Clinical and Paraclinical Findings

Clinical severity is determined by the degree of obstruction. Most of these patients are asymptomatic. The pulmonic part of the second heart sound (S2) may be accentuated only if there is pulmonary hypertension (PH) proximal to stenosis. An ejection systolic murmur is heard at the upper left sternal border (LSB) and transmitted to the back and axilla. A continuous murmur is often audible in patients with significant branch stenosis due to aortopulmonary collateral formation [3, 4].

In electrocardiography right ventricular (RV) hypertrophy is seen when obstruction is severe.

In chest radiography mild or moderate peripheral PA stenosis frequently creates normal findings. Obvious differences in vascularity among lung regions are unusual. When obstruction is severe and diffuse, right atrial and RV enlargement may be seen [4, 5].

Echocardiography is useful in making the diagnosis and also excluding the related lesions;

A. Alizadehasl, MD, FACC (✉)
Echocardiography Lab, Department of Cardiology, Rajaie Cardiovascular Medical and Research Center, Iran University of Medical Science, Tehran, Iran
e-mail: alizadeasl@gmail.com, alizadeasl@rhc.ac.ir

A. Sadeghpour, MD, FACC, FASE
Echocardiography Lab, Department of Cardiology, Adult Congenital Heart Disease Clinic, Rajaie Cardiovascular Medical and Research Center, Iran University of Medical Science, Tehran, Iran
e-mail: anita.sadeghpour@gmail.com, asadeghpour@rhc.ac.ir

Electronic supplementary material The online version of this chapter (doi: 10.1007/978-1-4471-6383-1_44) contains supplementary material, which is available to authorized users.

A. Sadeghpour et al. (eds.), *Comprehensive Approach to Adult Congenital Heart Disease*,
DOI 10.1007/978-1-4471-6383-1_44,

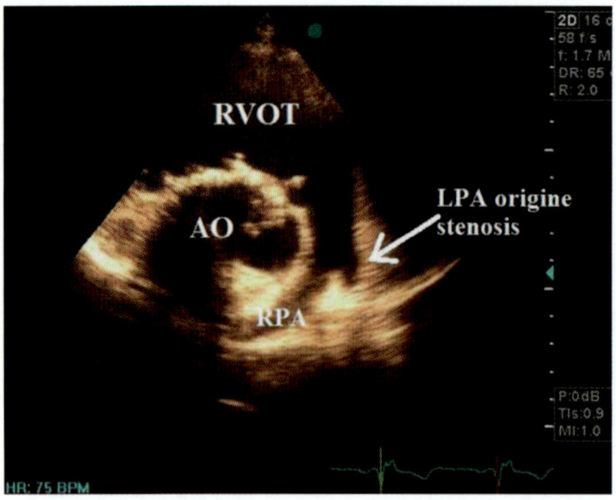

Fig. 44.1 Left PA origin stenosis detected in 2D echocardiography which should be confirmed by CFI and Doppler study. Echocardiography is useful in making the diagnosis of proximal stenosis of PA branches and also excluding the related lesions. *Ao* aorta, *RVOT* right ventricular outflow tract, *RPA* right pulmonary artery

but it is limited in imaging the distal PA branches [1, 6] (Fig. 44.1 and Videos 44.1 and 44.2).

RV pressure study can be evaluated by tricuspid valve regurgitation flow gradient CMR and spiral CT are valued diagnostic tests, cause they let a more detailed distal evaluation of the branch PAs. Though many patients need cardiac catheterization and angiography, these other techniques are outstanding for the initial study and for following the progress of the lesions' severity [6–8].

The radionuclide quantitative lung perfusion scan is valuable in instances with unilateral stenosis to define whether and which intervention is required.

Cardiac catheterization and angiocardiography permits the evaluation of RV pressure and the pressures in the pulmonary arterial tree, and also this method lets to precisely study the severity and extent of the stenosis [7, 8].

Management

Balloon dilation with or without stent for cases with significant isolated left PA stenosis is effective to relieve the obstruction; however, in cases with more severe and diffuse bilateral stenoses, the indications for intervention are subject to RV pressure. Interventions also depend on the part and extent of the lesion and the dilation capability of the stenosis. In some cases, several attempts at dilation are required to achieve any improvement in vessel caliber. As a rule, surgery has a little value in patients with diffuse peripheral PA stenosis and can certainly make the condition worse [1, 5, 9, 10].

References

1. Gyllenswärd Å, Lodin H, Lundberg Å, et al. Congenital multiple peripheral stenoses of the pulmonary artery. Pediatrics. 1957;19:399.
2. Arvidsson H, Karnell J, Moller T. Multiple stenoses of the pulmonary arteries associated with pulmonary hypertension, diagnosed by selective angiography. Actaradiology. 1955;44:209.
3. Luan LL, D'Silva JL, Gasul BM, et al. Stenosis of the right main pulmonary artery. Clinical, angiocardiographic and catheterization findings in ten patients. Circulation. 1960;21:1116.
4. Emery JL, Mithal A. The number of alveoli in the terminal respiratory unit of man during late intrauterine life and childhood. Arch Dis Child. 1960;35:544–7.
5. Mac Mahon HE, Lee H, et al. Congenital segmental coarctation of pulmonary arteries. An anatomic study. Am J Pathol. 1967;50:15–20.
6. Ishikawa H, Kondo Y, Yusa Y, et al. An autopsy case of ulcerative colitis associated with Takayasu's disease with a review of 13 Japanese cases. Gastroenterol Jpn. 1993;28:110–7.
7. Erkan F, Cavdar T. Pulmonary vasculitis in Behçet's disease. Am Rev Respir Dis. 1992;146:232–9.
8. Almog Y, Polliack G, DranitzkiElhalel M, et al. Bilateral pulmonary artery aneurysms in Behçet's disease. Eur Respir J. 1993;6:1067–9.
9. Gonon M, Soler M, Bollinger CT, Imhof E, Elsasser S, Dalquen P, et al. Schwere Hämoptoe bei pulmonaler Vaskulitis. Dtsch Med Wochenschr. 1993;118:457–62.
10. Hamurydan V, Yurdakul S, Moral F, et al. Pulmonary arterial aneurysms in Behçet's syndrome: a report of 24 cases. Br J Rheumatol. 1994;33:48–51.

45 Subpulmonary Right Ventricular Outflow Tract Obstruction and Double-Chambered Right Ventricle

Anita Sadeghpour and Azin Alizadehasl

Keywords
Right ventricular outflow tract obstruction (RVOTO) • Double- chambered right ventricle (DCRV) • Ventricular septal defect (VSD) • Sub-pulmonary obstruction • Right ventricular (RV) muscle bundles

Morphology and Associated Lesions

Similar to many other lesions related with congenital heart disease (CHD), the terminology that surrounds double-chambered right ventricle (DCRV) has evolved over the past several decades. DCRV was initially defined more than 130 years ago. A DCRV is formed by RV obstruction due to anomalous muscle bundles. Those muscle bundles run between an area located in the ventricular septum, beneath the level of the septal leaflet of the tricuspid valve, and the anterior wall of the RV. While this can happen in isolation, it is more often part of a combination of lesions that contains DCRV, a perimembranous outlet-type ventricular septal defect, pulmonary valve stenosis, and discrete subaortic stenosis with or without aortic valve prolapse [1, 2].

Clinical Features

Most patients with DCRV initially present with no symptoms. The most common reason for referral is the detection of a murmur. Clinically, patients with DCRV and no ventricular septal defect resemble patients with isolated pulmonary valve stenosis [1].

There is concordance between the presence of a ventricular septal defect and its clinical picture. Typically, the patient is diagnosed with a ventricular septal defect or pulmonary outflow tract obstruction and, later, may show signs of the progression of the outflow stenosis such as

A. Sadeghpour, MD, FACC, FASE (✉)
Echocardiography Lab, Department of Cardiology, Adult Congenital Heart Disease Clinic, Rajaie Cardiovascular Medical and Research Center, Iran University of Medical Science, Tehran, Iran
e-mail: anita.sadeghpour@gmail.com, asadeghpour@rhc.ac.ir

A. Alizadehasl, MD, FACC
Echocardiography Lab, Department of Cardiology, Rajaie Cardiovascular Medical and Research Center, Iran University of Medical Science, Tehran, Iran
e-mail: alizadeasl@gmail.com, alizadeasl@rhc.ac.ir

Electronic supplementary material The online version of this chapter (doi: 10.1007/978-1-4471-6383-1_45) contains supplementary material, which is available to authorized users.

cyanosis, fatigue, and reduced exercise tolerance. Therefore, most cases are discovered incidentally during the evaluation of a ventricular septal defect. If the obstruction is isolated, there may be only an ejection systolic murmur heard best in the upper left sternal border. If the ventricular septal defect is the predominant lesion, the right ventricular (RV) outflow tract murmur may not be valued. Before the routine use of echocardiography, the diagnosis was often made during follow-up for a ventricular septal defect when the pansystolic murmur diminished in intensity and a systolic ejection murmur emerged. The patients are usually pink unless there is progression of the RV outflow tract stenosis in the setting of a ventricular septal defect [1, 3, 4].

Paraclinic

Electrocardiography

The electrocardiogram (ECG) is similar to that of patients with isolated pulmonary valve stenosis beyond the newborn period. In cases with a nonrestrictive ventricular septal defect and mild subpulmonary stenosis, the ECG typically shows biventricular hypertrophy due to a left-to-right shunt and associated pulmonary hypertension. If the stenosis is more severe, RV hypertrophy will be seen [4].

Chest Radiography

Chest radiography (CXR) may disclose either a left-to-right shunt with augmented pulmonary vascular markings or a severe RV obstruction with lessened pulmonary vascularity. The usual arrangement contains atrial situs solitus, levocardia, and left aortic arch. Cardiomegaly may be seen in a number of patients. CXR is usually normal in those with isolated RV outflow stenosis, whereas those with a ventricular septal defect may have either increased or reduced pulmonary blood flow, depending on the severity of the stenosis [4–6].

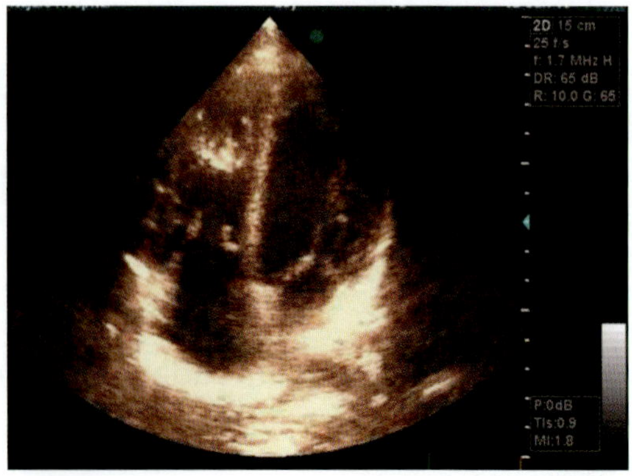

Fig. 45.1 Transthoracic echocardiography in 4 chambers shows an anomalous hypertrophied muscle bundle in the midportion of the right ventricle (Video 45.1)

Echocardiography

Echocardiography currently enables diagnosis on a two-dimensional Doppler echocardiogram. The level of subpulmonary obstruction, the degree of stenosis, and its relationship with the ventricular septal defect are appreciated best in a combination of subcostal right anterior oblique and precordial short-axis views (Figs. 45.1 and 45.2, Videos 45.2, 45.3, 45.4, 45.5 and 45.6). *Anomalous muscle bundles divided the RV into the high-pressure proximal chamber and a low-pressure distal chamber.*

Echocardiography can evaluate the presence of possible subaortic stenosis and aortic cusp prolapse. Color flow, pulsed, or continuous-wave Doppler assessment usually allows differentiation of the ventricular septal defect flow from that originating from the muscle bundles. Also, this permits an accurate evaluation of the hemodynamic effect of the subpulmonary obstruction. Transesophageal echocardiography has been used to define structures in older patients with poor windows [4, 6–8].

Cardiac Catheterization

This technique is seldom necessary. In older patients in whom the echocardiographic images of the subpulmonary region may be suboptimal, a combination of computed tomography or

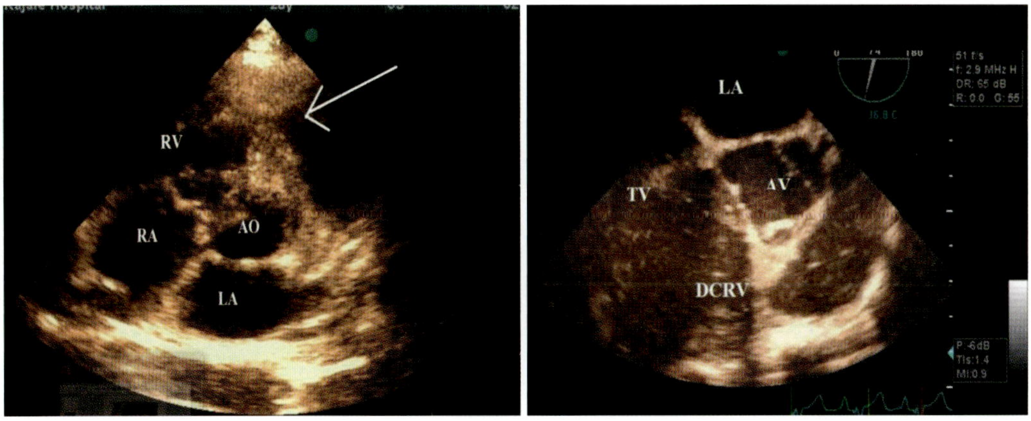

Fig. 45.2 Double-chamber RV as a variation of subpulmonary stenosis; the anomalous muscle bundle is shown by white arrow in the midportion of the RV (the junction of the inlet and outlet and proximal to the infundibulum)

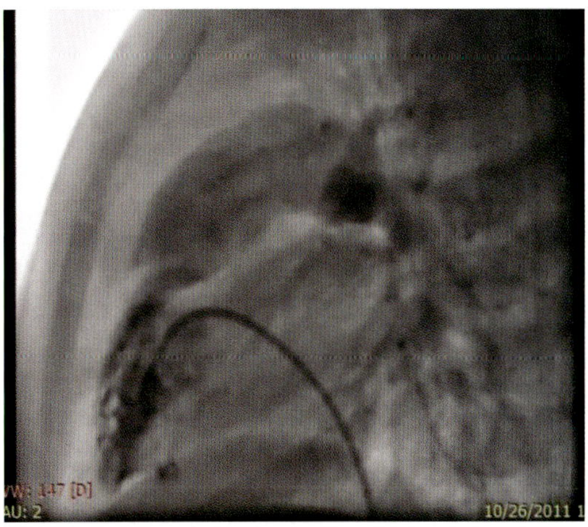

Fig. 45.3 Injection in severely hypertrabeculated RV shows two separate chambers. Main PA and its branches size are normal

magnetic resonance angiography and echocardiography is all that is usually needed (Fig. 45.3, Video 45.7) [5, 6].

Management

In the presence of a ventricular septal defect, a significant left-to-right shunt can be present, requiring anti-failure treatment, particularly if the muscle bundles are not sufficiently obstructive to diminish the pulmonary blood flow. Indeed, management is dictated by the severity of the subpulmonary stenosis and the presence of related lesions. In patients with isolated subpulmonary obstruction, surgery is indicated when the RV pressure is more than 2/3 of the systemic pressure. This includes the resection of the muscle bundles. For those cases with an associated ventricular septal defect, the decision is based on the size of the ventricular septal defect, degree of the related subaortic stenosis, presence of aortic valve prolapse, and severity of the subpulmonary stenosis. Overall, the outcome is excellent with a low rate of recurrence after the surgical resection of the obstructive muscle bundles. Rarely, the recurrence of the subaortic obstruction may happen [6–8].

References

1. Restivo A, Cameron AH, Anderson RH, et al. Divided right ventricle: a review of its anatomical varieties. Pediatr Cardiol. 1984;5(3):197–204.
2. Byrum CJ, Dick 2nd M, Behrendt DM, et al. Excitation of the double chamber right ventricle: electrophysiologic and anatomic correlation. Am J Cardiol. 1982; 49(5):1254–8.
3. Hubail ZJ, Ramaciotti C. Spatial relationship between the ventricular septal defect and the anomalous muscle bundle in a double-chambered right ventricle. Congenit Heart Dis. 2007;2(6):421–3.
4. Nagashima M, Tomino T, Satoh H, et al. Double-chambered right ventricle in adulthood. Asian Cardiovasc Thorac Ann. 2005;13(2):127–30.
5. Puvaneswary M, Indira N, Sreedhar M, et al. Double-chambered right ventricle: magnetic resonance imaging findings. Australas Radiol. 2005;49(2):170–4 [Medline].

6. Vogel M, Freedom RM, Brand A, et al. Ventricular septal defect and subaortic stenosis: an analysis of 41 patients. Am J Cardiol. 1983;52(10):1258–63.
7. Animasahun BA, Ekure EN, Njokanma OF. Double-chambered right ventricle: an uncommon congenital heart disease. Case report and literature review. Cardiovasc J Afr. 2011;22(5):274–7.
8. Romano MM, Furtado RG, Dias CG, et al. Double-chambered right ventricle in an adult patient diagnosed by transthoracic echocardiography. Cardiovasc Ultrasound. 2007;5:2.

Accessory Mitral Valve Tissue

46

Anita Sadeghpour and Azin Alizadehasl

Keywords

Accessory mitral valve tissue (AMVT) • Left ventricular outflow tract obstruction (LVOTO) • Echocardiography • Endocardial cushion

Accessory mitral valve tissue (AMVT) is an extremely rare congenital cardiac anomaly of embryologic development and growth of the endocardial cushion first described by McLean in 1963. The incidence of this anomaly is unknown. It is an unusual cause for subvalvular left ventricular outflow tract (LVOT) obstruction. The common clinical presentations are due to LVOT obstruction [1–3].

AMVT is a very rare clinical object. It may be diagnosed in both neonate-childhood and adulthood periods in patients usually symptomatic for exercise intolerance, dyspnea, chest pain, palpitations, fatigue, or syncope. Rarely can it be associated to thromboembolic accidents. Nevertheless, AMVT is frequently an incidental finding. However, it is very commonly associated with other cardiac and vascular congenital abnormalities [1, 4, 5].

Two-dimensional echocardiography, both transthoracic and transesophageal, is considered the main imaging modality for AMVT diagnosis, determination of the anatomic characteristics and functional significance, and also patient's follow-up (Fig. 46.1a, b). The AMVT exhibits an irregular parachute or sail-like feature that is attached to the chordae of the MV, anterior MV leaflet, accessory papillary muscle, or rarely the interventricular septum. Large, bulky, and redundant AMVT folded onto itself can appear as a bulbous, globular, or even cystic mass [4, 6, 7] (Videos 46.1, 46.2, and 46.3).

The recent introduction of 3-dimensional echocardiography permits a more realistic characterization of this entity and its associated anomalies [1, 2].

Surgery is indicated only in cases with significant LVOT obstruction and in cases undergoing correction of other cardiac malformations and anomalies or exploration of an intracardiac mass [1, 4, 6].

A. Sadeghpour, MD, FACC, FASE (✉)
Echocardiography Lab, Department of Cardiology, Adult Congenital Heart Disease Clinic, Rajaie Cardiovascular Medical and Research Center, Iran University of Medical Science, Tehran, Iran
e-mail: anita.sadeghpour@gmail.com, asadeghpour@rhc.ac.ir

A. Alizadehasl, MD, FACC
Echocardiography Lab, Department of Cardiology, Rajaie Cardiovascular Medical and Research Center, Iran University of Medical Science, Tehran, Iran
e-mail: alizadeasl@gmail.com, alizadeasl@rhc.ac.ir

Electronic supplementary material The online version of this chapter (doi: 10.1007/978-1-4471-6383-1_46) contains supplementary material, which is available to authorized users.

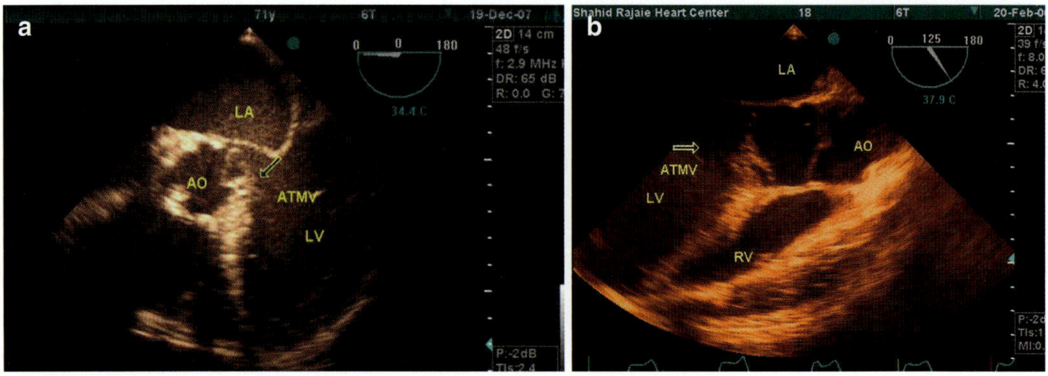

Fig. 46.1 (**a**, **b**) Showing accessory tissue mitral valve (ATMV) in transesophageal echocardiography long-axis view. *ATMV* accessory tissue mitral valve, *LA* left atrium, *LV* left ventricle, *AO* aorta

In conclusion in patients without rest and only an exertional mild LVOT obstruction and no other cardiac malformations, prophylactic resection of AMVT is not required, antibiotic prophylaxis for infective endocarditis may be indicated, and a regular follow-up is suggested to identify any progression in LVOT obstruction entity (Fig. 46.1a, b). Echocardiography particularly TEE plays a vital role in the diagnosis, treatment, and follow-up of patients with this rare congenital anomaly [6, 8, 9].

References

1. Yetkin E, Turhan H. Recurrence of cerebrovascular thromboembolic event in a woman with accessory mitral valve during puerperium period. Int J Cardiol. 2005;105:102–3.
2. Popescu BA, Ghiorghiu I, Apetrei E, et al. Subaortic stenosis produced by accessory mitral valve: the role of echocardiography. Echocardiography. 2005;22:39–41.
3. Oliver JM, Gonzales A, Gallego P, Sanchez-Recalde A, Benito F, Mesa JM. Discrete subaortic stenosis in adults (increased prevalence and slow rate of progression of the obstruction and aortic regurgitation). J Am Coll Cardiol. 2001;38:835–42.
4. Eiriksson H, Midgley FM, Karr SS, et al. Role of echocardiography in the diagnosis and surgical management of accessory mitral valve tissue causing left ventricular outflow tract obstruction. J Am Soc Echocardiogr. 1995;8:105–7.
5. Sono J, Mckay R, Arnold RM. Accessory mitral valve leaflet causing aortic regurgitation and left ventricular outflow tract obstruction (case report and review of published reports). Br Heart J. 1988;59:491–7.
6. Willens HJ, Levy R, Perez A. Diagnosis of accessory mitral valve tissue by transesophageal echocardiography. Echocardiography. 1994;11:39–45.
7. Prifti E, Frati G, Bonacchi M, Vanini V, Chauvaud S. Accessory mitral valve tissue causing left ventricular outflow tract obstruction(case reports and literature review). J Heart Valve Dis. 2001;10:774–8.
8. Garrett HE, Spray TL. Accessory mitral valve tissue (an increasingly recognized cause of left ventricular outflow tract obstruction). J Cardiovasc Surg (Torino). 1990;31:225–30.
9. Yoshimura N, Yamaguchi M, Oshima Y, Oka S, Ootaki Y, Tei T, et al. Clinical and pathological features of accessory valve tissue. Ann Thorac Surg. 2000;69:1205–8.

Parachute Deformity of Tricuspid Valve

47

Anita Sadeghpour and Azin Alizadehasl

Keywords

Parachute deformity of tricuspid valve • Sura-valvar ring • Subaortic stenosis • Coarctation • Shone complex • Parachute deformity of mitral valve

A parachute anomaly of an atrioventricular (AV) valve, as first described by Swan et al. (1949) and later correlated to particular associated malformations and abnormalities by Shone et al. (1963), has always referred only to the morphologically mitral valve (MV). A parachute deformity of an AV valve happens when all the chordae tendineae arise from a single papillary muscle or single muscle group. Of course, sometimes, the normal number of papillary muscles is present, but one papillary muscle is much bigger than its peers and demonstrates some characteristic features; and this type is known as a parachute-like asymmetric valve and has been well defined in the MV position and rarely in the tricuspid valve (TV). Also, rarely the dominant muscle may be directly attached to the AV valve leaflet with no separate chordae [1–4].

In addition, Shone et al. emphasized that the complex of supravalvular ring of the left atrium (LA), subaortic stenosis, and coarctation of the aorta, which they named the parachute MV complex, was related with the arterial side of the heart and vascular system. Also, Schiebler and associates detected a parachute anomaly affecting the right AV valve in congenitally corrected transposition of great arteries as did El Sayed et al, but of course the right AV valve in corrected transposition is the morphologically MV [3, 5, 6]

In fact the parachute abnormality of MV often occurs with left sided obstructive lesions though sometimes may happen as an isolated lesion. Symptoms depend on the severity of obstruction and associated lesions [1, 2, 5, 6].

Parachute abnormality of the TV has rarely been reported and its relationship with left to right shunts. Parachute anomaly of MV is a known entity and is usually associated with left-sided obstructive lesions. There has been only one report of parachute abnormality of the TV in association with right-sided stenotic lesions.

A. Sadeghpour, MD, FACC, FASE (✉)
Echocardiography Lab, Department of Cardiology, Adult Congenital Heart Disease Clinic, Rajaie Cardiovascular Medical and Research Center, Iran University of Medical Science, Tehran, Iran
e-mail: anita.sadeghpour@gmail.com, asadeghpour@rhc.ac.ir

A. Alizadehasl, MD, FACC
Echocardiography Lab, Department of Cardiology, Rajaie Cardiovascular Medical and Research Center, Iran University of Medical Science, Tehran, Iran
e-mail: alizadeasl@gmail.com, alizadeasl@rhc.ac.ir

Electronic supplementary material The online version of this chapter (doi: 10.1007/978-1-4471-6383-1_47) contains supplementary material, which is available to authorized users.

A. Sadeghpour et al. (eds.), *Comprehensive Approach to Adult Congenital Heart Disease*, DOI 10.1007/978-1-4471-6383-1_47, © Springer-Verlag London 2014

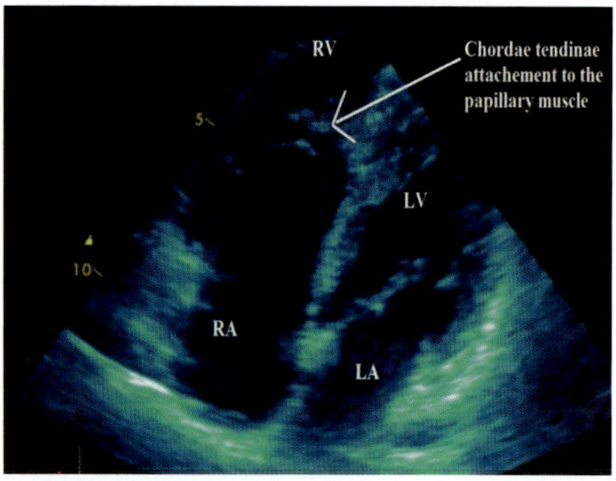

Fig. 47.1 Transthoracic echocardiography in 4-chamber view showing that all of the TV chordae tendineae are attached to a single papillary muscle (*arrow*). *LA* left atrium, *RA* right atrium, *LV* left ventricle, *RV* right ventricle

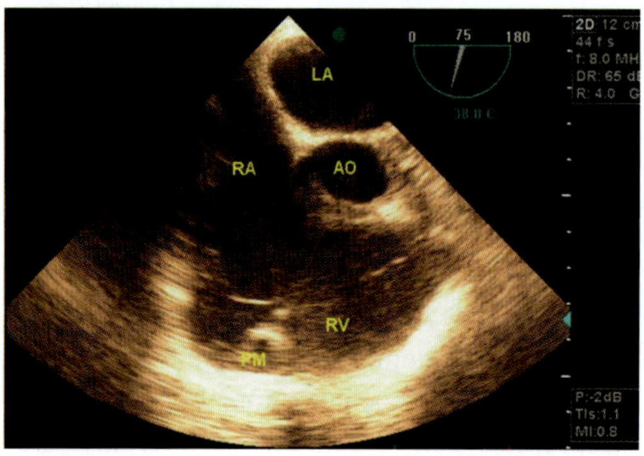

Fig. 47.2 Transesophageal echocardiography in RV inflow-outflow imaging of the same patient reveals that all of the TV chordae tendineae are attached to a single dominant papillary muscle. *LA* left atrium, *RA* right atrium, *AO* aorta, *RV* right ventricle, *PM* papillary muscle

Ariza et al. reported presence of parachute abnormality of the TV in association with tetralogy of Fallot that was manifested with congestive cardiac failure. Milo et al. have reported parachute anomaly of the TV in a patient with double outlet right ventricle [3, 7, 8].

Transthoracic echocardiography (Figs. 47.1 and 47.2) and occasionally transesophageal echocardiography are the main tools for the diagnosis of this anomaly and all associated lesions; and also, a patient that remains asymptomatic only needs to undergo serial echocardiography in order to study the severity of tricuspid regurgitation and sizes of the right heart chambers (Videos 47.1 and 47.2). We think that parachute anomalies of the TV are more common than published reports indicate. This is maybe because the clinical findings and pathological and anatomical features are masked by the severe anatomical malformations with which they are often associated [3, 8, 9].

References

1. Swan H, Trapnell JH, Denst J. Congenital mitral stenosis and systemic right ventricle with associated pulmonary vascular changes frustrating surgical repair of patent ductus arteriosus and coarctation of the aorta. Am Heart J. 1949;38:914–9.
2. Shone JD, Sellers RD, Anderson RC, et al. The developmental complex of "parachute mitral valve", supravalvular ring of left atrium, subaortic stenosis, and coarctation of aorta. Am J Cardiol. 1963;11:714–25.
3. Milo S, Stark J, Macartney FJ, et al. Parachute deformity of the tricuspid valve. Thorax. 1979;34(4):543e6.
4. Oosthoek PW, Wenink ACG, Macedo AJ, et al. The parachute-like asymmetric mitral valve and its two papillary muscles. J Thorac Cardiovasc Surg. 1997;114:9–15.
5. Schiebler GL, Edwards JE, Burchell HB, et al. Congenital corrected transposition of the great vessels: a study of 33 cases. Pediatrics. 1961;27:851488.
6. El S, Cleland H, Bentall WP, et al. Corrected transposition of the great arterial trunks: surgical treatment of the associated defects. J Thorac Cardiovasc Surg. 1962;44:443–58.
7. Ariza S, Cintado C, Castillo JA, et al. Parachute tricuspid valve associated with Fallot's tetralogy. Arch Mal Coeur Vaiss. 1979;72(3):317e20.
8. Marwah A, Suresh PV, Shah S, et al. Parachute tricuspid valve. Eur J Echocardiogr. 2006;7:226–7.
9. Maitre Azcarate MJ. Parachute deformity of the tricuspid valve. Thorax. 1980;35(3):240.

Pulmonary Vein Stenosis

48

Azin Alizadehasl and Anita Sadeghpour

Keywords

Pulmonary vein stenosis • Total anomalous pulmonary venous return • Pulmonary hypertension • Cardiovascular magnetic resonance imaging (CMR) • Ventricular septal defect (VSD)

Definition and Physiopathology

Congenital pulmonary vein stenosis (PVnS) can happen as a focal stenosis at the atrial connection site or complete hypoplasia in one or more of the pulmonary veins. Indeed, the primary form of PVnS with a pathological appearance similar to that in childhood cases has been reported rarely in unoperated adult patients [1, 2].

The related malformations comprise ventricular septal defect, atrial septal defect, tricuspid and mitral atresia, tetralogy of Fallot, and atrioventricular septal defect. Sometimes, PVnS is acquired after the surgical approach for the total anomalous pulmonary venous return. Pulmonary hypertension is one of the concerns about PVnS. In cases with unilateral PVnS, the symptoms are often absent [3, 4].

Paraclinical Aspects

The electrocardiogram (ECG) is frequently normal except for the presence of pulmonary hypertension, which leads to right ventricular hypertrophy [4].

Chest radiography in unilateral cases shows the oligemia of the involved lung and hyper-flow in the other one. In bilateral cases, pulmonary edema may be detected [1].

Echocardiography can frequently confirm the diagnosis of PVnS. Doppler color flow assessment of the right and left-sided pulmonary veins. Finding of high velocity turbulent flow pattern in pulmonary vein can further assist the diagnosis [1, 4].

Although it is possible to use echocardiography to study pulmonary hypertension, absolute Doppler gradients may not be helpful. Cardiovascular magnetic resonance imaging (CMR) is currently the gold standard for the diagnosis of PVnS inasmuch as it affords a detailed study of the anatomy and course of all

A. Alizadehasl, MD, FACC (✉)
Echocardiography Lab, Department of Cardiology, Rajaie Cardiovascular Medical and Research Center, Iran University of Medical Science, Tehran, Iran
e-mail: alizadeasl@gmail.com, alizadeasl@rhc.ac.ir

A. Sadeghpour, MD, FACC, FASE
Echocardiography Lab, Department of Cardiology, Adult Congenital Heart Disease Clinic, Rajaie Cardiovascular Medical and Research Center, Iran University of Medical Science, Tehran, Iran
e-mail: anita.sadeghpour@gmail.com, asadeghpour@rhc.ac.ir

A. Sadeghpour et al. (eds.), *Comprehensive Approach to Adult Congenital Heart Disease*, DOI 10.1007/978-1-4471-6383-1_48, © Springer-Verlag London 2014

the pulmonary veins. Accordingly, the combination of echocardiography and CMR can render invasive techniques unnecessary [4, 5].

Management

In unilateral PVnS without pulmonary hypertension, no treatment is necessary. Follow-up is, however, recommended because of the probability of the progression of the disease and the involvement of the other lung. In cases with bilateral stenoses, the mortality rate is practically 100 %. Stents generally can confer only short-term relief [5, 6].

References

1. Sadr IM, Tan PE, Kieran MW, et al. Mechanism of pulmonary vein stenosis in infants with normally connected veins. Am J Cardiol. 2000;86:577–9.
2. Omasa M, Hasegawa S, Bando T, et al. A case of congenital pulmonary vein stenosis in an adult. Respiration. 2004;71:92–4.
3. Breinholt JP, Hawkins JA, Minich L, et al. Pulmonary vein stenosis with normal connection: associated cardiac abnormalities and variable outcome. Ann Thorac Surg. 1999;68:164–8.
4. Hancock Friesen CL, Zurakowski D, Thiagarajan RR, et al. Total anomalous pulmonary venous connection: an analysis of current management strategies in a single institution. Ann Thorac Surg. 2005;79:596–606.
5. Caldarone CA, Najm HK, Kadletz M, et al. Relentless pulmonary vein stenosis after repair of total anomalous pulmonary venous drainage. Ann Thorac Surg. 1998;66:1514–20.
6. Ussia G, Marasini M, Zannini L, et al. Acquired pulmonary vein obstruction after open-heart surgery. Eur J Cardiothorac Surg. 2002;22:465–7.

Coronary Arteriovenous Fistula

49

Anita Sadeghpour and Azin Alizadehasl

Keywords
Coronary arteriovenous fistula (AVF) • Right coronary artery (RCA) • Left coronary artery (LCA) • Right ventricle (RV) • Right atrium (RA)

Morphology

Coronary arteriovenous fistula (AVF) is a communication between the coronary arteries and a cardiac chamber or vein. In about 55 % of patients, the right coronary artery (RCA) and its branches are the site of the fistula. The left coronary artery (LCA) develops this problem in nearly 35 % of cases. Among the chambers, the right ventricle (RV) is the most involved one, followed by the right atrium (RA) and to a lesser extent the coronary sinus. Coronary-to-pulmonary artery (PA) fistulas are rare [1, 2].

Clinical and Clinical Findings

Usually the myocardial blood flow is not compromised and the resulting shunt is small. Mostly patients are asymptomatic. Pulmonary hypertension and congestive heart failure are rare complications with an unusual large left-to-right shunt created by the coronary AVF. Also, bacterial endocarditis and rupture or thrombosis of the fistula or related dilated aneurysms should be contemplated. Loud, superficial, and continuous murmur at the lower or mid-sternal border is usually present [3].

The electrocardiogram (ECG) is usually normal except when there is a large shunt. Chest radiography is frequently normal and rarely reveals the enlargement of the chamber at fault.

In echocardiography, a significantly engorged feeding coronary artery may be noticed. Additionally, the entire course, entry site, and exit vessel or chamber might be found by Doppler and color flow echocardiography. Multiplane transesophageal echocardiography (TEE) can also

A. Sadeghpour, MD, FACC, FASE (✉)
Echocardiography Lab, Department of Cardiology, Adult Congenital Heart Disease Clinic, Rajaie Cardiovascular Medical and Research Center, Iran University of Medical Science, Tehran, Iran
e-mail: anita.sadeghpour@gmail.com, asadeghpour@rhc.ac.ir

A. Alizadehasl, MD, FACC
Echocardiography Lab, Department of Cardiology, Rajaie Cardiovascular Medical and Research Center, Iran University of Medical Science, Tehran, Iran
e-mail: alizadeasl@gmail.com, alizadeasl@rhc.ac.ir

Electronic supplementary material The online version of this chapter (doi: 10.1007/978-1-4471-6383-1_49) contains supplementary material, which is available to authorized users.

be helpful in this context (Figs. 49.1 and 49.2, Videos 49.1, 49.2, 49.3, and 49.4) [3–5].

If echocardiography proves a significant coronary AVF, a hemodynamic study via cardiac catheterization is required, and also coronary angiography can be employed to recognize the size and the anatomic characteristics of the fistula (Fig. 49.3, Video 49.5) [5].

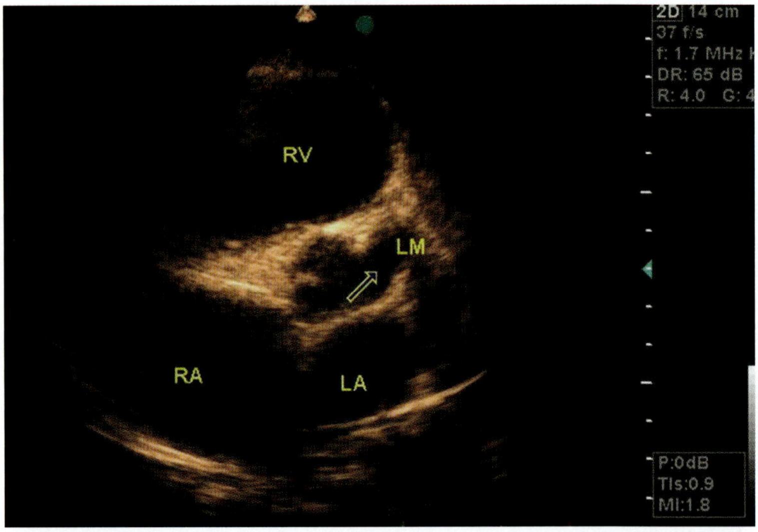

Fig. 49.1 Huge left main coronary artery in transthoracic echocardiography short-axis view (Video 49.1). *RV* right ventricle, *RA* right atrium, *LM* left main, *LA* left atrium, *Arrow* indicate the left main coronary artery

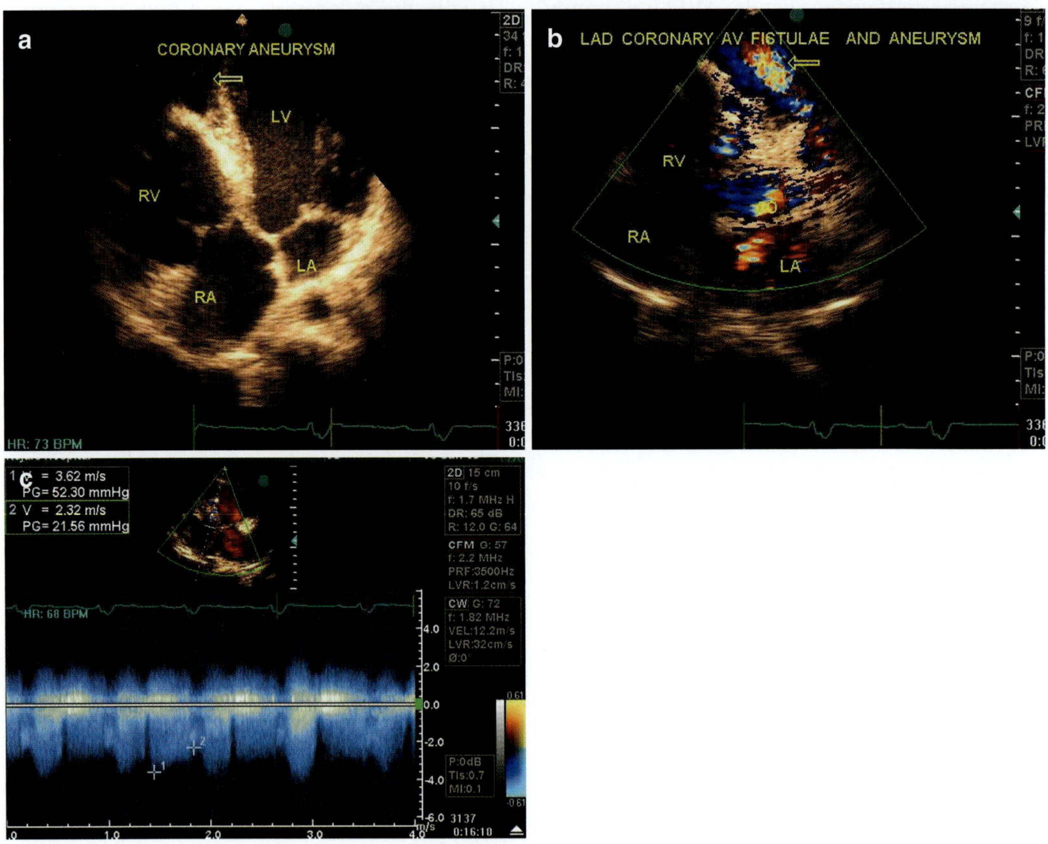

Fig. 49.2 (**a–c**) Off-axis transthoracic echocardiography showing coronary artery fistulae with aneurysmal formation and continuous turbulent flow which drains to the right ventricle (*RV*) (Videos 49.2, 49.3, and 49.4). LAD coronary AV fistula and aneurysm (*arrow*), *LV* left ventricle, *LA* left atrium, *RV* right ventricle, *RA* right atrium, *AO* aorta

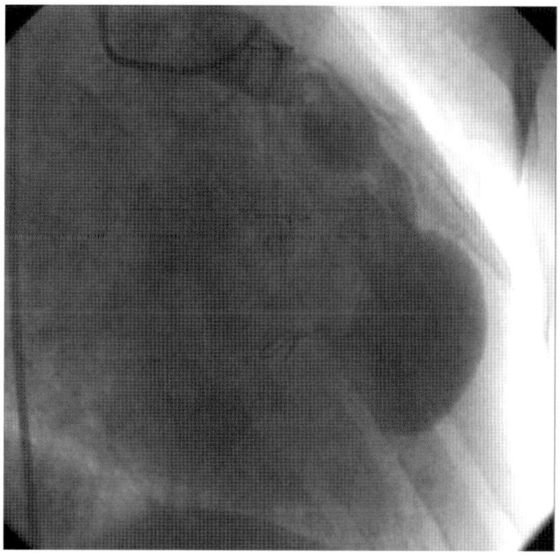

Fig. 49.3 Left coronary angiography showing aneurysmal dilatation of the left main and left anterior descending (*LAD*) descending coronary artery with fistulization to the right ventricle (*RV*) (Video 49.5)

Management

Untreated small fistulas have an excellent prognosis in the long term, but the larger ones can create premature coronary artery disease in the involved vessels. Coil embolization during catheterization time is the treatment of choice. The surgical approach is required for a few cases [3, 6, 7].

References

1. Padfield GJ. A case of coronary cameral fistula. Eur J Echocardiogr. 2009;10(5):718–20.
2. Cemri M, Sahinarslan A, Akinci S, et al. Dual coronary artery-pulmonary artery fistulas. Can J Cardiol. 2009;25(3):e95.
3. Schamroth C. Coronary artery fistula. J Am Coll Cardiol. 2009;53(6):523.
4. Liberthson RR, Sagar K, Berkoben JP, et al. Congenital coronary arterio-venous fistula. Report of 13 patients, review of the literature and delineation of management. Circulation. 1979;59(5):849–54.
5. Weymann A, Lembcke A, Konertz WF. Right coronary artery to superior vena cava fistula: imaging with cardiac catheterization, 320-detector row computed tomography, magnetic resonance imaging, and transesophageal echocardiography. Eur Heart J. 2009; 30(17):2146.
6. Chen ML, Lo HS, Su HY, et al. Coronary artery fistula: assessment with multi detector computed tomography and stress myocardial single photon emission computed tomography. Clin Nucl Med. 2009;34(2):96–8.
7. Saglam H, Koçogullari CU, Kaya E, et al. Congenital coronary artery fistula as a cause of angina pectoris. Turk Kardiyol Dern Ars. 2008;36(8):552–4.

Cor Triatriatum

50

Azin Alizadehasl and Anita Sadeghpour

Keywords
Cor triatrium • Sinister • Dexter • Fibro-muscular diaphragm • Pulmonary vein stenosis

Morphology

The failure of absorption of the common pulmonary vein creates this malformation and results in a left atrium (LA) divided by an abnormal fibromuscular diaphragm into a posterosuperior chamber receiving the pulmonary veins and an anteroinferior chamber having LA appendage and mitral orifice. The interrelation between the divided atrial chambers may be large, small, or absent, depending on the size of the opening in the membrane which defines the degree of obstruction to pulmonary venous return. Rises in both pulmonary venous pressures may result in an even severe pulmonary artery hypertension [1, 2].

A. Alizadehasl, MD, FACC (✉)
Echocardiography Lab, Department of Cardiology, Rajaie Cardiovascular Medical and Research Center, Iran University of Medical Science, Tehran, Iran
e-mail: alizadeasl@gmail.com, alizadeasl@rhc.ac.ir

A. Sadeghpour, MD, FACC, FASE
Echocardiography Lab, Department of Cardiology, Adult Congenital Heart Disease Clinic, Rajaie Cardiovascular Medical and Research Center, Iran University of Medical Science, Tehran, Iran
e-mail: anita.sadeghpour@gmail.com, asadeghpour@rhc.ac.ir

Clinical Findings

Cor triatriatum may be detected as an incidental finding in a patient who experiences echocardiography for another reason. In overall, this represents the unobstructed form that requires no early intervention. Cases with more severe obstruction present in a style similar to patients with congenital pulmonary vein stenosis [1, 3].

Electrocardiography

In unobstructed cases, this is normal. In those with significant obstruction, there is right ventricular (RV) hypertrophy due to the associated pulmonary artery hypertension. Sinus rhythm is the rule and atrial fibrillation is the exception. Peaked right atrial (RA) P waves are common. However, broad, notched left atrial P waves also happen and may be related to prolonged conduction in the accessory chamber (Fig. 50.1) [1, 4].

Electronic supplementary material The online version of this chapter (doi: 10.1007/978-1-4471-6383-1_50) contains supplementary material, which is available to authorized users.

A. Sadeghpour et al. (eds.), *Comprehensive Approach to Adult Congenital Heart Disease*,
DOI 10.1007/978-1-4471-6383-1_50, © Springer-Verlag London 2014

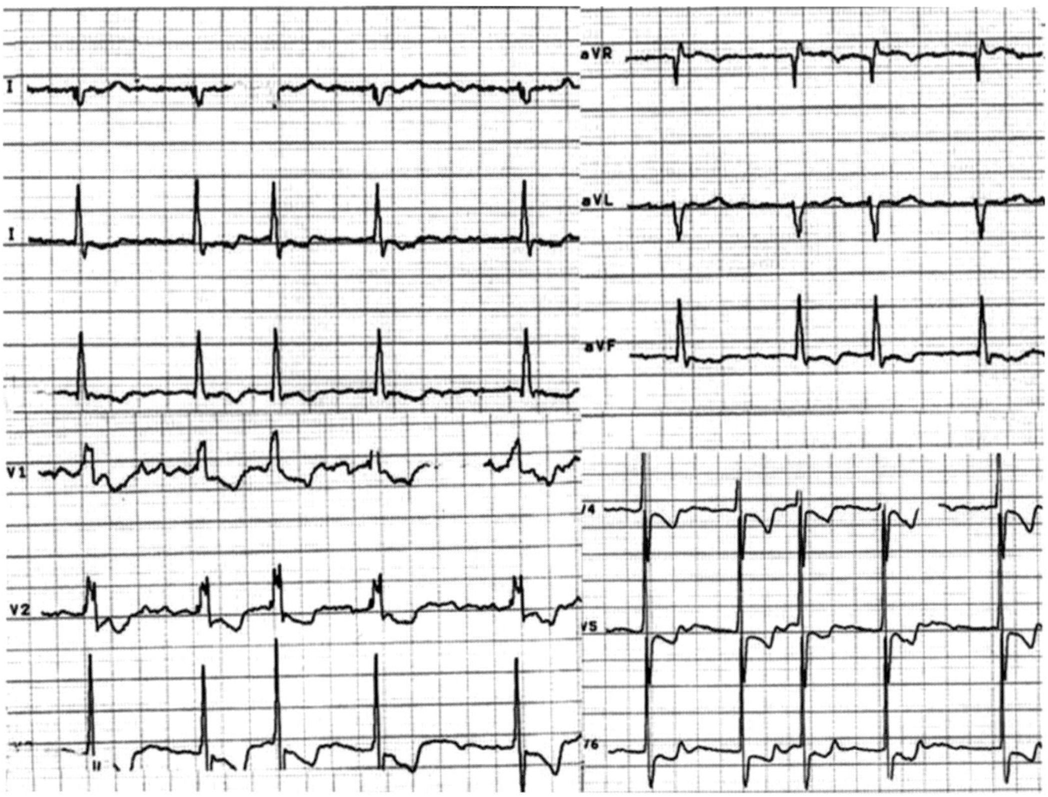

Fig. 50.1 Atrial fibrillation, right axis deviation, and right ventricular hypertrophy

Chest Radiography

This may be normal in those with mild obstruction or in those who demonstrate pulmonary edema with significant obstruction. The combination of pulmonary venous congestion without LA enlargement (LA appendage prominence) is a radiological feature of cor triatriatum (Fig. 50.2) [1, 5].

Echocardiography

The diagnosis is established by two-dimensional echocardiography or TEE, with further insight from three-dimensional reconstruction. The obstructive membrane is visualized in the parasternal long- and short-axis and four-chamber views and can be distinguished from a supravalvular mitral ring by its position superior to the LA appendage, which makes part of the distal chamber. Also present is diastolic fluttering of the mitral leaflets and high-velocity flow noticed by Doppler examination in the distal atrial chamber and at the mitral orifice [5, 6].

Associated abnormalities are common and found in 70 % of patients. These include atrial septal defect (ASD), patent foramen ovale (PFO), ventricular septal defect (VSD), persistence left superior vena cava (SVC), partial anomalous pulmonary venous return, patent ductus arteriosus, and aortic coarctation [5].

TEE can help to define the location of the membrane of the fibromuscular diaphragm and the size and number of fenestrations. There are three anatomic types of cor triatriatum: (1) diaphragmatic, (2) hourglass, and (3) tubular. Cor triatriatum can also be classified according to the size of the opening across the membrane: Group 1, no opening; Group II, one or more openings; and Group III, a wide opening and the size and number of fenestrations in the membrane are variable [7].

Turbulent color flow suggests obstruction. Pulsed Doppler is used to measure the gradient across the opening in the membrane. Three-dimensional echocardiography may provide additional information (Fig. 50.3, Videos 50.1, 50.2, 50.3, and 50.4) [5, 7].

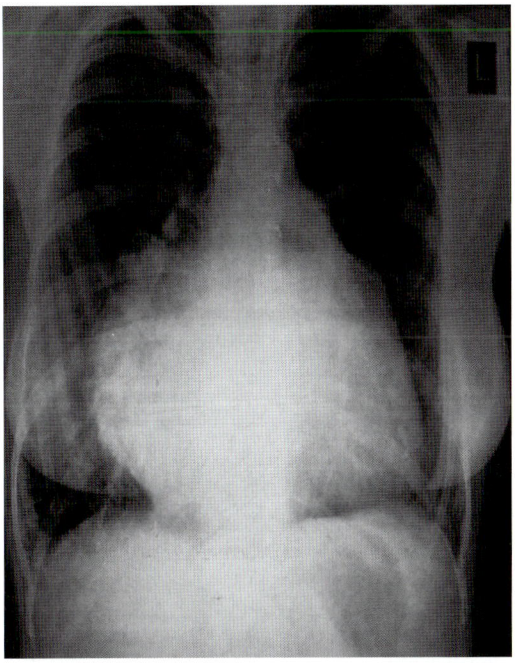

Fig. 50.2 Post-cardiac surgery cardiomegaly, left atrial enlargement without left atrial appendage prominence, right atrial and ventricular enlargement, and pulmonary venous congestion, differential diagnosis: (1) cor triatriatum, (2) mitral stenosis plus pulmonary hypertension, and (3) other left atrial obstructive lesions

Differential Diagnosis

The differential diagnosis contains prominent folds in the atrial wall, supravalvular mitral rings, and persistent left SVC. Further, the membrane may occasionally appear as an artifact. In cor triatriatum, the distinguishing feature of this type is that the membrane or fibromuscular diaphragm typically originates from the LA wall and lies between the left atrial appendage and the common pulmonary venous chamber [1, 4, 8].

Management

Surgical resection of the membrane is the treatment of choice for patients with significant obstruction. This results in symptom relief and a reduction in pulmonary artery pressure. In general, the outcome after surgery is good [8, 9].

Cor Triatriatum Dexter

Cor triatriatum dexter is an infrequent congenital heart disorder where the RA is divided into two chambers by a skin or membrane (partitioning of

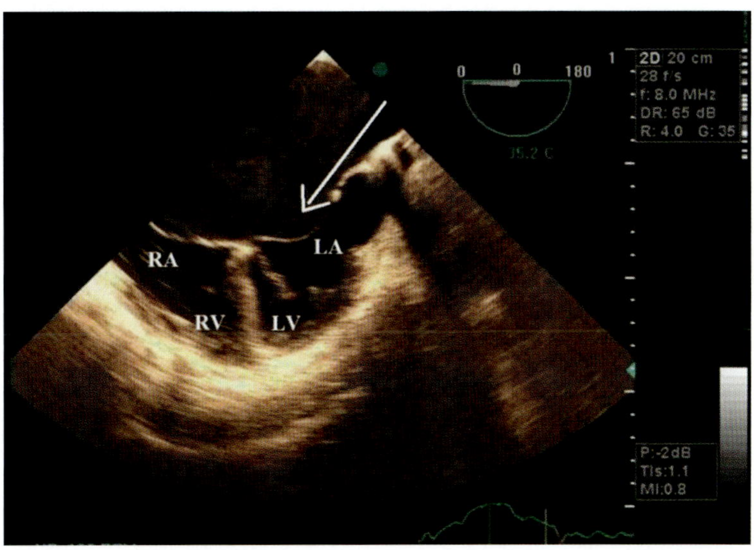

Fig. 50.3 Transesophageal echocardiography in 4-chamber view showing cor triatriatum with a small opening and significant smoky pattern (Videos 50.3 and 50.4). *LA* left atrium, *RA* right atrium, *LV* left ventricle, *RV* right ventricle

the RA to make a triatrial heart) that is formed by the persistence of the sinus venosus's right valve. Characteristically, the RA partition is caused by an exaggerated fetal eustachian and Thebesian valves, which form an incomplete septum transversely at the lower part of the RA together [10].

Unlike obstructive cor triatriatum sinister, which has a high mortality rate if not corrected, cor triatriatum dexter has very different clinical manifestations dependent on the degree of partitioning of the RA. If the septation is mild, the patient is asymptomatic, and this is an incidental finding in cardiac surgery for other abnormalities or during echocardiography. More severe septation can cause RV failure with significant elevated central venous pressures [10, 11].

Cor triatriatum dexter can happen as an isolated sporadic cardiac anomaly or related to other deformities, specially, of the right heart structures such as ASD, pulmonary valve stenosis or atresia, tricuspid valve disease, or Ebstein anomaly. Cyanosis is a very uncommon presentation of this disease; however, it is prominent when the membrane causes obstruction in RV inflow and most of the flow is directed to the LA through a PFO or ASD [10, 11].

Since many cases are asymptomatic, the diagnosis of cor triatriatum dexter frequently is determined at postmortem study. But antemortem diagnosis is possible by using angiography, echocardiography, contrast echocardiography, or cardiac MRI [11].

Asymptomatic cases are usually not treated unless they are experiencing cardiac surgery for other causes. In the past, the choice of treatment for symptomatic patients has been surgically resection of the membrane. In recent times, disruption of the membrane percutaneous catheter has been reported and has been recommended as a chosen alternative for surgery [12].

References

1. Jegier W, Gibbons JE, Wiglesworth FW. Cor triatriatum: clinical, hemodynamic and pathological studies surgical correction in early life. Pediatrics. 1963;31:255–67.
2. Talner CN. Report of the New England Regional Infant Cardiac Program, by Donald C Fyler, MD. Pediatrics. 1998;102(1 pt 2):258–9.
3. Borst H. Ein Cor triatriatum. Zentralble Allerg Pathol. 1905;16:812–5.
4. Humpl T, Reineker K, Manlhiot C, et al. Cor triatriatum sinistrum in childhood. A single institution's experience. Can J Cardiol. 2010;26(7):371–6.
5. Thakrar A, Shapiro MD, Jassal DS, et al. Cor triatriatum: the utility of cardiovascular imaging. Can J Cardiol. 2007;23(2):143–5.
6. Vallakati A, Nerella N, Chandra P, et al. Incidental diagnosis of cor triatriatum in 2 elderly patients. J Am Coll Cardiol. 2012;59(22):e43.
7. Schluter M, Langenstein BA, Thier W, et al. Transesophageal two-dimensional echocardiography in the diagnosis of cor triatriatum in the adult. J Am Coll Cardiol. 1983;2(5):1011–5.
8. Alphonso N, Norgaard MA, Newcomb A, et al. Cor triatriatum: presentation, diagnosis and long-term surgical results. Ann Thorac Surg. 2005;80(5):1666–71.
9. Ott DA, Cooley DA, Angelini P, et al. Successful surgical correction of symptomatic cor triatriatum dexter. J Thorac Cardiovasc Surg. 1979;78:573–5.
10. Hoye DJ, Wilson EC, Fyfe DA, et al. Cor triatriatum dexter: a rare cause of neonatal cyanosis. Anesth Analg. 2010;110:716–8.
11. Fiorilli R, Argento G, Tomasco B, et al. Cor triatriatum dexter diagnosed by transesophageal echocardiography. J Clin Ultrasound. 1995;23:502–4.
12. Mazzucco A, Bortolotti U, Gallucci V, et al. Successful repair of symptomatic cor triatriatum dexter in infancy. J Thorac Cardiovasc Surg. 1983;85:140–3.

Pulmonary Arteriovenous Malformations

51

Azin Alizadehasl and Anita Sadeghpour

Keywords
Pulmonary arteriovenous malformations • Pulmonary arteries • Pulmonary veins • Pulse oximetry • Echocardiogram with bubble contrast • Hereditary hemorrhagic telangiectasia (HHT)

Morphology

Pulmonary arteriovenous malformations (PAVMs) were first defined in 1897. They include abnormal communications between the pulmonary arteries and the pulmonary veins.

Most cases with PAVMs have the autosomal dominant hereditary hemorrhagic telangiectasia (HHT). PAVMs may also be acquired infrequently secondary to not only chronic infections like actinomycosis, schistosomiasis, and tuberculosis but also end-stage metastatic thyroid cancer. These arteriovenous malformations may form a communication between the pulmonary artery and the pulmonary vein or between a bronchial artery and the pulmonary vein. PAVMs happen twice as often in females as in males; however, a male predominance has been detected among newborns [1, 2].

Anatomy

About 53–70 % of PAVMs are detected in the lower lobes. Nearly 70 % of patients have unilateral disease and 36 % have multiple lesions, and 50 % of those with multiple lesions have bilateral disease. PAVMs might be microscopic (i.e., telangiectasia), although they are classically 1–5 cm [1, 3].

Pathogenesis

The exact pathogenesis of PAVMs is unknown. At the terminal arterial loops, a defect can appear, allowing the dilation of the thin-walled capillary sacs. Otherwise, PAVMs are the result of the partial resorption of the vascular septa separating the

A. Alizadehasl, MD, FACC (✉)
Echocardiography Lab, Department of Cardiology, Rajaie Cardiovascular Medical and Research Center, Iran University of Medical Science, Tehran, Iran
e-mail: alizadeasl@gmail.com, alizadeasl@rhc.ac.ir

A. Sadeghpour, MD, FACC, FASE
Echocardiography Lab, Department of Cardiology, Adult Congenital Heart Disease Clinic, Rajaie Cardiovascular Medical and Research Center, Iran University of Medical Science, Tehran, Iran
e-mail: anita.sadeghpour@gmail.com, asadeghpour@rhc.ac.ir

Electronic supplementary material The online version of this chapter (doi: 10.1007/978-1-4471-6383-1_51) contains supplementary material, which is available to authorized users.

A. Sadeghpour et al. (eds.), *Comprehensive Approach to Adult Congenital Heart Disease*,
DOI 10.1007/978-1-4471-6383-1_51, © Springer-Verlag London 2014

arterial and venous plexus, which normally have anastomosis during the growth and development of the fetus [1].

Clinical Findings

Symptoms begotten by PAVMs are frequently insidious as the malformations gradually enlarge.

Dyspnea (especially with exercise) may develop over many years. In severe instances, dyspnea in the upright position (platypnea) can be present. Noticeable cyanosis can be present if there is a major degree of desaturation. Hemoptysis and even rarely massive hemoptysis may happen. Less frequent complaints consist of chest pain, cough, headaches, dizziness, dysarthria, vertigo, syncope, and diplopia. The reason for these symptoms is not exactly clear, but they may be allied to hypoxemia or polycythemia or even paradoxical embolization across the PAVMs.

Murmurs over the site of the PAVMs are heard in cases with large PAVMs. These machinery murmurs are most audible through inspiration. Cyanosis and digital clubbing may be present [1, 2].

Pulse Oximetry

Pulse oximetry is a beneficial tool in the initial screening for PAVMs. Pulse oximetry must be performed in the supine and upright positions. Oxygen saturation <95 % is suggestive of either right-to-left shunting or concomitant pulmonary disease. With significant PAVMs, oxygen saturation classically declines in the upright position [1, 3].

Chest Radiography

Chest radiographs expose some abnormalities in many cases with large PAVMs. The typical abnormal finding is a round- or an oval-shaped mass of uniform density. The mass is often lobulated and most commonly is seen in the lower lobes of the lung [1, 2].

Echocardiography

Echocardiography, including transesophageal echocardiogram, is a helpful tool for excluding other causes of intracardiac right-to-left shunts [3, 4].

Echocardiogram with Bubble Contrast

A peripheral intravenous line is implanted, and a solution of 8 cc of normal saline mixed with 1 cc of the patient's blood and 1 cc of air is agitated to create microbubbles in the solution. The solution is then injected swiftly when the heart is imaged in four-chamber view (preferably). These microbubbles can produce a bright echo reflection.

The right atrium, followed by the right ventricle, is opacified normally, and then the microbubbles (< 50 microns in diameter) are filtered into the pulmonary capillary bed such that no bubbles are seen in the left heart. Be that as it may, in the presence of PAVMs, the bubbles pass through the malformation and are seen in the left atrium and the left ventricle. Any visible air should not be injected on the grounds that it could result in systemic air embolization.

PAVMs can be differentiated from intracardiac shunts based on the time of the appearance of the bubbles. In the left atrium, the appearance of the bubbles within one cardiac cycle implies intracardiac shunting, whereas bubbles that appear later denote PAVMs [3, 4] (Fig. 51.1a, b).

Nevertheless, other methods are required to confirm the result. Contrast-enhanced computed tomography (CT) scanning, radionuclide perfusion lung scanning, and even pulmonary angiography and magnetic resonance imaging (MRI) can be helpful in establishing the exact diagnosis [5, 6].

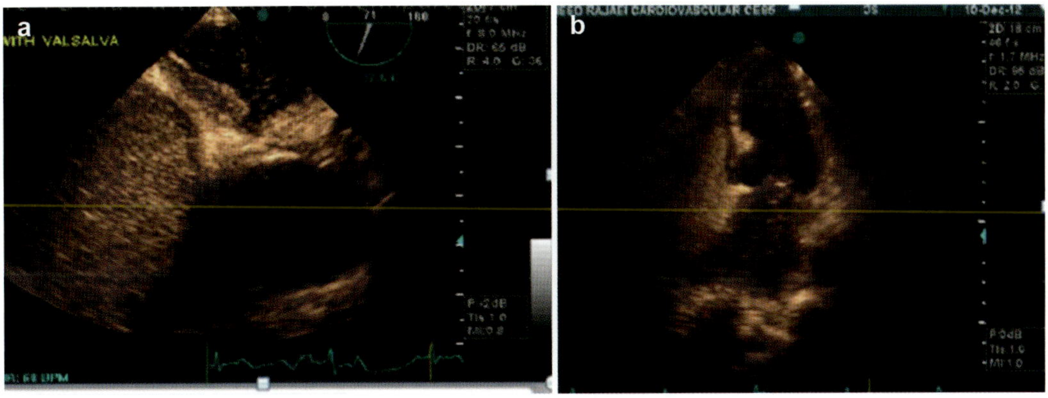

Fig. 51.1 (**a**, **b**) Right-hand agitated saline contrast study can differentiate PFO (*left image*) from PAVMs (*right image*) by the site and time of the bubble appearance in the left atrium (Videos 51.1 and 51.2)

Management

Catheter Intervention

Embolization therapy is the treatment of choice in that it is capable of totally occluding the PAVMs' feeding arteries.

Indications for embolotherapy consist of:

1. Progressive enlargement and dilatation of the lesions
2. Paradoxical embolization
3. Symptomatic hypoxemia
4. Feeding vessels ≥3 mm in size

Surgery is indicated in very rare cases [1, 4, 6].

References

1. Vaišnyte B, Vajauskas D, Palionis D, et al. Diagnostic methods, treatment modalities, and follow-up of extra cranial arterio-venous malformations. Medicina (Kaunas). 2012;48(8):388–98.
2. Al-Saleh S, Mei-Zahav M, Faughnan ME, et al. Screening for pulmonary and cerebral arteriovenous malformations in children with hereditary haemorrhagic telangiectasia. Eur Respir J. 2009;34(4):875–81.
3. Parra JA, Bueno J, Zarauza J, et al. Graded contrast echocardiography in pulmonary arteriovenous malformations. Eur Respir J. 2009;33:85–91.
4. Zukotynski K, Chan RP, Chow CM, et al. Contrast echocardiography grading predicts pulmonary arteriovenous malformations on CT. Chest. 2007;132(1): 18–23.
5. White Jr RI, Pollak JS. Pulmonary arteriovenous malformations: diagnosis with three-dimensional helical CT – a breakthrough without contrast media. Radiology. 1994;191(3):613–4.
6. Nawaz A, Litt HI, Stavropoulos SW, et al. Digital subtraction pulmonary arteriography versus multidetector CT in the detection of pulmonary arteriovenous malformations. J Vasc Interv Radiol. 2008;19(11): 1582–8.

Aortopulmonary Window

52

Anita Sadeghpour, Shadi Faghihi,
and Shabnam Mohammadzadeh

Keywords

Aortopulmonary window (AP window) • Aortopulmonary septal defect (APSD) • "T" artifact • Transthoracic echocardiography • Transesophageal echocardiography (TEE)

Embryopathy

Aortopulmonary septal defect (APSD) as an uncommon congenital heart defect is a defect in the septum between the aorta and pulmonary artery, resulting in a communication between the two arteries [1].

Mierop described three types of aortopulmonary septal defect (Fig. 52.1).

The three types of aortopulmonary septal defect are as follows:

A. Type I, proximal defect, midway between the semilunar valves and pulmonary bifurcation
B. Type II, distal defect with posterior border absent and aortic origin of right pulmonary artery
C. Type III, total defect, which is the combination of types I and II [2]

Associated lesions are PDA, *interrupted aortic arch* or severe coarctation, TOF and anomalous coronary from pulmonary artery, VSD, aortic atresia, double aortic arch, and other more complex heart diseases [1, 3].

Symptoms

Symptoms depend on the size of the defect, pulmonary vascular resistance (PVR), and associated anomalies.

- In a large defect with low PVR, it results in signs and symptoms of congestive heart failure (CHF) between the second and eighth weeks of life. Less commonly, the defect is small and shows an asymptomatic murmur.

A. Sadeghpour, MD, FACC, FASE (✉)
Echocardiography Lab, Department of Cardiology,
Adult Congenital Heart Disease Clinic,
Rajaie Cardiovascular Medical and Research Center,
Iran University of Medical Science, Tehran, Iran
e-mail: anita.sadeghpour@gmail.com,
asadeghpour@rhc.ac.ir

S. Faghihi, MD
Department of Cardiology,
Rajaie Cardiovascular Medical and Research Center,
Tehran, Iran

S. Mohammadzadeh, MD
Department of Cardiology,
Adult Congenital Heart Disease Clinic,
Moheb General Hospital, Tehran, Iran

Electronic supplementary material The online version of this chapter (doi: 10.1007/978-1-4471-6383-1_52) contains supplementary material, which is available to authorized users.

A. Sadeghpour et al. (eds.), *Comprehensive Approach to Adult Congenital Heart Disease*,
DOI 10.1007/978-1-4471-6383-1_52, © Springer-Verlag London 2014

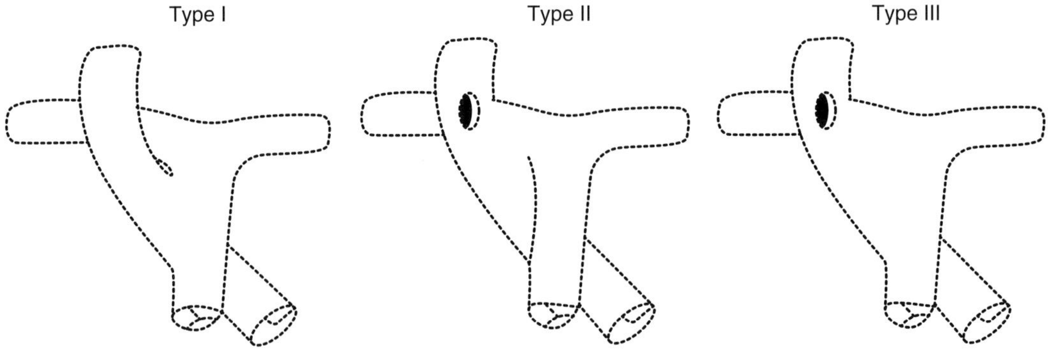

Fig. 52.1 Three types of aortopulmonary septal defect

- In a large, nonrestrictive defect with elevated PVR, CHF does not develop, and the patients may be asymptomatic and difficult to diagnose except after many years [4].

Sign

- In a large defect with low PVR, physical examination findings are tachypnea, tachycardia, and increased breathing effort, wide pulse pressure with bounding pulses, gallop rhythm, continuous murmur at the left upper sternal border, and hepatomegaly.
- In high PVR situations, findings may be subtler: single S2, cyanosis.
- In small defects, a continuous murmur may be the only one finding [4].

Electrocardiography

Criteria of right ventricular hypertrophy usually are present, although biventricular hypertrophy may be present in the presence of large defect. Rarely, the ECG is normal or shows only a mild degree of right ventricular hypertrophy with an rsR' pattern in the right precordial leads [1].

Radiography

The chest x-ray shows signs of a large left-to-right shunt like a moderately enlarged heart with prominent pulmonary vascular markings, prominent main PA segment. LA and LV borders are also prominent. The aortic knuckle is not prominent [1].

Echocardiography

Echocardiography can accurately diagnose the main and associated anomalies. The left atrium, LV, and PA are dilated. The right ventricle may be hypertrophied. The semilunar valves usually have normal relation and function. "T" artifact at the edges of the defect is the distinguishing sign from normal dropout. CFD can show flow through the defect.

Spectral Doppler shows abnormal, continuous forward flow in the pulmonary arteries. Significant diastolic flow reversal is found in both the proximal aortic arch and descending aorta. PAH can also be detected by echocardiography (Figs. 52.2, 52.3, and 52.4, Videos 52.1, 52.2, 52.3, and 52.4) [6].

Cardiac Catheterization

Cardiac catheterization usually is not required (according to the complete data obtained by echocardiography). The right ventricular and pulmonary arterial pressures usually are at systemic levels. The LA pressure may be elevated but the LV pressure is usually normal. Aortic systolic pressure usually is normal with decreased diastolic pressure and widened pulse pressure. The catheter often can direct to the main pulmonary

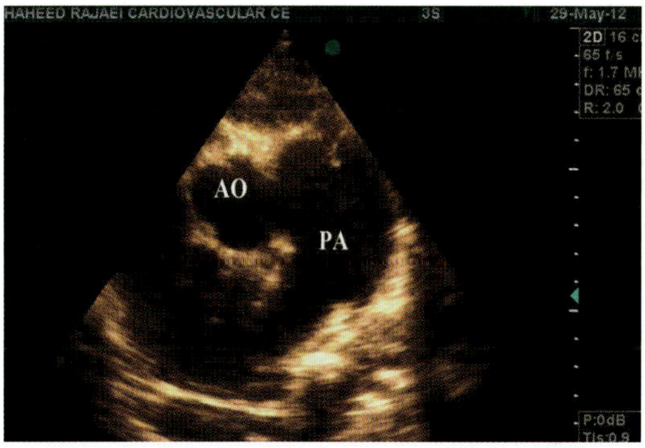

Fig. 52.2 Transthoracic echocardiography in short axis view showing "T" artifact at the edges of the defect suggestive for aortopulmonary septal defect that was confirmed by color flow imaging (Video 52.1). *AO* aorta, *PA* Pulmonary artery

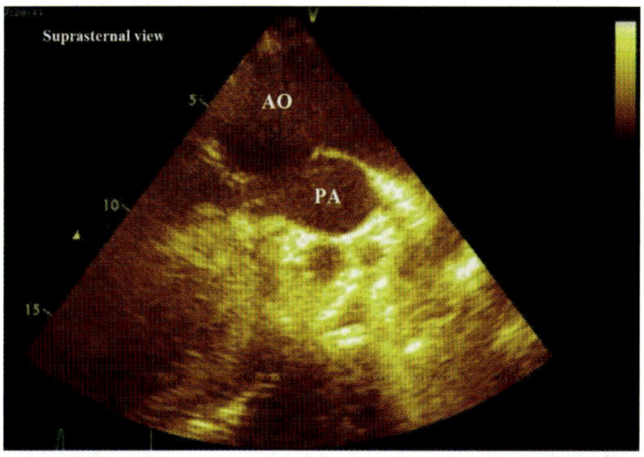

Fig. 52.3 Aortopulmonary septal defect in transthoracic echocardiography in suprasternal view (Video 52.2). *AO* aorta, *PA* Pulmonary artery

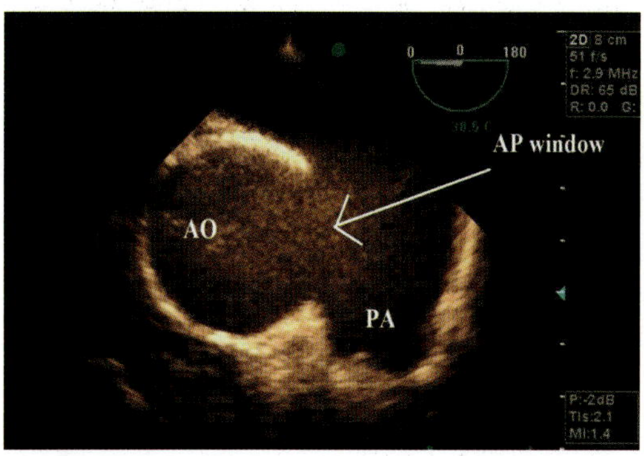

Fig. 52.4 Aortopulmonary septal defect in transesophageal echocardiography (Video 52.3 and 52.4). *AO* aorta, *PA* Pulmonary artery

artery through the defect. An ascending aorta or main pulmonary angiogram will demonstrate the defect. Aortogram can also show associated aortic abnormality [1]. The anomalous origin of a coronary artery from pulmonary arteries (if it exists) can be detected by PA angiogram (Fig. 52.5) [5].

Medical Therapy

Medical palliative therapy may be done before elective surgery. Surgical repair is obligatory to prevent the development of pulmonary hypertension. Digoxin and diuretics may have some symptomatic benefit before surgery. The benefit of vasodilator agents (e.g., angiotensin-converting enzyme inhibitors, phosphodiesterase inhibitors, nitrates) is uncertain.

Positive pressure ventilation with induced hypercarbia and limiting inspired oxygen concentration to 21 % may help limit pulmonary blood flow in infants with high pulmonary blood flow.

Reports of device closure of small aortopulmonary septal defects with efficient rims are existing [4].

Surgical Therapy

The aorta and pulmonary artery are divided, and the defects may be closed primarily or with patch [4].

Postoperative Care

Existence of complete repair should be confirmed postoperatively. Older infant or child is at risk for postoperative pulmonary hypertension that may require aggressive management with inhaled nitric oxide. Other drugs such as sildenafil or calcium channel blockers may be useful [4].

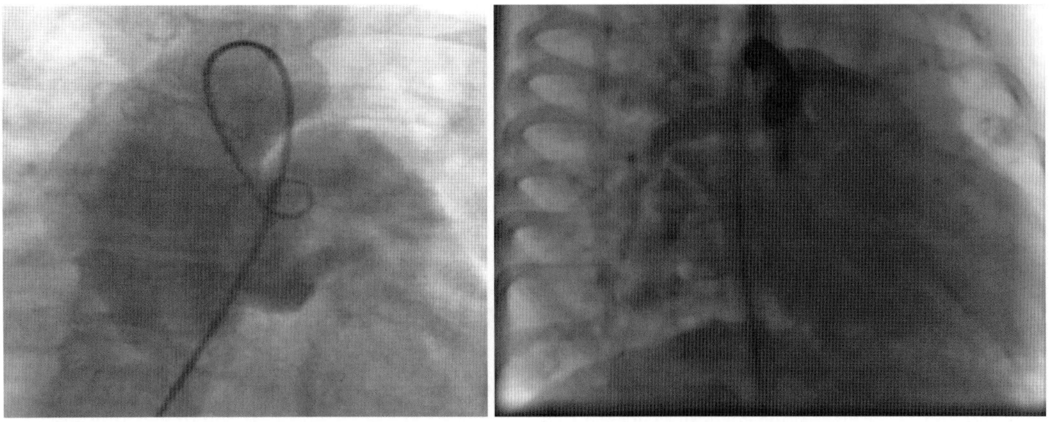

Fig. 52.5 AP window injection in AP view shows coincident AO and PA opacification and also indicates the high PAP (Video 52.5)

References

1. Allen HD, Driscoll DJ, et al. Moss and Adams' heart disease in infant, children and adolescent. 8th ed. Philadelphia: William's & Wilkins; 2013.
2. Mori K, Ando M, Takao A, et al. Distal type of aortopulmonary window. Report of 4 cases. Br Heart J. 1978;40:681–9.
3. Bertolini A, Dalmonate P, Bava GI, et al. Aortopulmonary septal defect. A review of literature and report of ten cases. J Cardiovasc Surg. 1994;35:207–13.
4. Love BA, Seib BM. http://Emedicine.medscape.com/article/893798-overview. Accessed on 5 Mar 2012.
5. Deveral PB, Lincoln J, Aberdeen E, et al. Aortopulmonary window. J Thorac Cardiovasc Surg. 1969;57:479–86.
6. Balaji S, Burch M, Sullivan ID. Accuracy of cross sectional echocardiography in diagnosis of aortopulmonary window. Am J Cardiol. 1991;67:650–3.

Crisscross Heart

53

Anita Sadeghpour and Azin Alizadehasl

Keywords
Criss cross heart • Supero-inferior ventricles • Transposition of great arteries (TGA) • Ventricular septal defect (VSD) • Echocardiography

Crisscross heart (CCH), or supero-inferior ventricles, is a rotational congenital heart defect (CHD) in which the pulmonary and systemic venous streams cross each other at the atrioventricular (AV) level without mixing. Its occurrence is <8/1000000 and accounts for less than 0.1 % of CHD [1–3].

AV structures are parallel to each other in the normal heart, if seen from the front, while in CCH the AV chambers are not parallel and angulated by as much as 90°. The atriums connect with the contralateral ventricles, and the ventricular chambers are placed in a supero-inferior position (the right ventricle (RV) superiorly and the left ventricle (LV) inferiorly positioned), regardless of whichever the AV connection is concordant or discordant. The diagnosis of CCH and its associated lesions are made by using 2-dimensional (2D) and color Doppler echocardiography [2–4].

In 1961, Lev and Rowlatt explained a rare arrangement of the cardiac chambers and inlets, that is, ventricular chambers placed in a supero-inferior style (the RV superiorly and the LV inferiorly). In 1974, Anderson et al. used the term CCH for this cardiac anomaly that produces the crossing of the pulmonary and systemic venous streams without mixing them at the AV level. Nowadays, some cases are described with situs solitus, situs inversus or isomerism, and mostly AV concordance. The physiology of CCH is determined by the concordant or discordant AV and VA connection and also the associated cardiac disease. CCH may be seen in three types, that is, normal hearts, complete transposition, and corrected transposition. Most patients with CCH have other anomalies such as transposition

A. Sadeghpour, MD, FACC, FASE (✉)
Echocardiography Lab, Department of Cardiology, Adult Congenital Heart Disease Clinic, Rajaie Cardiovascular Medical and Research Center, Iran University of Medical Science, Tehran, Iran
e-mail: anita.sadeghpour@gmail.com, asadeghpour@rhc.ac.ir

A. Alizadehasl, MD, FACC
Echocardiography Lab, Department of Cardiology, Rajaie Cardiovascular Medical and Research Center, Iran University of Medical Science, Tehran, Iran
e-mail: alizadeasl@gmail.com, alizadeasl@rhc.ac.ir

Electronic supplementary material The online version of this chapter (doi: 10.1007/978-1-4471-6383-1_53) contains supplementary material, which is available to authorized users.

DOI 10.1007/978-1-4471-6383-1_53, © Springer-Verlag London 2014

of the great vessels, ventricular septal defect, RV hypoplasia, subpulmonary stenosis, straddling of AV, and others [3, 4].

The diagnosis should be supposed by echocardiography when the parallel arrangement of the AV valves and inlets cannot be obtained, and importantly the two valves are not easily visualized simultaneously on a single apical 4-chamber view (Videos 53.1, 53.2, and 53.3). Color flow mapping can help in evaluating the AV and VA connections and also recognition of the crossover of the inflow streams. Previous studies reported that the failure to achieve a typical 4-chamber view was diagnostic key for differentiation of the CCH [4–6].

Surgical choices vary according to the sequential segmental examination and associated anomalies. In conclusion, CCH is a rare cardiac anomaly that can be identified by a transthoracic echocardiography by an attentive and alert echocardiographer to define the relationships of the cardiac chambers and connections and also associated cardiac anomalies [6, 7].

References

1. Attie F, Castellanos Muñoz L, Ovseyevitz J, Flores-Delgado I, Testelli RM, Buendía A, et al. Crossed atrioventricular connections. Am Heart J. 1980; 99:163–72.
2. Anderson RH, Lie JT, Sieg K, Hagler DJ, Ritter DG, Davis GD. A criss-cross heart. Detailed anatomic description and discussion of morphogenesis. Mayo Clin Proc. 1977;52:569–75.
3. Anderson RH, Shinebourne EA, Gerlis LH. Criss-cross atrioventricular relationships producing paradoxical atrioventricular concordance or discordance: their significance to nomenclature of congenital heart disease. Circulation. 1974;50:176–80.
4. Figueroa JR, Orellana JE, Castellanos LM, Antona CV, Hernández AB, Barrón JV. Echocardiographic segmental analysis in patients with an atrioventricular criss-cross. Rev Esp Cardiol. 2009;62:1055–9.
5. Araoz AP, Reddy PG, Thompson DP, Higgins BC. Magnetic resonance angiography of criss-cross heart. Circulation. 2002;105:537–8.
6. Yang YL, Wang XF, Cheng TO, Xie MX, Lü Q, He L, et al. Echocardiographic characteristics of the criss-cross heart. Int J Cardiol. 2010;140(2):133–7.
7. Robinson JP, Kumpeng V, MaCartney JF. Cross sectional echocardiographic and angiocardiographic correlation in crisscross hearts. Br Heart J. 1985;54:61–7.

Patent Foramen Ovale (PFO)

54

Azin Alizadehasl and Anita Sadeghpour

Keywords
Patent foramen ovale (PFO) • Fossa ovalis • Atrial septum pimum • Atrial septum secundum • Contrast echocardiography • Transient ischemic attack (TIA)

Definition and Epidemiology

A patent foramen ovale (PFO) is an anatomical communication between two atria with a possibility for right-to-left shunt. PFO is a flap-like opening between the atrial septa primum and secundum at the site of the fossa ovalis that persists after 1 year of age. In utero, the foramen ovale helps as a physiologic conduit for right-to-left shunting. After birth, once the pulmonary circulation is established, left atrial (LA) pressure increases, permitting functional closure of the foramen ovale. This is followed by an anatomical closure by the age of 1 year [1, 2].

PFO is identified in 10–15 % of patients by contrast transthoracic echocardiography (TTE), but autopsy studies demonstrate a 25–30 % prevalence of PFO. This difference is possibly due to the ability to directly visualize PFO at autopsy, but contrast echocardiography depends on detection of secondary physiologic phenomenon. The prevalence and size of PFO is similar in men and women. The prevalence of PFO reduces with age: 34 % up to age 30 years, 25 % for age 30–80 years, and 20 % for older than 80 years [2, 3].

A. Alizadehasl, MD, FACC (✉)
Echocardiography Lab, Department of Cardiology, Rajaie Cardiovascular Medical and Research Center, Iran University of Medical Science, Tehran, Iran
e-mail: alizadeasl@gmail.com, alizadeasl@rhc.ac.ir

A. Sadeghpour, MD, FACC, FASE
Echocardiography Lab, Department of Cardiology, Adult Congenital Heart Disease Clinic, Rajaie Cardiovascular Medical and Research Center, Iran University of Medical Science, Tehran, Iran
e-mail: anita.sadeghpour@gmail.com, asadeghpour@rhc.ac.ir

Clinical Findings

Most cases with isolated PFO are asymptomatic; however, these patients may have a history of stroke or transient ischemic attack (TIA) of indeterminate etiology. According to some references, some patients with PFO present with migraine or migraine-like symptoms. Other less frequent clinical appearances of PFO include the following: acute myocardial infarction and systemic embolism such as renal infarction and posttraumatic or postsurgical systemic fat embolism [2, 4].

Electronic supplementary material The online version of this chapter (doi: 10.1007/978-1-4471-6383-1_54) contains supplementary material, which is available to authorized users.

A. Sadeghpour et al. (eds.), *Comprehensive Approach to Adult Congenital Heart Disease*,
DOI 10.1007/978-1-4471-6383-1_54, © Springer-Verlag London 2014

Associated Cardiac Anomalies

The associated cardiac anomalies include atrial septal aneurysm (a redundant and mobile interatrial tissue in fossa ovalis), elongated Eustachian valve, Chiari network, ASD, and Ebstein anomaly [1, 2].

Echocardiography

In some cases, PFO is detectable with color flow Doppler imaging in TTE. A small flame of color flow may be seen in the middle area of the interatrial septum (Fig. 54.1, Videos 54.1 and 54.2).

Contrast TTE is usually needed to detect small PFO. After achieving optimal visualization of the interatrial septum on TTE or transesophageal echocardiography (TEE), a bolus of agitated saline is injected into an antecubital vein. Then, microbubbles appear in the right atrium (RA). The study is positive for PFO when the microbubbles appear in the LA within three cardiac cycles of their appearance in the RA [5–7] (Fig. 54.2, Video 54.3).

Valsalva maneuver increases RA pressure and accelerates right-to-left shunting. 2D TEE with contrast provides greater visualization of the interatrial septum and thus is preferred to contrast

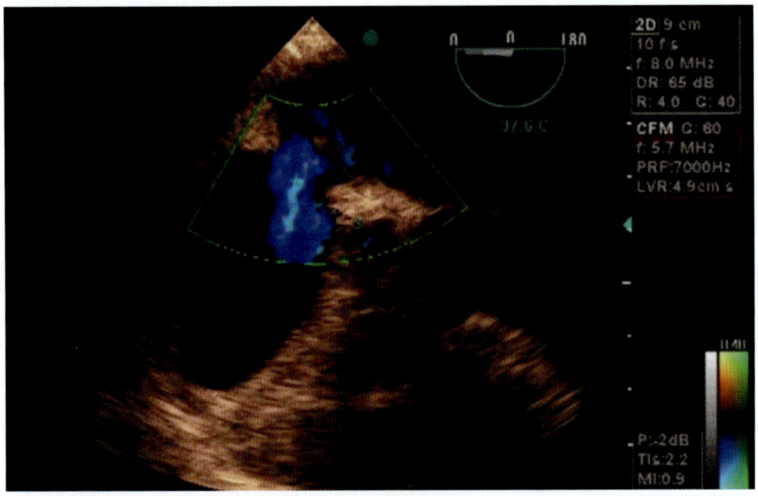

Fig. 54.1 A small flame of color flow may be seen in the middle area of the interatrial septum

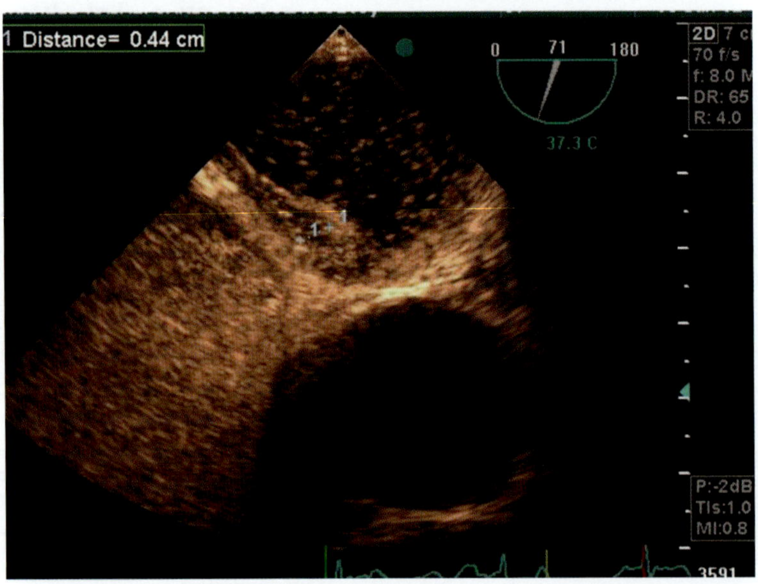

Fig. 54.2 Agitated saline injection into an antecubital vein showing many bubble passages from the interatrial septum within three cardiac cycles of their appearance in the RA suggestive of PFO

TTE for detecting PFO. When clinically indicated, 2D TEE with contrast is strongly suggested for patients whose findings on TTE are negative. A 3D TEE makes available direct visualization of the entire interatrial septum, PFO anatomy, and adjacent structures [6, 7].

Management

Most cases with a PFO as an isolated finding take no special management. No consensus is present on treatment of PFO in patients with TIA or stroke. When PFO is accompanied by an unexplained neurologic event, traditionally antiplatelet (often aspirin) therapy alone in low-risk patients or concomitant with warfarin in high-risk cases is used. With the use of warfarin, the international normalized ratio (INR) is maintained at 2–3. The first recurrence rate of stroke or TIA has been reported to be 3.4–3.9 % per year; however, in patients with atrial septal aneurysm and PFO, this risk increases to 9 %, whereas the rate of subsequent stroke or TIA recurrence in 2 years increases to 22 % [8, 9].

Percutaneous closure of PFO during cardiac catheterization is the treatment of choice. The indications are as follows:

1. Recurrent cryptogenic stroke due to supposed paradoxical embolism through PFO
2. Contraindications to anticoagulant therapy
3. Substitute to medical therapy or surgical closure as an alternative treatment
4. Cryptogenic stroke, TIA, or peripheral or coronary embolism due to supposed paradoxical embolism through a PFO that is related with hypercoagulability state
5. Divers with a PFO who are at risk of clinical events that are associated to paradoxical embolism through a PFO in decompression
6. Systemic deoxygenation due to right-to-left shunting through a PFO in the absence of severe pulmonary hypertension

And according to some references, there are two other indications for PFO closure:

7. Migraine headache accompanied by aura
8. Posttraumatic fat embolism with cerebral embolism through PFO

Surgical closure of PFO with double continuous sutures has resulted in the elimination of shunt across the PFO; the indications are as follows:

1. PFO more than 25 mm in dimension
2. Inadequate rims of tissue around the defect
3. Percutaneous device failure [8–10]

References

1. Kerut EK, Norfleet WT, Plotnick GD, et al. Patent foramen ovale: a review of associated conditions and the impact of physiological size. J Am Coll Cardiol. 2001;38(3):613–23.
2. Aslam F, Shirani J, Haque AA. Patent foramen ovale: assessment, clinical significance and therapeutic options. South Med J. 2006;99(12):1367–72.
3. Thaler DE, Ruthazer R, Di Angelantonio E, et al. Neuroimaging findings in cryptogenic stroke patients with and without patent foramen ovale. Stroke. 2013;44(3):675–80.
4. Agostoni P, Gasparini G, Destro G. Acute myocardial infarction probably caused by paradoxical embolus in a pregnant woman. Heart. 2004;90(3):e12.
5. Sievert H, Taaffe M. Patent foramen ovale: the jury is still out. Eur Heart J. 2004;25(5):361–2.
6. Maffe S, Dellavesa P, Zenone F, et al. Transthoracic second harmonic two- and three-dimensional echocardiography for detection of patent foramen ovale. J Am Coll Cardiol Intv. 2010;3(9):968–73.
7. Shanks M, Manawadu D, Vonder Muhll I, Khan K, Becher H, Choy J. Detection of patent foramen ovale by 3D echocardiography. JACC Cardiovasc Imaging. 2012;5(3):329–31.
8. Danzi GB, Sesana M, Capuano C, et al. Percutaneous closure of patent foramen ovale: pathophysiology, indications, and technique. Neurol Sci. 2003;24 Suppl 1: S17–9.
9. Meier B, Lock JE. Contemporary management of patent foramen ovale. Circulation. 2003;107(1):5–9.
10. Khositseth A, Cabalka AK, Sweeney JP, Fortuin FD, Reeder GS, Connolly HM, et al. Transcatheter Amplatzer device closure of atrial septal defect and patent foramen ovale in patients with presumed paradoxical embolism. Mayo Clin Proc. 2004;79(1):35–41.

Transcatheter Closure of the Atrial Septal Defect

55

Anita Sadeghpour and Azin Alizadehasl

Keywords
Percutaneous • Transcatheter closure of the atrial septal defect (ASD) • Ostium secundum ASD • ASD rims • Transesophageal echocardiography (TEE)

The atrial septal defect (ASD) is the second most common adult congenital heart disease, accounting for about 10 % of all congenital heart anomalies. Seventy percent of ASDs are of the ostium secundum type, and surgical repair is the standard of care for the other ASD types such as ostium primum and sinus venosus. Surgical correction was once the standard of care for the secundum ASD; however, over the past decades, many devices have been developed to treat the secundum ASD percutaneously. The benefits of the percutaneous approach have been well demonstrated in recent years [1, 2].

Indeed, the transcatheter method is evolving to become the new efficient standard of care for adults with the ASD. Similar to the surgical approach, this method results not only in symptomatic improvement and increase in exercise capacity but also in improvement in cardiac chamber anatomy and geometry and in cardiac hemodynamics. The authors of several studies have concluded that ASD closure in adults is safe and efficient with an outstanding long-term outcome in terms of clinical symptoms and hemodynamic improvement [2–4].

The American College of Cardiology and the American Heart Association (ACC/AHA) guidelines recommend that a secundum ASD >5 mm with Qp/Qs >1.5 or an ASD associated with right ventricular volume overload should be closed in the following scenarios: as long as the pulmonary artery pressure is 2/3 systemic pressure; pulmonary vascular resistance is <2/3 systemic vascular resistance; or the patient is responsive to either pulmonary vasodilator therapy or occlusion test of the defect. Indeed, ASD closure should be considered in all hemodynamically significant secundum ASDs regardless of the patient's age or symptoms. Contraindications are as follows: (1) presence of other congenital cardiac deformities such as anomalous pulmonary venous drainage or ostium primum, sinus

A. Sadeghpour, MD, FACC, FASE (✉)
Echocardiography Lab, Department of Cardiology, Adult Congenital Heart Disease Clinic, Rajaie Cardiovascular Medical and Research Center, Iran University of Medical Science, Tehran, Iran
e-mail: anita.sadeghpour@gmail.com, asadeghpour@rhc.ac.ir

A. Alizadehasl, MD, FACC
Echocardiography Lab, Department of Cardiology, Rajaie Cardiovascular Medical and Research Center, Iran University of Medical Science, Tehran, Iran
e-mail: alizadeasl@gmail.com, alizadeasl@rhc.ac.ir

A. Sadeghpour et al. (eds.), *Comprehensive Approach to Adult Congenital Heart Disease*,
DOI 10.1007/978-1-4471-6383-1_55, © Springer-Verlag London 2014

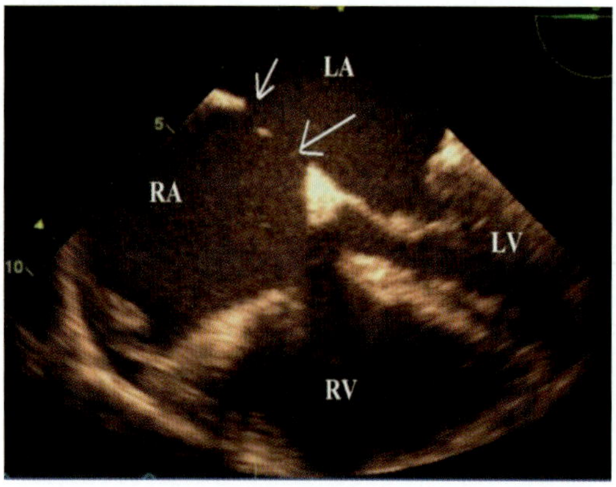

Fig. 55.1 Interatrial septum with two nearby adjacent defect which can be closed by a large device. *RV* right ventricle, *RA* right atrium, *LV* left ventricle, *LA* left atrium

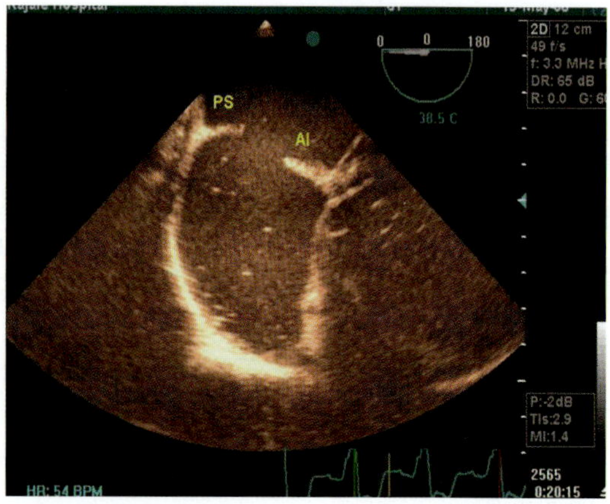

Fig. 55.2 Transesophageal echocardiography in four-chamber view showing the mitral or anteroinferior rim *AI* and posterosuperior *PS* rims

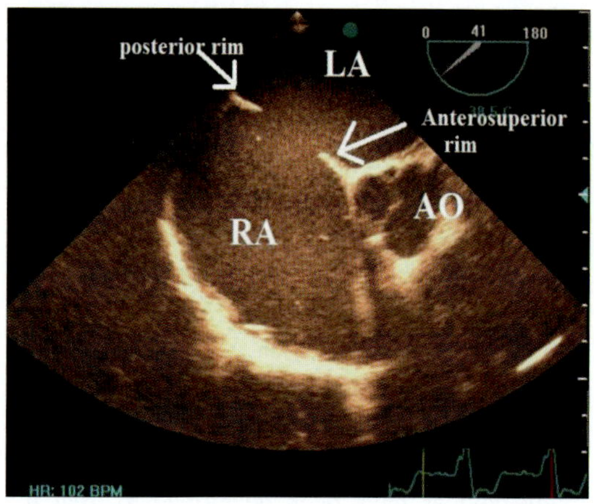

Fig. 55.3 Transesophageal echocardiography in short-axis view showing aortic (anterosuperior rim) and posterior rims. *AO* aorta, *RA* right atrium, *LA* left atrium

venosus, or coronary sinus ASDs which would need surgical correction (should be closed surgically) and (2) severe irreversible pulmonary hypertension and no evidence of a left-to-right shunt [2, 3].

Factors that decide appropriateness for transcatheter closure include the size of the defect and also the presence of adequate tissue rims around the defect. Precise imaging of the anatomic features of the ASD is critical for case selection, planning, and guidance during the procedure. This is accomplished using two-dimensional (2D) and three-dimensional (3D) echocardiography. Accordingly, pre-procedural transthoracic echocardiography (TTE) and transesophageal echocardiography (TEE) have the main role in establishing the initial ASD diagnosis, ASD location, ASD size, ASD number (single or multiple fenestrations, Fig. 55.1), pulmonary arterial and right ventricular dilatation, anterior systolic (paradoxical) or flat interventricular septal motion due to significant right ventricular volume overload, pulmonary artery pressure, (sometimes) direct visualization of the defect by 2D-echo imaging (particularly from a subcostal view of the interatrial septum), associated lesions such as mitral valve prolapse and anomalous pulmonary venous connection, measurement of the distance between the ASD and the mitral valve and the coronary sinus, and delineation of the ASD rims and their pliability [4–7].

TEE can provide detailed explanations about the ASD size and rimes (Figs. 55.2, 55.3, and 55.4). Conventionally, the rims of a secundum ASD are labeled as aortic (superoanterior), atrioventricular (AV) valve (mitral or inferoanterior), superior vena caval (SVC or superoposterior), inferior vena caval (IVC or inferoposterior), and posterior (from the posterior free wall of the atria).

Depending on the device, this technique is available only for patients with a secundum ASD with a stretched diameter < 41 mm and with adequate rims [6–9].

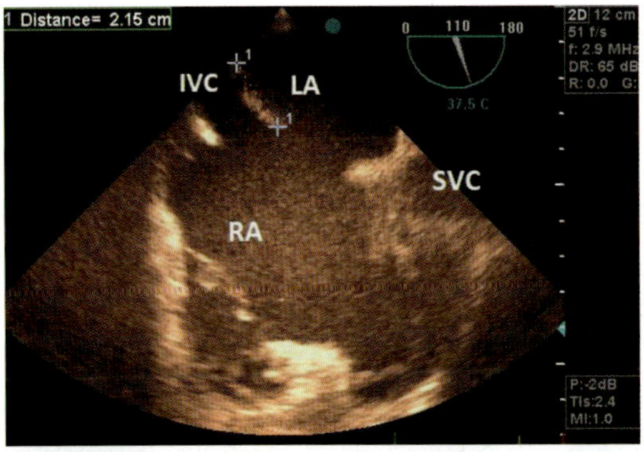

Fig. 55.4 Bicaval view showing superior vena caval (*SVC* or superoposterior) and inferior vena caval (*IVC* or inferoposterior, about 2.16 cm) rims. *RA* right atrium, *LA* left atrium

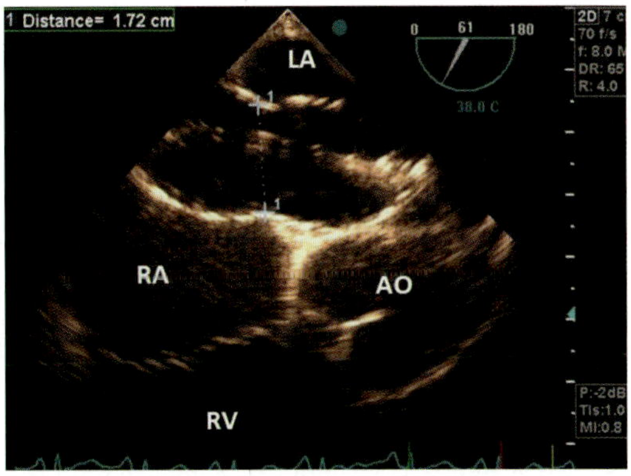

Fig. 55.5 Transesophageal echocardiography showing how to measure the balloon stretch diameter of the ASD. *RV* right ventricle, *RA* right atrium, *AO* aorta, *LA* left atrium

The Manifold Intra-procedural Benefits of TEE

- Confirming the position of the guide wire in the left atrium
- Measuring the balloon stretch diameter of the ASD (Fig. 55.5)
- Monitoring if the inflated balloon has closed the defect
- Detecting leaks around the balloon
- Guiding the release of the device
- Monitoring the Chiari network entanglement
- Monitoring thrombus on catheters [8–11]
- Providing adequate deployment and positioning of the left atrial disk (Fig. 55.6)
- Documenting the degree of the residual shunt through and around the device (Fig. 55.7)
- Guiding correct device placement and assessing leaks across the device

The Post-procedural Advantages of TEE

- Assessing leaks across the device immediately after implantation
- Assessing the adequacy of the occlusion
- Checking position stability during the wiggle maneuver
- Reviewing the device relation to the mitral valve, coronary sinus, and right upper pulmonary vein

Of course, occasionally, transient inferior ST elevation will be noted on electrocardiographic

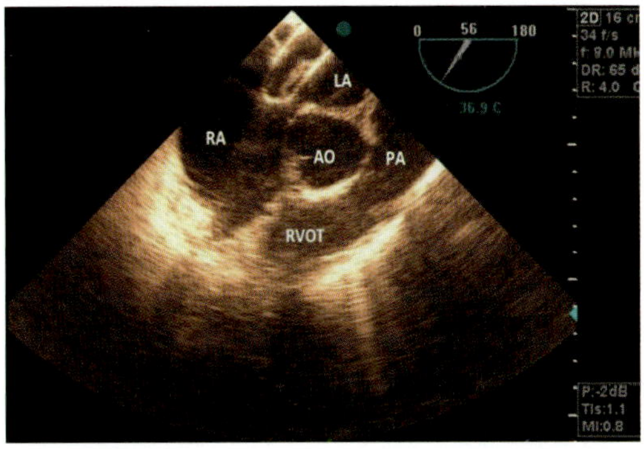

Fig. 55.6 Improper position and prolapse of the left atrial disk into the right atrium. *RV* right ventricle, *RA* right atrium, *AO* aorta, *LA* left atrium, *RVOT* right ventricular outflow tract

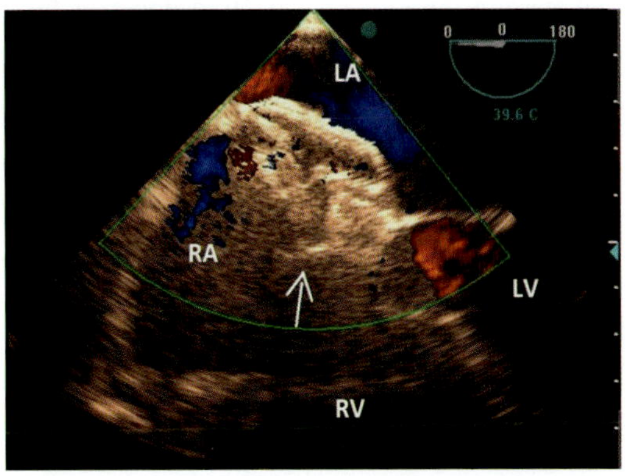

Fig. 55.7 Trivial shunts by color flow imaging around the edge of the device that frequently disappear on full release of the device. *RV* right ventricle, *RA* right atrium, *LV* left ventricle, *LA* left atrium, residual shunt

(ECG) monitoring during the procedure. This is thought to be caused by minor embolization, usually of air from the catheters, to the right coronary artery. TEE is ideally placed for the assessment and monitoring of any associated inferior regional wall motion abnormalities. In the intra-procedural time, it must be ensured that the deployed disk is unfolded properly, such that it attains an almost flat shape. If the device twists on loading into the catheter or if the delivery catheter is advanced too far into the left atrium, the left atrial disk is liable to catch against the left atrial free wall or appendage, causing twisting of the waist and a cobra-head malformation of the disk occurs. Trivial shunts on color flow mapping can also be detected around the edge of the device; they, however, frequently disappear on full release of the device, when its proper conformation is obtained. Any significant residual shunt more than this will need to be thoroughly delineated and discussed with the proceduralist [2, 3, 12, 13].

TEE also has benefits in the post-procedural: checking the device position (Figs. 55.8, 55.9, and 55.10), checking the device structural integrity, assessing residual shunts, checking the device relation to other structures such as the mitral valve or right upper pulmonary vein, and looking for potential complications such as thrombus and infection [8, 9, 14].

Recently, 3D echocardiography has been employed for precise evaluation of the ASD size and margins through "matrix" transducers, which permit acquisition of a pyramid-shaped volume of echocardiographic data (Fig. 55.11). To reach the highest resolution of the atrial septum and adjacent structures, a full-volume 3D dataset is achieved over 4 to 7 cardiac cycles. For transthoracic 3D views, the subcostal view is the view of choice because its projection is en face to the atrial septum. In cases with suboptimal windows, the low parasternal four-chamber view can be used. Note that 3D TEE overcomes the limitations of poor acoustic windows in adult patients (Fig. 55.12).

Real-time 3D imaging confirms the changing in the shape of the ASD during a single cardiac cycle, with the maximum size in diastole. During the procedure, live 3D or a 3D zoom mode is

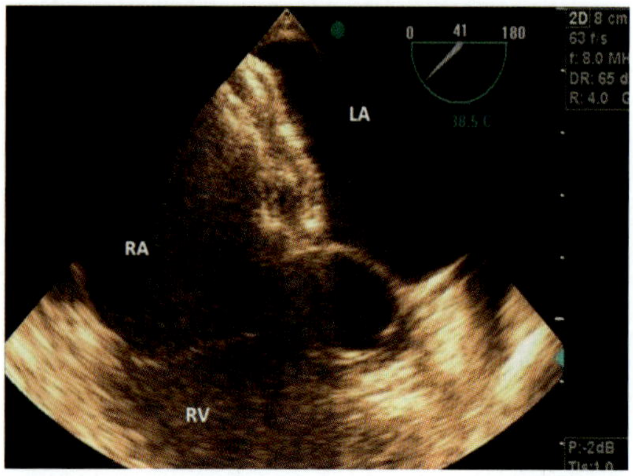

Fig. 55.8 Post-procedural evaluation of device showing proper size and well-seated ASD occluder. *RV* right ventricle, *RA* right atrium, *LA* left atrium

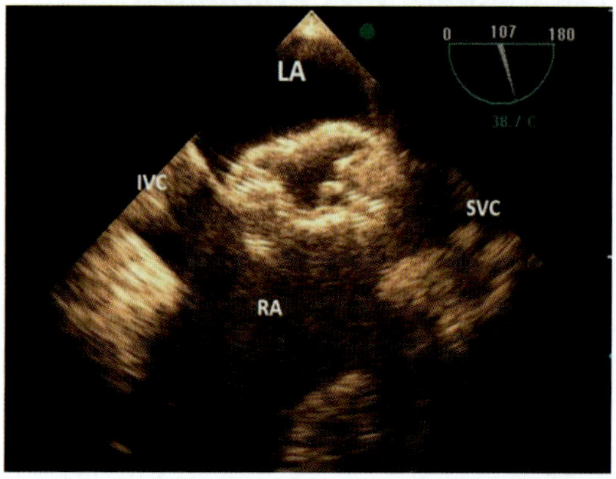

Fig. 55.9 Post-procedural evaluation of device showing oversize, well-seated ASD occluder. *RA* right atrium, *LA* left atrium, *IVC* inferior vena cava, *SVC* superior vena cava

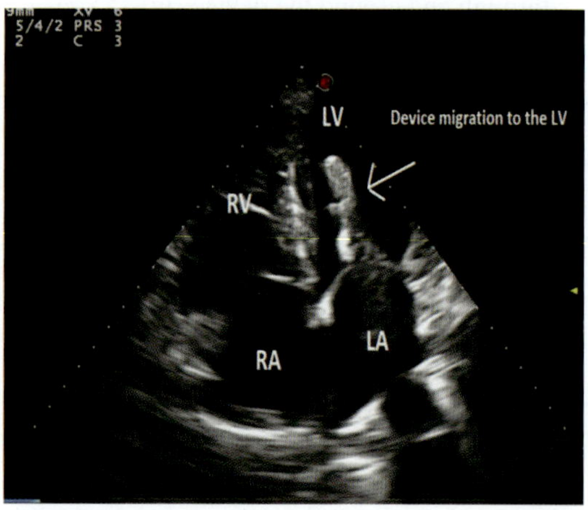

Fig. 55.10 Transthoracic echocardiography in four-chamber view showing migration of the device into the left ventricle. *RV* right ventricle, *RA* right atrium, *LV* left ventricle, *LA* left atrium

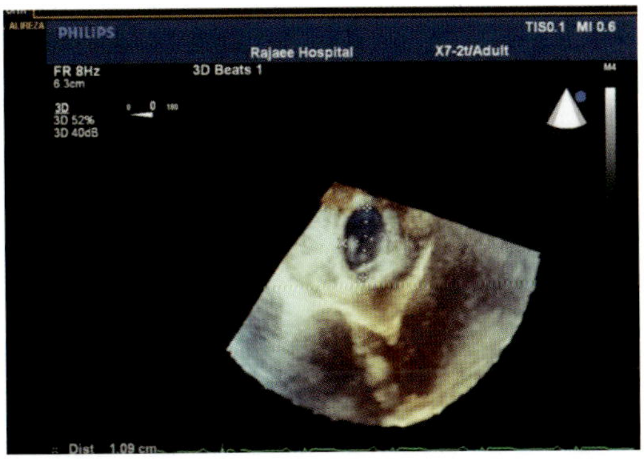

Fig. 55.11 Three-dimensional transesophageal echocardiography, showing precise anatomic detail of an atrial septal defect

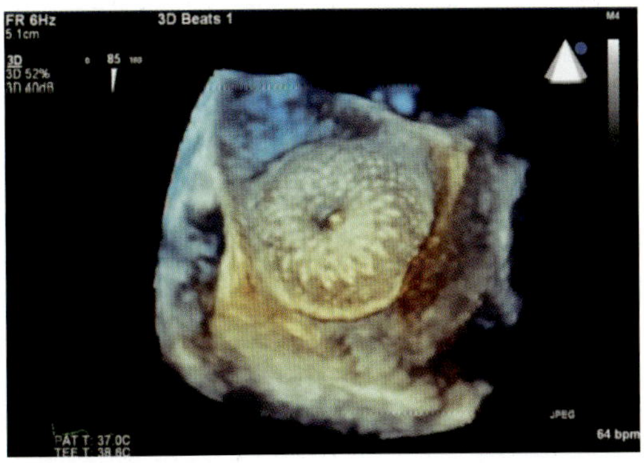

Fig. 55.12 Post-procedural evaluation of device by 3D TEE

used to observe the position of guide wires, sheaths, and devices in real time. Moreover, 3D echocardiography is principally helpful in cases with multiple ASDs to ensure the placement of the delivery sheath through the larger defect. Also, 3D echocardiography may be potentially helpful in cases with difficult ASDs by demonstrating the alignment of the disks against the septum during deployment [6, 9, 15, 16].

In conclusion, ASD device closure can be the first option for the management of the secundum ASD. Echocardiography plays a critical role in patient selection, guidance, and post-deployment evaluation for the transcatheter closure of the ASD. Understanding the echo-anatomic correlation by TEE is perhaps the most essential and basic requisite to ensure a successful procedure. Furthermore, 3D echocardiography is likely to further this understanding in the future, particularly in difficult cases such as multiple defects or defects with deficient margins.

References

1. Attie F, Rosas M, Granados N, et al. Surgical treatment for secundum atrial septal defects in patients >40 years old. A randomized clinical trial. J Am Coll Cardiol. 2001;38:2035–42.
2. Majunke N, Bialkowski J, Wilson N, et al. Closure of atrial septal defect with the Amplatzer septal occluder in adults. Am J Cardiol. 2009;103:550–4.
3. Patel A, Lopez K, Banerjee A, et al. Transcatheter closure of atrial septal defects in adults ≥40 years of age: immediate and follow-up results. J Interv Cardiol. 2007;20:82–8.
4. Jones TK, Latson LA, Zahn E, et al. Multicenter Pivotal Study of the HELEX Septal Occluder Investigators. Results of the U. S. multicenter pivotal study of the HELEX septal occluder for percutaneous closure of secundum atrial septal defects. J Am Coll Cardiol. 2007; 49:2215–21.
5. Berger F, Vogel M, Alexi-Meshkishvili V, et al. Comparison of results and complications of surgical and amplatzer device closure of atrial septal defects. J Thorac Cardiovasc Surg. 1999;118:678–80.
6. Knepp MD, Rocchini AP, Lloyd TR, et al. Long-term follow up of secundum atrial septal defect closure with the Amplatzer septal occluder. Congenit Heart Dis. 2010;5:32–7.
7. Humenberger M, Rosenhek R, Gabriel H, et al. Benefit of atrial septal defect closure in adults: impact of age. Eur Heart J. 2011;32:553–60.
8. Rosas M, Zabal C, Garcia-Montes J, et al. Transcatheter versus surgical closure of secundum atrial septal defect in adults: impact of age at Intervention. A concurrent matched comparative study. Congenit Heart Dis. 2007;2:148–55.
9. Khan AA, Tan JL, Li W, et al. The impact of transcatheter atrial septal defect closure in older population: a prospective study. JACC Cardiovasc Interv. 2010;3:276–81.
10. Swan L, Varma C, Yip J, et al. Transcatheter device closure of atrial septal defects in the elderly: technical considerations and short-term outcomes. Int J Cardiol. 2006;107:207–10.
11. Teo KS, Dundon BK, Molaee P, et al. Percutaneous closure of atrial septal defects leads to normalisation of atrial and ventricular volumes. J Cardiovasc Magn Reson. 2008;10:55.
12. Fang F, Yu CM, Sanderson JE, et al. Prevalence and determinants of incomplete right atrial reverse remodeling after device closure of atrial septal defects. Am J Cardiol. 2011;108:114–9.
13. Balint OH, Samman A, Haberer K, et al. Outcomes in patients with pulmonary hypertension undergoing percutaneous atrial septal closure. Heart. 2008;94: 1189–93.

14. Yong G, Khairy P, De Guise P, et al. Pulmonary arterial hypertension in patients with transcatheter closure of secundum atrial septal defects: a longitudinal study. Circ Cardiovasc Interv. 2009;2:455–62.
15. Jateganokar S, Scholtz W, Schmidt H, et al. Percutaneous closure of atrial septal defects: echocardiographic and functional results in patients older than 60 years. Circ Cardiovasc Interv. 2009;2:85–9.
16. Vaidyanathan B, Simpson JM, Kumar RK. Transesophageal echocardiography for device closure of atrial septal defects. J Am Coll Cardiol Imaging. 2009;2(10):1238–42.

Transcatheter Closure of the Ventricular Septal Defects

56

Azin Alizadehasl and Anita Sadeghpour

Keywords
Transcatheter closure of the ventricular septal defect (VSD) • Perimemberanous VSD • Transesophageal echocardiography (TEE) • Pulmonary vascular resistance • Arrhythmia

Introduction

The ventricular septal defect (VSD) is a common congenital heart defect (CHD) in both children and adults. Standard treatment for the VSD is open surgery, which is generally performed with minimal operative mortality but still carries some risks such as complete atrioventricular block (AVB) and residual shunt. Since the first report of transcatheter VSD closure in 1988, this catheter-based approach for the VSD (especially for the perimembranous VSD, which involves the membranous septum and accounts for approximately 70 % of cases) has been shown to be an alternative approach to surgical closure, with acceptable mortality and morbidity rates as well as promising results [1–3].

A. Alizadehasl, MD, FACC (✉)
Echocardiography Lab, Department of Cardiology, Rajaie Cardiovascular Medical and Research Center, Iran University of Medical Science, Tehran, Iran
e-mail: alizadeasl@gmail.com, alizadeasl@rhc.ac.ir

A. Sadeghpour, MD, FACC, FASE
Echocardiography Lab, Department of Cardiology, Adult Congenital Heart Disease Clinic, Rajaie Cardiovascular Medical and Research Center, Iran University of Medical Science, Tehran, Iran
e-mail: anita.sadeghpour@gmail.com, asadeghpour@rhc.ac.ir

Inclusion and Exclusion Criteria

The inclusion criteria for transcatheter VSD closure are comprised of the following:

1. Congenital perimembranous or muscular VSDs as shown by echocardiography
2. Maximum VSD diameter <20 mm by transthoracic echocardiography (TTE)
3. Defect located at the 9–11 o'clock positions of an analog clock in the short-axis parasternal view by TTE
4. Distance >1 mm between the perimembranous VSD and the aortic valve (AV)
5. Left-to-right shunt
6. Calculated pulmonary vascular resistance <8 Wood units

The exclusion criteria consist of the following:

1. Defects associated with other cardiac anomalies requiring a surgical approach
2. Irreversible pulmonary vascular disease (pulmonary vascular resistance >8 Wood units)

A. Sadeghpour et al. (eds.), *Comprehensive Approach to Adult Congenital Heart Disease*,
DOI 10.1007/978-1-4471-6383-1_56, © Springer-Verlag London 2014

3. Severe AV regurgitation
4. Severe AV prolapse
5. Right-to-left shunt [1, 3, 4]

Procedure

Catheterization procedure is done without tracheal intubation and under conscious sedation for patients younger than 10 years of age. Heparin (100 IU/kg) and antibiotics are administered intravenously during the procedure. Access is through the right femoral vein and also right femoral artery. Angiography in the left ventricle (LV) at a 55°/20° left anterior oblique cranial projection is used to profile the VSD. Location and size of the VSD and its relationship with the AV are studied. The diameter of the VSD is measured at the largest diastolic period, and an occluder device is selected according to this measurement. The defect is then passed from the LV with a 5-French partly cut pigtail catheter or a right Judkins catheter. An arteriovenous circuit is set up through the femoral vein approach on the same side. A long sheath (6–12 Fr) is advanced to the LV through the arteriovenous circuit and placed beneath the AV. Through the long sheath, the VSD occluder is deployed under fluoroscopic control and echocardiographic help and guidance. Angiography in the LV and ascending aorta is performed again to confirm complete occlusion and to detect any new-onset AV regurgitation.

Continuous electrocardiographic (ECG) monitoring is used during the first 24 h after the procedure. Aspirin (5 mg/kg daily) is administered for 6 months in all patients [1, 4–7].

Complications and Follow-up

During follow-up, a large number of patients having been reported to date (by Hijazi et al.) had excellent closure results with 100 % complete closure rate at 6-month follow-up. A series of six patients were also reported to have 100 % complete occlusion. The only complication reported

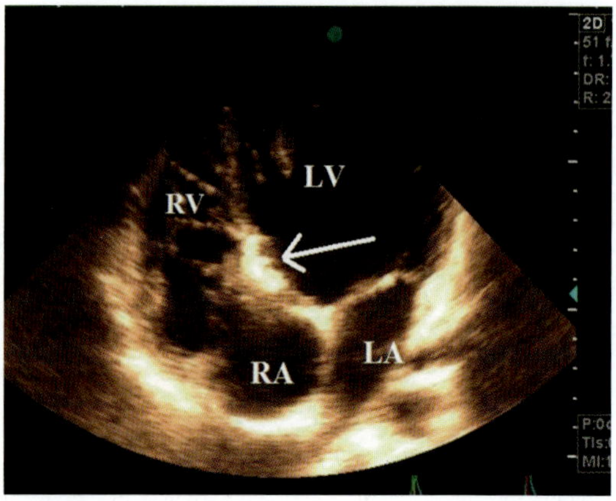

Fig. 56.1 *White arrow* showing VSD occluder with tricuspid valve entrapment. *LA* left atrium, *RA* right atrium, *LV* left ventricle, *RV* right ventricle

is transient arrhythmia, which occurred during or immediately after deployment [6, 7].

The most common complications associated with transcatheter VSD closure are heart rhythm disturbances. Other common adverse events include valvular regurgitation, device embolization, hemolysis, hematoma, and fever. These adverse events are generally manageable and do not outweigh the benefits. Many types of cardiac arrhythmia may take place during the transcatheter procedure. Bundle branch block and transient or permanent AVB are reported too. Complete AVB has been reported to be the most significant complication in both the early phase and follow-up period, with an incidence rate varying from 3.5 to 8.6 % [1, 8, 9].

Valvular regurgitation is another major consideration in the transcatheter closure of the perimembranous VSD. Impingement of the occluder on the valve leaflets may cause instant aortic or tricuspid regurgitation by interfering with the chordae tendineae (Figs. 56.1 and 56.2).

Thus, echocardiography and angiography are crucial for confirming correct device deployment. Other mechanisms may be associated with the improper placement of the occluder on the tricuspid septal leaflets, migration of the occluder, shape memory of Nitinol wires, or rupture of the chordae tendineae [1, 6, 10].

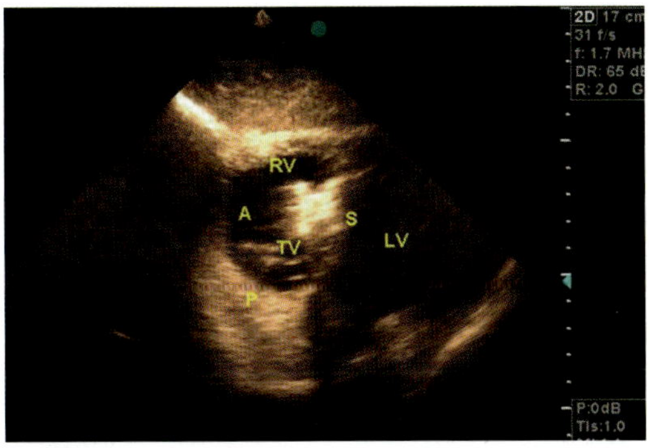

Fig. 56.2 Improper placement of the occluder on the tricuspid septal leaflets resulting impingement of the occluder on the tricuspid chordae tendineae. *RV* right ventricle, *TV* tricuspid valve, *LV* left ventricle, *P* posterior leaflet of TV, *A* anterior leaflet of TV, *S* septal leaflet of TV

References

1. Butera G, Chessa M, Carminati M. Percutaneous closure of ventricular septal defects. Cardiol Young. 2007;17:243–53.
2. Qin Y, Chen J, Zhao X, Liao D, Mu R, Wang S, Wu H, Guo H. Transcatheter closure of perimembranous ventricular septal defect using a modified double-disk occluder. Am J Cardiol. 2008;101:1781–6.
3. Hijazi ZM, Hakim F, Haweleh AA, Madani A, Tarawna W, Hiari A, Cao QL. Catheter closure of perimembranous ventricular septal defects using the new Amplatzer membranous VSD occluder: initial clinical experience. Catheter Cardiovasc Interv. 2002; 56:508–15.
4. Knauth AL, Lock JE, Perry SB, McElhinney DB, Gauvreau K, Landzberg MJ, Rome JJ, Hellenbrand WE, Ruiz CE, Jenkins KJ. Transcatheter device closure of congenital and postoperative residual ventricular septal defects. Circulation. 2004;110:501–7.
5. Fu YC, Bass J, Amin Z, Radtke W, Cheatham JP, Hellenbrand WE, Balzer D, Cao QL, Hijazi ZM. Transcatheter closure of perimembranous ventricular septal defects using the new Amplatzer membranous VSD occluder: results of the U.S. phase I trial. J Am Coll Cardiol. 2006;47:319–25.
6. Chessa M, Butera G, Negura D, Bussadori C, Giamberti A, Fesslova V, Carminati M. Transcatheter closure of congenital ventricular septal defects in adult: mid-term results and complications. Int J Cardiol. 2009;133:70–3.
7. Thanopoulos BD, Tsaousis GS, Konstadopoulou GN, et al. Transcatheter closure of muscular ventricular septal defects with the Amplatzer Ventricular Septal Defect Occluder: Initial clinical applications in children. J Am Coll Cardiol. 1999;33:1395–9.
8. Latiff HA, Alwi M, Kandhavel G, et al. Transcatheter closure of multiple muscular ventricular septal defects using Gianturco coils. Ann Thorac Surg. 1999;68: 1400–1.
9. Rodes J, Piechaud JF, Ouaknine R, Hulin S, Cohen L, Magnier S, Lecompte Y, Lefevre T. Transcatheter closure of apical ventricular muscular septal defect combined with arterial switch operation in a newborn infant. Catheter Cardiovasc Interv. 2000;49:173–6.
10. Hijazi ZM, Hakim F, Al-Fadley F, et al. Transcatheter closure of single muscular ventricular septal defects using the Amplatzer Muscular VSD Occluder: initial results and technical considerations. Catheter Cardiovasc Interv. 2000;49:167–72.

Indications of Surgery in Adult Congenial Heart Disease

57

Alireza Alizadeh Ghavidel

Keywords
Surgery • Adult congenital heart disease • Sternotomy • Peripheral cannulation • Jatene procedure

Introduction

Due to tremendous development in cardiothoracic surgery, over the past decades, 95 % of newborns with congenital heart disease (CHD) survive into adulthood. Although most of adult patients with CHD have undergone surgical intervention during childhood and also there have been recently remarkable advances in percutaneous transcatheter techniques to treat adult congenital heart disease (ACHD), a significant proportion of these patients will have to undergo cardiovascular surgery at some point in adulthood.

Surgeries may be considered in a number of patients with ACHD. These patients include those with prior palliative operations or residual defects. Patients with associated cardiac lesions who have not been operated due to missed diagnosis or lack of sever lesions may also need the surgery in adulthood.

The detailed management strategies in adults with various CHDs have been discussed in the related chapters, and this chapter provides an overview on indications for surgery in some types of ACHD.

Atrial Septal Defect

In the absence of symptoms or associated intracardiac lesions, small unrepaired atrial septal defects (ASDs) do not require surgical intervention [1]. These patients should be followed up continuously because LV compliance decreases with age, leading to increased left-to-right shunting and subsequent development of symptoms. However, in several specific conditions such as paradoxical embolism or maybe recent-onset atrial arrhythmias, ASD closure is indicated, regardless of the defect size. Larger ASDs are usually accompanied by RV enlargement and should be closed, even in asymptomatic patients. ASD closure is contraindicated in patients who develop severe irreversible pulmonary artery hypertension (i.e., Eisenmenger's physiology) [1].

In patients with paroxysmal or persistent atrial fibrillation or flutter, a concomitant Maze procedure during ASD closure may be advised [1]. The type of the ASD may also determine the treatment strategy. For example, patients with sinus venosus,

A. Alizadeh Ghavidel, MD
Cardiac Surgery Ward, Department of Cardiac Surgery, Rajaie Cardiovascular Medical and Research Center, Iran University of Medical Science, Tehran, Iran
e-mail: aaghavidel@gmail.com, aghavidel@rhc.ac.ir

A. Sadeghpour et al. (eds.), *Comprehensive Approach to Adult Congenital Heart Disease*, DOI 10.1007/978-1-4471-6383-1_57, © Springer-Verlag London 2014

ostium primum, and coronary sinoseptal ASD have been shown to have better results with surgical closure than with percutaneous intervention. However, in patients with ostium secundum ASD, closure can be performed either surgically or using a percutaneous device. In several conditions, the anatomical characteristics of the ASD such as multiple ASDs, fenestrated septum primum, inadequate septal rim, and redundant or aneurysmal septum primum preclude the use of a device. Furthermore, in patients with concomitant lesions which need surgery such as significant tricuspid regurgitation or Maze procedure requiring atrial arrhythmias, the surgical closure of the ASD should be considered.

Patent Foramen Ovale

The patent foramen ovale (PFO) should be closed in patients experiencing recurrent cryptogenic stoke on anticoagulation. In patients with prior exposure to changes in atmosphere pressure that increases the risk of paradoxical air embolism, the PFO should also be closed [1].

Atrioventricular Septal Defect

Adult patients with untreated complete atrioventricular septal defects usually suffer from severe pulmonary artery hypertension and severe pulmonary vascular disease; surgical repair, therefore, has no benefit in such cases. All patients with partial atrioventricular septal defects must be surgically treated unless severe pulmonary artery hypertension exists. Low surgical mortality and good survival rates have been reported for these patients [2].

Occasionally, surgery is indicated in adult patients with this anomaly for the repair of residual defects or valve regurgitation.

Ventricular Septal Defect

Usually small ventricular septal defects (VSDs) with Qp/Qs <1.5 are not considered for surgical repair. Untreated small VSDs are not uneventful during long-term follow-up, and the recent mortality and morbidity rates of surgical repair have been low; consequently, the percutaneous or surgical closure of small VSDs may be the right option in selected patients [3].

Moderate-sized VSDs usually have a significant shunt (Qp/Qs >1.5) and should be closed either by interventional or surgical repair. Large VSDs should be repaired unless there is irreversible pulmonary artery hypertension or Eisenmenger's physiology.

Patent Ductus Arteriosus

The surgical closure of a large patent ductus arteriosus (PDA) is rarely indicated in adult patients since most of these patients have Eisenmenger's physiology (net right-to-left shunt). Currently, most small- or moderate-sized PDAs are closed by percutaneous intervention using different occlusive devices. Distorted, aneurysmal, or severely calcified PDAs are not suitable for percutaneous closure and surgery is usually recommended. Patients with an enlarged LV or left atrium (LA), pulmonary hypertension, or net left-to-right shunting and patients with previous endarteritis are also recommended to undergo PDA closure (class I, level of evidence C) [1].

Tetralogy of Fallot

The total correction of the tetralogy of Fallot (TOF) is indicated in adulthood, with the exception of patients with severe left ventricular (LV) or right ventricular (RV) dysfunction. Post-TOF repair complications are not uncommon. There are different indications for surgical re-interventions in patients with previous TOF repair, including [1]:

1. Severe pulmonary regurgitation in patients with clinical cardiac symptoms or exercise intolerance may indicate pulmonary valve replacement (class I, level of evidence B).
2. Severe pulmonary regurgitation after TOF repair along with moderate RV dysfunction or enlargement; new-onset sustained, moderate to severe tricuspid regurgitation; or symptomatic

atrial/ventricular arrhythmia may indicate pulmonary valve replacement (class IIa, level of evidence B and C).
3. Residual right outflow tract stenosis in post-TOF repair patients with peak gradient >50 mmHg or right-to-left ventricular pressure >0.7 may indicate surgical re-intervention (class IIa, level of evidence C).
4. Symptomatic residual VSD with Qp/Qs >1.5 may indicate VSD closure (class IIa, level of evidence B).
5. Severe aortic insufficiency in symptomatic patients after TOF total correction may indicate valve repair/replacement if more than mild LV dysfunction exists (class IIa, level of evidence C).
6. Multiple residual defects in combination with RV dysfunction or enlargement may indicate surgical re-intervention (class IIa, level of evidence C).

Ebstein's Anomaly

Patients with Ebstein's anomaly may be considered for surgical intervention for tricuspid valve repair or replacement and simultaneous closure of an ASD, if present. However, these operations should only be carried out in patients who have symptoms or exhibit any of decreased exercise capacity, cyanosis, paradoxical emboli, deteriorating cardiomegaly (as evident on chest X-ray), and increasing RV dilation or decreasing RV systolic function.

Surgical re-repair or replacement of the tricuspid valve may be considered for adult patients with Ebstein's anomaly if they have [1]:

1. Symptoms, poor exercise capacity, or New York Heart Association (NYHA) functional class III–IV
2. Severe post-repair tricuspid regurgitation with progressive RV dilation, RV systolic function reduction, or development or deterioration of atrial and/or ventricular arrhythmias
3. Dysfunction of the bioprosthetic tricuspid valve in association with significant combined regurgitation and stenosis
4. Predominant bioprosthetic valve stenosis (MG >12–15 mmHg)

Surgery may be considered earlier with lesser degrees of bioprosthetic stenosis if patients have symptoms or decreased exercise tolerance.

Coarctation of the Aorta

Interventional repair of the coarctation of aorta may consist of surgery or percutaneous catheter-based therapy. Patients with trans-coarctation gradient ≥20 mmHg and luminal obstruction ≥55 % at the coarctation site need interventional repair. Surgery may also be considered in patients with gradient <20 mmHg across the coarctation site and luminal narrowing <50 %, if radiologic findings document the presence of a significant collateral flow. However, controversy continues over the most efficient type of therapy for native aortic coarctation in adults. In patients with native coarctation, surgery is preferred if the coarctation is tubular or long segment, and there are concomitant proximal arch hypoplasia, aneurysms, dissection, or significant ectasia. Recurrent coarctation in patients with long re-coarctation segment or associated aortic arch hypoplasia is also an indication for reparative surgery [1].

Cor Triatriatum

Cor triatriatum is rarely seen in adults. These patients usually present with dyspnea, pulmonary hypertension or pulmonary edema, and atrial fibrillation similar to mitral stenosis. Symptomatic patients should be subjected to surgical repair.

Bicuspid Aortic Valve

Patients with bicuspid aortic valve (BAV) and aortic stenosis without aortic insufficiency are usually good candidates for percutaneous balloon valvotomy. Surgery is indicated when percutaneous intervention fails or when significant aortic insufficiency occurs. Indications for intervention in patients with BAV and severe aortic stenosis include [4]:

1. Patients with related symptoms (syncope, angina)

2. Patients candidate for other valve surgery or coronary artery bypass grafting (CABG)
3. Patients with systolic dysfunction [left ventricular ejection fraction (LVEF) <50 %] (class I, level of evidence B)

Surgical or percutaneous intervention may be considered for asymptomatic patients with severe aortic stenosis and abnormal exercise tolerance test (class IIa, level of evidence B).

Surgery should be performed when there is severe aortic insufficiency in symptomatic patients, asymptomatic cases with resting LVEF ≤50 %, asymptomatic patients with resting LVEF >50 % and severe LV enlargement (left ventricular end-diastolic diameter >70 mm or left ventricular end-systolic diameter >50 mm or left ventricular end-systolic diameter >25 mm/m^2), and patients who need other cardiac valve surgery (class I, level of evidence B).

The key points in patients with BAV and dilated ascending aorta are:

1. Patients with BAV and dilated ascending aorta (diameter >40 mm) should be subjected to close follow-up and annual cardiac imaging studies.
2. Surgical root reconstruction should be performed for patients with ascending aorta diameter >50 mm or high aneurysmal dilatation rate (> 5 mm/year).
3. Ascending aorta repair or replacement may be considered for patients with BAV candidate for aortic valve surgery when the diameter of the ascending aorta is 35–49 mm.

Subaortic Stenosis

Surgical indications in patients with subaortic stenosis according to the American College of Cardiology/American Heart Association (ACC/AHA) guideline for adult congenital heart disease (ACHD) include [1]:

1. Patients with peak gradient (PG) >50 mmHg or mean gradient (MG) >30 mmHg on Doppler echocardiography (class I, level of evidence C)
2. Patients with PG <50 mmHg or MG <30 mmHg and progressive aortic insufficiency and LV end-systolic diameter ≥50 mm or LVEF <55 % (class I, level of evidence C)

Surgery may also be considered in cases with PG <50 mmHg or MG <30 mmHg if the patient has LV hypertrophy or has a plan for pregnancy or is involved in vigorous sport (class IIa, level of evidence C).

Supravalvular Aortic Stenosis

Percutaneous intervention has no role in the management of supravalvular aortic stenosis and surgery is the only option for these patients. Surgery should be considered in symptomatic cases with discrete or diffuse supra-aortic stenosis who have PG >70 mmHg or MG >50 mmHg by Doppler echocardiographic study [1].

Surgery is also recommended for lesser degrees of stenosis if the patient has related symptoms or LV hypertrophy or dysfunction and in a symptomatic patient intending to become pregnant or a patient active in sport [1].

Rupture of Valsalva Sinus Aneurysm

Prompt surgery should be performed in all patients with rupture of Valsalva sinus aneurysm with or without concomitant VSD or aortic insufficiency [1, 5]. Hemodynamic disturbance and acute heart failure symptoms are frequently seen in these patients.

Symptomatic or enlarging unruptured Valsalva sinus should be surgically treated. Surgical repair may be considered for asymptomatic cases with small- to moderate-sized aneurysm of the Valsalva sinus when the patient undergoes aortic valve or root surgery for any other indication.

Persistent Truncus Arteriosus

The surgical repair of truncus regurgitation is usually performed during the neonatal period or 10–15 years after previous repair; therefore, the presentation of truncus arteriosus in adults is unusual.

Isolated Pulmonary Valve Stenosis

Severe pulmonary valve stenosis is not common in childhood. Infrequently, less degrees of pulmonary valve stenosis present in adult patients, and percutaneous balloon valvotomy is the first line of interventional therapy. Surgery is usually recommended for patients with other cardiac problems requiring surgery (VSD, tricuspid regurgitation). The indications of the surgery in patients with isolated pulmonary valve stenosis include [1, 6]:

1. Residual pulmonary valve stenosis after balloon valvotomy; PG >50 mmHg for symptomatic and PG >70 mmHg for asymptomatic patients
2. Dysplastic or complex RV outflow tract obstruction and concomitant severe pulmonary regurgitation that precludes percutaneous balloon valvotomy

Peripheral Pulmonary Artery Stenosis

Patients with peripheral artery stenosis >50 % of the diameter, patients with related symptoms, or patients with systolic RV pressure >50 mmHg should be considered for interventional therapy (class I, level of evidence B) [1].

Percutaneous catheter-based intervention is the treatment of choice in these patients, and surgery should be performed only in patients with concomitant cardiac lesions or in those amenable to percutaneous intervention.

Double-Chambered Right Ventricle

Double-chambered right ventricle is very uncommon in adulthood. In contrast to children, the clinical presentation usually includes chest pain, syncope, and dyspnea on exertion. Surgery is indicated for symptomatic patients. Also, patients with signs of myocardial ischemia or gradient ≥40 mmHg should be considered for surgery.

Coronary Artery Fistula

Any coronary arteriovenous fistula should be closed in patients with related symptoms, regardless of the size of the fistula and shunting, either by percutaneous or by surgical intervention (class I, level of evidence C) [1]. The clinical findings and symptoms usually include myocardial ischemia, arrhythmia, unexplained ventricular dysfunction, or enlargement or endarteritis.

The percutaneous or surgical closure of a large coronary arteriovenous fistula should be performed in all patients (even asymptomatic cases) (class I, level of evidence C) [1].

Asymptomatic patients with a small fistula and a nonsignificant left-to-right shunt are not candidates for interventional closure and may be followed up every 3–5 years.

Dextro-transposition of the Great Arteries [1, 7]

Reconstructive surgery or catheter-based intervention may be considered for residual and/or recurrent lesions in adults with prior surgery for dextro-transposition of the great arteries (D-TGA). The type of the previous surgery and also the specific characteristics of the current lesion may determine the preferred method of treatment. Herein, the indications of reoperation after different surgical procedures are presented.

After Arterial Switch Repair

Surgery is indicated for repairing supravalvular and branch pulmonary valve stenosis either when it occurs alone or when it happens in association with valvular and subvalvular stenosis. Patients with LV outflow tract obstruction should only undergo surgery if LV pressure rises to suprasystemic values or obstruction-related symptoms develop. The size of the obstruction per se, even if moderate or severe, as estimated by pressure gradient, may not predict LV function properly. Patients with severe RV outflow tract obstruction should undergo reoperation if they have peak-to-peak gradient >50 mmHg or RV/LV ratio >0.7. Patients with severe pulmonary regurgitation who have concomitant significant RV dilatation or dysfunction should undergo pulmonary valve repair or replacement.

Other conditions occurring late after arterial switch may also need surgical intervention such as coronary ostial stenosis causing myocardial ischemia and neoaortic root dilation. In the latter, valve-sparing root replacement may be suitable in the absence of aortic valve dysfunction. Nevertheless, in patients with more than mild aortic regurgitation, aortic root replacement with aortic valve replacement or aortic valve repair may be advisable.

After Atrial Baffle Procedure

d-TGA patients with previous atrial baffle operation should undergo surgical intervention in the following conditions:

1. If they exhibit moderate to severe systemic (morphological tricuspid) atrioventricular valve regurgitation in the absence of significant ventricular dysfunction
2. If they develop baffle leak in association with any of left-to-right shunt ratio >1.5:1, right-to-left shunt with at rest or exertional arterial deoxygenation, symptoms, and the increasing ventricular enlargement
3. If they have superior/inferior vena cava or pulmonary venous pathway obstructions not amenable to percutaneous intervention
4. If they have severe subpulmonary stenosis with symptoms

After Rastelli Procedure

d-TGA adults with previous Rastelli procedure may undergo reoperations for several purposes, including conduit and/or valve replacement, conduit regurgitation treatment, residual VSD closure relief, branch pulmonary artery stenosis repair, permanent pacing, Maze procedure (for patients with intermittent or chronic atrial tachyarrhythmia undergoing cardiac reoperation for any cause), and heart transplantation. Be that as it may, each of these operations has its own specific indications, which are depicted in Table 57.1.

Table 57.1 Indications for reoperation after Rastelli procedure [1, 7]

Conduit and/or valve replacement
Conduit obstruction
Peak-to-peak gradient >50 mmHg
Right ventricular/left ventricular pressure ratio >0.7
Subaortic (baffle) obstruction
Mean gradient >50 mmHg
Presence of concomitant severe aortic regurgitation
Treatment of severe conduit regurgitation
Presence of symptoms
Declining exercise tolerance
Severely depressed right ventricular function
Severe right ventricular enlargement
Development/progression of atrial or ventricular arrhythmias
More than moderate tricuspid regurgitation
Surgical closure of residual ventricular septal defect
Qp/Qs >1.5:1
Systolic pulmonary artery pressure >50 mmHg
Increasing left ventricular size from volume overload
Decreasing right ventricular function from pressure overload
Right ventricular outflow tract obstruction
Peak instantaneous gradient >50 mmHg
or
Pulmonary artery pressure <two thirds of systemic pressure
or
Pulmonary valve resistance <two thirds of systemic vascular resistance
and
A net left-to-right shunt of 1.5:1
or
A decrease in pulmonary artery pressure with pulmonary vasodilators (oxygen, nitric oxide, or prostaglandins)

Moreover, adults with branch pulmonary artery stenosis who are not amenable to percutaneous treatment should undergo surgical intervention after Rastelli repair of d-TGA. Intermittent or chronic atrial tachyarrhythmia in adults with d-TGA can be treated effectively with a concomitant Maze procedure during reoperation for any reason.

Congenitally Corrected Transposition of the Great Arteries [1, 7]

Surgery is indicated in adults with unrepaired congenitally corrected transposition of the great arteries (CCTGA) if it is associated with severe atrioventricular valve regurgitation. Patients in whom the LV is functioning at systemic pressures may also be considered for anatomical reconstruction with atrial and arterial level switch/Rastelli repair. Moreover, patients with VSD should undergo simple surgical VSD closure if the LV-to-aorta baffling is not feasible for the VSD or if the VSD is restrictive. Rarely, LV dysfunction and severe LV outflow obstruction necessitate surgery for the purpose of LV-to-pulmonary artery conduit. Other hemodynamic disturbances that are indications of operation in CCTGA patients are outlined in Table 57.2.

Surgery may also be required in patients with associated pathologies such as systemic atrioventricular valve regurgitation, systemic ventricle dysfunction, and rarely pulmonary overcirculation resulting in the development of symptoms. Surgery is usually considered prior to the decline of systemic ventricle ejection fraction <45 %.

Table 57.2 Hemodynamic indications for operation in congenitally corrected transposition of the great arteries [1, 7]

Moderate or deteriorating systemic atrioventricular valve regurgitation
Conduit obstruction after anatomic repair, if associated with
Systemic or nearly systemic right ventricular pressures
and/or
Right ventricular dysfunction
Conduit obstruction after nonanatomic repair, if associated with
Systemic or suprasystemic left ventricular pressures
Moderate or severe aortic regurgitation/neoaortic regurgitation, if associated with
Development of ventricular dysfunction
or
Deteriorating ventricular dilatation

Reoperation should also be undertaken in the following conditions:

1. Systemic atrioventricular valve repair or replacement in patients who have previously undergone a nonanatomic repair
2. Conduit replacement and resection of LV outflow obstruction in patients in whom a Rastelli operation has been performed for the anatomical repair. Selected patients of this group may need aortic or mitral valve repair/replacement.

Tricuspid Atresia/Single Ventricle

Reoperation should be considered in adult patients with prior Fontan repair for single-ventricle physiology if any of the following criteria is met [1, 8]:

1. Unintended residual ASD that results in a right-to-left shunt with symptoms and/or cyanosis not amenable to transcatheter closure
2. Hemodynamically significant residual systemic artery-to-pulmonary artery shunt, residual surgical shunt, or residual ventricle-to-pulmonary artery connection not amenable to transcatheter closure
3. Moderate to severe systemic atrioventricular valve regurgitation
4. Significant (> 30 mmHg peak to peak) subaortic obstruction
5. Fontan pathway obstruction
6. Development of venous collateral channels or pulmonary arteriovenous malformation not amenable to transcatheter management
7. Pulmonary venous obstruction
8. Rhythm abnormalities such as complete atrioventricular block or sick sinus syndrome requiring epicardial pacemaker insertion
9. Creation or closure of a fenestration not amenable to transcatheter intervention

For patients with recurrent atrial fibrillation or flutter without hemodynamically significant anatomic abnormalities, reoperation for Fontan conversion may be useful [1]. This operation includes the revision of an atriopulmonary connection to an intracardiac lateral tunnel, intra-atrial conduit, or extracardiac conduit. In these patients, a concomitant Maze procedure should also be considered [1].

References

1. Warnes CA, Williams RG, Bashore TM, et al. ACC/AHA 2008 guidelines for the management of adults with congenital heart disease: a report of the American College of Cardiology/American Heart Association Task Force on Practice Guidelines (Writing Committee to Develop Guidelines on the Management of Adults With Congenital Heart Disease). J Am Coll Cardiol. 2008;52(23):e143–263.
2. Bergin ML, Warnes CA, Tajik AJ, et al. Partial atrioventricular canal defect: long-term follow-up after initial repair in patients>or=40 years old. J Am Coll Cardiol. 1995;25(5):1189–94.
3. Soufflet V, Van de Bruaene A, Troost E, et al. Behavior of unrepaired perimembranous ventricular septal defect in young adults. Am J Cardiol. 2010;105(3):404–7.
4. Vahanian A, Alfieri O, Andreotti F, et al. Guidelines on the management of valvular heart disease (version 2012): the Joint Task Force on the Management of Valvular Heart Disease of the European Society of Cardiology (ESC) and the European Association for Cardio-Thoracic Surgery (EACTS). Eur J Cardiothorac Surg. 2012;42(4):S1–44.
5. Takach TJ, Reul GJ, Duncan JM, et al. Sinus of Valsalva aneurysm or fistula: management and outcome. Ann Thorac Surg. 1999;68(5):1573–7.
6. Peterson C, Schilthuis JJ, Dodge-Khatami A, et al. Comparative long-term results of surgery versus balloon valvuloplasty for pulmonary valve stenosis in infants and children. Ann Thorac Surg. 2003;76(4):1078–82.
7. Baumgartner H, Bonhoeffer P, De Groot NM, et al. ESC Guidelines for the management of grown-up congenital heart disease (new version 2010). Eur Heart J. 2010;31(23):2915–57.
8. Fontan F, Baudet E. Surgical repair of tricuspid atresia. Thorax. 1971;26:240–8.

Index

A. Sadeghpour et al. (eds.), *Comprehensive Approach to Adult Congenital Heart Disease*,
DOI 10.1007/978-1-4471-6383-1, © Springer-Verlag London 2014

D

F

G

H

Plomería

Nivel uno

QUINTA EDICIÓN

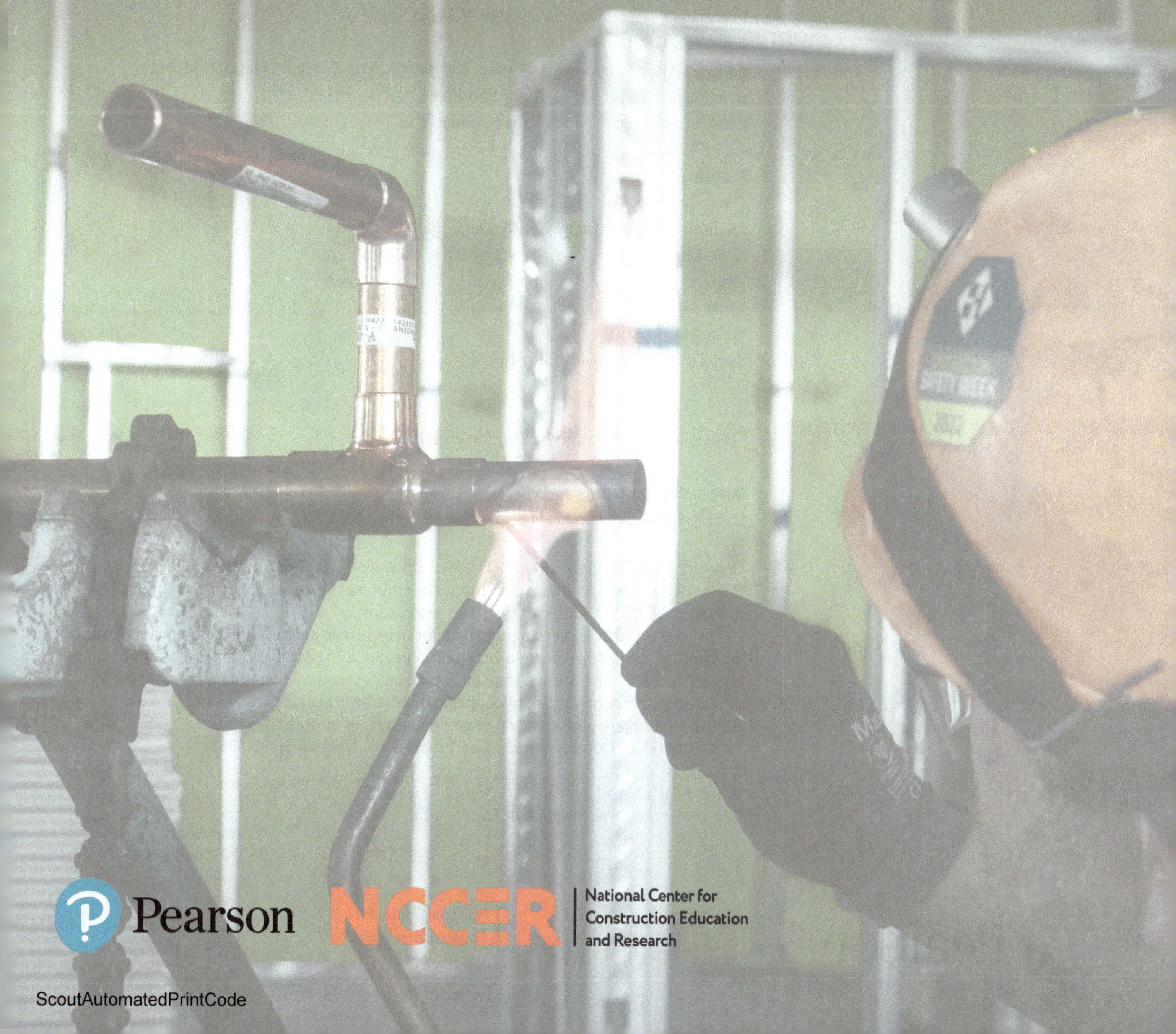

Pearson

NCCER National Center for Construction Education and Research

ScoutAutomatedPrintCode

NCCER

Presidente y director ejecutivo: Boyd Worsham
Vicepresidenta de innovación y progreso: Jennifer Wilkerson
Directora de educación: Lisa Strite
Gerente de proyectos de traducción Plomería: Yesenia Tejas
Director de proyectos sénior: Chris Wilson
Directora de producción sénior: Erin DuRant
Jefe de redacción técnica: Gary Ferguson
Redactoras técnicas: Natalie Hasty, Karyn Redmond
Directora de arte: Carrie Pelzer
Artista de producción: Judd Ivines
Gerenta de proyectos de pruebas y evaluaciones: Elizabeth Schlaupitz
Coordinadora de contenidos digitales y licencias: Amanda Smith
Especialista en permisos: Rachel Roque
Diseñadora de instrucción: Windy Wang
Gerente de autoedición: Eric Caraballoso
Especialistas en producción: Daphney Milian, Olga Trofymenko
Gestora de contenido digital: Kelly Beck
Coordinadoras de contenidos digitales: Yesenia Tejas
Editor jefe: Graham Hack
Editores: Alfonso Fernandez-Galán, Karina Kuchta, Zi Meng, Hannah Murray
Coordinadora de proyectos: Chelsi Santana
Asistentes de producción: Edward Fortman

Pearson

Directora de gestión de proyectos: Vanessa Price
Productora sénior de contenido: Alexandrina B. Wolf
Coordinadora de soluciones de empleabilidad: Mónica Pérez
Productores de contenido: Alma Dabral

Redacción: NCCER
Tecnologías de contenidos: Gnostyx

Fuentes del texto: Palatino LT Pro y Helvetica Neue

Imagen de la portada

Foto de portada proporcionada por: Amanda Smith, NCCER.

10 9 8 7 6 5 4 3 2 1
Código de impresión automatizado de Scout

Edición rústica
ISBN-13: 978-0-13-823079-1

Pearson

NCCER | National Center for Construction Education and Research

PRÓLOGO

Para el alumno

La mayoría de las personas creen que los plomeros solo van a los hogares a destapar un desagüe o instalar un electrodoméstico. Sin embargo, también instalan, realizan el mantenimiento y reparan muchos tipos de caños y sistemas de drenaje diferentes. Por ejemplo, algunos sistemas transportan agua a una planta municipal de tratamiento de agua y, de allí, a edificios residenciales, comerciales y públicos. Otros desechan residuos, suministran gas a estufas y hornos o transportan diversos líquidos y aire comprimido a través de sistemas a alta presión. Las tuberías de las centrales eléctricas transportan el vapor que mueve las turbinas. En plantas de fabricación, como cervecerías y destilerías, las tuberías se utilizan para trasladar material a través de diversos procesos de producción.

La plomería y los oficios relacionados constituyen una de las ocupaciones del sector de la construcción con la mayor cantidad de puestos, que provee unos 505,000 empleos. Esta profesión sigue creciendo y se espera que, para 2030, haya unas 55,000 oportunidades laborales disponibles. La plomería es uno de los oficios de la construcción mejores pagados. De hecho, según la encuesta sobre salarios del oficio de la construcción de 2022 del NCCER, el salario promedio de un plomero es de USD 73,320.

Lo nuevo en *Plomería, nivel uno*

La quinta edición revisada de *Plomería, nivel uno* tiene un nuevo formato con el objetivo de brindar una mejor experiencia tanto para el aprendiz como para el instructor. El NCCER se enorgullece de publicar esta edición con nuestro diseño de sistemas de enseñanza más reciente, que vincula los objetivos de aprendizaje con el contenido de cada módulo. En *Plomería, nivel uno* se introdujeron importantes mejoras en el diseño y actualizaciones globales de contenido. Se ha incorporado lo último en tecnologías para la unión de caños, así como los equipos relacionados, junto con una serie de herramientas manuales y accionadas por una fuente de energía nueva y mejorada. Los factores medioambientales relacionados con la plomería se abordan en varias de las secciones *Iniciativa verde*. A su vez, los doce módulos incluyen imágenes y gráficos nuevos y actualizados.

Le deseamos éxito en este programa de capacitación. Si tiene comentarios acerca de cómo el NCCER podría mejorar este libro, complete el formulario de *Online Curriculum Feedback Form* usando el código QR que se encuentra en esta página. En el NCCER, nos interesa recibir y agradecemos los comentarios de nuestros clientes. Puede enviar los suyos por correo electrónico a la dirección **support@nccer.org**. Para indicar que el comentario se refiere a este título, escriba *#PlumbingL1* en el asunto cuando lo envíe.

En nuestro sitio web, **www.nccer.org**, encontrará información sobre nuestros productos y cursos de capacitación más recientes.

Nos interesa recibir sus comentarios. Puede enviarnos sus opiniones a **curriculum@nccer.org** o enviar comentarios y consultas generales a **info@nccer.org**.

ESCANÉAME

Planes de estudios estandarizados del NCCER

El NCCER es una fundación educativa sin fines de lucro 501(c)(3) fundada en 1996 por las empresas de construcción y las asociaciones nacionales de construcción más importantes y progresistas del mundo. Fue fundada para abordar la escasez de mano de obra que enfrenta la industria y para desarrollar procesos de capacitación y planes de estudios estandarizados. En la actualidad, el NCCER está financiado por cientos de empresas líderes en la construcción y el mantenimiento, fabricantes y asociaciones nacionales. Los planes de estudios estandarizados del NCCER fueron desarrollados por el NCCER en asociación con Pearson, el editorial de educación más importante del mundo.

Estas son algunas características de los planes de estudios estandarizados del NCCER:

- historial de éxito comprobado en el sector;
- planes de estudios elaborados por la industria y para la industria;
- estandarización nacional que ofrece portabilidad de las habilidades laborales adquiridas y los créditos de capacitación;
- cumplimiento de los requisitos de la Oficina de Programas para Aprendices en relación con la capacitación en el aula (*CFR 29:29*);
- información bien ilustrada, actualizada y práctica.

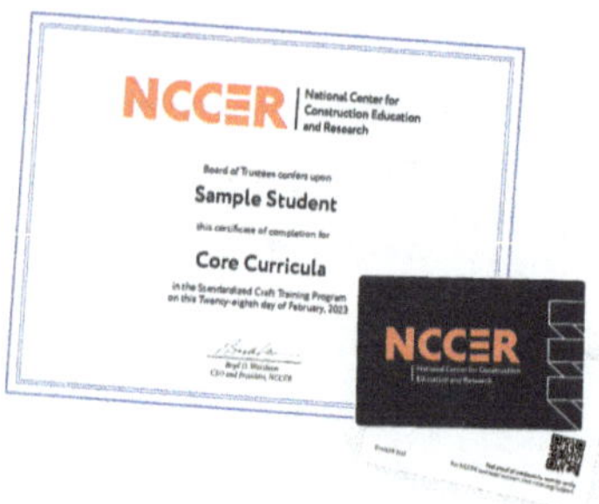

El centro también cuenta con el Registro del NCCER, que proporciona expedientes, certificados y tarjetas a las personas que han logrado completar un nivel de capacitación de un oficio de los planes de estudios del NCCER. *Los programas de capacitación deben ser dictados por un centro acreditado patrocinador de programas de capacitación del NCCER para recibir estas certificaciones.*

Insignias en línea

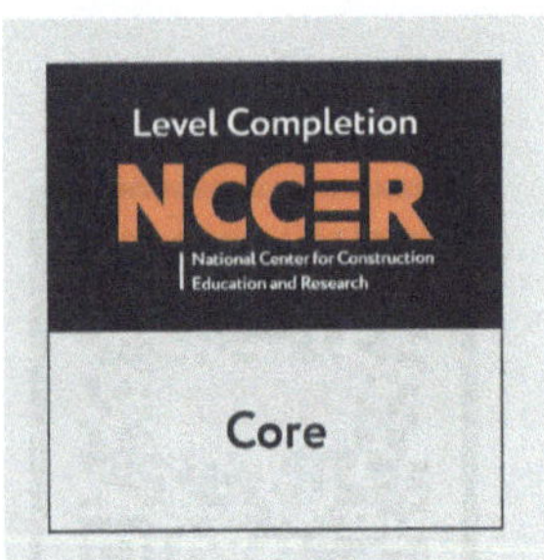

¡Muestre sus credenciales reconocidas por la industria en línea con las insignias digitales del NCCER!

El NCCER ahora ofrece credenciales en línea. Transforme sus conocimientos, habilidades y logros en insignias que pueda compartir en las plataformas de redes sociales, enviar a su red de contactos y agregar a su currículum. Para obtener más información, visite **www.nccer.org**.